Toxic Metals, Chronic Diseases and Related Cancers

Toxic Metals, Chronic Diseases and Related Cancers

Editor

Soisungwan Satarug

MDPI • Basel • Beijing • Wuhan • Barcelona • Belgrade • Manchester • Tokyo • Cluj • Tianjin

Editor
Soisungwan Satarug
The University of Queensland
Centre for Health Services Research
Translational Research Institute
Australia

Editorial Office
MDPI
St. Alban-Anlage 66
4052 Basel, Switzerland

This is a reprint of articles from the Special Issue published online in the open access journal *Toxics* (ISSN 2305-6304) (available at: https://www.mdpi.com/journal/toxics/special issues/metals diseases).

For citation purposes, cite each article independently as indicated on the article page online and as indicated below:

LastName, A.A.; LastName, B.B.; LastName, C.C. Article Title. *Journal Name* **Year**, *Volume Number*, Page Range.

ISBN 978-3-0365-4171-6 (Hbk)
ISBN 978-3-0365-4172-3 (PDF)

Contents

About the Editor

Soisungwan Satarug

Dr. Soisungwan Satarug completed her B.S. degree in Medical Technology at Chiang Mai University in Thailand; M.S. degree in Biochemistry at Mahidol University in Thailand; M.C.H. degree in Nutrition at the University of Queensland in Australia; and Ph.D. degree in Biochemistry at the University of Arizona in the USA. She received postdoctoral fellowship training in metabolic activation of carcinogens and carcinogenesis in the USA, Japan, Germany, and France. She was a research scientist at the National Research Centre for Environmental Toxicology in Brisbane, Australia, where she investigated environmental exposure to toxic metals as part of the Australia National Cadmium Minimization Program. Currently, she is a research advisor at the Kidney Disease Research Collaborative, Translational Research Institute, University of Queensland, in Brisbane, Australia. Her research interests revolve around the interplay of nutrition, genetics, and the environment in human disease.

toxics

MDPI

Editorial

Editorial to Special Issue Toxic Metals, Chronic Diseases and Related Cancers

Soisungwan Satarug

Kidney Disease Research Collaborative, Centre for Health Services Research, Translational Research Institute, Brisbane, QLD 4102, Australia; sj.satarug@yahoo.com.au

Citation: Satarug, S. Editorial to Special Issue Toxic Metals, Chronic Diseases and Related Cancers. *Toxics* 2022, *10*, 125. https://doi.org/10.3390/toxics10030125

Received: 10 February 2022
Accepted: 3 March 2022
Published: 5 March 2022

In this Special Issue, entitled "Toxic Metals, Chronic Diseases and Related Cancers", there are 19 published manuscripts, including reports of environmental exposure monitoring [1,2] and food safety surveillance [3,4]; reviews focusing on health risks of chronic exposure to cadmium and lead [5], experimental studies on the toxicity of cadmium, lead or mercury in gonads [6], and evidence that cadmium exposure may be one of the environmental factors contributing to hyperglycemia, insulin resistance and diabetes [7]; a mathematical model of the oral glucose tolerance test [8]; epidemiological studies examining health impacts of cadmium, lead, and mercury [9–15]; and reports concerning the immunotoxicity of high exposure to lead [16], the effects of cadmium on protein reabsorption by kidney tubular epithelial cells [17], the cytotoxicity of hexavalent chromium [18], and the carcinogenicity of aluminum in vivo [19].

Environmental Monitoring

To assess the health impact of a hazardous waste incinerator in Constantí, Catalonia, Spain, Esplugas et al. quantified elemental composition (As, Be, Cd, Cr, Hg, Mn, Ni, Pb, Sn, Tl and V) of scalp hair samples from schoolchildren living in close proximity to the incinerator and compared data to those recorded for schoolchildren in other areas [1]. Arsenic, beryllium and thallium were not detected, but cadmium and vanadium were found in 39% and 24.5% of samples, respectively. In order of high to low, the elemental contents of samples analyzed were Pb > Hg > Ni > Sn > Mn > Cr. These elemental contents were similar or lower than those reported for scalp hair samples from other areas [1]. In the most recent autopsy series describing tissue metal content, García et al. report that cadmium was detected in 30%, 30%, 100%, and 100% of brain, bone, liver and kidney samples, while lead was detected in 50%, 95%, 80%, and 85% of brain, bone, liver and kidney samples, respectively [2]. Preferential accumulations of cadmium in kidneys and lead in bone were evident [2].

Food Safety Surveillance and Mortality from Kidney Failure

Horiguchi et al. report cadmium intake levels among women living in two areas of Japan with recognized cadmium pollution in excess of the current tolerable intake level of 0.83 μg/kg bw/d [3]. In one area where rice cadmium content ranged from below 0.02 to 0.971 mg/kg, the average cadmium intake was 55.7 μg/d (1.03 μg/kg body weight per day). In the other area, where rice cadmium content varied between 0.008 and 0.687 mg/kg/d, the average cadmium intake was 48.7 μg/d (0.86 μg/kg bw/d). The percentage of rice samples containing cadmium above the Codex safety standard of 0.4 mg/kg was 8.2% in one area and 5.8% in the other.

In another Japanese area polluted by cadmium, 12 of 22 villages produced rice with cadmium contents above the 0.4 mg/kg standard. In a 35-year follow-up study of 2602 residents in this area (1169 men and 1433 women), Nishijo et al. found that lifetime cadmium intake $\geq$ 1 g was associated with a 49% increase in mortality from kidney failure among women. They also found that urinary cadmium levels $\geq$ 10 μg/g creatinine at baseline (35 years earlier) were associated with a 33% increase in all-cause mortality in women. Of note, a lifetime cadmium intake of 1 g is half of a "tolerable" lifetime intake guideline of 2 g.

Clinical Kidney Function (GFR) Deterioration

A review by Satarug et al. summarizes dietary sources and urine- and blood-based exposure measures of cadmium and lead, the two most prevalent toxic metals in humans. The review also examines the health risks of chronic exposure to cadmium and lead and the pathogenesis of cadmium-induced GFR reduction [5]. An evolving body of evidence links these metals to chronic kidney disease and mortality from cancer and heart disease [5]. Chronic kindey disease is defined as a fall of GFR below 60 ml/min/1.73m^2 or an increment of albumin-to-creatinine ratio to 30 mg/ g creatinine in women and to $\geq$ 20 mg/ g creatinine in men that persists for at least three months.

In a prospective cohort study of 601 Mexican children, Rodríguez-López et al. report means for cadmium intake of 4.4 µg/d at baseline and 8.1 µg/d after nine years [10]. The respective percentages of intake levels exceeding a tolerable level at baseline and at nine years of the cohort were 64% and 16%. A dietary transition to sweets, lettuce, and sandwiches as the main cadmium sources was seen at 4 years of age which coincided with a rise of an obesity prevalence from 18% to 46.8% at 9 years of age. Because a tolerable intake guideline was on a body weight basis, the % of intake levels exceeding a tolerable range fell while mean intake rose. Cadmium intake levels among children 8–12 years old showed a marginally inverse association with estimated glomerular filtration rate (eGFR).

Satarug et al. report a significant effect on eGFR of low environmental exposure to cadmium and lead among 392 Thai subjects (mean age 34.9 years) [11]. The mean for eGFR in subjects with urinary cadmium in the fourth quartile was, respectively, 4.65 and 4.94 mL/min/1.73 m^2 lower than those with urine cadmium in the first quartile (p = 0.021) and the second quartile (p = 0.011). In an in-depth analysis of data from 704 persons, of which 172, 310, and 222 were drawn, respectively, from the low, moderate, and high exposure areas of Thailand, a decrease in eGFR was the result of loss of intact nephrons due to extensive injury to kidney tubular cells caused by cadmium [12]. An elevation of β_2-microglobulin (β_2MG) excretion was speculatively due to effects of cadmium on both tubular reabsorption and nephron number.

Fujishiro et al. report that reabsorption of β_2MG and metallothionein (MT) by immortalized cells derived from human proximal tubule dropped after incubation with cadmium for 3 days [17]. A similar result was seen when S1 and S2 cell culture models of mouse proximal tubule were tested. Renal reuptake of iron (bound to transferrin) occurring at proximal tubule did not seem to be affected by cadmium. However, reabsorption of albumin and transferrin by these cells was not affected by cadmium. A question remains with regard to the specificity of this cadmium effect. A recent study suggested that reabsorption of β_2MG and MT may occur mainly at the distal tubule and collecting duct, where other receptor-mediated endocytosis systems are expressed [20].

Reproductive Health, Low Infant Birthweight, and Abnormal Growth

A review by Massányi et al. summarizes experimental studies showing the effects of cadmium, lead or mercury on the function of gonads, where female gametes (oocytes), male gametes (spermatozoa), and sex hormones are formed [6]. The reported effects of cadmium in ovaries include reduced follicular growth, follicular atresia, and prolonged estrus cycle. In testes, notable effects of cadmium are degeneration of the seminiferous tubules, disorganization of germinal epithelium in seminiferous tubules and abnormal spermatogenesis [6]. It is argued that low environmental exposure to cadmium, lead or mercury may contribute to the worldwide decline of human fertility which currently stands at 15% of childbearing age couples.

The Mediterranean diet is rich in iron and selenium, elements that in theory can reduce cadmium absorption. Gonzalez-Nahm et al. undertook a prospective cohort study of 185 mother–infant pairs of central North Carolina, USA to assess whether a Mediterranean diet during pregnancy modified the effect of prenatal cadmium exposure on birth outcomes [9]. The 25th, 50th, and 75th percentile levels of prenatal blood cadmium levels among cohort participants were 0.12, 0.24 and 0.46 μg/L, respectively. For the entire group, prenatal blood cadmium levels $\geq$ 0.46 μg/L were associated with low infant birthweight ($\leq$2500 g). In a subgroup analysis, the effect size of cadmium in Mediterranean diet adherence and non-adherence groups was similar. In this study, maternal adherence to a Mediterranean diet pattern did not mitigate the effect of cadmium on infant birthweight. However, the effect size observed was large (β = −210; 95% CI: −332, −88; p = 0.008), and it warrants further research to find dietary patterns that can diminish the absorption of dietary cadmium during pregnancy.

In a study of 311 children (151 girls and 160 boys), aged 3–7 years, from a coastal area of Thailand, Yimthiang et al. report a 2-fold increase in the risk of stunted growth among children who had high blood lead levels ($\geq$5 μg/dL) [14]. Milk consumption reduced the risk of abnormal growth by 43%. It is likely that calcium in milk reduced lead absorption by competing with lead for the metal transporters responsible for the absorption of lead. Another protective mechanism of milk might be due to organic substances that chelate lead and reduce its absorption. The authors also link high blood lead in children to parental occupations, such as fishing net production, that involved the use of lead weights.

Insulin Resistance and Diabetes

A review by Buha et al. discusses the evidence that cadmium exposure may contribute to hyperglycemia, insulin resistance and diabetes [7]. The authors describe various obstacles in their effort to derive an exposure limit for the insulin resistance associated with chronic low environmental exposure to cadmium. The predicaments are analogous to research into the threshold levels for endocrine-disrupting chemicals. The authors argue that a hazard-based, no-threshold approach should be applied when glucose homeostasis and insulin resistance are considered [7].

To overcome the limitation of a conventional approach to studying a complex physiological process in which many organs and tissues are involved, Rocca et al. use mathematical modeling to interpret oral glucose tolerance test data [8]. With a model incorporating four ordinary differential equations, they show that perinatal exposure to low-level cadmium in mother's milk reduced pancreatic β-cell sensitivity to glucose [8]. A review by Mari et al. presents an in-depth discussion on mathematical modeling to investigate complex physiological processes [21].

Stroke, Hyperlipdemia, and Liver Injury

In a case–control study of 92 stroke patients and 83 controls who were residents of the Canary Islands of Spain, Medina-Estévez et al. observed an association between high blood lead and an increase in risk of stroke by 65% when a univariate analysis was used [13]. In a multivariate analysis, high blood lead was associated with a 91% increase in risk of stroke after controlling for other stroke risk factors (smoking, hypertension, dyslipidemia and coronary cardiopathy). In contrast, high blood levels of gold and cerium were associated with a decrease in risk of stroke by 19% and 50%, respectively. The authors suggest that higher blood gold and cerium levels may explain the lower incidence of stroke in both men and women in the Canary Islands, compared to other regions of Spain. Further research is required, given that gold and cerium, like lead, are cumulative elemental chemicals, and little is known about their sources and effects in the body.

Lee et al. assessed the potential health effect of mercury intake among 6454 participants in the Korean National Environmental Health Survey [14]. They found higher means for blood mercury in women than men (3.70 vs. 2.63 μg/L), and noted that high blood mercury was associated, respectively, with 10.5% and 34.5% increases in risk of hyperlipidemia and liver injury (elevated plasma levels of liver enzymes).

Immunosuppression and Cancer

Pukanha et al. assessed immunotoxicity of occupational exposure to high levels of lead using white blood cells samples from a group of boatyard workers ($n = 14$) and an age-matched control group of farmers ($n = 16$) [16]. The median blood lead concentration was 37.1 μg/dL in workers and 4.3 μg/dL in controls. Compared to controls, workers had 8.4% fewer active phagocytic cells and 33.9% fewer cytotoxic T (Tc) cells, but the percentage of regulatory T (Treg) cells was higher by a factor of 2.7. In all subjects, blood lead levels showed positive correlations with the percentages of Treg cells ($r = 0.843$, $p < 0.001$) and interleukin-4 ($r = 0.473$, $p = 0.041$) while showing an inverse correlation with the percentages of Tc cells ($r = -0.563$, $p = 0.015$). Thus, chronic high exposure to lead may suppress cellular immunity while causing a shift towards humoral immunity. The immunosuppressive conditions accompanying lead exposure may increase the risks of infection and cancer.

Ma et al. employed classic molecular techniques to identify a specific molecular entity responsible for the cytotoxicity of hexavalent chromium in human liver cell line L02 [18]. It was shown that mitochondrial fission and fragmentation seen in L02 hepatocytes treated with chromium was mediated by Dynamin-Related Protein 1 (DRP1). A translocation of DRP1 from the cytoplasm to mitochondrial inner membrane occurred following excessive production of reactive oxygen species induced by chromium treatment.

García-Alegría et al. evaluated the effects of aluminum (as $AlCl_3$) alone or in combination with N-nitroso-N-methylurea (NMU), a chemical used in experimental induction of breast cancer [19]. Aluminum was administered to Sprague Dawley rats by gavage 5 days/week for 90 days, at a dose of 10 mg/day/kg of body weight, while NMU was administered via intraperitoneal route 50 and 70 days of age, at a dose of 50 mg/kg of body weight. Unexpectedly, aluminum accumulation was higher in mammary gland tissue from the group treated with aluminum only (38.2 vs. 12.3 μg/g). Based on an analysis of transcript levels, the involvement of SCL11A2 (divalent metal transporter 1) in the uptake of aluminum in mammary gland tissue was unlikely. Aluminum treatment alone induced minimum-to-moderate intraductal cell proliferation, lymph node hyperplasia, and serous gland adenoma.

Environmental exposure is estimated to account for 70–90% of the risks of acquiring chronic ailments. Presently, chronic kidney disease affects 8% to 16% of the world population, while the global prevalence of infertility among childbearing age couples is around 15%. Collectively, data presented in this Special Issue indicate that environmental exposure to toxic metals may contribute to these looming statistics. Alarming evidence suggests that exposure to cadmium may affect every stage of life, and that exposure in early life may determine susceptibility to certain diseases in adulthood. Prevention of these outcomes requires avoidance of further environmental contamination, minimization of exposure, and reduction of toxic metals in food crops to the lowest achievable levels.

Funding: This research received no external funding.

Acknowledgments: The author thanks Kenneth R. Phelps for his insightful comments and for editing the English.

Conflicts of Interest: The author has no conflict of interest to declare.

References

1. Esplugas, R.; Mari, M.; Marquès, M.; Schuhmacher, M.; Domingo, J.L.; Nadal, M. Biomonitoring of Trace Elements in Hair of Schoolchildren Living Near a Hazardous Waste Incinerator—A 20 Years Follow-Up. *Toxics* **2019**, *7*, 52. [CrossRef] [PubMed]
2. García, F.; Marquès, M.; Barbería, E.; Torralba, P.; Landin, I.; Laguna, C.; Domingo, J.L.; Nadal, M. Biomonitoring of Trace Elements in Subjects Living Near a Hazardous Waste Incinerator: Concentrations in Autopsy Tissues. *Toxics* **2020**, *8*, 11. [CrossRef] [PubMed]
3. Horiguchi, H.; Oguma, E.; Sasaki, S.; Miyamoto, K.; Hosoi, Y.; Ono, A.; Kayama, F. Exposure Assessment of Cadmium in Female Farmers in Cadmium-Polluted Areas in Northern Japan. *Toxics* **2020**, *8*, 44. [CrossRef] [PubMed]
4. Nishijo, M.; Nogawa, K.; Suwazono, Y.; Kido, T.; Sakurai, M.; Nakagawa, H. Lifetime Cadmium Exposure and Mortality for Renal Diseases in Residents of the Cadmium-Polluted Kakehashi River Basin in Japan. *Toxics* **2020**, *8*, 81. [CrossRef] [PubMed]
5. Satarug, S.; Gobe, G.C.; Vesey, D.A.; Phelps, K.R. Cadmium and Lead Exposure, Nephrotoxicity, and Mortality. *Toxics* **2020**, *8*, 86. [CrossRef]

6. Massányi, P.; Massányi, M.; Madeddu, R.; Stawarz, R.; Lukáč, N. Effects of Cadmium, Lead, and Mercury on the Structure and Function of Reproductive Organs. *Toxics* **2020**, *8*, 94. [CrossRef]
7. Buha, A.; Đukić-Ćosić, D.; Ćurčić, M.; Bulat, Z.; Antonijević, B.; Moulis, J.-M.; Goumenou, M.; Wallace, D. Emerging Links between Cadmium Exposure and Insulin Resistance: Human, Animal, and Cell Study Data. *Toxics* **2020**, *8*, 63. [CrossRef]
8. Rocca, A.; Fanchon, E.; Moulis, J.-M. Theoretical Modeling of Oral Glucose Tolerance Tests Guides the Interpretation of the Impact of Perinatal Cadmium Exposure on the Offspring's Glucose Homeostasis. *Toxics* **2020**, *8*, 30. [CrossRef]
9. Gonzalez-Nahm, S.; Nihlani, K.; House, J.S.; Maguire, R.L.; Skinner, H.G.; Hoyo, C. Associations between Maternal Cadmium Exposure with Risk of Preterm Birth and Low Birth Weight: Effect of Mediterranean Diet Adherence on Affected Prenatal Outcomes. *Toxics* **2020**, *8*, 90. [CrossRef]
10. Rodríguez-López, E.; Tamayo-Ortiz, M.; Ariza, A.C.; Ortiz-Panozo, E.; Deierlein, A.L.; Pantic, I.; Tolentino, M.C.; Estrada-Gutiérrez, G.; Parra-Hernández, S.; Espejel-Núñez, A.; et al. Early-Life Dietary Cadmium Exposure and Kidney Function in 9-Year-Old Children from the PROGRESS Cohort. *Toxics* **2020**, *8*, 83. [CrossRef]
11. Satarug, S.; Gobe, G.C.; Ujjin, P.; Vesey, D.A. A Comparison of the Nephrotoxicity of Low Doses of Cadmium and Lead. *Toxics* **2020**, *8*, 18. [CrossRef]
12. Satarug, S.; Vesey, D.A.; Ruangyuttikarn, W.; Nishijo, M.; Gobe, G.C.; Phelps, K.R. The Source and Pathophysiologic Significance of Excreted Cadmium. *Toxics* **2019**, *7*, 55. [CrossRef] [PubMed]
13. Medina-Estévez, F.; Zumbado, M.; Luzardo, O.P.; Rodríguez-Hernández, Á.; Boada, L.D.; Fernández-Fuertes, F.; Santandreu-Jimenez, M.E.; Henríquez-Hernández, L.A. Association between Heavy Metals and Rare Earth Elements with Acute Ischemic Stroke: A Case-Control Study Conducted in the Canary Islands (Spain). *Toxics* **2020**, *8*, 66. [CrossRef] [PubMed]
14. Lee, S.; Cho, S.-R.; Jeong, I.; Park, J.B.; Shin, M.-Y.; Kim, S.; Kim, J.H. Mercury Exposure and Associations with Hyperlipidemia and Elevated Liver Enzymes: A Nationwide Cross-Sectional Survey. *Toxics* **2020**, *8*, 47. [CrossRef] [PubMed]
15. Yimthiang, S.; Waeyang, D.; Kuraeiad, S. Screening for Elevated Blood Lead Levels and Related Risk Factors among Thai Children Residing in a Fishing Community. *Toxics* **2019**, *7*, 54. [CrossRef]
16. Pukanha, K.; Yimthiang, S.; Kwanhian, W. The Immunotoxicity of Chronic Exposure to High Levels of Lead: An Ex Vivo Investigation. *Toxics* **2020**, *8*, 56. [CrossRef]
17. Fujishiro, H.; Yamamoto, H.; Otera, N.; Oka, N.; Jinno, M.; Himeno, S. In Vitro Evaluation of the Effects of Cadmium on Endocytic Uptakes of Proteins into Cultured Proximal Tubule Epithelial Cells. *Toxics* **2020**, *8*, 24. [CrossRef]
18. Ma, Y.; Zhang, Y.; Xiao, Y.; Xiao, F. Increased Mitochondrial Fragmentation Mediated by Dynamin-Related Protein 1 Contributes to Hexavalent Chromium-Induced Mitochondrial Respiratory Chain Complex I-Dependent Cytotoxicity. *Toxics* **2020**, *8*, 50. [CrossRef]
19. García-Alegría, A.M.; Gómez-Álvarez, A.; Anduro-Corona, I.; Burgos-Hernández, A.; Ruíz-Bustos, E.; Canett-Romero, R.; González-Ríos, H.; López-Cervantes, J.G.; Rodríguez-Martínez, K.L.; Astiazaran-Garcia, H. Genotoxic Effects of Aluminum Chloride and Their Relationship with N-Nitroso-N-Methylurea (NMU)-Induced Breast Cancer in Sprague Dawley Rats. *Toxics* **2020**, *8*, 31. [CrossRef]
20. Zavala-Guevara, I.P.; Ortega-Romero, M.S.; Narváez-Morales, J.; Jacobo-Estrada, T.L.; Lee, W.-K.; Arreola-Mendoza, L.; Thévenod, F.; Barbier, O.C. Increased Endocytosis of Cadmium-Metallothionein through the 24p3 Receptor in an In Vivo Model with Reduced Proximal Tubular Activity. *Int. J. Mol. Sci.* **2021**, *22*, 7262. [CrossRef]
21. Mari, A.; Tura, A.; Grespan, E.; Bizzotto, R. Mathematical Modeling for the Physiological and Clinical Investigation of Glucose Homeostasis and Diabetes. *Front. Physiol.* **2020**, *11*, 575789. [CrossRef] [PubMed]

toxics

MDPI

Article

Biomonitoring of Trace Elements in Hair of Schoolchildren Living Near a Hazardous Waste Incinerator—A 20 Years Follow-Up

Roser Esplugas [1], Montse Mari [2], Montse Marquès [1], Marta Schuhmacher [2], José L. Domingo [1] and Martí Nadal [1,*]

[1] Laboratory of Toxicology and Environmental Health, School of Medicine, IISPV, Universitat Rovira i Virgili, 43201 Reus, Catalonia, Spain; roser.esplugas@urv.cat (R.E.); montserrat.marques@urv.cat (M.M.); joseluis.domingo@urv.cat (J.L.D.)

[2] Environmental Engineering Laboratory, Departament d'Enginyeria Quimica, Universitat Rovira i Virgili, 43007 Tarragona, Catalonia, Spain; montserrat.mari@urv.cat (M.M.); marta.schuhmacher@urv.cat (M.S.)

* Correspondence: marti.nadal@urv.cat; Tel.: +34-977-758-930

Received: 26 August 2019; Accepted: 27 September 2019; Published: 1 October 2019

Abstract: Since 1998, a monitoring program is periodically performed to assess the environmental and human health impact of air chemicals potentially emitted by a hazardous waste incinerator (HWI) located in Constantí (Catalonia, Spain). In 2017, samples of hair were collected from 94 schoolchildren (aged 10–13 years) living nearby and the levels of 11 trace elements (As, Be, Cd, Cr, Hg, Mn, Ni, Pb, Sn, Tl and V) were determined. The concentrations showed the following descending order: Pb > Hg > Ni > Sn > Mn > Cr. In turn, As, Be and Tl were not detected, while Cd and V were found only in a few samples. Some metal levels were significantly, positively correlated. Some significant differences were also noticed according to the gender and the specific zone of residence. Finally, the levels of trace elements showed fluctuations through time. Cr and Pb showed a significant decrease in comparison to the concentrations obtained in the baseline study (1998). According to the current results, metal emissions from the HWI are not relevant in terms of human health impact since their levels were similar and even lower than those reported in other contaminated areas.

Keywords: Trace elements; hair; children; hazardous waste incinerator; Constantí (Catalonia, Spain)

1. Introduction

To date, there is only a hazardous waste incinerator (HWI) in Spain, which is located in Constantí (Tarragona County, Catalonia). Being built in 1996–1998, it started to operate in 1999. At the building time, a large pre-operational monitoring program was initiated, not only as an additional measure of environmental control but also responding to the demands of residents and public authorities. The study was focused on two chemicals of special concern: polychlorinated dibenzo-*p*-dioxins and dibenzofurans (PCDD/Fs) as well as metals and metalloids. One of the main goals of this program was aimed at assuring that the facility would not be a relevant source of environmental pollution and its operations should not affect the health of the population living nearby. The initial surveillance program was designed to evaluate the impact on the environment, through the monitoring of soil and vegetation [1,2], while the impact on the residents was assessed through the monitoring of biological tissues such as blood, breast milk and hair [3–8]. Furthermore, the dietary intake of PCDD/Fs and metals by the local population was also evaluated [9,10].

The location of this HWI, which is situated near a chemical/petrochemical industrial complex, a municipal waste incinerator and in a zone with heavy traffic, can mean additional toxic emissions. Considering that there exist many emission sources in the area, the environmental surveillance of metals and metalloids is clearly a need for public health. The non-occupationally population is exposed to trace elements mainly through the diet including water [11], being inhalation and transdermal absorption minor exposure pathways [12]. The effects of a chronic/acute exposure to trace elements are varied, including cancer (e.g., arsenic [As], cadmium [Cd], chromium [Cr], nickel [Ni]), skin lesions (e.g., As, beryllium [Be], tin [Sn]), neurological disorders (e.g., mercury [Hg], manganese [Mn], thallium [Tl]), learning disability (e.g., lead [Pb]) or respiratory problems (e.g., vanadium [V]) among others [13–17]. Furthermore, it should be taking to account that the synergistic effect of the co-exposure to different metals and metalloids can also lead to cumulative adverse health effects [18,19].

The monitoring program has been continuously conducted since 1999. While information of the environmental levels of pollutants has been quite recurrent in the last 20 years [20], data on the concentrations of trace elements in the same biomonitors (i.e., hair, blood and autopsy tissues) have been updated every 4–5 years [21–24].

Despite the traditional approach for human biomonitoring is based on the analysis of blood and urine, human hair is also a very useful and valuable biological matrix [25]. The levels of metals in hair are up to 10-fold higher than those usually found in blood or urine [26]. The concentrations of heavy metals in hair can be modulated by endogenous factors including metabolic pathways, as well as exogenous impregnations such as air pollutants [27]. More interestingly, hair samples allow an easy sampling and storage, being a non-invasive method.

The biomonitoring of children is more complex than that of adults. However, results are undoubtedly of great interest [28], as children are more susceptible to metal exposure, since they have higher absorption rates in relation to their body weight. Moreover, they have low capacity of detoxification and excretion, as well as behavioural patterns that the environmental pollution can potentially affect more easily [29,30].

Being part of a large biological surveillance program, this study was aimed at identifying whether there are any health risks for the population living close to the HWI. More specifically, the purpose of the present study was to measure the concentration of As, Be, Cd, Cr, Hg, Mn, Ni, Pb, Sn, Tl and V in hair of schoolchildren who live near the facility. A detailed analysis of the correlation between metals and the differences according to the sex and specific zones of residence was also carried out. Furthermore, temporal trends were determined by comparing these data with those of previous surveys.

2. Materials and Methods

2.1. Sample Collection

Between June and September of 2017, hair samples were obtained from 94 schoolchildren (44 boys and 50 girls aged 10–13 years). About 2–3 cm of hair was cut from an area close to the occipital region of the scalp. Only naturally coloured hair was selected in order to avoid biased results. The participants were classified in 3 groups according to the area of residence: (1) urban (named as *downtown*), (2) close to an important chemical/petrochemical complex (named as *CH/PCH complex*) and (3) near a large oil refinery, the HWI and a municipal incinerator (named as *refinery/HWI/MI*) (Figure 1). A consent form according to the declaration of Helsinki was signed by the tutors of each participant. The study protocol, 07/2017, was reviewed and approved by the Ethical Committee for Human Studies of the Pere Virgili Health Research Institute (IISPV), Reus/Tarragona, Spain in March 30, 2017 [22,23].

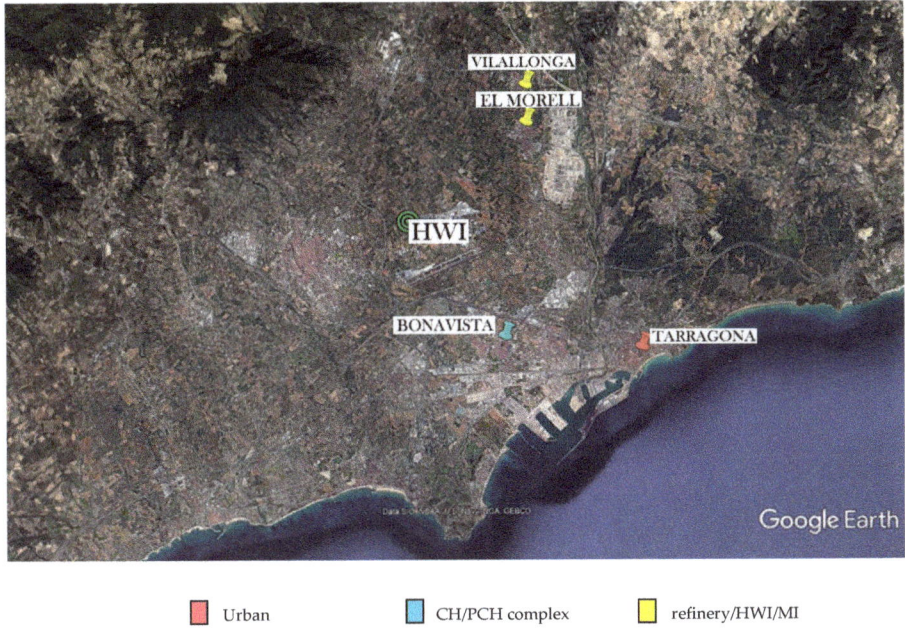

Urban CH/PCH complex refinery/HWI/MI

Figure 1. Sampling area.

2.2. Pre-treatment and Chemical Analysis

Hair samples were washed with 1% Triton X-100 (E. Merck, Darmstadt, Germany) in an ultrasounds bath for 20 minutes in order to remove external contamination. Then, the soap was removed with distilled water and samples were 3 times-washed with Milli-Q water. Around 150 mg of sample were placed in hermetic Teflon bombs and digested with 2 mL of 65% nitric acid (Suprapur, E. Merck, Darmstadt, Germany) for 12 hours at 110 °C. Samples were then filtered, diluted to 10 mL of Milli-Q water and stored at −20 °C.

The concentrations of As, Be, Cd, Cr, Hg, Mn, Ni, Pb, Sn, Tl and V in hair samples were analysed according to previous studies conducted in our laboratory [6,31–33] using inductively coupled plasma-mass spectrometry (ICP-MS, Perkin Elmer Elan 6000). Each sample was tested by duplicate, being *Lobster Hepatopancreas* employed as quality control (*NRC Canada*, *TORT-2*) every 5 samples. Blanks used during the digestion were also run every 5 samples. The limits of detection (LODs) were 0.03 μg/g for Be, Cd, Pb and Tl; 0.07 μg/g for As, Cr, Mn, Ni, Sn and V; and 0.13 μg/g for Hg.

2.3. Statistical Analysis

All data were analysed by using the statistical package SPSS 25.0. Values with a *Z*-score above 2.5 and under −2.5 were considered as outliers. In addition, a visual inspection of the boxplot was also conducted to verify these outliers. Non-detected levels of metals were assumed as to be one-half of the respective LOD (ND = ½ LOD). Only trace elements with values 70% (or more) above the LOD were considered for further statistical evaluation. To assess the distribution of the values, the Kolmogorov-Smirnov test was used. Correlations between metal concentrations were performed employing the Spearman correlation coefficient. The Student's t-test was used to compare differences of metal levels between boys and girls. In turn, ANOVA and subsequent T3 Dunnett's post-hoc tests were employed to assess differences between groups according to the zones of residence and the significance in the temporal evolution. The level of statistical significance was established at $p < 0.05$.

3. Results

The concentrations of the 11 analysed elements in 94 samples of hair from schoolchildren living in Tarragona County are shown in Table 1. Arsenic, Be and Tl were not detected, whereas Cd and V were only detected in 37 and 23 samples, respectively. In previous campaigns of the monitoring program, traces of Cd and V were only found in very few samples of hair [6,31–33]. Although the information relative to these elements is shown, they are excluded from the statistical analysis.

Table 1. Metal concentrations (μg/g) in hair of 94 school children living in Tarragona County (2017).

Metal	Mean ± SD	Median	Recovery (%)	Interquartile Range	LOD	Maximum
As	ND	-	81.6	-	0.07	
Be	ND	-	42.3	-	0.03	
Cd	0.04 ± 0.05	0.02	85.0	0.02	0.03	0.44
Cr	0.14 ± 0.05	0.13	92.3	0.00	0.07	0.44
Hg	0.73 ± 0.56	0.59	86.9	0.62	0.13	2.70
Mn	0.30 ± 0.16	0.25	86.4	0.23	0.07	0.77
Ni	0.54 ± 0.53	0.36	73.3	0.48	0.07	2.66
Pb	1.44 ± 1.89	0.93	73.9	1.52	0.03	11.86
Sn	0.41 ± 0.34	0.32	47.1	0.42	0.07	1.64
Tl	ND	ND	88.9	-	0.03	-
V	0.07 ± 0.08	0.07	104.2	0.16	0.07	0.43

ND = not detected, LOD = limit of detection. Data are given as mean ± SD.

Lead presented the highest mean concentration (1.44 μg/g), ranging from undetected values to 11.9 μg/g. Mercury also presented relatively high levels, with a mean and a range of 0.73 and 0.13–2.70 μg/g, respectively. The mean concentrations of Sn, Mn and Cr were 0.41, 0.30 and 0.14 μg/g, respectively. Finally, Cd and V were detected only in a few samples. Both metals exhibited the lowest concentrations (0.04 and 0.07 μg/g, respectively). When evaluating the correlation between metal levels (Table 2), a weak but significant positive correlation, was found between Mn and Ni, Pb ($p < 0.01$) and Sn ($p < 0.05$) and also between Ni and both Cr and Sn ($p < 0.01$).

Table 2. Correlations between metal concentrations in hair of 94 schoolchildren living in Tarragona County (2017).

Metal	Cr	Hg	Mn	Ni	Pb	Sn	V
Cd	0.085	0.028	0.261	0.345	0.533	0.375	0.181
Cr		0.061	0.177	0.271 **	0.198	0.091	0.180
Hg			−0.057	−0.130	0.077	0.047	0.164
Mn				0.405 **	0.291 **	0.234 *	0.128
Ni					0.158	0.299 **	0.286
Pb						0.158	0.106
Sn							0.268

Spearman correlation coefficient (r) is shown. * and ** means significant differences at $p < 0.05$ and $p < 0.01$ (bilateral), respectively.

When metal concentrations were assessed according to the sex of the schoolchildren, significant differences were found in the levels of Hg, Ni, Pb and Sn (Figure 2). Thus, girls exhibited significant lower levels of Hg (0.61 μg/g vs. 0.88 μg/g, ($p < 0.05$)) and Pb (1.03 μg/g vs. 1.89 μg/g, $p < 0.05$) and significant higher concentrations of Ni (0.69 μg/g vs. 0.36 μg/g, $p < 0.01$) and Sn (0.54 μg/g vs. 0.28 μg/g, $p < 0.001$) than boys. Finally, Cd, Cr and Mn did not show significant differences between girls and boys.

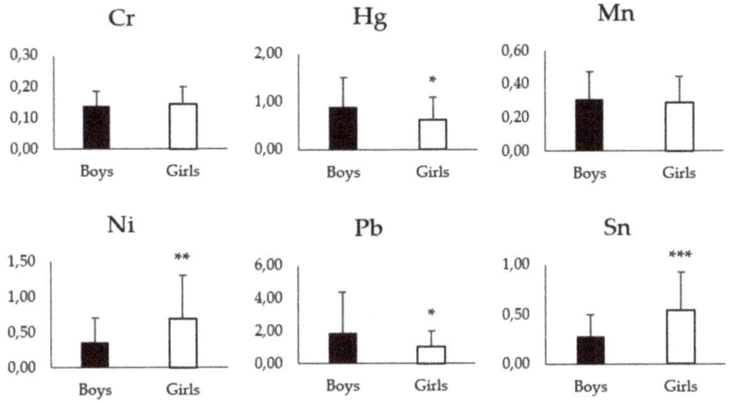

Figure 2. Metal concentrations (µg/g) in hair of schoolboys ($n = 44$) and girls ($n = 50$) living in Tarragona County (2017). Data are given as mean ± SD. Statistics: non-parametric t-test. Significant differences between both groups at: $^{*}p < 0.05$, $^{**}p < 0.01$ and $^{***}p < 0.001$.

Mercury was identified as the only element showing significant differences in the levels in hair according to the specific zones of residence (Table 3). Significantly higher concentrations of Hg were found in the children living in Tarragona downtown with respect to those living in the remaining two evaluated areas ($p < 0.01$), both of them with industrial characteristics.

Table 3. Metal concentrations (µg/g) in hair of school children living in Tarragona County according to the specific zones of residence (2017).

Metal	Downtown	CH/PCH Complex	Refinery/HWI/MI
As	ND	ND	ND
Be	ND	ND	ND
Cd	0.03 ± 0.03	0.04 ± 0.09	0.04 ± 0.03
Cr	0.14 ± 0.05	0.15 ± 0.07	0.13 ± 0.03
Hg	1.07 ± 0.64 ^{a}	0.54 ± 0.45 ^{b}	0.56 ± 0.40 ^{b}
Mn	0.26 ± 0.15	0.29 ± 0.20	0.33 ± 0.15
Ni	0.42 ± 0.41	0.55 ± 0.61	0.63 ± 0.56
Pb	1.08 ± 0.85	1.55 ± 2.93	1.73 ± 1.82
Sn	0.47 ± 0.37	0.27 ± 0.26	0.44 ± 0.34
Tl	ND	ND	ND
V	0.10 ± 0.10	0.07 ± 0.08	0.04 ± 0.03

ND = not detected. Data are given as mean ± SD. Statistics: ANOVA and T3 Dunnett's post-hoc test. Data not showing a common superscript ($^{a, b, c}$) indicate significant differences between zones (downtown, CH/PCH complex and refinery/HWI/MI) at $p < 0.05$.

The temporal trends of metal concentrations in hair of schoolchildren are summarized in Table 4. The results of the current study are compared with those of previous surveys, including the baseline study (1998) and the intermediate campaigns (2002, 2007 and 2012). A significant decrease of Cd in recent years was noted when compared to the baseline results ($p < 0.001$). Chromium levels significantly increased in 2007 and 2012 in comparison to previous years ($p < 0.001$) but the concentration of this element notably decreased in 2017 ($p < 0.001$), being this reduction significant in contrast to the previous surveys. Despite Ni concentrations were significantly lower in 2002 ($p < 0.001$), they have remained nearly constant through time. Furthermore, although Pb concentrations decreased significantly after the baseline survey ($p < 0.001$), in 2017 they raised again, being significantly higher than those observed in 2007 and 2012 ($p < 0.01$). Tin showed significantly lower concentrations in the period 2002–2012 ($p < 0.001$), while current values are comparable to those found in 1998. Mercury was the only element which did not exhibit significant differences between surveys. Finally, V was found at relatively low concentrations, being detected in only 23 samples in 2017 but contrasting with data from previous surveys, where it was never detected.

Table 4. Metal concentrations (μg/g) in hair of school children living in Tarragona County obtained in the studies conducted in 1998, 2002, 2007, 2012 and 2017.

Metal	1998	2002	2007	2012	2017
As	ND	ND	ND	ND	ND
Be	ND	ND	ND	ND	ND
Cd	0.18 ± 0.14 [a]	ND	0.02 ± 0.01 [b]	0.02 ± 0.01 [b]	0.04 ± 0.05
Cr	0.36 ± 0.52 [a]	0.37 ± 0.21 [a]	1.31 ± 1.14 [b]	0.98 ± 0.22 [b]	0.14 ± 0.05 [c]
Hg	0.67 ± 0.42	0.70 ± 0.45	0.56 ± 0.53	0.58 ± 0.23	0.73 ± 0.56
Mn	0.26 ± 0.17 [ac]	0.16 ± 0.23 [b]	0.21 ± 0.24 [ab]	0.20 ± 0.23 [b]	0.30 ± 0.16 [c]
Ni	0.65 ± 0.54 [a]	0.27 ± 0.22 [b]	0.48 ± 0.58 [a]	0.53 ± 0.73 [a]	0.54 ± 0.53 [a]
Pb	5.81 ± 3.86 [a]	0.86 ± 2.02 [bc]	0.58 ± 0.68 [b]	0.63 ± 0.78 [b]	1.44 ± 1.89 [c]
Sn	0.37 ± 0.45 [a]	0.13 ± 0.10 [b]	0.16 ± 0.18 [b]	0.20 ± 0.29 [b]	0.41 ± 0.34 [a]
Tl	ND	ND	ND	ND	ND
V	ND	ND	ND	ND	0.07 ± 0.08

ND= not detected. Data are given as mean ± SD. Statistics: ANOVA and T3 Dunnett's post-hoc test. Data not showing a common superscript ([a, b, c]) indicate significant differences between years (1998, 2002, 2007, 2012 and 2017) at $p < 0.05$.

4. Discussion

Some metals were significantly and positively correlated: Mn with Ni, Pb and Sn and also Ni with Cr and Sn. This kind of correlations has been previously reported in the scientific literature. In Russia, Semenova et al. [34] also found a positive correlation between Pb and Mn in hair of children living in the vicinity of abandoned mines in the South Urals, while Drobyshev et al. [35] reported positive correlations of Al, Cu, Fe, Ni and V, when analysing the concentrations of trace elements in children (aged 7–9) of St. Petersburg.

The body growth, physiology, the presence of specific sexual hormones and metabolizing enzymes, along with lifestyle and physical activity contribute to exhibit differences in the accumulation and excretion processes of metals between boys and girls [36]. Sex can play a role, being suggested that females are more vulnerable to exposure to trace metals than males, particularly at higher levels of exposure [37]. Some authors have even reported higher concentrations of trace elements in hair of girls than in boys [14,38]. In agreement with these findings, girls living in Tarragona County showed significantly higher levels of Ni and Sn than boys. However, Hg and Pb were found at lower levels in girls, when compared to boys. Further research is required to better understanding the sex differences in metal levels in hair, especially highlighting if changes can be applied to all the trace elements or there exist variabilities among metals.

It has been largely described that the profile of hair metal composition depends on local environmental conditions [39]. When we analysed the differences in metal levels between zones of residence, it was observed that children living in Tarragona downtown presented higher levels of Hg than those living near the CH/PCH complex or near the refinery/HWI/MI. Since the environmental concentrations of Hg are not increased in this area according to data from soils and vegetation [40,41], traffic could be even more important than the industrial activity, in terms of Hg exposure. However, it must be remarked that dietary intake plays a key role in human exposure to metals. Food consumption is the most contributive pathway of exposure to metals and metalloids [42]. As suggested by Castaño et al. [15], the relationship between the zone of residence and Hg concentrations could be attributed to the nutritional habits of children, which are invariably different according to their socio-economic status.

The temporal profile of metal concentrations in hair of schoolchildren has revealed some interesting findings. Thus, the significant reduction of Pb since 1998 may be attributed to their removal from gasoline, as this element -as an additive- was banned in 2001. In fact, the benefits of this legislative measure, in terms of environmental pollution by Pb, have been largely observed [43]. However, an accurate assessment of the temporal trends of metal concentrations in hair should be conducted also using data from other biological tissues, which are not currently available. Furthermore, changes in the dietary habits of the population living in Tarragona County should be also considered. In 2012, an increase in the dietary exposure to Hg and Cr was reported [44]. In turn, a spectacular decrease in the intake of both elements occurred recently (unpublished data), which was also found for PCDD/Fs [45].

The concentrations of trace elements in hair of schoolchildren were compared with those of recent studies found in the scientific literature (Table 5). Most of these investigations are focused on areas with important industrial or mining activities or even in urban zones [11,14,26,30,34–37,46,47]. The different results might be attributed to the differences among the respective geographical areas. Furthermore, despite the mean Cr concentration is similar to most levels found in recent literature, Cr concentrations in the urban area of Madrid were approximately 5-fold higher than those of the present study [46]. The mean level of Hg was also higher than the concentrations found in other locations, such as toxic waste disposal sites of Russia [35] and different urban areas [14,47]. In contrast, Hg concentrations in children from Tarragona County were lower than those found in other Spanish studies focused on assessing urban and industrial/mining areas [26,46]. The current Mn values were lower than elsewhere, differing notably from those found in Sardinia (Italy) and Russia [34,35,37]. In contrast, higher Ni levels were found when our data are compared with those of other studies, excepting those reported by Xie et al. [30] in Shaoguan Guangdong (China) and Evrenoglou et al. [14] in Athens (Greece). In turn, Pb levels were higher than those found in hair of children living in some mining, volcanic, sub-urban and urban areas [14,26,34,36,47] but lower than values from children living near certain mining zones, as well as near to toxic waste disposal sites and cement plants [11,30,34,35,37]. The individual characteristics of the geographic areas where the children live would probably be the responsible of the observed variability in Ni and Pb levels among studies.

Thus, the trace element levels obtained in our study, which are similar and even lower than those reported in other contaminated areas, suggest that metal emissions from the HWI are not relevant in terms of human health impact. Nevertheless, additional studies in combination with information from other biological tissues, as well as the dietary intake of metals, are clearly needed for a complete identification of potential health risks.

Table 5. Summary of recently published metal concentrations (μg/g) in hair of children in different countries.

City, Country	Zone	Age (years)	Sex	As	Be	Cd	Cr	Hg	Mn	Ni	Pb	Sn	Tl	V	Reference
Constantí, Tarragona, Spain	HWI, industrial, urban	7–13	Both	ND	ND	0.04	0.14	0.73	0.30	0.54	1.44	0.41	ND	0.07	Present study
Karabash, Russia *	copper smelter	14	Both	0.06		0.07	0.16		0.72	0.21	1.96				Skalny et al. [11]
Varna, Russia *	control locations	14	Both	0.06		0.04	0.26		0.53	0.23	1.43				Skalny et al. [11]
Tomino, Russia *	control locations	14	Both	2.04		0.12	0.14		0.60	0.30	5.44				Skalny et al. [11]
Kifisia Athens, Greece	urban	11–12	Both	0.031		0.03		0.49		0.92	1.36				Evrenoglou et al. [14]
Philadelphia, Athens, Greece	urban	11–12	Both	0.035		0.03		0.52		1.38	3.31				Evrenoglou et al. [14]
Kryoneri, Athens, Greece	sub-urban	11–12	Both	0.026		0.03		0.36		0.62	0.80				Evrenoglou et al. [14]
Huelva, Spain	living near industrial/mining areas	6–9	Both	0.07		<0.003		1.28	0.26		<0.09				Molina-Villalba et al. [26]
Shaoguan Guangdong, Tielong, China	cement plant and ex-mining area	≤15	Both	1.13		0.19	0.17			1.21	10.88				Xie et al. [30]
Rural settlements Tubinsk, Russia	vicinity of abandoned mines in South Urals	7–14	Both			0.05			1.43	0.24	2.74				Semenova et al. [34]
Ishmurzino, Russia	vicinity of abandoned mines in South Urals	7–14	Both			0.30			1.21	0.30	1.97				Semenova et al. [34]
Semenovsk, Russia	vicinity of abandoned mines in South Urals	7–14	Both			0.03			2.38	0.45	0.91				Semenova et al. [34]
Leningradskaya Oblast,' St. Petersburg, Russia	controls from a non-urban settlement	7–9	Both	0.04		0.16	0.25	0.22	3.41	0.42	2.51			0.05	Drobyshev et al. [35]
Leningradskaya Oblast,' St. Petersburg, Russia	proximity to the toxic waste disposal grounds	7–9	Both	0.03		0.14	0.31	0.14	2.93	0.39	3.82			0.05	Drobyshev et al. [35]
Pace del Mela, Sicily *#	industrial	11–14	Both	0.03		0.01	0.10		0.40	0.10	0.80			0.10	Tamburo et al. [36]
Gela, Butera and Niscemi, Sicily *#	polymetallic mining area	11–14	Both	0.04		0.02	0.10		0.20	0.10	0.40				Tamburo et al. [36]
Palermo, Sicily *#	urban	11–14	Both	0.0003		0.02	0.20		0.20	0.04	0.80			0.10	Tamburo et al. [36]
Small towns around Etna, Sicily *#	volcanic	11–14	Both	0.03		0.01	0.10		0.30	0.10	0.40			0.20	Tamburo et al. [36]
Sardinia, Italy	mining areas	11–13	Both	3.60		3.60	0.70		1.60	4.90	13.10			1.20	Varrica et al. [37]
Alcalá de Henares, Madrid, Spain	urban	6–9	Both	ND	ND	0.52	0.66	1.10	0.30	0.42	1.48	1.29	ND	0.44	Peña-Fernández et al. [46]
Flix, Spain	urban	12–13	Boys	0.08	0.004	ND		0.47	0.13	0.26	0.80	0.23	ND	0.19	Torrente et al. [47]
Flix, Spain	urban	12–13	Girls	0.09	0.004	0.02		0.47	0.19	0.53	0.59	0.33	ND	0.17	Torrente et al. [47]

ND = Non-detected.* Metal concentration is expressed as median. # Metal levels were measured in scalp hair.

5. Conclusions

The presence of Cd, Pb, Hg, Ni, Sn, Mn, Cr and V in hair of schoolchildren living near the HWI of Constantí (Tarragona County, Catalonia, Spain) was confirmed in this study. Some significant differences according to the sex were noted, while Hg was the only metal with significant differences according to the zone of residence of the schoolchildren. The levels of Cr and Pb decreased since 1998, when the biomonitoring program was started and despite Mn, Ni, Pb and Sn showed higher levels in 2017 when compared to some previous surveys, their concentrations were even lower than those reported in recent literature. The present results indicate that the current emissions of metals by the HWI do not pose direct health risks of immediate concern. The follow-up monitoring program should be continued in order to assure there are no changes in human exposure to trace elements in the vicinity of the HWI.

Author Contributions: Conceptualization, M.S. and J.L.D.; methodology, M.M. (Montse Mari) and M.M. (Montse Marquès); software, M.M. (Montse Mari); validation, R.E. and M.N.; formal analysis, R.E. and M.M. (Montse Marquès); investigation, R.E., M.M. (Montse Mari), M.S., J.L.D. and M.N.; resources, M.M. (Montse Mari); data curation, R.E.; writing—original draft preparation, R.E.; writing—review and editing, M.N.; visualization, M.S.; supervision; project administration, M.M. (Montse Marquès) and J.L.D; funding acquisition, J.L.D.

Funding: This study was funded by Sarpi Constantí SL, Catalonia, Spain.

Acknowledgments: The authors appreciate the technical assistance of Anabel Díez for the sampling and the analytical treatment, as well all the schoolchildren and their families, who provided all the samples.

Conflicts of Interest: The authors declare no conflict of interest.

References

1. Schuhmacher, M.; Granero, S.; Llobet, J.M.; de Kok, H.A.; Domingo, J.L. Assessment of baseline levels of PCDD/F in soils in the neighbourhood of a new hazardous waste incinerator in Catalonia, Spain. *Chemosphere* **1997**, *35*, 1947–1958. [CrossRef]
2. Llobet, J.M.; Schuhmacher, M.; Domingo, J.L. Observations on metal trends in soil and vegetation samples collected in the vicinity of a hazardous waste incinerator under construction (1996–1998). *Toxicol. Environ. Chem.* **2000**, *77*, 119–129. [CrossRef]
3. Schuhmacher, M.; Domingo, J.L.; Llobet, J.M.; Lindström, G.; Wingfors, H. Dioxin and dibenzofuran concentrations in adipose tissue of a general population from Tarragona, Spain. *Chemosphere* **1999**, *38*, 2475–2487. [CrossRef]
4. Schuhmacher, M.; Domingo, J.L.; Llobet, J.M.; Lindström, G.; Wingfors, H. Dioxin and dibenzofuran concentrations in blood of a general population from Tarragona, Spain. *Chemosphere* **1999**, *38*, 1123–1133. [CrossRef]
5. Schuhmacher, M.; Domingo, J.L.; Llobet, J.M.; Kiviranta, H.; Vartiainen, T. PCDD/F concentrations in milk of nonoccupationally exposed women living in southern Catalonia, Spain. *Chemosphere* **1999**, *38*, 995–1004. [CrossRef]
6. Granero, S.; Llobet, J.M.; Schuhmacher, M.; Corbella, J.; Domingo, J.L. Biological monitoring of environmental pollution and human exposure to metals in Tarragona, Spain. I. *Trace Elem. Electrolytes* **1998**, *15*, 39–43.
7. Llobet, J.M.; Granero, S.; Schuhmacher, M.; Corbella, J.; Domingo, J.L. Biological monitoring of environmental pollution and human exposure to metals in Tarragona, Spain. II. Levels in autopsy tissues. *Trace Elem. Electrolytes* **1998**, *15*, 44–49.
8. Llobet, J.M.; Granero, S.; Torres, A.; Schuhmacher, M.; Domingo, J.L. Biological monitoring of environmental pollution and human exposure to metals in Tarragona, Spain. III. Blood levels. *Trace Elem. Electrolytes* **1998**, *15*, 76–80.
9. Domingo, J.L.; Schuhmacher, M.; Granero, S.; Llobet, J.M. PCDDs and PCDFs in food samples from Catalonia, Spain. An assessment of dietary intake. *Chemosphere* **1999**, *38*, 3517–3528. [CrossRef]
10. Llobet, J.M.; Granero, S.; Schuhmacher, M.; Corbella, J.; Domingo, J.L. Biological monitoring of environmental pollution and human exposure to metals in Tarragona, Spain. IV. Estimation of the dietary intake. *Trace Elem. Electrolytes* **1998**, *15*, 136–141.

11. Skalny, A.V.; Zhukovskaya, E.V.; Kireeva, G.N.; Skalnaya, M.G.; Grabeklis, A.R.; Radysh, I.V.; Shakieva, R.A.; Nikonorov, A.A.; Tinkov, A.A. Whole blood and hair trace elements and minerals in children living in metal-polluted area near copper smelter in Karabash, Chelyabinsk region, Russia. *Environ. Sci. Pollut. Res.* **2018**, *25*, 2014–2020. [CrossRef] [PubMed]
12. Linares, V.; Perelló, G.; Nadal, M.; Gómez-Catalán, J.; Llobet, J.M.; Domingo, J.L. Environmental versus dietary exposure to POPs and metals: A probabilistic assessment of human health risks. *J. Environ. Monit.* **2010**, *12*, 681–688. [CrossRef] [PubMed]
13. Sakakibara, M.; Sera, K. Current Mercury Exposure from Artisanal and Small-Scale Gold Mining in Bombana, Southeast Sulawesi, Indonesia—Future Significant Health Risks. *Toxics* **2017**, *5*, 7. [CrossRef]
14. Evrenoglou, L.; Partsinevelou, S.A.; Stamatis, P.; Lazaris, A.; Patsouris, E.; Kotampasi, C.; Nicolopoulou-Stamati, P. Children exposure to trace levels of heavy metals at the north zone of Kifissos River. *Sci. Total Environ.* **2013**, *443*, 650–661. [CrossRef] [PubMed]
15. Castaño, A.; Pedraza-Díaz, S.; Cañas, A.I.; Pérez-Gómez, B.; Ramos, J.J.; Bartolomé, M.; Pärt, P.; Soto, E.P.; Motas, M.; Navarro, C.; et al. Mercury levels in blood, urine and hair in a nation-wide sample of Spanish adults. *Sci. Total Environ.* **2019**, *670*, 262–270. [CrossRef]
16. Jiang, F.; Ren, B.; Hursthouse, A.; Deng, R.; Wang, Z. Distribution, source identification and ecological-health risks of potentially toxic elements (PTEs) in soil of thallium mine area (southwestern Guizhou, China). *Environ. Sci. Pollut. Res.* **2019**, *26*, 16556–16567. [CrossRef]
17. Quansah, R.; Armah, F.A.; Essumang, D.K.; Luginaah, I.; Clarke, E.; Marfoh, K.; Cobbina, S.J.; Nketiah-Amponsah, E.; Namujju, P.B.; Obiri, S.; et al. Association of Arsenic with Adverse Pregnancy Outcomes/Infant Mortality: A Systematic Review and Meta-Analysis. *Environ. Health Perspect.* **2015**, *123*, 412–421. [CrossRef]
18. Bartrem, C.; Tirima, S.; Von Lindern, I.; Von Braun, M.; Worrell, M.C.; Mohammad Anka, S.; Abdullahi, A.; Moller, G. Unknown risk: Co-exposure to lead and other heavy metals among children living in small-scale mining communities in Zamfara State, Nigeria. *Int. J. Environ. Health Res.* **2014**, *24*, 304–319. [CrossRef]
19. Anyanwu, B.; Ezejiofor, A.; Igweze, Z.; Orisakwe, O. Heavy Metal Mixture Exposure and Effects in Developing Nations: An Update. *Toxics* **2018**, *6*, 65. [CrossRef]
20. Marquès, M.; Nadal, M.; Díaz-Ferrero, J.; Schuhmacher, M.; Domingo, J.L. Concentrations of PCDD/Fs in the neighborhood of a hazardous waste incinerator: Human health risks. *Environ. Sci. Pollut. Res.* **2018**, *25*, 26470–26481. [CrossRef]
21. Domingo, J.L.; García, F.; Nadal, M.; Schuhmacher, M. Autopsy tissues as biological monitors of human exposure to environmental pollutants. A case study: Concentrations of metals and PCDD/Fs in subjects living near a hazardous waste incinerator. *Environ. Res.* **2017**, *154*, 269–274. [CrossRef] [PubMed]
22. Schuhmacher, M.; Mari, M.; Nadal, M.; Domingo, J.L. Concentrations of dioxins and furans in breast milk of women living near a hazardous waste incinerator in Catalonia, Spain. *Environ. Int.* **2019**, *125*, 334–341. [CrossRef] [PubMed]
23. Nadal, M.; Mari, M.; Schuhmacher, M.; Domingo, J.L. Monitoring dioxins and furans in plasma of individuals living near a hazardous waste incinerator: Temporal trend after 20 years. *Environ. Res.* **2019**, *173*, 207–211. [CrossRef] [PubMed]
24. Nadal, M.; García, F.; Schuhmacher, M.; Domingo, J.L. Metals in biological tissues of the population living near a hazardous waste incinerator in Catalonia, Spain: Two decades of follow-up. *Environ. Res.* **2019**, *176*, 108578. [CrossRef]
25. Chojnacka, K.; Michalak, I.; Zielińska, A.; Górecka, H.; Górecki, H. Inter-relationship between elements in human hair: The effect of gender. *Ecotoxicol. Environ. Saf.* **2010**, *73*, 2022–2028. [CrossRef] [PubMed]
26. Molina-Villalba, I.; Lacasaña, M.; Rodríguez-Barranco, M.; Hernández, A.F.; Gonzalez-Alzaga, B.; Aguilar-Garduño, C.; Gil, F. Biomonitoring of arsenic, cadmium, lead, manganese and mercury in urine and hair of children living near mining and industrial areas. *Chemosphere* **2015**, *124*, 83–91. [CrossRef]
27. Jursa, T.; Stein, C.; Smith, D. Determinants of Hair Manganese, Lead, Cadmium and Arsenic Levels in Environmentally Exposed Children. *Toxics* **2018**, *6*, 19. [CrossRef] [PubMed]
28. Taraškevičius, R.; Zinkutė, R.; Gedminienė, L.; Stankevičius, Ž. Hair geochemical composition of children from Vilnius kindergartens as an indicator of environmental conditions. *Environ. Geochem. Health* **2018**, *40*, 1817–1840. [CrossRef]

29. Vella, C.; Attard, E. Consumption of Minerals, Toxic Metals and Hydroxymethylfurfural: Analysis of Infant Foods and Formulae. *Toxics* **2019**, *7*, 33. [CrossRef]
30. Xie, W.; Peng, C.; Wang, H.; Chen, W. Health risk assessment of trace metals in various environmental media, crops and human hair from a mining affected area. *Int. J. Environ. Res. Public Health* **2017**, *14*, 1595. [CrossRef]
31. Nadal, M.; Bocio, A.; Schuhmacher, M.; Domingo, J.L. Monitoring metals in the population living in the vicinity of a hazardous waste incinerator: Levels in hair of school children. *Biol. Trace Elem. Res.* **2005**, *104*, 203–213. [CrossRef]
32. Ferré-Huguet, N.; Nadal, M.; Schuhmacher, M.; Domingo, J.L. Monitoring Metals in Blood and Hair of the Population Living Near a Hazardous Waste Incinerator: Temporal Trend. *Biol. Trace Elem. Res.* **2009**, *128*, 191–199. [CrossRef] [PubMed]
33. Martorell, I.; Nadal, M.; Vilavert, L.; Garcia, F.; Schuhmacher, M.; Domingo, J.L. Concentrations of trace elements in the hair of children living near a hazardous waste incinerator in Catalonia, Spain. *Trace Elem. Electrolytes* **2015**, *32*, 43–51. [CrossRef]
34. Semenova, I.N.; Rafikova, Y.S.; Khasanova, R.F.; Suyundukov, Y.T. Analysis of metal content in soils near abandoned mines of Bashkir Trans-Urals and in the hair of children living in this territory. *J. Trace Elem. Med. Biol.* **2018**, *50*, 664–670. [CrossRef] [PubMed]
35. Drobyshev, E.J.; Solovyev, N.D.; Ivanenko, N.B.; Kombarova, M.Y.; Ganeev, A.A. Trace element biomonitoring in hair of school children from a polluted area by sector field inductively coupled plasmamass spectrometry. *J. Trace Elem. Med. Biol.* **2017**, *39*, 14–20. [CrossRef] [PubMed]
36. Tamburo, E.; Varrica, D.; Dongarrà, G. Gender as a key factor in trace metal and metalloid content of human scalp hair. A multi-site study. *Sci. Total Environ.* **2016**, *573*, 996–1002. [CrossRef]
37. Varrica, D.; Tamburo, E.; Milia, N.; Vallascas, E.; Cortimiglia, V.; De Giudici, G.; Dongarrà, G.; Sanna, E.; Monna, F.; Losno, R. Metals and metalloids in hair samples of children living near the abandoned mine sites of Sulcis-Inglesiente (Sardinia, Italy). *Environ. Res.* **2014**, *134*, 366–374. [CrossRef]
38. Sanna, E.; Floris, G.; Vallascas, E. Town and gender effects on hair lead levels in children from three Sardinian Towns (Italy) with different environmental backgrounds. *Biol. Trace Elem. Res.* **2008**, *124*, 52–59. [CrossRef]
39. Tamburo, E.; Varrica, D.; Dongarrà, G. Coverage intervals for trace elements in human scalp hair are site specific. *Environ. Toxicol. Pharmacol.* **2015**, *39*, 70–76. [CrossRef]
40. Giné-Bordonaba, J.; Vilavert, L.; Nadal, M.; Schuhmacher, M.; Domingo, J.L. Monitoring environmental levels of trace elements near a hazardous waste incinerator human health risks after a decade of regular operations. *Biol. Trace Elem. Res.* **2011**, *144*, 1419–1429. [CrossRef]
41. Vilavert, L.; Nadal, M.; Schuhmacher, M.; Domingo, J.L. Concentrations of metals in soils in the neighborhood of a hazardous waste incinerator: Assessment of the temporal trends. *Biol. Trace Elem. Res.* **2012**, *149*, 435–442. [CrossRef] [PubMed]
42. González, N.; Calderón, J.; Rúbies, A.; Timoner, I.; Castell, V.; Domingo, J.L.; Nadal, M. Dietary intake of arsenic, cadmium, mercury and lead by the population of Catalonia, Spain: Analysis of the temporal trend. *Food Chem. Toxicol.* **2019**, *132*, 110721. [CrossRef] [PubMed]
43. Schuhmacher, M.; Bellés, M.; Rico, A.; Domingo, J.L.; Corbella, J. Impact of reduction of lead in gasoline on the blood and hair lead levels in the population of Tarragona Province, Spain, 1990–1995. *Sci. Total Environ.* **1996**, *184*, 203–209. [CrossRef]
44. Domingo, J.L.; Perelló, G.; Giné Bordonaba, J. Dietary intake of metals by the population of Tarragona County (Catalonia, Spain): Results from a duplicate diet study. *Biol. Trace Elem. Res.* **2012**, *146*, 420–425. [CrossRef] [PubMed]
45. González, N.; Marquès, M.; Nadal, M.; Domingo, J.L. Levels of PCDD/Fs in foodstuffs in Tarragona County (Catalonia, Spain): Spectacular decrease in the dietary intake of PCDD/Fs in the last 20 years. *Food Chem. Toxicol.* **2018**, *121*, 109–114. [CrossRef] [PubMed]

46. Peña-Fernández, A.; González-Muñoz, M.J.; Lobo-Bedmar, M.C. Evaluating the effect of age and area of residence in the metal and metalloid contents in human hair and urban topsoils. *Environ. Sci. Pollut. Res.* **2016**, *23*, 21299–21312. [CrossRef]
47. Torrente, M.; Gascon, M.; Vrijheid, M.; Sunyer, J.; Forns, J.; Domingo, J.; Nadal, M. Levels of Metals in Hair in Childhood: Preliminary Associations with Neuropsychological Behaviors. *Toxics* **2013**, *2*, 1–16. [CrossRef]

toxics MDPI

Article

Biomonitoring of Trace Elements in Subjects Living Near a Hazardous Waste Incinerator: Concentrations in Autopsy Tissues

Francisco García [1,2], Montse Marquès [1], Eneko Barbería [2], Pilar Torralba [2], Inés Landin [2], Carlos Laguna [2], José L. Domingo [1] and Martí Nadal [1,*]

1 Laboratory of Toxicology and Environmental Health, School of Medicine, IISPV, Universitat Rovira i Virgili, Sant Llorenç 21, 43201 Reus, Catalonia, Spain; francisco.garcia@urv.cat (F.G.); montserrat.marques@urv.cat (M.M.); joseluis.domingo@urv.cat (J.L.D.)

2 Institut de Medicina Legal i Ciències Forenses, Divisió de Tarragona, Rambla del President Lluís Companys 10, 43005 Tarragona, Catalonia, Spain; eneko.barberia@urv.cat (E.B.); mariapilar.torralba@xij.gencat.cat (P.T.); mariaines.landin@urv.cat (I.L.); carlosjavier.laguna@xij.gencat.cat (C.L.)

* Correspondence: marti.nadal@urv.cat; Tel.: +34-977758930

Received: 21 January 2020; Accepted: 8 February 2020; Published: 11 February 2020

Abstract: The only hazardous waste incinerator (HWI) in Spain started to operate in 1999. Twenty years later, the levels of 11 trace elements (As, Be, Cd, Cr, Hg, Mn, Ni, Pb, Sn, Tl and V) were analyzed in five different autopsy tissues (kidney, liver, brain, bone and lung) from 20 individuals who had been living near the facility. In 2019, As, Be, Tl and V were not detected in any of the analyzed tissues, while Hg could be only quantified in very few samples. The highest levels of Cd and Pb were found in kidney and bone, respectively, while those of Mn were observed in liver and kidney. In turn, the mean concentrations of Cr and Sn were very similar in all tissues. A consistent temporal trend (1998–2019) was only found for Cr and Pb. On the one hand, the mean Cr concentrations in kidney and bone have increased progressively since 1998. In contrast, the mean levels of Pb decreased significantly over time, probably due to ban of Pb as gasoline additive. The data global analysis indicates that the emissions of trace elements by the HWI have not increased the exposure and/or accumulation of these elements in individuals living near the facility.

Keywords: trace elements; autopsy tissues; hazardous waste incinerator; temporal trends

1. Introduction

In 2016, the total waste generated in the EU-28 by all economic activities and households amounted to 2538 million tons, being 100.7 million tons classified as hazardous waste (HW), which means 4% of the total [1]. According to EU statistics, in the period 2010–2016 there was an increasing trend of around 5% in the generation of HW in the EU-28. Although landfilling is still the most predominant practice used to manage HW in the EU, recycling is also relatively important, as up to 37.8% of the total amount was recycled. Other alternatives include backfilling and incineration, either with or without energy recovery. The percentages of HW that is incinerated vary across the EU, with Norway, Denmark and Portugal presenting the highest rates (34%, 19% and 12%). In contrast, the contribution of incineration to HW management in countries, such as Malta, Greece or Bulgaria is nominal.

In 2016, only 3.6% of the HW generated in Spain was incinerated. Currently, Spain counts with only one HW incinerator (HWI), which is located in Constantí (Tarragona, Catalonia, Spain). This facility has been continuously operating for 20 years since 1999, when it started its regular operations. In the 1996–1998 period, a pre-operational surveillance program was conducted to assess potential temporal changes that could occur regarding the exposure to environmental pollutants potentially emitted by the plant. The baseline survey included the analysis of polychlorinated dibenzo-*p*-dioxins and dibenzofurans (PCDD/Fs) and a number of trace elements, two groups of pollutants of high concern for the population, and whose levels in stack air must be periodically controlled [2]. The contents of PCDD/Fs and trace elements were determined in a wide range of environmental and biological samples [3–9]. Because diet is the most important route of exposure to these chemicals [10–12], the dietary intake by the local population was also evaluated [13,14]. The biomonitoring was based on the analysis of 11 trace elements in samples of hair from schoolchildren, blood from general population, as well as samples of autopsy tissues from individuals who had been residing near the plant for at least the last 10 years [3–5]. Since then, the concentrations of the same chemicals in the same matrices have been updated every 5 years [15–17]. Recently, we have reported the levels of As and a number of metals in human hair and blood of the population living in the neighborhood of the HWI [18,19].

In the present study, the concentrations of trace elements were determined in samples of autopsy tissues collected in 2019 from subjects who had been living near the HWI of Constantí. The temporal trends in the pollutant levels were also established by comparing the current results with those found in the baseline (1998) and the previously performed (2002–2007–2013) studies. Finally, the concentrations of these elements in autopsy tissues were correlated with those found in other biomonitors (human hair and blood) from non-occupationally exposed individuals living in the same area.

2. Materials and Methods

2.1. Sampling

In 2019, autopsy tissue samples were collected from 20 individuals who—at the time of death—had been residing near the Constantí HWI at least during the previous 10 years. These individuals were not occupationally exposed, being five of them smokers. The samples were collected in close collaboration with forensic doctors from the Tarragona Division of the Institute of Legal Medicine and Forensic Sciences of Catalonia. Samples were obtained from 19 men and one woman, with an average age of 56 years. From each subject, samples (1 g) of the following tissues were obtained: kidney, liver, brain, bone tissue, and lung. One hundred samples (five tissues per individual) were collected. Autopsies and sample collection were performed within the first 24 h after the death. Samples were stored in hermetically sealed polyethylene containers and frozen at −20 °C for processing [20–22]. The protocol of the biological surveillance program, number 07/2017, was reviewed and approved by the Ethical Committee for Clinical Research (CEIm) of the Pere Virgili Health Research Institute (IISPV), Reus/Tarragona, Spain, in 20 March 2017. Furthermore, the specific protocol for the biomonitoring study of autopsy tissues, number PR164/19, was complementarily evaluated and approved by the Clinical Research Ethics Committee (CEIC) of the Bellvitge University Hospital, Barcelona, Spain, in 9 May 2019.

2.2. Chemical Analysis

The concentrations of arsenic (As), beryllium (Be), cadmium (Cd), chromium (Cr), mercury (Hg), manganese (Mn), nickel (Ni), lead (Pb), tin (Sn), thallium (Tl) and vanadium (V) were determined in all samples. In order to obtain fully comparable data, the same experimental procedure as that used in previous studies of the surveillance program [21,22], was followed. Briefly, 0.5 g of each sample were treated in Teflon vessels containing 5 mL of nitric acid (65%, Suprapur, E. Merck, Darmstadt, Germany) during 8 h at room temperature. Afterwards, samples were heated for 8 h more at 80 °C. After cooling, samples were filtrated, made up to 25 mL with deionized water and properly stored −20 °C until the chemical determination. The analysis of the 11 trace elements was conducted by means of inductively coupled plasma-mass spectrometry (ICP-MS) using an Elan 6000 instrument (Perkin Elmer, Waltham, MA, USA). The limits of detection (LODs) were 0.025 μg/g for Cd, Pb and Tl; 0.05 μg/g for Mn; 0.10 μg/g for As, Be and Hg; 0.25 μg/g for Ni; and 0.50 μg/g for Cr, Sn and V. The quality of the experimental procedure was controlled and assured by analyzing reference materials

(Lobster Hepatopancreas, TORT 2, NRC Canada, Ottawa, ON, Canada) and blanks in every batch of samples Reproducibility was assured as reported in previous investigations [22]. Recovery percentages ranged between 84% and 121%.

2.3. Statistics

When any of the analyzed metals could not be detected, a concentration equivalent to one-half of their respective detection limit was assumed (ND = 1/2 LOD). Statistical significance of the results was first assessed by applying the Levene test to verify the homoscedasticity of the data. Depending on whether the variance followed a normal distribution or not, a variance analysis (ANOVA) or the Mann-Whitney U-test was subsequently performed. A probability lower than 0.05 ($p < 0.05$) was considered significant. Pearson correlations in the concentrations among the five evaluated tissues, as well as with those of human hair and blood [18,19], were also carried out.

3. Results

Data regarding the concentrations of trace elements in samples of autopsy tissues collected in 2019 are summarized in Table 1. The levels of As, Be, Tl and V were below their respective detection limits (<0.10, <0.10, <0.025 and <0.50 μg/g, respectively) in all tissues. Mercury could be only detected in one sample of liver and three of kidney, with its levels being under the detection limit in the remaining 96 samples. Cadmium showed the highest levels in kidney, with a mean concentration of 11.10 μg/g, while in other organs the concentrations were much lower (range: 0.02–0.76 μg/g). The average Cr concentration in the five analyzed tissues was very similar, with values ranging from 0.29 to 1.02 μg/g. In turn, Mn could be quantified in all tissues, with relatively higher levels in liver and kidney (1.16 and 0.82 μg/g, respectively). Lead showed higher values in bone (mean: 1.00 μg/g; range: <0.025–5.39 μg/g) than in the other evaluated tissues. Finally, Sn was also detected in the five tissues, with similar levels in all (range: 0.78–1.94 μg/g).

Table 1. Concentration (in μg/g) of trace elements in samples of autopsy tissues collected in 2019 from subjects who had been living near the HWI of Constantí.

Tissue		Mean	±	St. Dev.	Median	Min	Max	Detection Rate (%)
LIVER	**As**		<0.10		-	ND	ND	0
	Be		<0.10		-	ND	ND	0
	Cd	0.76	±	0.61	0.64	0.13	2.77	100
	Cr	0.47	±	0.17	0.54	<0.50	0.74	65
	Hg	0.06	±	0.04	0.05	<0.10	0.23	5
	Mn	1.16	±	0.28	1.18	0.62	1.83	100
	Ni	0.14	±	0.06	0.13	<0.25	0.35	10
	Pb	0.23	±	0.42	0.08	<0.025	1.80	80
	Sn	1.33	±	0.52	1.21	0.88	3.30	100
	Tl		<0.025		-	ND	ND	0
	V		<0.50		-	ND	ND	0
KIDNEY	**As**		<0.10		-	ND	ND	0
	Be		<0.10		-	ND	ND	0
	Cd	11.10	±	8.17	8.06	0.83	44.35	100
	Cr	0.29	±	0.11	0.25	<0.50	0.58	15
	Hg	0.08	±	0.09	0.05	<0.10	0.34	15
	Mn	0.82	±	0.23	0.87	0.32	1.22	100
	Ni	0.21	±	0.23	0.13	<0.25	1.08	15
	Pb	0.15	±	0.17	0.09	<0.025	0.65	85
	Sn	1.04	±	0.28	1.08	0.70	1.94	100
	Tl		<0.025		-	ND	ND	0
	V		<0.50		-	ND	ND	0

Table 1. *Cont.*

Tissue		Mean	±	St. Dev.	Median	Min	Max	Detection Rate (%)
	As		<0.10		-	ND	ND	0
	Be		<0.10		-	ND	ND	0
	Cd	0.02	±	0.02	0.01	<0.025	0.06	30
	Cr	0.32	±	0.12	0.25	<0.50	0.58	25
	Hg		<0.10		-	ND	ND	0
BRAIN	**Mn**	0.25	±	0.15	0.21	0.16	0.86	100
	Ni	0.16	±	0.11	0.13	<0.25	0.58	10
	Pb	0.08	±	0.12	0.02	<0.025	0.47	50
	Sn	0.78	±	0.25	0.72	0.54	1.60	100
	Tl		<0.025		-	ND	ND	0
	V		<0.50		-	ND	ND	0
	As		<0.10		-	ND	ND	0
	Be		<0.10		-	ND	ND	0
	Cd	0.02	±	0.02	0.01	<0.025	0.07	30
	Cr	1.02	±	0.24	1.00	0.63	1.52	100
	Hg		<0.10		-	ND	ND	0
BONE	**Mn**	0.05	±	0.04	0.03	<0.05	0.16	40
	Ni		<0.25		-	ND	ND	0
	Pb	1.00	±	1.33	0.54	<0.025	5.39	95
	Sn	1.94	±	0.64	1.73	1.07	3.51	100
	Tl		<0.025		-	ND	ND	0
	V		<0.50		-	ND	ND	0
	As		<0.10		-	ND	ND	0
	Be		<0.10		-	ND	ND	0
	Cd	0.13	±	0.18	0.04	<0.025	0.62	65
	Cr	0.30	±	0.12	0.25	<0.50	0.62	15
	Hg		<0.10		-	ND	ND	0
LUNG	**Mn**	0.08	±	0.04	0.07	<0.05	0.15	75
	Ni	0.15	±	0.07	0.13	<0.25	0.40	10
	Pb	0.05	±	0.11	0.01	<0.025	0.42	35
	Sn	1.31	±	0.33	1.20	0.91	2.11	100
	Tl		<0.025		-	ND	ND	0
	V		<0.50		-	ND	ND	0

Table 2 shows the concentrations of the metals analyzed in autopsy samples (brain, bone, kidney, liver, and lung) in the 1998 (baseline), 2003, 2007, 2013, and 2019 surveys, as well as the percentage variation in the periods 1998–2019 and 2013–2019. Between 1998 and 2019, a significant decrease in Cd, Hg and Pb concentrations was noticed (20%, 70% and 91%, respectively), while only Cd showed a significant reduction between the campaigns performed in 2013 and 2019 (45%; $p < 0.001$).

In kidney, a significant increase in Cr levels, as well as in those of Hg and Sn, was observed between the baseline (1998) and the current (2019) studies. In contrast, none of the evaluated elements showed a significant change of concentration between 2013 and 2019. In 2019, the mean concentrations of As, Be, Hg, Tl and V in brain were lower than their respective detection limits. Regarding Cr, a non-significant decrease (44%) was observed in the period 2013–2019, while a non-significant increase was noted between 1998 and 2019 ($p > 0.05$). Lead was the only element for which a significant change in concentration was observed in kidney, with a significant reduction (94%; $p < 0.001$) between the baseline (1998) and the current (2019) surveys.

In bone, most elements showed a decrease of their concentrations with respect to those found in the baseline study, with significant reductions in Cd, Pb and Sn (50%, 75% and 74%, respectively). In contrast, Cr showed a significant increase, from 0.51 to 1.02 μg/g, between 1998 and 2019. With respect to the previous survey, conducted in 2013, the levels of Sn significantly increased ($p < 0.001$) and those of Mn significantly decreased ($p < 0.05$).

Table 2. Mean concentration (μg/g) of trace elements in autopsy tissues collected between 1998 and 2019. Temporal trends.

Tissue		1998	2003	2007	2013	2019	% Variation 1998–2019	% Variation 2013–2019
LIVER	As	<0.05	<0.05	0.07	<0.05	<0.10	-	-
	Be	<0.02	<0.05	<0.03	<0.05	<0.10	-	-
	Cd	0.95	1.36	0.8	1.38	0.76	−20 ***	−45 **
	Cr	0.26	<0.25	0.63	0.66	0.47	81	−29
	Hg	0.2	0.14	0.14	<0.05	0.06	−70 *	-
	Mn	1.28	1.07	0.99	1.45	1.16	−9	−20
	Ni	0.09	<0.1	0.07	<0.10	0.14	56	-
	Pb	2.56	0.3	0.35	0.18	0.23	−91 ***	28
	Sn	5.06	0.19	0.07	<0.05	1.33	−74	-
	Tl	<0.02	<0.01	<0.01	<0.03	<0.025	-	-
	V	<0.12	<0.25	<0.25	<0.10	<0.50	-	-
KIDNEY	As	<0.05	<0.05	0.06	<0.05	<0.10	-	-
	Be	<0.02	<0.05	<0.03	<0.05	<0.10	-	-
	Cd	17.52	17.46	14.72	21.15	11.1	−37	−48
	Cr	0.09	<0.25	0.42	0.66	0.29	222 ***	−56 **
	Hg	0.33	0.23	0.3	0.15	0.08	−76 *	−47 *
	Mn	1.01	0.74	0.78	1.09	0.82	−19	−25
	Ni	<0.01	<0.10	<0.05	<0.10	0.21	-	-
	Pb	<0.02	0.06	0.77	0.1	0.15	-	50
	Sn	1.66	0.17	0.05	<0.05	1.04	−37 *	-
	Tl	<0.02	<0.01	<0.01	<0.03	<0.025	-	-
	V	<0.12	<0.25	<0.25	<0.10	<0.50	-	-
BRAIN	As	<0.05	<0.05	<0.05	<0.05	<0.10	-	-
	Be	<0.02	<0.05	<0.03	<0.05	<0.10	-	-
	Cd	0.03	0.02	0.32	<0.05	0.02	−33	-
	Cr	0.22	<0.25	0.45	0.57	0.32	45	−44
	Hg	<0.05	<0.05	0.1	<0.05	<0.10	-	-
	Mn	0.22	0.03	0.24	0.33	0.25	14	−24
	Ni	<0.01	<0.10	0.36	<0.05	0.16	-	-
	Pb	1.41	0.06	0.1	<0.05	0.08	−94 ***	-
	Sn	1.32	0.09	0.03	<0.05	0.78	−41	-
	Tl	<0.02	<0.01	<0.01	<0.05	<0.025	-	-
	V	<0.12	<0.25	0.28	<0.05	<0.50	-	-
BONE	As	0.06	<0.05	0.19	<0.05	<0.10	-	-
	Be	<0.02	<0.05	0.03	<0.05	<0.10	-	-
	Cd	0.04	0.05	0.04	<0.03	0.02	−50 **	-
	Cr	0.51	<0.25	1.39	1.38	1.02	100 ***	−26
	Hg	<0.05	<0.05	0.05	<0.05	<0.10	-	-
	Mn	0.06	<0.03	0.25	0.13	0.05	−17	−62 *
	Ni	0.64	1.16	1.53	<0.10	<0.25	-	-
	Pb	3.99	2.11	2.66	1.39	1	−75 ***	-28
	Sn	7.4	0.34	0.31	0.17	1.94	−74 ***	1041 ***
	Tl	<0.02	<0.01	<0.01	<0.03	<0.025	-	-
	V	<0.12	<0.25	<0.25	<0.10	<0.50	-	-
LUNG	As	<0.05	<0.05	0.14	<0.05	<0.10	-	-
	Be	<0.02	<0.05	<0.03	<0.05	<0.10	-	-
	Cd	0.42	0.18	0.27	0.26	0.13	−69	−50
	Cr	0.33	0.25	0.58	0.64	0.3	−9	−53 *
	Hg	<0.05	<0.05	<0.05	<0.05	<0.10	-	-
	Mn	0.13	0.04	0.3	0.21	0.08	−38	−62 **
	Ni	0.08	0.12	0.07	<0.10	0.15	88 **	-
	Pb	2.27	0.13	0.08	0.05	0.05	−98 ***	0
	Sn	2.16	0.2	0.07	<0.05	1.31	−39	-
	Tl	<0.02	<0.01	<0.01	<0.03	<0.025	-	-
	V	<0.12	<0.25	0.58	<0.10	<0.50	-	-

* $p < 0.05$; ** $p < 0.01$; *** $p < 0.001$.

In lung, most trace elements presented a reduction of their concentration over time. However, the difference between 1998 and 2019 were only significant for Pb ($p < 0.001$). In contrast, Ni levels significantly increased (88%; $p < 0.01$). With respect to our most recent study (2013), none of the trace elements showed an increase of concentration in lung, while significant decreases were noted for Cr and Mn ($p < 0.05$ and $p < 0.01$, respectively).

Some fluctuations in the concentrations of trace elements in the analyzed human tissues were found. However, a general trend was not observed after 20 years of continuous operation of the plant. When considering the whole assessment period (1998–2019), no changes were observed for any metal, excepting Cr and Pb. On one hand, between 1998 and 2019, Cr concentration increased in all tissues excepting lung. However, the increase was only significant in kidney and bone. It must be recalled that Cr is a highly toxic metal, being one of the chemical forms (Cr^{6+}) fully recognized as carcinogenic [23,24]. On the other hand, the mean Pb levels in autopsy tissues were significantly lower in 2019 than in 1998, with the only exception of kidney, an organ where Pb could not be detected in the baseline survey. This fact would be closely related to the banning of Pb as a gasoline additive, introduced in the early 2000s [25].

The concentrations of trace elements in five autopsy tissues according to sex are depicted in Figure 1. Unfortunately, a proper statistical study could not be performed, since 19 out of the 20 subjects were men. Therefore, scientifically valid conclusions cannot be extracted from such a poorly representative number of samples. Anyway, the most notable finding is that the only recruited woman had higher levels of Pb than the mean of men in liver (1.80 vs. 0.15 µg/g) and kidney (0.51 vs. 0.13 µg/g), while in the other tissues, Pb concentrations were higher in men. In addition, the levels of Cr were higher in the tissue samples corresponding to men than those from women.

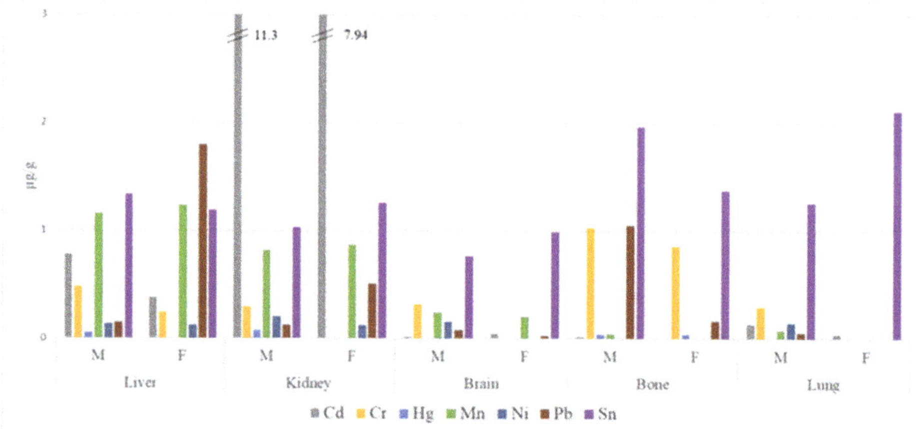

Figure 1. Concentrations (in µg/g) of trace elements in samples of autopsy tissues collected in 2019 according to the sex of the subjects (M: male; F: female).

Table 3 presents the mean concentrations of the trace elements analyzed in autopsy tissues according to age. Three age groups were considered: <35 ($n = 3$), 35–65 ($n = 10$), and >65 ($n = 7$). Due to the relatively small number of samples, a statistical comparison among groups could not be conducted. However, the data may be indicative to set age-specific trends. A correlation study of the metal concentrations in the autopsy tissues was also performed, taking into account that each subject provided five different tissues (brain, bone, kidney, liver, and lung). Notwithstanding, none of the individuals showed a general increase in the body burdens of trace elements, as Pearson correlations among tissues were not statistically significant.

Table 3. Concentrations (μg/g) of trace elements in samples of autopsy tissues collected in 2019 according to the age of the subjects.

Tissue		<35 years (n = 3)			35–65 years (n = 10)			>65 years (n = 7)		
		Mean	±	St. Dev.	Mean	±	St. Dev.	Mean	±	St. Dev.
	As		<0.10			<0.10			<0.10	
	Be		<0.10			<0.10			<0.10	
	Cd	0.99	±	0.53	0.55	±	0.34	0.96	±	0.86
	Cr	0.47	±	0.19	0.46	±	0.19	0.48	±	0.16
	Hg		<0.10			<0.10			0.08	
LIVER	Mn	1.32	±	0.45	1.06	±	0.24	1.24	±	0.25
	Ni	0.13	±	0.00	0.14	±	0.05	0.16	±	0.08
	Pb	0.23	±	0.28	0.33	±	0.58	0.08	±	0.09
	Sn	2.03	±	1.20	1.20	±	0.30	1.21	±	0.11
	Tl		<0.025			<0.025			<0.025	
	V		<0.50			<0.50			<0.50	
	As		<0.10			<0.10			<0.10	
	Be		<0.10			<0.10			<0.10	
	Cd	5.50	±	3.54	12.98	±	8.99	10.81	±	7.94
	Cr	0.33	±	0.15	0.28	±	0.10	0.29	±	0.11
	Hg	0.15	±	0.17	0.08	±	0.09		<0.10	
KIDNEY	Mn	1.04	±	0.34	0.84	±	0.20	0.69	±	0.22
	Ni		<0.25		0.25	±	0.31	0.18	±	0.14
	Pb	0.06	±	0.10	0.20	±	0.22	0.11	±	0.08
	Sn	0.85	±	0.18	1.15	±	0.31	0.96	±	0.22
	Tl		<0.025			<0.025			<0.025	
	V		<0.50			<0.50			<0.50	
	As		<0.10			<0.10			<0.10	
	Be		<0.10			<0.10			<0.10	
	Cd	0.03	±	0.02	0.02	±	0.02	0.02	±	0.01
	Cr	0.34	±	0.15	0.33	±	0.14	0.29	±	0.10
	Hg		<0.10			<0.10			<0.10	
BRAIN	Mn	0.22	±	0.05	0.29	±	0.20	0.21	±	0.03
	Ni	0.13	±	0.00	0.17	±	0.14	0.16	±	0.09
	Pb	0.11	±	0.11	0.05	±	0.04	0.12	±	0.19
	Sn	0.73	±	0.10	0.79	±	0.32	0.80	±	0.17
	Tl		<0.025			<0.025			<0.025	
	V		<0.50			<0.50			<0.50	
	As		<0.10			<0.10			<0.10	
	Be		<0.10			<0.10			<0.10	
	Cd	0.10	±	0.16	0.16	±	0.21	0.10	±	0.14
	Cr	0.37	±	0.21	0.28	±	0.08	0.30	±	0.14
	Hg		<0.10			<0.10			<0.10	
LUNG	Mn	0.10	±	0.03	0.07	±	0.05	0.08	±	0.04
	Ni		<0.25		0.15	±	0.09	0.15	±	0.06
	Pb		<0.025		0.06	±	0.13	0.07	±	0.10
	Sn	1.30	±	0.30	1.26	±	0.33	1.38	±	0.36
	Tl		<0.025			<0.025			<0.025	
	V		<0.50			<0.50			<0.50	
	As		<0.10			<0.10			<0.10	
	Be		<0.10			<0.10			<0.10	
	Cd		<0.025		0.03	±	0.02	0.02	±	0.01
	Cr	0.70	±	0.06	1.06	±	0.31	1.11	±	0.12
	Hg		<0.10			<0.10			<0.10	
BONE	Mn	0.05	±	0.02	0.04	±	0.07	0.06	±	0.05
	Ni	0.13	±	0.00	0.13	±	0.00	0.13	±	0.00
	Pb	0.06	±	0.07	0.43	±	0.34	2.23	±	1.69
	Sn	2.39	±	0.69	1.80	±	0.36	1.94	±	0.61
	Tl		<0.025			<0.025			<0.025	
	V		<0.50			<0.50			<0.50	

4. Discussion

In recent years, a number of scientific studies on the concentrations of metals in humans—for occupationally and non-occupationally exposed populations—have been published [26]. Recently, Dudek-Adamska et al. [27] analyzed the concentrations of Cr in samples of blood and internal organs collected at autopsy from 21 female and 39 male non-occupationally exposed subjects in Southern Poland. Reference ranges of Cr in brain, liver, kidney and lung were 4.7–136, 11–506, 2.9–298 and 13–798 ng/g, respectively. The concentrations corresponding to individuals living near the HWI of Constantí would be within that range, but in the upper side for liver, kidney and lung. In turn, the mean levels of Cr in brain for the population of the current study was 2-fold higher than for the Polish residents. In Sweden, Akerstrom et al. [28] studied the relationship between Hg in kidney, blood, and urine in environmentally exposed individuals, and its implications for biomonitoring. The mean concentration of Hg in kidney from 152 healthy kidney donors (65 men and 87 women) was reported to be 0.33 μg/g, a value 4-times higher than that observed in the autopsied subjects who had been living near the HWI here assessed.

The analysis of trace elements in autopsy tissues is part of a large surveillance program on the HWI. In 2017, the concentrations of the same elements in samples of human hair from schoolchildren and of blood from an adult population, all of them living near the facility, were determined [18,19]. The temporal decrease of Pb in autopsy tissues was also observed in the other biomonitors. In 2017, the mean concentration of Pb in human hair from schoolchildren was 1.44 μg/g, being significantly lower than the value found in the baseline survey (5.81 μg/g). In blood, the mean Pb level in 2017 was 12.98 μg/kg, with a significant ($p < 0.05$) reduction with respect to the previous (2012) study but non-significant ($p > 0.05$) compared to the baseline survey. In addition, the notable increase of Cr observed in some autopsy tissues was also detected in blood [19], where values increased from undetected levels to 6.29 μg/kg. In contrast, Cr levels in human hair did not increase through time [18]. Since the biological concentrations of environmental contaminants in the human body are highly dependent on the dietary intake, food levels of the same pollutants are also periodically monitored. In our last study, corresponding to data on foodstuffs samples collected in 2013 [29], the estimated dietary intake of Cr and Hg was found to progressively and significantly increase with respect to the baseline study.

Some toxic habits, such as smoking or alcohol consumption, have been pointed out as potential sources of toxic elements (i.e., Cd, Pb) [20], whose exposure is related to adverse health effects, including the probability to develop cancer [30]. In the present study, a correlation between smoking and the burdens of the toxic elements analyzed in the five human tissues was not found. However, the reduced number of samples (n = 5 smokers out of 20 subjects) makes difficult to establish any conclusion in this sense.

5. Conclusions

The analysis of the temporal trends of the concentrations of a number of trace elements in five autopsy tissues indicates that there have been fluctuations through time, when comparing the results of the campaign performed in 2019 with those corresponding to the baseline survey (1998). Furthermore, no significant changes were noted between 2013 and 2018 for most elements. A general increasing or decreasing tendency was not found, with the only exceptions of Pb and Cr. On one hand, the mean blood levels of Pb were significantly reduced compared to the baseline (1998) study, mainly due to the effect of banning Pb as a gasoline additive, introduced in the early 2000's. On the other hand, the average Cr concentration in most tissues is still higher than that found in the baseline study, although the difference was only significant in kidney and bone. In contrast, the 5 analyzed autopsy tissues showed significantly lower concentrations than the levels found in the previous campaign (2013), when a generalized increase, not only in autopsy tissues, but also in some environmental samples, was noticed. That rise was also supported by the increase in the dietary intake of Cr estimated for the adult population living near the HWI.

In any case, the levels of trace elements obtained in the present study are similar to those reported recently in various studies of different countries. The global analysis of the data clearly indicates that air emissions of the HWI have not a significant exposure or accumulation of these elements in individuals living in the area near the facility. Moreover, the temporal changes may be more directly related to differences in the dietary exposure of the population.

Author Contributions: Conceptualization, J.L.D. and M.N.; methodology, F.G., E.B., P.T., I.L., C.L., M.N.; software, M.M., M.N.; validation, F.G., J.L.D.; formal analysis, F.G., E.B., P.T., M.M.; investigation, F.G., I.L., C.L.; resources, F.G., J.L.D.; data curation, F.G., M.N.; writing—original draft preparation, M.M., M.N.; writing—review and editing, M.M., J.L.D.; visualization, F.G., J.L.D.; supervision, F.G., M.N.; project administration, M.N.; funding acquisition, J.L.D. All authors have read and agreed to the published version of the manuscript.

Funding: This study was funded by Sarpi Constantí SL, Catalonia, Spain.

Acknowledgments: The authors appreciate the technical assistance of Jordi Sierra and Anabel Díez for the analytical treatment, as well all the relatives of the individuals who provided the autopsy tissue samples.

Conflicts of Interest: The authors declare no conflict of interest.

References

1. Eurostat. *Waste Statistics*; European Commission: Brussels, Belgium, 2020. Available online: https://ec.europa.eu/eurostat/statistics-explained/index.php?title=Waste_statistics (accessed on 20 January 2020).
2. Rovira, J.; Mari, M.; Nadal, M.; Schuhmacher, M.; Domingo, J.L. Environmental monitoring of metals, PCDD/Fs and PCBs as a complementary tool of biological surveillance to assess human health risks. *Chemosphere* **2010**, *80*, 1183–1189. [CrossRef]
3. Granero, S.; Llobet, J.M.; Schuhmacher, M.; Corbella, J.; Domingo, J.L. Biological monitoring of environmental pollution and human exposure to metals in Tarragona, Spain. I. Levels in hair of school children. *Trace Elem. Electrol.* **1998**, *15*, 39–43.
4. Llobet, J.M.; Granero, S.; Schuhmacher, M.; Corbella, J.; Domingo, J.L. Biological monitoring of environmental pollution and human exposure to metals in Tarragona, Spain. II. Levels in autopsy tissues. *Trace Elem. Electrol.* **1998**, *15*, 44–49.
5. Llobet, J.M.; Granero, S.; Torres, A.; Schuhmacher, M.; Domingo, J.L. Biological monitoring of environmental pollution and human exposure to metals in Tarragona, Spain. III. Blood levels. *Trace Elem. Electrol.* **1998**, *15*, 76–80.
6. Llobet, J.M.; Schuhmacher, M.; Domingo, J.L. Observations on metal trends in soil and vegetation samples collected in the vicinity of a hazardous waste incinerator under construction (1996–1998). *Toxicol. Environ. Chem.* **2000**, *77*, 119–129. [CrossRef]
7. Schuhmacher, M.; Domingo, J.L.; Llobet, J.M.; Kiviranta, H.; Vartiainen, T. PCDD/F concentrations in milk of non-occupationally exposed women living in southern Catalonia, Spain. *Chemosphere* **1999**, *38*, 995–1004. [CrossRef]
8. Schuhmacher, M.; Domingo, J.L.; Llobet, J.M.; Lindström, G.; Wingfors, H. Dioxin and dibenzofuran concentrations in blood of a general population from Tarragona, Spain. *Chemosphere* **1999**, *38*, 1123–1133. [CrossRef]
9. Schuhmacher, M.; Domingo, J.L.; Llobet, J.M.; Lindstrom, G.; Wingfors, H. Dioxin and dibenzofuran concentrations in adipose tissue of a general population from Tarragona, Spain. *Chemosphere* **1999**, *38*, 2475–2487. [CrossRef]
10. Sirot, V.; Traore, T.; Guérin, T.; Noël, L.; Bachelot, M.; Cravedi, J.P.; Mazur, A.; Glorennec, P.; Vasseur, P.; Jean, J.; et al. French infant total diet study: Exposure to selected trace elements and associated health risks. *Food Chem. Toxicol.* **2018**, *120*, 625–633. [CrossRef]
11. González, N.; Calderón, J.; Rúbies, A.; Timoner, I.; Castell, V.; Domingo, J.L.; Nadal, M. Dietary intake of arsenic, cadmium, mercury and lead by the population of Catalonia, Spain: Analysis of the temporal trend. *Food Chem. Toxicol.* **2019**, *132*, 110721. [CrossRef]
12. González, N.; Marquès, M.; Nadal, M.; Domingo, J.L. Occurrence of environmental pollutants in foodstuffs: A review of organic vs. conventional food. *Food Chem. Toxicol.* **2019**, *125*, 370–375. [CrossRef] [PubMed]

13. Domingo, J.L.; Schuhmacher, M.; Granero, S.; Llobet, J.M. PCDDs and PCDFs in food samples from Catalonia, Spain. An assessment of dietary intake. *Chemosphere* **1999**, *38*, 3517–3528. [CrossRef]
14. Llobet, J.M.; Granero, S.; Schuhmacher, M.; Corbella, J.; Domingo, J.L. Biological monitoring of environmental pollution and human exposure to metals in Tarragona, Spain. IV. Estimation of the dietary intake. *Trace Elem. Electrol.* **1998**, *15*, 136–141.
15. Nadal, M.; García, F.; Schuhmacher, M.; Domingo, J.L. Metals in biological tissues of the population living near a hazardous waste incinerator in Catalonia, Spain: Two decades of follow-up. *Environ. Res.* **2019**, *176*, 108578. [CrossRef] [PubMed]
16. Nadal, M.; Mari, M.; Schuhmacher, M.; Domingo, J.L. Monitoring dioxins and furans in plasma of individuals living near a hazardous waste incinerator: Temporal trend after 20 years. *Environ. Res.* **2019**, *173*, 207–211. [CrossRef] [PubMed]
17. Schuhmacher, M.; Mari, M.; Nadal, M.; Domingo, J.L. Concentrations of dioxins and furans in breast milk of women living near a hazardous waste incinerator in Catalonia, Spain. *Environ. Int.* **2019**, *125*, 334–341. [CrossRef] [PubMed]
18. Esplugas, R.; Mari, M.; Marquès, M.; Schuhmacher, M.; Domingo, J.L.; Nadal, M. Biomonitoring of trace elements in hair of schoolchildren living near a hazardous waste incinerator - A 20 years follow-up. *Toxics* **2019**, *7*, 52. [CrossRef]
19. Esplugas, R.; Serra, N.; Marquès, M.; Schuhmacher, M.; Nadal, M.; Domingo, J.L. Trace elements in blood of the population living near a hazardous waste incinerator in Catalonia, Spain. *Biol. Trace Elem. Res.* **2020**. [CrossRef]
20. Garcia, F.; Ortega, A.; Domingo, J.L.; Corbella, J. Accumulation of metals in autopsy tissues of subjects living in Tarragona County, Spain. *J. Environ. Sci. Health A* **2001**, *36*, 1767–1786. [CrossRef]
21. Bocio, A.; Nadal, M.; Garcia, F.; Domingo, J.L. Monitoring metals in the population living in the vicinity of a hazardous waste incinerator: Concentrations in autopsy tissues. *Biol. Trace Elem. Res.* **2005**, *106*, 41–50. [CrossRef]
22. Mari, M.; Nadal, M.; Schuhmacher, M.; Barbería, E.; García, F.; Domingo, J.L. Human exposure to metals: Levels in autopsy tissues of individuals living near a hazardous waste incinerator. *Biol. Trace Elem. Res.* **2014**, *159*, 15–21. [CrossRef] [PubMed]
23. Kim, J.; Seo, S.; Kim, Y.; Kim, D.H. Review of carcinogenicity of hexavalent chrome and proposal of revising approval standards for an occupational cancers in Korea. *Ann. Occup. Environ. Med.* **2018**, *30*, 7. [CrossRef] [PubMed]
24. Proctor, D.M.; Suh, M.; Campleman, S.L.; Thompson, C.M. Assessment of the mode of action for hexavalent chromium-induced lung cancer following inhalation exposures. *Toxicology* **2014**, *325*, 160–179. [CrossRef] [PubMed]
25. Nadal, M.; Schuhmacher, M.; Domingo, J.L. Metal pollution of soils and vegetation in an area with petrochemical industry. *Sci. Total Environ.* **2004**, *321*, 59–69. [CrossRef] [PubMed]
26. Domingo, J.L.; García, F.; Nadal, M.; Schuhmacher, M. Autopsy tissues as biological monitors of human exposure to environmental pollutants. A case study: Concentrations of metals and PCDD/Fs in subjects living near a hazardous waste incinerator. *Environ. Res.* **2017**, *154*, 269–274. [CrossRef]
27. Dudek-Adamska, D.; Lech, T.; Konopka, T.; Kościelniak, P. Chromium in postmortem material. *Biol. Trace Elem. Res.* **2018**, *186*, 370–378. [CrossRef]
28. Akerstrom, M.; Barregard, L.; Lundh, T.; Sallsten, G. Relationship between mercury in kidney, blood, and urine in environmentally exposed individuals, and implications for biomonitoring. *Toxicol. Appl. Pharm.* **2017**, *320*, 17–25. [CrossRef]
29. Perelló, G.; Nadal, M.; Domingo, J.L. Dietary exposure to metals by adults living near a hazardous waste incinerator in Catalonia, Spain: Temporal trend. *Trace Elem. Electrol.* **2015**, *32*, 133–141. [CrossRef]
30. Laniyan, T.A.; Adewumi, A.J. Health risk assessment of heavy metal pollution in groundwater around an exposed dumpsite in Southwestern Nigeria. *J. Health Pollut.* **2019**, *9*, 191210.

toxics

MDPI

Article

Exposure Assessment of Cadmium in Female Farmers in Cadmium-Polluted Areas in Northern Japan

Hyogo Horiguchi [1,2,*], Etsuko Oguma [1,2], Satoshi Sasaki [3], Kayoko Miyamoto [4], Yoko Hosoi [2], Akira Ono [1,5] and Fujio Kayama [2]

1 Department of Hygiene, Kitasato University School of Medicine, Kanagawa 252-0374, Japan; oguma@med.kitasato-u.ac.jp (E.O.); a-ono@furukawadenchi.co.jp (A.O.)
2 Department of Environmental and Preventive Medicine, School of Medicine, Jichi Medical University, Tochigi 329-0498, Japan; yk_hosoi2005@yahoo.co.jp (Y.H.); kayamafujio@gmail.com (F.K.)
3 Department of Social and Preventive Epidemiology, School of Public Health, The University of Tokyo, Tokyo 113-0033, Japan; stssasak@m.u-tokyo.ac.jp
4 Department of Registered Dietitian, Koyo Nursing Nutrition College, Koyo Gakuen, Ibaraki 306-0013, Japan; kayokomy@nifty.com
5 Environmental Promotion Department, The Furukawa Battery Co., Ltd., Fukushima 972-8501, Japan
* Correspondence: hhyogo@med.kitasato-u.ac.jp

Received: 14 April 2020; Accepted: 12 June 2020; Published: 17 June 2020

Abstract: Akita prefecture is located in the northern part of Japan and has many cadmium-polluted areas. We herein performed an exposure assessment of cadmium in 712 and 432 female farmers in two adjacent cadmium-polluted areas (A and B, respectively), who underwent local health examinations from 2001–2004. We measured cadmium concentrations in 100 food items collected from local markets in 2003. We then multiplied the intake of each food item by its cadmium concentration in each subject to assess cadmium intake from food and summed cadmium intake from all food items to obtain the total cadmium intake. Median cadmium intake levels in areas A and B were 55.7 and 47.8 μg/day, respectively, which were both higher than that of the general population and were attributed to local agricultural products, particularly rice. We also calculated weekly cadmium intake per body weight and compared it to the previous provisional tolerable weekly intake reported by the Joint FAO (Food and Agriculture Organization)/WHO (World Health Organization) expert committee on food additives or current tolerable weekly intake in Japan of 7 μg/kg BW/week. Medians in areas A and B were 7.2 and 6.0 μg/kg BW/week, respectively. Similar estimated values were also obtained by the Monte Carlo simulation. These results demonstrated that the cadmium exposure levels among the farmers were high enough to be approximately the tolerable weekly intake.

Keywords: cadmium; food; farmer; PTWI (provisional tolerable monthly intake); TWI (tolerable weekly intake); Monte Carlo simulation

1. Introduction

Humans are exposed on a daily basis to cadmium (Cd), a toxic heavy metal, mainly through the consumption of food containing Cd. Cd absorbed via food accumulates in the kidneys and may cause renal tubular dysfunction, called Cd nephropathy, in the inhabitants of Cd-polluted areas [1]. The most severe case of Cd toxicity is itai-itai disease, which is characterized by osteomalacia and renal anemia. It develops among patients with Cd nephropathy [2]. The heaviest Cd-polluted area in Japan was along the Jinzu River basin of Toyama prefecture, at which agricultural fields were contaminated by a large amount of Cd derived from an upstream mine. A large number of inhabitants in this area developed Cd nephropathy and 200 patients with itai-itai disease were officially recognized by 2020.

Although the Cd-polluted area in Toyama was completely restored in 2011, large but scattered Cd-polluted areas still remain in Akita prefecture, which is located in the northern part of Japan, due to the previous activities of mines and smelters [3]. Pollution levels are particularly high in the northern area of Akita prefecture, in which we performed local health examinations on female farmers as part of the Japanese multi-centered environmental toxicant study (JMETS) [4,5]. JMETS aimed for risk assessment of Cd by targeting females, who are generally more vulnerable to Cd toxicity than males. Health examinations were sequentially performed in two adjacent areas: the area along Yoneshiro River in Odate city in 2001–2002 (area A) [4] and that upstream of the river in Kazuno city and Kosaka town in 2003–2004 (area B) [5] (Figure 1). Cd pollution levels were higher in area B than in area A because area B was directly affected by two large mines and their affiliated smelters, while area A was secondarily contaminated through irrigation from the river that runs from area B. These studies revealed that many farmers were exposed to high levels of Cd through the consumption of self-harvested rice contaminated by Cd, some of whom had Cd nephropathy [4–6].

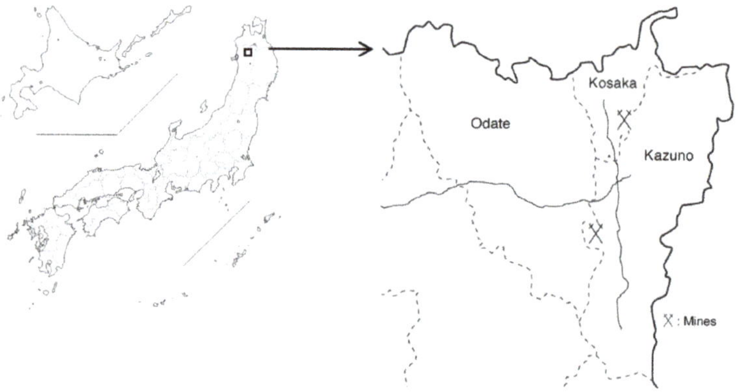

Figure 1. A map of area A (Odate city) and area B (Kazuno city and Kosaka town) in Akita, and their location in Japan (cited from CraftMAP). The thick solid line, dotted lines, and thin solid lines indicate the prefectural boundary, boundaries of municipalities, and courses of the river, respectively.

The provisional tolerable monthly intake (PTMI) of Cd reported by the Joint FAO (Food and Agriculture Organization)/WHO (World Health Organization) expert committee on food additives (JECFA) is now 25 μg/kg/month and was amended from the provisional tolerable weekly intake (PTWI) of 7 μg/kg/week in 2010 [7]. In Japan, the tolerable weekly intake (TWI) of Cd of 7 μg/kg/week remains in effect and was set by the Food Safety Commission of Japan (FSCJ) in 2008. In our previous study on area A in 2001, we performed dietary exposure assessments on Cd in subjects undergoing health examinations and obtained weekly Cd intake levels for comparisons with the PTWI of Cd at that time [4]. The findings revealed that 33–51% of subjects had Cd intake levels in excess of the PTWI. However, the exposure assessment was performed using a simplified method based on Cd concentrations in rice and miso, fermented soybean paste, and the consumption of these two foods to estimate individual Cd intake according to average Japanese Cd intake levels. Therefore, a more detailed exposure assessment of Cd is needed in this area to clarify the actual status of dietary Cd exposure in its inhabitants. A similar exposure assessment of Cd in area B, in which Cd pollution was heavier than in area A, needs to be conducted.

In the present study, we collected 100 types of local food items in 2 Cd-polluted areas in Akita, measured their Cd concentrations, and assessed Cd exposure levels in the subjects of previous local health examinations using an individual food analysis method based on Cd concentrations in individual food items and the intake amounts of these food items by subjects obtained from diet surveys conducted at health examinations. We also performed the Monte Carlo simulation [8] to evaluate the probabilistic distribution of the Cd intake levels of these subjects in order to confirm the assessment. We demonstrated that Cd intake levels in these subjects were approximately PTWI or TWI, which showed that subjects exposed to Cd were at risk of adverse effects.

2. Materials and Methods

2.1. Sampling and Handling of Food Items

We selected approximately 80 local food items from the table of food groups of the Japan's National Health and Nutrition Survey provided by the Ministry of Health, Labor, and Welfare, that were eaten at a high frequency in diet surveys from health examinations conducted on local female farmers in area A in 2001–2002 [4]. We then deleted food items in which Cd concentrations were undetectable in the study on the absorption rate of dietary Cd among female farmers conducted in the winter of 2002–2003 [9]. We added food items that were assumed to have high Cd concentrations, such as seaweed, shellfish, mollusks, and livers, based on a previous study [10]. In November and December 2003, we purchased these food items at local markets in areas A and B based on the recommendations of a local female farmer who was familiar with traditional dietary patterns. We collected 100 food items for the measurement of Cd concentrations. We aimed to collect three of each food item in each area; however, this number increased or decreased depending on the inventory status. Therefore, the number of purchases ranged between 1 and 10, with an average of six. We collected 100 g of the edible portions of each food item and stored them at room temperature, 4 °C, or −20 °C depending on their perishability until the measurement of Cd concentrations.

2.2. Measurement of Cd Concentrations

The measurement of Cd concentrations in food items, except for rice, was conducted by Japan Food Research Laboratories (Tokyo, Japan). Next, 10 to 20 g of the edible portion of food, which was precisely measured in a Kjeldahl flask, was added to 200 mL of nitric acid (HNO_3) and heated. After the vigorous reaction was completed, 5 mL of sulfuric acid (H_2SO_4) was added to the flask and heated again until the color changed to light yellow. After cooling, the inside of the flask was washed well with deionized water (less than 1 µs/cm of conductance) and heated again until H_2SO_4 was released as white smoke. The residual was then dissolved in an appropriate quantity of deionized water to make a sample solution. The solution was moved to a separatory funnel and 10 mL of 50% diammonium hydrogen citrate and Thymol blue indicator (0.1 g of Thymol blue in 100 mL of ethyl alcohol) were then added. After neutralization with ammonium solution, the volume of the solution was increased to 100 mL by the addition of deionized water, and this was followed by 5 mL of 3% ammonium pyrrolidine-N-dithiocarbamate (APDC) solution/ammonium sulfate and 10 mL of butyl acetate with shaking for 5 min. After being left to stand, the butyl acetate layer was collected for the measurement of Cd concentrations using a flame atomic absorption spectrometer (AA-890, Nippon Jarrell-Ash Co., Ltd., Tokyo, Japan). The original standard Cd solution (Kanto Chemical Co., Inc., Tokyo, Japan) was diluted with 1% hydrochloric acid (HCl) to make 0.4 and 0.8 µg/mL standard Cd solutions. Quality control was achieved in the analysis using sugar (commercial products) added with Cd as an alternative to certified reference materials. Its additional recovery was maintained within 90–110%. The detection limits for cereals, other food items, and drinking water were 0.01 mg/kg, 0.005 mg/kg, and 0.001 mg/L, respectively.

2.3. Health Examinations and Diet Surveys

Health examinations performed on female farmers in areas A and B in 2001–2004 were described previously [4.5]. In the present study, we used data obtained on age, height, weight, and the results of a diet history questionnaire (DHQ) from 725 and 438 subjects in areas A and B, respectively. DHQ is designed to assess food and nutrient intake levels in the previous month based on the quantity and semiquantitative frequency of the consumption of 110 food items commonly eaten in Japan [11].

Estimates of intake for food, energy, and selected nutrients were calculated using an ad hoc computer algorithm for DHQ based on Standard Tables of Food Composition in Japan, which has already been validated [12,13]. We used data obtained on individual food intake levels to calculate Cd intake levels. Among subjects, 12 and 6 with extremely low or high energy intake levels (≤1000 or ≥3500 kcal/day) were excluded in areas A and B, respectively, in addition to one whose consumption of rice was zero in area A, resulting in 712 and 432 subjects for analyses.

2.4. Calculation of Cd Intake Levels

We calculated the Cd intake levels of individual subjects by multiplying the intake of each food item by its Cd concentration and then summed Cd intake levels from all foods consumed. However, the food items for which intake levels were assessed by DHQ and those for which Cd concentrations were measured were not always in one-to-one correspondence. Therefore, we adjusted mismatches for reconciliation, as described below. Regarding boiled barley-rice, which is assumed to consist of 70% rice and 30% wheat, the Cd concentrations of rice and wheat flour, respectively, were multiplied. Since the intake levels of udon (wheat noodles) and soba (buckwheat noodles) were collectively assessed by DHQ, they were divided into two halves, each of which was multiplied by the Cd concentration of udon or soba. The intake levels of various noodles, including Chinese noodles or spaghetti, which were separately assessed by DHQ, were multiplied by the Cd concentration of udon, assuming that these foods were similarly made of wheat flour. The intake levels of butter rolls, croissants, pizza, pancakes, and okonomiyaki (Japanese-style pancakes) were also multiplied by the Cd concentration of white bread, while those of snack foods, Japanese sweets, cakes, cookies, and doughnuts were multiplied by the Cd concentration of manju (Japanese sweet bun). Regarding sweet potatoes, taro, yams, and Chinese yams, which were assessed collectively by DHQ, the average Cd concentration of sweet potatoes, taro, and yams was used. The average Cd concentration of silken and cotton tofu was used for tofu (soybean curd). The average Cd concentration of spinach, garland chrysanthemum, Japanese mustard spinach, Bok choy (Chinese cabbage), and Japanese leek was used for leafy green vegetables, which were collectively assessed by DHQ. Concerning the intake of wakame seaweed, the Cd concentration of raw wakame seaweed was used. The intake of mushrooms was evenly divided into shiitake mushroom and other mushrooms, and the Cd concentrations of shiitake mushroom and maitake mushroom were multiplied. Regarding the intake of shrimp and fish eggs, the average Cd concentrations of prawns and shrimp and of cod and salmon roe, respectively, were used. Since the intake of shellfish included oysters and other shellfish in DHQ, the Cd concentrations of oysters with innards and the average Cd concentrations of scallops without innards, Japanese littleneck clams, and freshwater clams were respectively multiplied. The average Cd concentration of beef liver, pork liver, chicken liver, Hinai chicken liver, and the innards of Hinai chicken was used for the intake of liver. Food items for which Cd concentrations were not detected, such as animal meat, eggs, milk, and green tea (after brewing), were not included in the calculation of total Cd intake. Cd intake from garlic, okra, belvedere fruit, kelp, hijiki seaweed, agar-agar, mozuku seaweed, and scallops with innards was also excluded because they were not evaluated by DHQ; however, their Cd concentrations were measured. The arithmetic means (AMs) of the Cd concentrations of these food items from both areas were multiplied by their corresponding food intake, while rice Cd concentrations in individual subjects, which were obtained in previous health examinations, were used to calculate individual Cd intake from rice. When a subject consumed brown rice, the Cd concentration of which is generally reduced by 10% due to polishing [14], the Cd concentration adjusted to be equivalent to polished rice was multiplied for calculations. One rice sample was missing in area A, which was substituted with the geometric mean (GM) of the Cd concentration in rice. The Cd concentrations of some foods with masses that are changed by cooking were corrected using the table of mass changes in individual food items from the Standard Tables of Food Compositions in Japan (7th edition, Japanese Ministry of Education, Culture, Sports, Science and Technology).

2.5. Statistical Analysis

Age, height, weight, total energy intake, and rice intake, which followed a normal distribution, were presented as AMs with arithmetic standard deviations (SDs) and differences in their mean values were analyzed by the Student's *t*-test. Since Cd concentrations in rice followed a clear lognormal distribution with large numbers and the distribution of Cd concentrations in other food items was not clear because of small numbers, rice and other food items were shown as GMs and AMs, respectively. Cd intake levels with skewed distributions were presented as medians with 25th and 75th percentiles and differences in their median values were analyzed by the median test. The χ^2 test was used to compare the proportions of Cd intake per body weight above the PTWI or TWI. Regarding multiple comparisons, the Steel-Dwass test was performed to compare the medians of age-classified Cd intake. The judgment of outliers was made using the Smirnov-Grubbs test. After the exclusion of outliers, the Monte Carlo simulation was performed on weekly Cd intake levels with 10,000 repetitions of the calculation based on the supposition of a lognormal distribution. Statistical analyses were performed using IBM SPSS Statistics V25 (SPSS Japan, Tokyo, Japan) based on the basic management of data by Mac Excel Tokei ver. 2.0 (Esumi, Tokyo, Japan).

3. Results

Food items and their Cd concentrations, divided into 10 subgroups, are listed in Tables 1–10. Cd concentrations in rice and rice products were high (Table 1). The average Cd concentrations in rice, 0.158 and 0.109 mg/kg, were lower than the safety standard of 0.4 mg/kg; however, 8.2 and 5.8% of rice had Cd concentrations that were above the safety standard in areas A and B, respectively. Among cereals, tubers, and roots, while the Cd concentrations of wheat flour and its products were not high, taro (satoimo in Japanese) had a high Cd concentration of 0.289 mg/kg (Table 2). The Cd concentrations of soybeans, including edamame, were high, whereas those of their processed foods were not, except for miso (Table 3). Cd was detected in all vegetables investigated, among which spinach, Japanese parsley, garland chrysanthemum, Japanese mustard spinach, and belvedere fruit showed high Cd concentrations (Table 4). Shiitake mushroom and seaweed (wakame, kombu, nori, and hijiki in Japanese) had markedly high Cd concentrations (Tables 5 and 6). Among fish and shellfish, salted squid guts, scallops with innards, oysters with innards, and freshwater clams, all of which had innards, had very high Cd concentrations, while fish meat itself did not (Table 7). Cd was not detected in many livestock food items, such as meat, eggs, and milk, except for the innards (Table 8). Cd was not detected in fruit (Table 9). High Cd concentrations were found in chocolate and tea leaves (Table 10). Cd was not detected in brewed tea.

We then calculated Cd intake levels by subjects who underwent health examinations, multiplied Cd concentrations in food items by individual food intake, and showed the results obtained in subgroups. The backgrounds of subjects in areas A and B, the food intake levels for whom were used to calculate Cd intake levels, are shown in Table 11. No significant differences were observed in age, energy intake, or rice intake between the 2 areas, whereas significant differences were noted in height ($p = 0.047$) and weight ($p = 0.047$), but were biologically negligible.

Cd intake from seaweed, fish, and shellfish was combined into one subgroup as seafood and that from livestock food was included in the subgroup as others, while that from fruit was excluded from calculations (Table 12). Among the subgroups, Cd intake from the subgroup of rice and rice products was the highest in both areas, and accounted for approximately 40–50% of the total Cd intake. Cd intake levels from the subgroups of vegetables and seafood were higher than those in the other subgroups. Cd intake from the subgroup of rice and rice products was significantly higher in area A than in area B, while those from other subgroups were similar between the two areas, except for vegetables, with Cd intake being significantly lower in area A than in area B. The median total Cd intake levels in areas A and B were 55.7 and 47.8 μg/day, respectively, with the former being significantly higher than the latter.

Table 1. Cadmium (Cd) concentrations in rice and rice products. Data are presented as arithmetic means, except for rice, which are presented as geometric means (GMs).

Food Items	*n*	Cd (mg/kg)	Ranges
Rice (area A)	711 *	0.158 (GM)	<0.02–0.971
Rice (area B)	432	0.109 (GM)	0.008–0.687
Kiritampo; pounded rice skewer	6	0.063	0.070–0.102
Glutinous rice	10	0.098	0.02–0.32
Rice cakes	5	0.069	0.017–0.182
Rice crackers	4	0.091	0.017–0.263

*: One sample is missing.

Table 2. Cadmium (Cd) concentrations in cereals, tubers, and roots. Data are presented as arithmetic means.

Food Items	*n*	Cd (mg/kg)	Ranges
White bread	6	0.018	0.016–0.023
Ampan, bean-jam bun	6	0.010	0.010–0.014
Wheat flour *	3	0.021	0.019–0.024
Udon; wheat noodles	6	0.005	0.005–0.007
Soba; buckwheat noodles	6	0.019	0.007–0.034
Sesame seeds	6	0.055	0.021–0.11
Sweet potato	6	0.008	0.005–0.016
Potato	6	0.034	0.005–0.098
Taro	6	0.289	0.036–0.795
Yams, Chinese yams	7	0.061	0.005–0.167
Potato chips *	3	0.059	0.029–0.114

*: Only from area A.

Table 3. Cadmium (Cd) concentrations in soybeans and soybean products. Data are presented as arithmetic means.

Food Items	*n*	Cd (mg/kg)	Ranges
Soybeans	4	0.115	0.05–0.25
Silken tofu	5	0.015	0.009–0.028
Cotton tofu	6	0.027	0.013–0.052
Deep-fried tofu	6	0.051	0.033–0.083
Natto; fermented soybeans	6	0.028	0.011–0.055
Miso; soybean paste	6	0.123	0.026–0.259
Edamame; soybeans in the pod	6	0.155	0.085–0.293
Soy sauce	4	0.019	0.015–0.026

Table 4. Cadmium (Cd) concentrations in vegetables. Data are presented as arithmetic means.

Food Items	*n*	Cd (mg/kg)	Ranges
Carrot	6	0.047	0.013–0.107
Spinach	6	0.064	0.030–0.122
Tomato	5	0.012	0.005–0.022
Squash	6	0.016	0.008–0.024
Broccoli	6	0.012	0.005–0.027
Japanese white radish	6	0.009	0.005–0.023
Onions	5	0.016	0.005–0.031
Cabbage	6	0.008	0.006–0.011
Chinese cabbage	6	0.020	0.011–0.038
Burdock	6	0.063	0.017–0.212

Table 4. *Cont.*

Food Items	*n*	Cd (mg/kg)	Ranges
Dropwort Japanese parsley	6	0.010	0.005–0.019
Eggplant	6	0.017	0.005–0.028
Garland chrysanthemum	5	0.074	0.006–0.244
Japanese mustard spinach	5	0.065	0.009–0.23
Bok choy (Chinese cabbage)	5	0.029	0.01–0.101
Green pepper	5	0.006	0.005–0.009
Garlic	6	0.051	0.01–0.142
Okra	3	0.023	0.012–0.043
Belvedere fruit	6	0.069	0.041–0.095
Japanese leek *	3	0.032	0.005–0.083
Pickled vegetables	10	0.022	0.009–0.095
Smoked daikon pickles	6	0.024	0.017–0.035

*: Only from area A.

Table 5. Cadmium (Cd) concentrations in mushrooms. Data are presented as arithmetic means.

Food Items	*n*	Cd (mg/kg)	Ranges
Raw shiitake mushroom	7	0.374	0.065–0.527
Maitake mushroom	6	0.043	0.023–0.108

Table 6. Cadmium (Cd) concentrations in seaweed and seaweed products. Data are presented as arithmetic means.

Food Items	*n*	Cd (mg/kg)	Ranges
Wakame seaweed (raw)	6	0.253	0.069–0.544
Wakame seaweed (dried) *	3	4.64	4.11–5.06
Kelp (konbu seaweed)	6	0.682	0.119–1.78
Laver (nori seaweed)	4	0.413	0.209–0.66
Hijiki seaweed	5	1.066	0.693–1.53
Agar-agar *	3	0.024	0.014–0.033
Mozuku seaweed	6	0.006	0.005–0.01

*: Only from area A.

Table 7. Cadmium (Cd) concentrations in fish and shellfish. Data are presented as arithmetic means.

Food Items	*n*	Cd (mg/kg)	Ranges
Salmon	6	<0.005	
Tuna	6	0.009	0.005–0.013
Cod	6	<0.005	
Horse mackerel	6	0.012	0.007–0.015
Mackerel	6	0.012	0.005–0.018
Sandfish without eggs	6	0.012	0.009–0.017
Sandfish with eggs	6	0.014	0.01–0.018
Squid	6	0.032	0.018–0.081
Salted squid guts	5	2.36	0.978–6.57
Octopus	6	0.007	0.005–0.011
Prawn	7	0.055	0.005–0.17
Shrimp *	2	0.022	0.009–0.035
Cod roe	6	0.008	0.005–0.015
Salmon roe	3	<0.005	

Table 7. *Cont.*

Food Items	*n*	Cd (mg/kg)	Ranges
Scallops without innards	5	0.0408	0.012–0.103
Scallops with innards	5	3.635	0.684–5.54
Oysters with innards	6	0.680	0.486–1.03
Japanese littleneck clam	4	0.160	0.028–0.305
Freshwater clam	4	0.375	0.235–0.55
Hampen (fish minced and steamed)	6	0.005	0.005–0.006
Dried whitebait	6	0.010	0.005–0.02
Broiled eel	6	0.008	0.005–0.011

*: Only from area B.

Table 8. Cadmium (Cd) concentrations in livestock food. Data are presented as arithmetic means.

Food Items	*n*	Cd (mg/kg)	Ranges
Beef	6	<0.005	
Pork	5	<0.005	
Chicken	4	<0.005	
Hinai chicken	5	<0.005	
Horse meat	3	0.006	0.005–0.007
Beef liver *	1	0.021	
Pork liver	4	0.024	0.016–0.028
Chicken liver	5	0.015	0.01–0.022
Hinai chicken liver *	2	0.039	0.033–0.044
Innards of Hinai chicken	6	0.021	0.008–0.066
Sausage	3	0.006	0.005–0.008
Egg	6	<0.005	
Milk	6	<0.005	

*: Only from area A.

Table 9. Cadmium (Cd) concentrations in fruit. Data are presented as arithmetic means.

Food Items	*n*	Cd (mg/kg)	Ranges
Apple	6	<0.005	
Apple juice	6	<0.005	
Kiwi fruit	5	<0.005	

Table 10. Cadmium (Cd) concentrations in others. Data are presented as arithmetic means.

Food Items	*n*	Cd (mg/kg)	Ranges
Manju; sweet bun	10	0.022	0.010–0.127
Chocolate *	3	0.042	0.03–0.084
Curry roux *	3	0.015	0.012–0.018
Flavor seasonings *	1	0.025	
Ketchup	3	0.016	0.016–0.017
Japanese green tea leaves *	3	0.026	0.009–0.049
Nutritional supplement drink *	3	<0.005	
Well water *	7	<0.005	

*: Only from area A.

Table 11. Backgrounds of female farmers who underwent health examinations in areas A and B.

Backgrounds	Area A (n = 712)		Area B (n = 432)	
	Mean ± SD	Ranges	Mean ± SD	Ranges
Age	57.4 ± 11.3	21–79	57.2 ± 9.3	35–82
Height (cm)	152.0 ± 6.2	130–180	152.8 ± 5.9 *	132–169
Weight (kg)	54.5 ± 8.0	34–92	55.5 ± 8.5 *	33–94
Energy intake (kcal/day)	1933.7 ± 463.7	1000–3440	1923.8 ± 459.0	1047–3451
Rice intake (g/day)	371.8 ± 118.9	78.6–1120	359.0 ± 105.3	30–880

*: $p < 0.05$ versus area A (unpaired Student's t-test).

Table 12. Daily cadmium intake per person (μg/day) in female farmers in areas A and B.

Subgroups of Cadmium Intake	Area A (n = 712)		Area B (n = 432)	
	Median (25–75th Percentile)	Ranges	Median (25–75th Percentile)	Ranges
Total cadmium intake	55.7 (40.5–75.4)	10.6–301	47.8 (34.2–64.5) *	10.2–187
Rice and rice products	28.3 (17.1–44.7)	0.1–289	19.4 (9.9–37.4) *	0.1–154
Cereals, tubers, and roots	2.4 (1.5–4.3)	0–40.7	2.3 (1.4–3.8)	0–13.8
Soybeans and soybean products	3.4 (2.3–4.6)	0.2–22.6	3.4 (2.5–4.5)	0.3–11.1
Vegetables	6.2 (3.9–9.0)	0.5–26.2	6.8 (4.3–9.4) *	0.7–29
Mushrooms	2.8 (1.1–4.4)	0–39.3	2.6 (0.8–4.4)	0–24.6
Seafood **	6.1 (3.4–10.9)	0.3–46.5	6.3 (3.9–9.9)	0.4–52.2
Others ***	0.5 (;0.3–0.9)	0–6.1	0.5 (0.3–0.9)	0–5.4

*: $p < 0.05$ versus area A (median test). **: including seaweed, fish, and shellfish. ***: including manju, livestock food, chocolate, and flavor seasonings.

We then compared the results obtained with Cd intake by the general population in Japan (Figure 2) [15,16]. Cd intake has been gradually decreasing in Japan: 31.1 μg/day (16.2 μg/day from rice and 14.9 μg/day from other food items) in 1981, 21.1 μg/day (7.8 μg/day from rice and 13.3 μg/day from other food items) in 2007, and 17.8 μg/day (5.7 μg/day from rice and 12.1 μg/day from other food items) in 2015. This was mainly attributed to a reduction in Cd intake from rice. Cd intake levels from rice and rice products in areas A (28.3 μg/day) and B (19.4 μg/day) were 3.6- and 2.5-fold higher, respectively, than that (7.8 μg/day) by the general population in 2007, while Cd intake levels from other food items in areas A and B (approximately 24.0 μg/day) were 1.8-fold higher than that (13.3 μg/day) by the general population. Total Cd intake levels in areas A and B were approximately 2.5-fold higher than that by the general population.

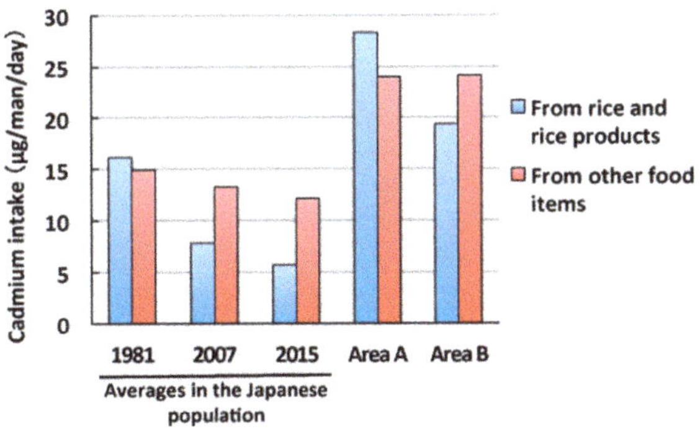

Figure 2. Cadmium intake levels per person from rice and rice products and from others in female farmers in cadmium-polluted areas A and B in Akita, Japan, shown by medians, and comparisons with average cadmium intake in the Japanese population.

We also calculated weekly Cd intake per body weight, using individual values of body weight, to compare the PTWI of JECFA at that time or the current TWI in Japan of 7 μg/kg BW/week. Median weekly Cd intake levels were 7.2 and 6.0 μg/kg BW/week in areas A and B, respectively, with both being approximately PTWI or TWI (Table 13). The distributions of weekly Cd intake levels in areas A and B were shown in histograms (Figure 3). The exclusion of data obtained from two subjects in area A that were extremely large and considered to be outliers resulted in similar distributions in both areas that skewed to the higher side. The percentages of subjects with weekly Cd intake levels above PTWI or TWI were 51.7 and 38.0% in areas A and B, respectively ($p < 0.05$, χ^2 test) (Table 13).

Table 13. Weekly cadmium intake per body weight (μg/kg BW/week) in female farmers in areas A and B and their distribution.

Weekly Cadmium Intake	Area A (n = 712)	Area B (n = 432)
Median	7.2	6.0 *
25–75th percentiles	5.2–9.7	4.4–8.5
Ranges	1.5–42	1.3–26
<7 μg/kg/week	344 (48.3%)	268 (62.0%)
≥7 μg/kg/week	368 (51.7%)	164 (38.0%)

*: $p < 0.05$ versus area A (median test).

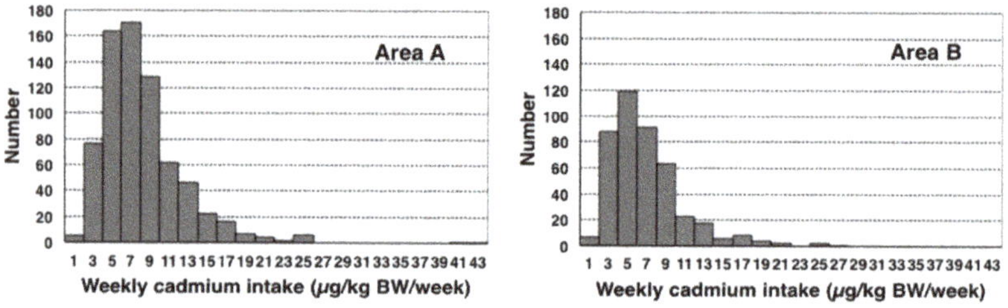

Figure 3. Distribution of weekly cadmium intake per body weight in female farmers in cadmium-polluted areas A and B in Akita, Japan.

We further divided weekly Cd intake per body weight into age-classified groups and examined differences between them (Table 14). In area A, weekly Cd intake per body weight was higher in subjects aged 40 or older than in younger subjects, while no significant differences were observed between age-classified groups in area B. Weekly Cd intake per body weight in subjects aged 50 or older was above PTWI or TWI in area A.

Table 14. Age-classified weekly cadmium intake per body weight (μg/kg BW/week) in female farmers in areas A and B.

Age Groups (Mean Age ± SD)	n	Median	25–75th Percentile
	Area A (n = 712)		
20–29 years (25.0 ± 3.0)	27	3.6	2.4–5.9
30–39 years (35.0 ± 3.2)	27	4.8	3.5–7.2
40–49 years (45.4 ± 2.9)	109	6.3 *	4.5–8.7
50–59 years (54.6 ± 2.9)	213	7.1 *	5.4–9.5
60–69 years (64.6 ± 2.8)	278	8.1 *	6.0–11
70 years– (72.8 ± 2.2)	58	7.8 *	6.0–11
	Area B (n = 432)		
30–39 years (36.8 ± 1.5)	14	6.3	4.5–14
40–49 years (45.8 ± 2.7)	85	5.1	3.2–7.7
50–59 years (54.6 ± 2.8)	151	5.7	3.9–7.5
60–69 years (63.9 ± 2.8)	143	6.8	5.2–9.0
70 years– (73.1 ± 2.8)	39	6.6	5.5–11

*: $p < 0.05$ versus 20–29 years (Steel-Dwass test).

We then performed the Monte Carlo simulation using the same data and the results obtained are shown in Figure 4. We excluded 2 outliers in area A, which markedly skewed their probability density distributions. As a result, we obtained estimated median weekly Cd intake levels of 7.0 and 6.0 μg/kg BW/week in areas A and B, respectively (Table 15), which were similar to the results described above.

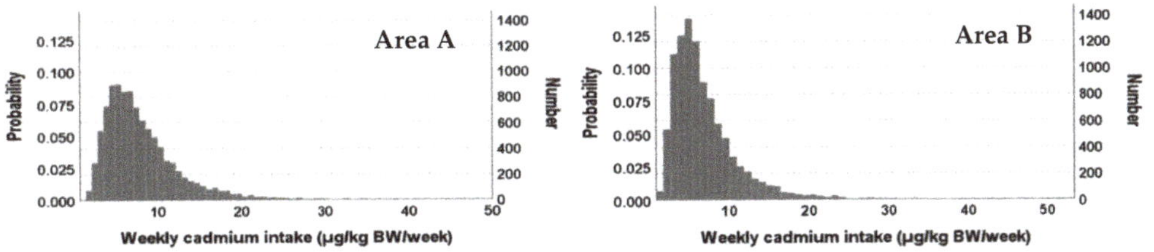

Figure 4. Probability density distributions of weekly cadmium intake per body weight in female farmers in cadmium-polluted areas A and B in Akita, Japan, estimated using the Monte Carlo simulation.

Table 15. Results of the Monte Carlo simulation for weekly cadmium intake per body weight (μg/kg BW/week) in female farmers in areas A and B.

Weekly Cadmium Intake	Area A (n = 710) *	Area B (n = 432)
Median	7.0	6.0
5–95th percentiles	3.1–17.0	2.6–15.9
Ranges	1.2–70.9	0.9–103

*: Two outliers were excluded.

4. Discussion

In the present study, we collected food items from local markets in two Cd-polluted areas in Akita, Japan, measured their Cd concentrations, and attempted to accurately assess Cd intake levels in local female farmers who had been exposed to high Cd levels by calculating individual Cd intake based on data obtained from diet surveys performed in health examinations. The present results demonstrated that Cd intake was approximately 2.5-fold higher in our subjects than in the general population. Furthermore, weekly Cd intake per body weight, which was confirmed by the Monte Carlo simulation, were approximately the same as the PTWI of JECFA or TWI of Japan, while 38.0–51.7% of subjects had weekly Cd intake per body weight that was above it.

The high Cd intake levels observed among our subjects may be attributed to high Cd concentrations in local agricultural products, particularly rice. Although Cd concentrations in rice in these areas (GMs of 0.158 and 0.109 mg/kg in areas A and B, respectively) were lower than the safety standard (0.4 mg/kg), they were markedly higher than the median rice Cd concentrations in Japan (0.06 mg/kg in 1997 and 1998 and 0.05 mg/kg in 2009 and 2010) [16], and there were rice that had Cd concentrations above the safety standard (8.2 and 5.8% in areas A and B, respectively). Although the intake of Cd was higher in area A than in area B, the actual accumulated levels of Cd in subjects were higher in area B than in area A, as demonstrated by their blood and urinary Cd levels (for example, urinary Cd levels in 70–79-year-old subjects were 4.90 and 9.34 μg/g cr. in areas A and B, respectively, and 2.99 μg/g cr. in control subjects) [5]. Since the biological half-life of Cd in humans is very long (10–30 years), blood and urinary Cd levels are stable indicators of the accumulation of Cd in the human body, particularly when the level of Cd that accumulates is high [1]. This discrepancy may have been due to the timing of the initiation of measures in rice farming to lower Cd absorption from the soil in 2002, namely, the flooding of paddy fields before and after heading during August [5,17]. Actually, the rates of rice with Cd concentration above the safety standard in these areas were decreased after that according to the results of intensive inspections targeted for Cd-polluted rice fields by Akita prefecture (Akita Prefect. Department of of Agriculture, Forestry, and Fisheries) (Supplemental Table S1).

More recently, our own investigations on farmers in the areas show that the median of Cd concentration in their self-harvested rice from 2010 to 2018 was 0.096 mg/kg and 0.7% of them were above the safety standard ($n = 599$) (unpublished data). These results indicate the flooding of paddy fields have effectively lowered Cd concentrations in rice from 2002 in these areas. The health examination in area A was performed in 2001–2002, at the initiation of the flooding of paddy fields, while that in area B was performed in 2002–2003, just after the flooding of paddy fields had started. Therefore, Cd intake levels may have been higher in area B than in area A before the start of the flooding of paddy fields.

Cd intake levels from food items other than rice and rice products, which remained constant independent of the flooding of rice paddy fields, were also higher in these areas in Akita than the average in Japan (Figure 2) [15]. Although total Cd intake other than rice and rice products in these areas was nearly twice the average in Japan in 2007; those from other food items varied [15]. Cd intake from cereals, tubers, and roots was 2.3–2.4 μg/day in these areas, which is similar to the average in Japan of 2.7 μg/day. On the other hand, Cd intake from soybeans and soybean products was 3.4 μg/day in these areas, which was approximately 3-fold higher than the average in Japan of 1.1 μg/day. Cd intake from vegetables and seafood in the general Japanese population was reported in the classification as "brightly colored vegetables", "vegetables, seaweeds", and "seafood" by the Ministry of Agriculture, Forestry, and Fisheries. Therefore, we compared total Cd intake from vegetables and seafood in areas A and B with total Cd intake from "brightly colored vegetables", "vegetables, seaweeds", and "seafood" in the general Japanese population; the former, 12.3–13.1 μg/day, was higher than the latter, 8.2 μg/day. In addition, Cd intake from mushrooms in these areas, 2.6–2.8 μg/day, which was absent from the report by the Ministry of Agriculture, Forestry, and Fisheries of Japan, significantly contributed to total Cd intake. These comparisons revealed that agricultural products in these areas contained high Cd concentrations due to Cd contamination in the local farmland, and the consumption of these products was a significant contributor to Cd overexposure among local farmers.

Among agricultural products, Cd concentrations were high in sesame seeds, taro (satoimo in Japanese), yams (yamaimo in Japanese), soybeans, carrot, spinach, burdock (gobo in Japanese), garland chrysanthemum (shungiku in Japanese), Japanese mustard spinach (komatsuna in Japanese), garlic, belvedere fruit (tomburi in Japanese), and shiitake mushroom. Among seafood, many types of seaweed (such as wakame, kombu, and hijiki in Japanese), salted squid guts, scallops (hotate in Japanese) and oysters (kaki in Japanese) with innards, Japanese littleneck clam (asari in Japanese), and freshwater clam (shijimi in Japanese) showed very high Cd concentrations. On the other hand, Cd concentrations were generally low in livestock food and fruit. These results are consistent with previous findings showing that Cd concentrations were high in tubers, soybeans, brightly colored vegetables, and seafood, particularly seaweed, and the innards of squid or shellfish in Japan [10,15].

Median weekly Cd intake levels in our subjects were 7.2 and 6.0 μg/kg BW/week in areas A and B, respectively, which were approximately the PTWI of JECFA at that time or the current TWI in Japan of 7 μg/kg BW/week. In our previous study on area A, we estimated weekly Cd intake levels to be between 5.70–6.72 μg/kg BW/week, which was consistent with the present results, based on 2 assumptions: all food items other than rice may be contaminated by Cd at the same percentage contribution as rice (50%) or at a constant level (15.0 μg/day) [4]. In addition, the percentage of subjects with weekly Cd intake levels higher than 7 μg/kg BW/week in area A, 51.7%, in the present study was similar to previously estimated percentages, 33–51%. These results indicate that previously estimated Cd intake levels, based only on Cd concentrations in rice and miso, were not inaccurate, and that local farmers in Cd-polluted areas in Akita exposed to Cd were at risk of adverse effects. Weekly Cd intake per body weight was above the PTWI or TWI in older subjects in area A, suggesting a higher risk of developing renal tubular dysfunction among the elderly. There were no age-classified subgroups above the PTWI or TWI in area B, but actually the older subjects might had been exposed to much higher levels of Cd like in area A before the start of the flooding of paddy fields.

Two methods are generally employed in exposure assessments of chemicals in food: a total diet study (TDS) and individual food analysis. There are two approaches in TDS: a market basket method and duplicate portion study [5,18]. In the market basket method, which assesses chemical intake in divided food groups, the average intake of a chemical in a certain population may be calculated; however, the concentration of this chemical in individual food items remains unknown. On the other hand, the duplicate portion study, which measures chemical concentrations in whole meals, provides information on actual chemical intake by individuals, but does not give stable results on chemical intake. We simultaneously performed a duplicate portion study in area A on 17 female farmers for three days to support the present results, and obtained a smaller median Cd intake of 19.0 μg/day that ranged between 9.8–63.1 μg/day (unpublished data). In contrast, the individual food analysis, adopted in the present study, allowed us to identify the source foods of chemical intake and calculate the average intake of a chemical in a population, similar to the market basket method. The individual food analysis generally cannot exclude uncertainties due to processing and cooking foodstuffs. However, Cd itself does not increase or diminish in foodstuffs by processing and cooking. Furthermore, mass changes in individual foods were included in the calculation of Cd intake based on the tables of mass changes in individual food, from the Standard Tables of Food Compositions in Japan (7th edition, Japanese Ministry of Education, Culture, Sports, Science, and Technology). Furthermore, a probabilistic assessment, the Monte Carlo simulation, may be performed using individual Cd concentrations in food items.

The National Institute of Health Sciences previously investigated Cd intake by the general Japanese population using the market basket method [15] and an assessment of Cd intake based on the individual food analysis, similar to the present study, was not previously performed in Japan. Cd intake in the Jinzu River basin of Toyama, the heaviest Cd-polluted area in Japan, was reported to be as high as 600 μg/day in 1968 using the market basket method [19]. On the other hand, in Kosaka town in Akita, the intake of Cd from rice by local residents, assessed from Cd concentrations in rice, was 100.6 μg/day in 1974–1976 [20], 92 μg/day in 1978, and 55 μg/day in 1999–2000 using the duplicate portion study [19]; the latter was similar to the present results. These findings indicate that Cd intake in Cd-polluted areas in Akita has been decreasing for decades, and are consistent with the present results. Cd intake in Cd-polluted areas in Akita is still higher than those by the general Japanese population and Western counties. Recent Cd intake by general populations assessed using the market basket method was 4.63 μg/day or 0.54 μg/kg body weight/week in U.S.A. [21], 0.16 μg/kg body weight/week in France [22], 0.77 μg/kg body weight/week in Spain [23], 1 μg/kg body weight/week in Sweden [24], 5.00 μg/day in Italy [25], 0.85μg/kg body weight/week in Belgium [26], and 13.5 μg/day in Denmark [27]. Although Cd intake in Eastern Asian countries, where rice is consumed as a staple food, is generally high, such as 32.7 μg/day in China [28] and 22.0 μg/day in Korea [29], Cd intake levels remain higher in Akita.

There are some limitations in the present study. The data used in this study were obtained in 2001–2003. Nevertheless, the results obtained remain important, even after approximately 20 years, because few Cd-polluted areas remain in Japan. Furthermore, data were collected at the start of the flooding of paddy fields, which has successfully decreased Cd exposure levels in farmers in these areas; therefore, these data will never be obtained again in the future.

Furthermore, the subjects examined were females and therefore the Cd intake by male farmers remains unknown. Cd intake levels by males may be higher than those by females based on differences in the amount of food consumed. However, since females are generally more vulnerable to Cd toxicity than males, such as higher intestinal Cd absorbability in females than in males, it is not inappropriate to use the results of the present study for risk assessments of Cd in the general population. In area B, the results of the Cd exposure assessment did not reflect previous Cd intake because of the flooding of paddy fields. However, the Cd intake level in area B was still higher than that by the general population. In DHQ, which assesses general nutritional intake, some food items that showed markedly higher Cd concentrations were absent, such as kelp and hijiki. Therefore, we were unable to include Cd intake from these foods in total Cd intake, which may have led to the underestimation of Cd exposure. The Japanese government provides Cd intake values by the general population as averages. Although median values in Cd-polluted areas cannot be statistically compared to these averages, the differences are large enough to identify areas at risk of health problems.

5. Conclusions

We performed an exposure assessment of Cd in female farmers, who are more vulnerable to Cd toxicity than males in Cd-polluted areas in Akita, Japan. Participants underwent local health examinations during 2001–2004, using the individual food analysis method with the Monte Carlo simulation. Results showed that Cd intake was higher than that by the general population, which was derived from local agricultural products, particularly rice, and also that their exposure levels to Cd were approximately the PTWI of JECFA or TWI of Japan.

Supplementary Materials: The following are available online at http://www.mdpi.com/2305-6304/8/2/44/s1, Table S1: Annual trend of rates of rice with a cadmium concentration above the safety standard (0.4 mg/kg) in the intensive inspections targeted for 3 cadmium-polluted areas in Akita prefecture, Japan, around the start of the flooding of paddy fields (2002).

Author Contributions: Formulating study protocols, F.K., H.H., and E.O.; collecting food items, H.H. and E.O.; health examinations, F.K., H.H., E.O., Y.H., S.S., and K.M.; advising about the diet study, S.S.; data curation, H.H.; statistical analyses, H.H. and A.O.; writing—original draft preparation, H.H.; visualization, H.H. and A.O.; funding acquisition, F.K. and H.H. All authors have read and agreed to the published version of the manuscript.

Funding: This research project was supported by grants mainly from the Ministry of Health, Labor, and Welfare and the Ministry of Agriculture and Forestry of Japan, and in part from CREST-JST and a Grant-in-Aid for Scientific Research (B) [20H03945] from the Ministry of Education, Science, and Culture of Japan.

Acknowledgments: The authors express special gratitude to JA Akita Kita and Kosaka Municipal Government as well as the subjects of this study for their corporation, to Shin Hasebe and Hinako Togashi for their guidance when collecting food items from local markets, to Koji Matsuno for measuring Cd concentrations in samples for the duplicate portion study, and Kentaro Murakami and Hitomi Okubo for helping with diet surveys.

Conflicts of Interest: The authors declare no conflicts of interest.

References

1. Nordberg, G.F.; Nogawa, K.; Nordberg, M. Cadmium. In *Handbook on the Toxicology of Metals*, 4th ed.; Nordberg, G.F., Fowler, B.A., Nordberg, M., Eds.; Academic Press: Burlington, MA, USA, 2015; pp. 667–716.
2. Aoshima, K. Recent clinical and epidemiological studies of *itai-itai* disease (cadmium-Induced renal tubular osteomalacia) and cadmium nephropathy in the Jinzu River basin in Toyama prefecture, Japan. In *Cadmium Toxicity*; Himeno, S., Aoshima, K., Eds.; Springer: Singapore, 2019; pp. 23–37.
3. Horiguchi, H. Cadmium exposure and its effects on the health status of rice farmers in Akita prefecture. In *Cadmium Toxicity*; Himeno, S., Aoshima, K., Eds.; Springer: Singapore, 2019; pp. 75–83.
4. Horiguchi, H.; Oguma, E.; Sasaki, S.; Miyamoto, K.; Ikeda, Y.; Machida, M.; Kayama, F. Dietary exposure to cadmium at close to the current provisional tolerable weekly intake does not affect renal function among female Japanese farmers. *Environ. Res.* **2004**, *95*, 20–31. [CrossRef]
5. Horiguchi, H.; Oguma, E.; Sasaki, S.; Okubo, H.; Murakami, K.; Miyamoto, K.; Hosoi, Y.; Murata, K.; Kayama, F. Age-relevant renal effects of cadmium exposure through consumption of home-harvested rice in female Japanese farmers. *Environ. Int.* **2013**, *56*, 1–9. [CrossRef]
6. Sasaki, T.; Horiguchi, H.; Arakawa, A.; Oguma, E.; Komatsuda, A.; Sawada, K.; Murata, K.; Yokoyama, K.; Matsukawa, T.; Chiba, M.; et al. Hospital-based screening to detect patients with cadmium nephropathy in cadmium-polluted areas in Japan. *Environ. Health Prev. Med.* **2019**, *24*, 8. [CrossRef] [PubMed]
7. WHO (World Health Organization). Cadmium. In *Evaluation of Certain Food Additives and Contaminants*; WHO Technical Report Series 960; WHO: Geneva, Italy, 2011; pp. 149–162.
8. Gibney, M.J.; van der Voet, H. Introduction to the Monte Carlo project and the approach to the validation of probabilistic models of dietary exposure to selected food chemicals. *Food Addit. Contam.* **2003**, *20* (Suppl. 1), S1–S7. [CrossRef] [PubMed]
9. Horiguchi, H.; Oguma, E.; Sasaki, S.; Miyamoto, K.; Ikeda, Y.; Machida, M.; Kayama, F. Comprehensive study of the effects of age, iron deficiency, diabetes mellitus, and cadmium burden on dietary cadmium absorption in cadmium-exposed female Japanese farmers. *Toxicol. Appl. Pharmacol.* **2004**, *196*, 114–123. [CrossRef]

10. Ishizaki, A.; Fukushima, M.; Sakamoto, M. Distribution of Cd in biological materials. 2. Cadmium and zinc contents of foodstuffs. *Jpn. J. Hyg.* **1970**, *25*, 207–222, (In Japanese with an English abstract). [CrossRef]
11. Sasaki, S.; Yanagibori, R.; Amano, K. Self-administered diet history questionnaire developed for health education: A relative validation of the test-version by comparison with 3-day diet record in women. *J. Epidemiol.* **1998**, *8*, 203–215. [CrossRef]
12. Sasaki, S.; Yanagibori, R.; Amano, K. Validity of a self-administered diet history questionnaire for assessment of sodium and potassium: Comparison with single 24-hour urinary excretion. *Jpn. Circ. J.* **1998**, *62*, 431–435. [CrossRef]
13. Sasaki, S.; Ushio, F.; Amano, K.; Morihara, M.; Todoriki, O.; Uehara, Y.; Toyooka, E. Serum biomarker-based validation of a self-administered diet history questionnaire for Japanese subjects. *J. Nutr. Sci. Vitaminol.* **2000**, *46*, 285–296. [CrossRef]
14. Masironi, R.; Koirtyohann, S.R.; Pierce, J.O. Zinc, copper, cadmium and chromium in polished and unpolished rice. *Sci. Total Environ.* **1977**, *7*, 27–43. [CrossRef]
15. Ministry of Agriculture, Forestry and Fisheries. Cadmium Concentrations in Agricultural Products in Japan. (In Japanese). Available online: https://www.maff.go.jp/j/syouan/nouan/kome/k_cd/jitai_sesyu/01_inv.html (accessed on 31 March 2020).
16. Aoshima, K.; Horiguchi, H. Historical lessons on cadmium environmental pollution problems in Japan and current cadmium exposure situation. In *Cadmium Toxicity*; Himeno, S., Aoshima, K., Eds.; Springer: Singapore, 2019; pp. 3–19.
17. Arao, T.; Ishikawa, S.; Murakami, M.; Abe, K.; Maejima, Y.; Makino, T. Heavy metal contamination of agricultural soil and countermeasures in Japan. *Paddy Water Environ.* **2010**, *8*, 247–257. [CrossRef]
18. Ministry of Agriculture, Forestry and Fisheries. The Guideline for Total Diet Study. (In Japanese). Available online: https://www.maff.go.jp/j/syouan/seisaku/risk_analysis/tds/ (accessed on 31 March 2020).
19. Ikeda, M.; Ezaki, T.; Tsukahara, T.; Moriguchi, J. Dietary cadmium intake in polluted and non-polluted areas in Japan in the past and in the present. *Int. Arch. Occup. Environ. Health* **2004**, *77*, 227–234. [CrossRef] [PubMed]
20. Haga, Y.; Kobayasi, T.; Otani, H.; Miura, H.; Kato, A.; Saruta, T. Environmental and medical investigation on the pollution of heavy metal, No.6. *Rep. Akita Pref. Inst. Public Health* **1978**, *22*, 135–139. (In Japanese)
21. Kim, K.; Melough, M.M.; Vance, T.M.; Noh, H.; Koo, S.I.; Chun, O.K. Dietary Cadmium Intake and Sources in the US. *Nutrients* **2018**, *11*, 2. [CrossRef]
22. Arnich, N.; Sirot, V.; Rivière, G.; Jean, J.; Noël, L.; Guérin, T.; Leblanc, J.C. Dietary exposure to trace elements and health risk assessment in the 2nd French Total Diet Study. *Food Chem. Toxicol.* **2012**, *50*, 2432–2449. [CrossRef]
23. Marín, S.; Pardo, O.; Báguena, R.; Font, G.; Yusà, V. Dietary exposure to trace elements and health risk assessment in the region of Valencia, Spain: A total diet study. *Food Addit. Contam. Part A Chem. Anal. Control Expo. Risk Assess* **2017**, *34*, 228–240. [CrossRef]
24. Sand, S.; Becker, W. Assessment of dietary cadmium exposure in Sweden and population health concern including scenario analysis. *Food Chem. Toxicol.* **2012**, *50*, 536–544. [CrossRef]
25. Filippini, T.; Cilloni, S.; Malavolti, M.; Violi, F.; Malagoli, C.; Tesauro, M.; Bottecchi, I.; Ferrari, A.; Vescovi, L.; Vinceti, M. Dietary intake of cadmium, chromium, copper, manganese, selenium and zinc in a Northern Italy community. *J. Trace Elem. Med. Biol.* **2018**, *50*, 508–517. [CrossRef]
26. Vromman, V.; Waegeneers, N.; Cornelis, C.; De Boosere, I.; Van Holderbeke, M.; Vinkx, C.; Smolders, E.; Huyghebaert, A.; Pussemier, L. Dietary cadmium intake by the Belgian adult population. *Food Addit. Contam. Part A Chem. Anal. Control Expo. Risk Assess* **2010**, *27*, 1665–1673. [CrossRef] [PubMed]
27. Vacchi-Suzzi, C.; Eriksen, K.T.; Levine, K.; McElroy, J.; Tjønneland, A.; Raaschou-Nielsen, O.; Harrington, J.M.; Meliker, J.R. Dietary Intake Estimates and Urinary Cadmium Levels in Danish Postmenopausal Women. *PLoS ONE* **2015**, *10*, e0138784. [CrossRef] [PubMed]

28. Xiao, G.; Liu, Y.; Dong, K.F.; Lu, J. Regional characteristics of cadmium intake in adult residents from the 4th and 5th Chinese Total Diet Study. *Environ. Sci. Pollut. Res. Int.* **2020**, *27*, 3850–3857. [CrossRef] [PubMed]
29. Kim, H.; Lee, J.; Woo, H.D.; Kim, D.W.; Choi, I.J.; Kim, Y.I.; Kim, J. Association between dietary cadmium intake and early gastric cancer risk in a Korean population: A case-control study. *Eur. J. Nutr.* **2019**, *58*, 3255–3266. [CrossRef] [PubMed]

toxics

MDPI

Article

Lifetime Cadmium Exposure and Mortality for Renal Diseases in Residents of the Cadmium-Polluted Kakehashi River Basin in Japan

Muneko Nishijo [1,*], Kazuhiro Nogawa [2], Yasushi Suwazono [2], Teruhiko Kido [3], Masaru Sakurai [4] and Hideaki Nakagawa [4]

1 Department of Public Health, Kanazawa Medical University, Uchinada, Ishikawa 920-0293, Japan
2 Department of Occupational and Environmental Medicine, Graduate School of Medicine, Chiba University, Chuoku, Chiba 260-8670, Japan; nogawa@chiba-u.jp (K.N.); suwa@faculty.chiba-u.jp (Y.S.)
3 Department of Community Health Nursing, School of Health Sciences, Kanazawa University, Kanazawa, Ishikawa 920-0942, Japan; tkido@staff.kanazawa-u.ac.jp
4 Department of Social and Environmental Medicine, Kanazawa Medical University, Uchinada, Ishikawa 920-0293, Japan; m-sakura@kanazawa-med.ac.jp (M.S.); hnakagaw@kanazawa-med.ac.jp (H.N.)
* Correspondence: ni-koei@kanazawa-med.ac.jp; Tel.: +81-76-286-2211

Received: 29 August 2020; Accepted: 25 September 2020; Published: 1 October 2020

Abstract: Very few studies have investigated the dose–response relationship between external cadmium (Cd) exposure and mortality. We aim to investigate the relationship between lifetime Cd intake (LCd) and mortality in the Cd-polluted Kakehashi River basin in Japan. Mortality risk ratios for a unit of increase of LCd and urinary Cd were analyzed using Cox's proportional model. LCd was estimated based on residency and Cd in rice produced in their living areas. In men, mortality for all causes was significantly increased for a 10-μg/g Cr increase in urinary Cd, but not for a 1-g increase in LCd. In women, mortality risks for all causes and renal diseases, particularly renal failure, were significantly increased for a 10-μg/g Cr increase in urinary Cd. Similarly, mortality risks for renal diseases and renal failure were significantly increased for a 1-g increase of LCd in women. Comparing the contribution of two exposure markers to increased mortality in women, LCd was more effective for increasing mortality risks for renal diseases and renal failure, while urinary Cd contributed more to increased mortality risk for all causes. LCd may show a better dose–response relationship with mortality risk for renal diseases in women.

Keywords: cadmium; mortality; lifetime cadmium intake; renal diseases; urinary cadmium; a follow-up study

1. Introduction

The kidney is a target organ of external cadmium (Cd), and renal tubular dysfunction is the most prevalent adverse health effect induced by Cd exposure. Significant associations between renal tubular dysfunction, indicated by increasing urinary low molecular protein and Cd exposure markers such as urinary Cd, were reported in residents of Cd-polluted areas in Japan [1].

Cd in rice (RCd) is believed to be a good exposure marker in Japan because Tsuchiya and Iwao (1978) [2] reported that Japanese residents took half or two-thirds of Cd from rice in a study conducted in the 1970s. Nogawa et al. (1989) [3] showed a prevalence of renal tubular dysfunction indicated by an increase in urinary β2–microglobulin (β2–MG) ≥1000 μg/g creatinine (g Cr) with increasing residential duration (years) as well as RCd produced in the communities, suggesting that lifetime Cd intake (LCd), defined from both factors of RCd and residential duration, is a useful indicator of external dose to show the dose–response relationship, with health effects induced by Cd exposure.

Significant dose–response relationships between LCd and urinary metallothionein in the Cd-polluted Kakehashi River basin [4,5] and between LCd and urinary glucoproteinuria in the Jinzu River basin [6] were reported in residents that were environmentally exposed to Cd in Japan.

In our previous studies, following-up subjects from the Kakehashi River basin who participated in health impact surveys in 1981–1982 for 9 and 15 years, we reported increased mortality for all causes, cardiovascular diseases, and renal diseases in the subjects with Cd-induced renal tubular dysfunction indicated by urinary β2-MG, protein, glucose, amino acids, and retinol-binding protein [7–12]. An investigation of the relationship between the urinary Cd levels and mortality in the 15- and 22-year follow-up studies showed increased mortality for all causes, including renal diseases and heart failure, among subjects with urinary Cd levels ≥10 μg/g Cr in the 1981–1982 survey compared with subjects with Cd levels <3 μg/g Cr [13,14].

Relationships between LCd and mortality have been reported in the inhabitants of the Cd-polluted Jinzu River basin in three studies [15–17], but these relationships have not been demonstrated among residents of the Kakehashi River basin in our previous studies. Therefore, we extended the follow-up period to 35 years and analyzed dose–response relationships between LCd and mortality for causes of deaths to clarify the effect of environmental Cd exposure on mortality risks, particularly for renal diseases.

2. Materials and Methods

The Kakehashi River basin is one of the Cd-polluted areas in Japan, and it includes 700 ha of rice paddy fields. The pollution was due to mining activity that included a full-scale operation near the Kakehashi River that started in 1930 and continued until mining ceased in 1971. Rice with Cd > 0.4 (ppm) was detected in 12 of 22 villages in this area, and restoration of polluted paddy fields was undertaken from 1977 to 1988.

A total of 2602 subjects ≥50 years of age (1169 men and 1433 women) living in the Cd-polluted Kakehashi River basin, whose residential periods were ascertained in the 1981–1982 health impact survey, were enrolled in the present follow-up study (82% participant rate). LCd was estimated for them from RCd levels produced in their living communities and residential period (days) until 1981–1982 using the following formula: LCd = (RCd × 333.5 g + 34 μg) × residential period in Kakehashi River basin + 50 μg × residential period in nonexposed areas [3] on the assumption of 333.5 g for daily rice intake obtained by duplicated diet method, 34 μg for daily Cd intake from food other than rice from the polluted area [18], and 50 μg for daily Cd intake from nonpolluted areas [19].

Their mean levels of age, LCd, urinary Cd, and urinary β2–MG, examined at the survey in 1981–1982, with test results by *t*-test to compare them between sexes, are shown in Table 1. At this time, urinary Cd and β2-MG were transformed to log10 values for analysis because of the improvement of distribution. Positive rates for urinary Cd and urinary β2–MG are also shown in Table 1. Significantly greater mean values of LCd, urinary Cd, and urinary β2–MG and greater positive rates of urinary Cd and β2–MG were found in women compared with men.

Cd in urine samples was measured by flameless atomic absorption spectrometry after ashing with HNO3, HsSO4, and HClO4 and extraction with ammonium pyrrolidine dithiocarbamate (APDC) and methyl isobutyl ketone (MIBK) [20]. Freeze-dried standard reference material for toxic elements in urine (The National Bureau of Standards, Washington, DC, USA) was used to test the accuracy and precision of the analytical method of urinary Cd. Cd concentration corrected by Cr in urine was used for analysis.

Table 1. Levels of external cadmium (Cd) exposure and renal dysfunction examined in the 1981–1982 health impact survey and the follow-up rates and period until 2016.

Exposure and Renal Markers	Men		Women		p-Value
	Mean, N	SD, (%)	Mean, N	SD, (%)	
Test resultsin 1981-2					
N	1169		1433		
Age	62.5	9.1	62.9	9.4	0.281
Lifetime Cd intake (g)	2.74	1.63	2.48	1.65	0.000
Urinary Cd (μg/gCr) [1,2]	4.6	1.9	7.2	1.8	0.000
Rate of Cd ≥10 (μg/gCr)	137	(11.9)	411	(29.3)	0.000
Urinary ß2–MG (μg/gCr) [1]	166.1	6.3	252.6	6.7	0.000
Rate of ß2-MG ≥1000 (μg/gCr)	174	(14.9)	268	(18.7)	0.001
Follow-up study					
N (follow-up rate)	1135	(97.1)	1361	(95.0)	
Follow-up period (months)	222	123.4	256	128.4	0.000

[1] Geometrical mean and geometrical standard deviation, [2] Participants were 1121 men and 1333 women. N: number of subjects, SD: standard deviation.

A 35-year prospective follow-up survey of subjects was conducted from the day of their initial examination at the health impact survey in 1981–1982 until November 2016. The survival status (alive or dead), the date of death, place of residence (still residing or not in the target area), and the date of death, if applicable, were determined for 2527 residents (1149 men and 1378 women) from family registry records of all subjects with the cooperation of the Prefecture Public Health Office and City Municipal Office. Then, individual causes of death were ascertained from vital statistics by linking them to health survey data, with survival status based on birthday, death day, gender, and address after getting the permission of the Ministry of Health in Japan. The final number of subjects available for mortality analysis was 2496 (1135 men and 1361 women, 96% follow-up rate) and their mean follow-up period (months) are shown in Table 1. Causes of deaths were classified according to the 9th and 10th Revised International Classification of Diseases. The study protocol was approved by the Ethics Committee of Kanazawa Medical University (No-212, 17 June 2014).

Increased mortality risks for all causes and major causes of deaths, including renal diseases and renal failure, associated with a 1-g increase of LCd or a 10-μg/gCr (1 of log10 transformed value) increase of urinary Cd were investigated after adjusting for age using Cox's proportional hazard model. This model is one of regression analysis used for investigating associations between the survival time from the date of the baseline survey to the endpoint of subjects and relevant factors. In addition, to investigate which exposure marker, LCd or urinary Cd, contributed more to increased mortality for all causes and renal diseases, the stepwise elimination method based on Wald was used in Cox's mortality risk analysis. The SPSS (version 21.0) software package for Windows (SPSS Inc., Armonk, NY, USA) was used for statistical analysis.

3. Results

3.1. Mortality Risk Ratios and Cd Exposure Markers in Men

Hazard ratios for all causes, major causes of deaths, and renal diseases for a 10-μg/g Cr increase of urinary Cd and those for a 1-g increase of LCd after controlling for age in men are shown in Table 2. For men, the hazard ratio for all causes of deaths was significantly increased for a 10-μg/g Cr increase of urinary Cd, albeit no major causes of deaths were found to contribute to increased mortality. For a 1-g increase of LCd, no significantly increased mortality risks for all causes and no causes of death were noted in men (Table 2).

Table 2. Dose–response relationships between hazard ratios and Cd exposure markers in men.

Causes of Deaths	D	HR	95%CI	*p*-Value
Urinary Cd (+10 μg/gCr)				
All causes	890	1.35	1.06, 1.71	0.014
Malignant neoplasms	253	1.17	0.74, 1.84	0.496
Cardiovascular diseases	125	1.39	0.74, 2.61	0.300
Cerebrovascular diseases	117	1.17	0.61, 2.23	0.633
Respiratory diseases	151	1.07	0.60, 1.90	0.819
Renal diseases	25	2.94	0.70, 12.3	0.140
Renal failure	22	2.73	0.59, 12.7	0.202
Lifetime Cd Intake (+1 g)				
All causes	903	0.97	0.94, 1.02	0.210
Malignant neoplasms	254	0.98	0.90, 1.06	0.417
Cardiovascular diseases	129	0.98	0.88, 1.09	0.680
Cerebrovascular diseases	118	0.92	0.83, 1.03	0.148
Respiratory diseases	152	0.94	0.85, 1.04	0.214
Renal diseases	26	1.20	0.94, 1.52	0.141
Renal failure	23	1.12	0.87, 1.43	0.390

D: number of deaths, HR: hazard ratio, CI: confidence interval, N: number of subjects $n = 1121$ for urinary Cd, $n = 1135$ for lifetime Cd intake.

3.2. Mortality Risk Ratios and Cd Exposure Markers in Women

In women, hazard ratio was significantly increased for all causes for 10 μg/g Cr increase of urinary Cd. For renal diseases, particularly for renal failure, hazard ratios were significantly increased for10 μg/g Cr increase of urinary Cd in women (Table 3). Although hazard ratio for all causes was not significantly increased for 1 g increase of LCd, mortality risks for renal diseases and renal failure were significantly increased for 1 g increase of LCd in women (Table 3). These results in women indicate that increasing dose of Cd exposure may increase mortality for renal diseases, particularly renal failure. At the same time, however, they rise a question which exposure marker, urinary Cd or LCd, is a better marker to contribute to increasing risk for renal disease deaths.

Table 3. Dose–response relationships between hazard ratios and Cd exposure markers in women.

Causes of Deaths	D	HR	95% CI	*p*-Value
Urinary Cd (+10 μg/gCr)				
All causes	873	1.34	1.04, 1.71	0.019
Malignant neoplasms	186	1.18	0.66, 2.10	0.572
Cardiovascular diseases	157	1.31	0.76, 2.26	0.330
Cerebrovascular diseases	132	1.05	0.55, 1.98	0.894
Respiratory diseases	109	1.25	0.66, 2.35	0.490
Renal diseases	32	5.23	1.97, 13.9	0.001
Renal failure	23	5.12	1.65, 15.9	0.005
Lifetime Cd Intake (+1 g)				
All causes	889	0.99	0.95, 1.03	0.696
Malignant neoplasms	187	0.97	0.88, 1.06	0.460
Cardiovascular diseases	160	1.00	0.92, 1.10	0.970
Cerebrovascular diseases	133	1.00	0.90, 1.11	0.971
Respiratory diseases	113	0.90	0.80, 1.01	0.067
Renal diseases	34	1.49	1.20, 1.85	0.000
Renal failure	23	1.48	1.14, 1.93	0.003

D: number of deaths, HR: hazard ratio, CI: confidence interval, N: number of subjects. $n = 1333$ for urinary Cd, $n = 1361$ for lifetime Cd intake.

3.3. Comparisons of Mortality From Renal Diseases between Men and Women at Different Cd Exposure Levels

Crude mortality rates for renal diseases in six groups with a 1-g difference of LCd (a) and in three groups with a 10-μg difference of urinary Cd (b) in men and women are illustrated in Figure 1.

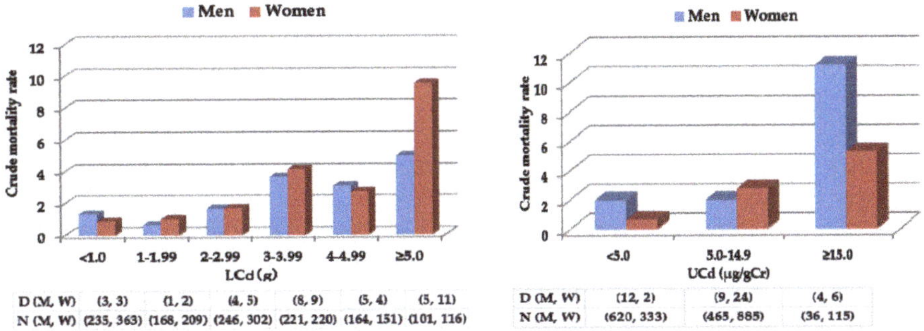

Figure 1. Crude mortality rates (%) for renal diseases and Cd exposure levels indicated by (**a**) LCd (+1 g) and (**b**) UCd (urinary Cd; +10 μg/g Cr). D (M, W): number of deaths for men and women; *n* (M, W): number of subjects of men and women.

Crude mortality from renal diseases was higher in men in the lowest exposure group, indicated by LCd (Figure 1a) or urinary Cd (Figure 1b), suggesting that factors other than Cd exposure, such as smoking and hypertension, relevant to chronic kidney disease (CKD), might influence mortality. While we found more deaths for renal diseases in the highest LCd group (LCd ≥ 5 g) in women compared men (Figure 1a), no stable result was obtained in the highest urinary Cd group (urinary Cd ≥ 10 μg/gCr), because of the small number of male subjects. These results suggest that mortality risk ratios for renal diseases might be changed, particularly in men, if relevant factors other than age could be controlled for in the analysis using Cox's proportional model.

3.4. Comparisons of Effects on Mortality between Urinary Cd and LCd in Women

To investigate which Cd exposure marker contributed to increased mortality from all causes and renal diseases, including renal failure, the stepwise elimination method was used for mortality risk analysis with three explanatory valuables, namely, urinary Cd, LCd, and age in women (Table 4). For all causes of deaths, age and urinary Cd were selected as factors that significantly increased mortality risks in women. However, age and LCd were selected as factors increasing mortality from renal diseases and renal failure in women, suggesting that LCd may be a good marker to show a better dose–effect relationship with mortality risk for renal diseases, including renal failure, compared with urinary Cd.

Table 4. Dose–response relationships between hazard ratios and Cd exposure markers in women.

Causes of Deaths	HR	95% CI	*p*-Value
All causes			
Age	1.15	1.14, 1.16	0.000
Urinary Cd (+10 μg/gCr)	1.33	1.04, 1.70	0.021
Renal diseases			
Age	1.12	1.07, 1.18	0.000
Lifetime Cd Intake (+1 g)	1.46	1.17, 1.82	0.001
Renal failure			
Age	1.18	1.10, 1.26	0.000
Lifetime Cd Intake (+1 g)	1.49	1.14, 1.93	0.003

D: number of deaths, HR: hazard ratio, CI: confidence interval, Number of subjects = 1333.

4. Discussion

In a 35-year follow-up study, an increase in LCd mortality from renal diseases, particularly for renal failure, in women ≥50 years of age, living in the environmentally contaminated Kakehashi River basin in Japan, suggests a dose–response relationship between the external dose of Cd and mortality from renal diseases in women.

Previously, we conducted follow-up studies of residents of the Kakehashi River basin in Japan who had participated in a health impact survey in 1981–1982 and reported the poor life prognosis of subjects associated with an increase in urinary Cd in a 15-year follow-up study [13] and a 22-year follow-up study [14]. In particular, for renal diseases, the mortality ratio was significantly higher in women in the higher urinary Cd group, with a 10- [13] or 20-μg/g Cr cut-off level [14] compared with the lower Cd-exposure group, albeit no dose–response relationships were shown between urinary Cd and mortality risks for renal diseases. In the present study, however, a 10-μg/g Cr increase of urinary Cd increased mortality not only for all causes but also for renal diseases.

LCd was used as an external Cd exposure maker to reflex the Cd exposure dose from the environment over a lifetime. In the present study, an increase in LCd was significantly associated with increased mortality from renal diseases in women, albeit no association was found in our previous 22-year follow-up. In women, we detected 26 deaths from renal diseases, which increased the statistical power in the present 35-year follow-up, and 14 deaths from renal diseases in the previous 22-year follow-up. Moreover, LCd was selected from two Cd exposure markers as a factor that contributed to increased mortality from renal diseases, suggesting that LCd showed a better dose–response relationship with mortality from renal diseases during a long time observation compared with urinary Cd. Since urinary Cd shows a sharp increase with increasing external Cd exposure only before the occurrence of renal tubular dysfunction [21,22], LCd might reflex the Cd dose that induces fatal renal diseases more than urinary Cd among subjects with a high prevalence of renal tubular dysfunction.

In the Jinzu River basin, Toyama, in Japan, where itai-itai disease is endemic, an increased mortality risk associated with LCd intake was suggested in residents who participated in the health survey in 1967 [15,16]. Recently, it was reported that an increase of LCd increased the mortality for all causes, renal disease, and the toxic effects of Cd (itai-itai disease) in the 26-year follow-up of female participants to the health impact survey in the Jinzu River basin conducted in 1979–1984 [17]. These results from the Jinzu River basin are consistent with our present results, indicating that LCd dose-dependently increased mortality over long time observation, particularly for renal diseases in women, albeit their follow-up period was shorter than ours. As their mean (SD) of LCd was 3.5 (1.9) g for men and 3.0 (1.5) g for women [17] and much higher than our values, 2.7 (1.6) g for men and 2.5 (1.6) g for women, this suggests heavier Cd contamination in rice in the Jinzu River basin. Although their hazard ratio for renal diseases for a 1-g increase of LCd was 1.25 and lower than that (1.49) in our present study of the Kakehashi River basin, direct causes of deaths might be renal failure in some cases diagnosed as the toxic effects of Cd (itai-itai disease), suggesting an underestimation of the mortality risk ratio for renal diseases in the Jinzu River basin. Moreover, increased mortality associated with an increase in LCd was also observed for all causes in the Jinzu River basin in women because of the much higher rate of death for specific causes of death to Cd exposure, such as renal diseases and the toxic effects of Cd (14.1%), compared with our results in the Kakehashi River basin (3.8%).

The association between LCd and mortality for renal diseases was significant only in women in both Cd-polluted areas, suggesting that women who took Cd from rice for a long time have more risk of dying from renal failure compared with men who took Cd at the same level. Since Cd absorption is higher in women because of lower body iron stores [23,24], we compared urinary Cd, uncorrected by Cr, in each LCd category, but no significant difference was found in any categories between men and women. However, urinary-uncorrected ß2–MG increased with increasing levels of LCd and was significantly higher in women compared with men when LCd $\geq$ 4.5 g. These findings suggest that renal tubular dysfunction may aggravate women more than men and cause renal failure deaths in women that are highly exposed to Cd.

In the study by Nogawa et al. [17], mortality was analyzed with three covariates, including age, smoking status at present, and hypertension history, while we performed our analysis with only one covariate of age, which is a limitation of our present study. However, no effects of smoking status or hypertension history were observed on mortality from renal diseases and the toxic effects of Cd of residents of the Jinzu River basin, suggesting that the confounding factors of smoking status and hypertension history may be limited in the association between mortality from renal diseases and LCd in the women of our study. In addition, the strength of the present study may be analyzing the effects of urinary Cd and LCd and internal and external Cd exposure markers on mortality at the same time in the same population. We showed that an increase in urinary Cd also increased mortality from renal diseases in women, as well as an increase in LCd, surely indicating the fatal renal toxic effects of environmental Cd exposure on women.

In Cd-polluted areas other than Japan, studies to investigate the dose relationship between mortality and external Cd exposure are limited. Only in Belgium, significantly higher lung cancer risk (incidence of fatal cancer) was reported for a doubling of Cd concentration in the soil of residential areas in a prospective population-based study from 1985 to 2004, which targeted the Flemish population who participated in the Cd in Belgium Study (CadmiBel) [25]. In almost all studies to investigate mortality risks for all causes [26], for cancer [27,28], and for cardiovascular diseases [29,30], internal Cd exposure markers such as urinary Cd or blood Cd were used as exposure markers because the exposure level is within background levels in their targeted population and it was difficult to estimate LCd.

5. Conclusions

A dose–response relationship between the external dose of Cd over a lifetime and mortality for renal diseases was found in women living in the Cd-polluted Kakehashi River basin, suggesting clear evidence of the impact of environmental Cd exposure on increased mortality from renal diseases in women.

Author Contributions: Conceptualization, M.N. and Y.S.; data curation, K.N. and M.S.; formal analysis, M.S.; funding acquisition, T.K.; methodology, K.N.; project administration, T.K. and H.N.; supervision, H.N.; writing—original draft, M.N.; writing—review and editing, Y.S. All authors have read and agreed to the published version of the manuscript.

Funding: This work was supported by a grant for aid from the Agency of Environment for Health Effects due to Heavy Metal Exposure 2009–2012 and 2013–2015, 2016–2018.

Acknowledgments: We thank the staff of Minami-Kaga Prefecture Public Health Office and Komatsu City Municipal Office in Ishikawa Prefecture, Japan, for their collaboration in the follow-up survey.

Conflicts of Interest: The authors declare no conflict of interest. The founding sponsors had no role in the design of the study; in the collection, analyses, or interpretation of data; in the writing of the manuscript, and in the decision to publish the results.

References

1. Frieberg, L. Cadmium and health. In *Advances in the Prevention of Environmental Cadmium Pollution and Countermeasures*; Nogawa, K., Kurachi, M., Kasuya, M., Eds.; Eiko Laboatory: Kanazawa, Japan, 1999; pp. 5–12.
2. Tsuchiya, K.; Iwao, S. Results and evaluation on cadmium intake of Cd-exposed inhabitants in Akita, Ishikawa and Nagasaki Prefectures. *Kankyo Hoken Rep.* **1978**, *44*, 86–115. (In Japanese)
3. Nogawa, K.; Honda, R.; Kido, T.; Tsuritani, I.; Yamada, Y.; Ishizaki, M.; Yamaya, H. A dose-response analysis of cadmium in the general environment with special reference to total cadmium intake limit. *Environ. Res.* **1989**, *48*, 7–16. [CrossRef]
4. Kido, T.; Shaikh, Z.A.; Kito, H.; Honda, R.; Nogawa, K. Dose-response relationship between dietary cadmium intake and metallothioneinuria in a population from a cadmium-polluted area of Japan. *Toxicology* **1991**, *66*, 271–278. [CrossRef]
5. Kido, T.; Shaikh, Z.A.; Kito, H.; Honda, R.; Nogawa, K. Dose-response relationship between total cadmium intake and metallothioneinuria using logistic regression analysis. *Toxicology* **1993**, *80*, 207–215. [CrossRef]
6. Kobayashi, E.; Okubo, Y.; Suwazono, Y.; Kido, T.; Nishijo, M.; Nakagawa, H.; Nogawa, K. Association between total cadmium intake calculated from the cadmium concentration in household rice and mortality

among inhabitants of the cadmium-polluted Jinzu River basin of Japan. *Toxicol. Lett.* **2002**, *129*, 85–91. [CrossRef]
7. Nakagawa, H.; Nishijo, M.; Morikawa, Y.; Tabata, M.; Senma, M.; Kitagawa, Y.; Kawano, S.; Ishizaki, M.; Sugita, N.; Nishi, M.; et al. Urinary ß2-microglobulin concentration and mortality in a cadmium-polluted area. *Arch. Environ. Health* **1993**, *48*, 428–435. [CrossRef]
8. Nakagawa, H.; Nishijo, M.; Morikawa, Y.; Tabata, M.; Miura, K.; Takahara, H.; Okumura, Y.; Yoshita, K.; Kawano, S.; Nishi, M.; et al. Increased urinary beta2-microglobulin and mortality rate by cause of death in a Cadmium-polluted area. *Environ. Health Prev. Med.* **1996**, *1*, 144–148. [CrossRef]
9. Nishijo, M.; Nakagawa, H.; Morikawa, Y.; Tabata, M.; Senma, M.; Kitagawa, Y.; Kawano, S.; Sugita, N.; Nishi, M.; Kido, T.; et al. Prognostic factors of renal dysfunction induced by environmental cadmium pollution. *Environ. Res.* **1994**, *64*, 112–121. [CrossRef]
10. Nishijo, M.; Nakagawa, H.; Morikawa, Y.; Tabata, M.; Senma, M.; Miura, K.; Takahara, H.; Kawano, S.; Nishi, M.; Mizukoshi, K.; et al. Mortality of inhabitants in an area polluted by cadmium: 15 year follow up. *Occup. Environ. Med.* **1995**, *52*, 181–184. [CrossRef]
11. Nishijo, M.; Nakagawa, H.; Morikawa, Y.; Kuriwaki, J.; Miura, K.; Kido, T.; Nogawa, K. Mortality in a cadmium polluted area in Japan. *Biometals* **2004**, *17*, 535–538. [CrossRef]
12. Nishijo, M.; Morikawa, Y.; Nakagawa, H.; Tawara, K.; Miura, K.; Kido, T.; Ikawa, A.; Kobayashi, E.; Nogawa, K. Causes of death and renal tubular dysfunction in residents exposed to cadmium in the environment. *Occup. Environ. Med.* **2006**, *63*, 545–550. [CrossRef] [PubMed]
13. Nakagawa, H.; Nishijo, M.; Morikawa, Y.; Miura, K.; Tawara, K.; Kuriwaki, J.; Kido, T.; Ikawa, K.; Kobayashi, E.; Nogawa, K. Urinary Cadmium and mortality among inhabitants of a cadmium polluted area in Japan. *Environ. Res.* **2006**, *100*, 323–329. [CrossRef] [PubMed]
14. Li, Q.; Nishijo, M.; Nakagawa, H.; Morikawa, Y.; Sakurai, M.; Nakamura, K.; Kido, T.; Nogawa, K.; Dai, M. Dose-response relationship between urinary cadmium and mortality in habitants of a cadmium-polluted area: A 22-year follow-up study in Japan. *Chin. Med. J.* **2011**, *124*, 3504–3509. [PubMed]
15. Kobayashi, E.; Okubo, Y.; Suwazono, Y.; Kido, T.; Nogawa, K. Dose-response relationship between total cadmium intake calculated from the cadmium concentration in rice collected from each household of farmers and renal dysfunction in inhabitants of the Jinzu River basin, Japan. *J. Appl. Toxicol.* **2002**, *22*, 431–436. [CrossRef] [PubMed]
16. Matsuda, K.; Kobayashi, E.; Okubo, Y.; Suwazono, Y.; Kido, T.; Nishijo, M.; Nakagawa, H.; Nogawa, K. Total cadmium intake and mortality among residents in the Jinzu River Basin, Japan. *Arch. Environ. Health* **2003**, *58*, 218–222. [CrossRef] [PubMed]
17. Nogawa, K.; Suwazono, Y.; Nishijo, M.; Sakurai, M.; Ishizaki, M.; Morikawa, Y.; Watanabe, Y.; Kido, T.; Nakagawa, H. Increase of lifetime cadmium intake dose-dependently increased all cause of mortality in female inhabitants of the cadmium-polluted Jinzu River basin, Toyama, Japan. *Environ. Res.* **2018**, *164*, 379–384. [CrossRef] [PubMed]
18. Ishikawa prefecture, Department of Health. *Report on the Health Examination of the Inhabitants in the Kakehashi Riber Basin, Ishikawa, Japan*; Ishikawa Prefecture, Department of Health: Kanazawa, Japan, 1976; pp. 79–84. (in Japanese)
19. Yamagata, N. Cadmium in the environment and in humans. In *Cadmium Studies in Japan: A Review*; Tsuchiya, K., Ed.; Kodansha Ltd.: Tokyo, Japan; Elsevier/North-Holland Biomedical Press: Amsterdam, The Netherlands, 1978; pp. 19–37.
20. Honda, R.; Nogawa, K.; Kobayashi, E.; Ishizaki, A. A simplified determination of urinary cadmium by flameless atomic absorption spectrometry using a heated graphite atomizer. *Hokuriku J. Public Health* **1979**, *6*, 13–19.
21. Nordberg, G.F. Cadmium metabolism and toxicity. *Environ. Physiol. Biochem.* **1972**, *2*, 7–36.
22. Bernard, A.; Goret, A.; Buchet, J.P.; Roels, H.; Lauwerys, R. Significance of cadmium level in blood and urine during long-term exposure of rats to cadmium. *J. Toxicol. Environ. Health* **1980**, *6*, 175–184. [CrossRef]
23. Kim, D.W.; Kim, K.Y.; Choi, B.S.; Youn, P.; Ryu, D.Y.; Klaassen, C.D.; Park, J.D. Regulation of metal transporters by dietary iron, and the relationship between body iron levels and cadmium uptake. *Arch. Toxicol.* **2007**, *81*, 327–334. [CrossRef]
24. Ruy, D.Y.; Lee, S.J.; Park, D.W.; Choi, B.S.; Klaassen, C.D.; Park, J.D. Dietary iron regulates intestinal cadmium absorption through iron transporters in rats. *Toxicol. Lett.* **2004**, *152*, 19–25. [CrossRef]

25. Nawrot, T.; Plusquin, M.; Hogervorst, J.; Roels, H.A.; Celis, H.; Thijs, L.; Vangronsveld, J.; Van Hecke, E.; Staessen, J.A. Environmental exposure to cadmium and risk of cancer: A prospective population-based study. *Lancet. Oncol.* **2006**, *7*, 119–126. [CrossRef]
26. Moberg, L.; Nilsson, P.M.; Samsioe, G.G.; Sallsten, G.L.; Barregard, L.G.; Engström, G.; Borgfeldt, C. Increased blood cadmium levels were not associated with increased fracture risk but with increased total mortality in women: The Malmö Diet and Cancer Study. *Osteoporos. Int.* **2017**, *28*, 2401–2408. [CrossRef] [PubMed]
27. McElroy, J.A.; Shafer, M.M.; Trenthan-Dietz, A.; Hampton, J.M.; Newcomb, P.A. Cadmium exposure and breast cancer risk. *J. Natl. Cancer Inst.* **2006**, *98*, 869–873. [CrossRef] [PubMed]
28. Adams, S.V.; Passarelli, M.N.; Newcomb, P.A. Cadmium exposure and cancer mortality in the Third National Health and Nutrition Examination Survey cohort. *Occup. Environ. Med.* **2012**, *69*, 153–156. [CrossRef] [PubMed]
29. Menke, A.; Muntner, P.; Silbergeld, E.K.; Platz, E.A.; Guallar, E. Cadmium levels in urine and mortality among U.S. adults. *Environ. Health Perspect.* **2009**, *117*, 190–196. [CrossRef]
30. Tellez-Plaza, M.; Navas-Acien, A.; Menke, A.; Crainiceanu, C.M.; Pastor-Barriuso, R.; Guallar, E. Cadmium exposure and all-cause and cardiovascular mortality in the U.S. general population. *Environ. Health Perspect.* **2012**, *120*, 1017–1022. [CrossRef]

toxics MDPI

Review

Cadmium and Lead Exposure, Nephrotoxicity, and Mortality

Soisungwan Satarug [1,*], Glenda C. Gobe [1,2,3], David A. Vesey [1,4] and Kenneth R. Phelps [5]

1 Kidney Disease Research Collaborative, The University of Queensland Faculty of Medicine and Translational Research Institute, Woolloongabba, Brisbane 4102, Australia; g.gobe@uq.edu.au (G.C.G.); David.Vesey@health.qld.gov.au (D.A.V.)
2 School of Biomedical Sciences, The University of Queensland, Brisbane 4072, Australia
3 NHMRC Centre of Research Excellence for CKD.QLD, UQ Faculty of Medicine, Royal Brisbane and Women's Hospital, Brisbane 4029, Australia
4 Department of Nephrology, Princess Alexandra Hospital, Brisbane 4075, Australia
5 Stratton Veteran Affairs Medical Center and Albany Medical College, Albany, NY 12208, USA; Kenneth.Phelps@va.gov
* Correspondence: sj.satarug@yahoo.com.au

Received: 12 August 2020; Accepted: 11 October 2020; Published: 13 October 2020

Abstract: The present review aims to provide an update on health risks associated with the low-to-moderate levels of environmental cadmium (Cd) and lead (Pb) to which most populations are exposed. Epidemiological studies examining the adverse effects of coexposure to Cd and Pb have shown that Pb may enhance the nephrotoxicity of Cd and vice versa. Herein, the existing tolerable intake levels of Cd and Pb are discussed together with the conventional urinary Cd threshold limit of 5.24 µg/g creatinine. Dietary sources of Cd and Pb and the intake levels reported for average consumers in the U.S., Spain, Korea, Germany and China are summarized. The utility of urine, whole blood, plasma/serum, and erythrocytes to quantify exposure levels of Cd and Pb are discussed. Epidemiological studies that linked one of these measurements to risks of chronic kidney disease (CKD) and mortality from common ailments are reviewed. A Cd intake level of 23.2 µg/day, which is less than half the safe intake stated by the guidelines, may increase the risk of CKD by 73%, and urinary Cd levels one-tenth of the threshold limit, defined by excessive $ß_2$-microglobulin excretion, were associated with increased risk of CKD, mortality from heart disease, cancer of any site and Alzheimer's disease. These findings indicate that the current tolerable intake of Cd and the conventional urinary Cd threshold limit do not provide adequate health protection. Any excessive Cd excretion is probably indicative of tubular injury. In light of the evolving realization of the interaction between Cd and Pb, actions to minimize environmental exposure to these toxic metals are imperative.

Keywords: cadmium; chronic kidney disease; lead; mortality; nephrotoxicity; threshold limit; tolerable intake level

1. Introduction

Cadmium (Cd) and lead (Pb) are metals that have no biologic role in humans [1–4]. All of their perceptible effects are toxic [1–4]. Indeed, Cd and Pb are two of ten chemicals listed by the World Health Organization (WHO) as environmental pollutants of major public health concern [5]. Tissues and organs accumulate Cd and Pb because no excretory mechanism has evolved to eliminate these metals [6–8]. Consequently, tissue levels of Cd and Pb increase with age, as do risks of common ailments that are often viewed as outcomes of aging. Although the highest concentrations of Cd and Pb are found, respectively, in kidneys and bone, toxic effects of these metals are not confined to diseases of the kidney and skeleton [1–4,9,10]. It has been estimated that dietary intake of Cd, Pb, inorganic arsenic, and methylmercury have resulted in 56,000 deaths and more than 9 million disability-adjusted life-years worldwide [11]. For the nonsmoking population of adults, diet is the main exposure source of Cd and Pb [2,12–16].

Oxidative stress and inflammation have been identified as common toxic mechanisms of Cd and Pb even though neither metal undergoes a change in valence (redox inert) [17–22]. Both are primarily divalent [22–24]. In addition, Cd has a similar ionic radius to that of calcium (Ca) and electronegativity similar to that of zinc (Zn), and both Cd and Pb exhibit higher affinity than Zn for sulphur-containing ligands (Cd > Pb > Zn) [23–26]. Consequently, displacement of Zn and Ca and disruption of Zn and Cu homeostasis are other plausible toxic mechanisms [27–35]. All sulphur-containing amino acids, peptides and proteins with functional thiol (-SH) groups are potential ligands (molecular targets) for Cd and Pb. Examples include glutathione (GSH), numerous enzymes, zinc-finger transcription factors, and the metal-binding protein metallothionein (MT) [23,24,36]. Through Zn displacement, Pb impairs the activity of delta-aminolevulinic acid dehydratase (δ-ALAD), an enzyme required for the biosynthesis of heme, which is the functional group of hemoglobin, nitric oxide synthase, and cytochromes of the mitochondrial respiratory chain and xenobiotic metabolism [37]. Inhibition of the calcium-permeable acid-sensing ion channel may be the mechanism that accounts for the neurotoxicity of Pb [38,39].

The goal of this review is to provide an update on health risks associated with the low-to-moderate levels of environmental Cd and Pb to which most populations are exposed. High-dose exposure, which is relatively rare, is outside the scope of this review. We sought to establish dose–response relationships between ingested amounts of these toxic metals and parameters of tubular cell injury that have been associated with loss of glomerular filtration. This information is relevant to public health policy regarding advisable exposure limits. We discuss the interim safe intake level for Pb, the current tolerable dietary intake level for Cd, and the concept of the threshold level of urinary Cd. We describe the main dietary sources of Cd and Pb and the estimated intake levels of these metals among average and high consumers of tainted food. We highlight the utility of blood and urinary levels of Cd and Pb as indicators of internal accumulation of the metals. A connection is elaborated between Cd-induced tubulopathy and a decrease in glomerular filtration rate (GFR) to levels commensurate with chronic kidney disease (CKD). Epidemiologic data linking Cd and Pb exposure to enhanced CKD risk are summarized, as are data from longitudinal studies showing that Cd and Pb exposure may increase mortality from cancer and cardiovascular disease.

2. Health Risk Assessment of Chronic Exposure to Cadmium and Lead

2.1. The Critical Target of Toxicity

Long-term chronic exposure to Cd and Pb has been associated with distinct pathologies in nearly every tissue and organ throughout the body [1–4,14,25]. However, in health risk assessment, the kidney was considered to be the critical target of Cd toxicity [1,8], while the brain was the critical target of Pb toxicity [3,4,25]. Accordingly, dietary intake estimates associated with a significant increase in the risk of nephrotoxicity of Cd or neurotoxicity of Pb were used to derive a tolerable intake level. One method to evaluate whether a given food contaminant poses a health risk is to compare dietary intake estimated by total diet studies with the provisional tolerable weekly intake (PTWI), as established by the Joint Expert Committee on Food Additives and Contaminants (JECFA) of the Food and Agriculture Organization (FAO) and the WHO of the United Nations (FAO/WHO).

2.2. Tolerable Intake Levels

The PTWI for a chemical was defined as an estimate of the amount of a given chemical that can be ingested weekly over a lifetime without an appreciable health risk. The PTWI figures were first provided for Cd and Pb in 1989 and then amended in 1993 and 2010 [40,41]. The 1993 PTWI figures for Cd and Pb were 7 and 25 μg per kg body weight per week, respectively. In 2010, the PTWI for Cd was amended to a tolerable monthly intake (TMI) level of 25 μg per kg body weight per month. This intake level is equivalent to 0.83 μg per kg body weight per day or 58 μg per day for a 70-kg person [41]. The model for deriving PTWI and TMI of Cd was based on elevated β_2-microglobulin (β_2MG) excretion as the sole evidence of nephrotoxicity [41]. In Section 3.1, we provide current Cd intake levels in various countries and their sources.

For Pb, the previously established PTWI of 25 μg per kg body weight per week was withdrawn because it did not afford health protection [41]. A new tolerable Pb intake level could not be established as dose–response analyses indicated that no threshold levels exist for neurotoxicity of Pb. Thus, no amount of Pb intake is safe, and no tolerable Pb intake level has been officially identified. However, the U.S. Food and Drug Administration (FDA) has proposed a dietary Pb intake level of 12.5 μg/day as an interim safe intake level for the general population of adults [42,43]. This intake level corresponds to a blood concentration of Pb ($[Pb]_b$) of 0.5 μg/dL, which has not been found to be associated with an adverse effect in adults in any epidemiologic studies. In Section 3.1, we provide current Pb intake levels in various countries and their sources.

2.3. Urinary Cd Threshold Level

A urinary Cd excretion rate (E_{Cd}) of 5.24 μg/g creatinine was adopted as a threshold limit [41]. However, the established threshold level is questionable. Chronic environmental exposure to low-level Cd, producing urinary Cd one-tenth of the conventional threshold, has been associated with deterioration of kidney function, as assessed with estimated GFR (eGFR) [44–46]. A urinary Cd concentration ($[Cd]_u$) as low as 1 μg/L, corresponding to blood Cd concentration ($[Cd]_b$) of 0.5 μg/L, was associated with an increased risk of eGFR less than 60 mL/min/1.73 m^2 [44,47]. It can be argued that risk of nephrotoxicity of any toxicants, Cd and Pb included, should be based on eGFR, which is a reliable measure of kidney function and diagnosis and staging of CKD [48–50]. A dose–response analysis of urinary Cd and eGFR, rather than of urinary Cd and β_2MG, indicates that Cd-induced nephrotoxicity occurs at a much lower E_{Cd} than previously thought [12,51–54]. We believe that the established TMI for Cd is not protective of kidneys, just as the 1993 PTWI for Pb does not prevent neurotoxicity. The 1993 PTWI for Pb has now been withdrawn [41]. In Section 4.3.4. we provide an in-depth analysis of β_2MG excretion in Cd nephropathy.

3. Exposure Sources and Dietary Intake Estimates

For the general nonsmoking population of adults, the diet is the major exposure source of both Cd and Pb. In this section, both natural and anthropogenic sources of Cd and Pb in the human diet are highlighted. In addition, a reliable dietary assessment and food safety monitoring method, such as a total diet study, is discussed, and estimated intake levels of Cd and Pb derived from recent total diet studies in various countries are provided.

3.1. Environmental Sources of Cadmium and Lead

Volcanic emissions, fossil fuel and biomass combustion, and cigarette smoke are sources of Cd and Pb released as CdO and PbO [55–59]. Experimental studies have shown that inhaled CdO and PbO are more bioavailable than oral Cd and Pb [60–63]. Typically, potable water is not a source of Cd or Pb, except in cases where significant amounts of Pb plumbing have been used, as occurred in the recent Flint, Michigan, water crisis [64,65].

Years of production and industrial use of Cd and Pb have mobilized these metals from nonbioavailable geologic matrices to biologically accessible sources from which they can enter food chains [55]. Like all other metals, Cd and Pb are not biodegradable and thus can persist indefinitely in the environment [55]. The use of contaminated phosphate fertilizers has also added these toxic metals to agricultural soils [6,7], causing a further increase in Cd and Pb in the food chain [66–68]. Livestock that graze on contaminated pastures can accumulate Cd in the kidney and liver at levels that make these organs unsafe for human consumption [69]. In Pb-exposed cattle, blood Pb levels correlated with levels of Pb in liver, bone and kidney, but not in brain or skeletal muscle (beef) [70]. Of note, a detectable amount of Pb was found in beef at a blood Pb concentration of 4.57 µg/dL. This blood Pb level was close to the exposure limit for neurotoxicity of Pb in children (5 µg/dL) [71]. Molluscs and crustaceans accumulate Cd and are also notorious hyperaccumulators of other metals [72–75]. For most species, fish muscle does not appear to be a significant source of Cd and Pb, but there are exceptions, as indicated in Section 3.1 [76].

In a similar manner to molluscs and crustaceans, plants have the propensity to concentrate Cd and Pb from the soil. Plants have evolved multiple metal detoxification mechanisms, including an array of metal-binding ligands such as MT, phytochelatins (PCs), other low-molecular-weight thiols, GSH, cysteine, γ-glutamylcysteine, and cysteinylglycine [77–79]. As Cd exerts toxicity in the "free" ion or unbound state, complexes of Cd and metal-binding ligands, such as CdMT and CdPC, are viewed as detoxified forms [80]. Accordingly, the various types of metal-binding ligands render plants capable of tolerating levels of Cd and Pb that are toxic to animals and humans.

Owing to their phylogenic characteristics, tobacco, rice, other cereal grains, potatoes, salad vegetables, spinach, and Romaine lettuce accumulate Cd more efficiently than other plants [81]. An outbreak of "itai-itai" disease, a severe form of Cd poisoning from contaminated rice, serves as a reminder of the health threat from Cd contamination of a staple food crop [82].

3.2. Total Diet Studies and Dietary Intake Estimates

Reliable methodology is vitally important to assess the levels of contaminants in commonly eaten foods and to set food safety standards. The total diet study has been widely used by authorities to estimate intake levels and identify sources of Cd and Pb in the human diet [83–87]. It is also known as the "market basket survey" because samples of foodstuffs are collected from supermarkets and retail stores to determine levels of nutrients, food additives, pesticide residues and contaminants [2,83–87]. It serves as a food safety monitoring program that provides a basis to define a maximally permissible concentration of a given contaminant in a specific food group.

In a typical total diet study, an intake level of a given contaminant from a study food item (rice as an example) is computed based on an amount of the food item consumed per day and the concentration of a contaminant in the rice samples that are analyzed in a study. The median and 90th percentile concentration levels of a contaminant are used to represent the intake levels of a contaminant by average and high consumers, respectively [88].

Table 1 summarizes most recent total diet studies showing intake levels of Cd among adult consumers in China [89–91], Korea [92,93], Germany [94], Spain [95,96] and the U.S. [97–99] along with the list of foods that contributed significantly to total intake of the metal. Table 1 summarizes also food products that contributed significantly to total intake of Pb and the estimated intake levels of the metal among adult consumers in China [89–91], Korea [92], Germany [100], Spain [95] and the U.S. [84]. Furthermore, Cd intake levels estimated for consumers in Sweden [88] France [101], Belgium [102] and a region with Cd pollution of Japan [103] are provided.

Table 1. Estimated intake levels of cadmium and lead and their sources.

Countries	Estimated Intake Levels as μg Per Day and Dietary Sources	
	Cadmium (Atomic Weight 112.4)	Lead (Atomic Weight 207.2)
China [89,90] 67% of population	Average consumers: 32.7 μg/day. Rice and vegetables as the main sources for most Chinese. Potato was the main source in Mongolia. High Cd foods: Nori, peanuts, squid, cuttlefish, and mushrooms.	Average consumers: 35.1 μg/day. Cereals, meats, vegetables, and beverages and water together contributed to 73.26% of total intake. High Pb foods: Kelp, nori, processed and preserved soybean, meat, and fungus. products.
Korea [92] $n = 4867$	Average consumers: 12.6 μg/day. Sources: Grain and grain-based products (40.4%), vegetables and vegetable products (16.5%), and fish and shellfish (17.9%). High Cd foods: Seaweed, shellfish and crustaceans, molluscs, nuts and seeds, and flavourings, with median values of 594, 186, 155, 15.7, and 6.23 μg/kg, respectively.	Average consumers: 9.8 μg/day. High Pb foods: Seaweed, shellfish and crustaceans, molluscs, fish, and sugar and sugar products, with respective median values of 94.2, 91.4, 62.4, 8.13, and 4.61 μg/kg, while the median value for beverages (fruit juice, carbonated fruit juice, carbonated drinks, sports drinks, and coffee) was 11.0 μg/kg.
Germany [94,100] $n = 15{,}371$	Average consumers: 14.6 μg/day. High consumers: 23.5 μg/day. Sources: Cereals and vegetables, beverages, fruits and nuts, and dairy products (milk included). High Cd foods: Cereals, oily seeds and fruits, and vegetables.	Average consumers: 37.1 μg/day. High consumers: 50.4 μg/day. Sources: Beverages, vegetables, fruits and nuts and cereals. High Pb foods: Meat (offal included), fish (seafood), vegetables and cereals.
Spain [95] $n = 1281$	Average consumers: 7.7 μg/day. Sources: Cereals and fish contributed to 38% and 29% of total intake. High Cd foods: Cereals (16.25 μg/kg), fish group (11.40 μg/kg).	Average consumers: 14.7 μg/day. Cereals contributed to 49% of total intake. High Pb foods: Sweeteners and condiments, vegetable oils, meat, and fish, with respective median levels of 32.5, 15.25, 14.90 and 13.21 μg/kg.
U.S. [84,97] $n = 14{,}614$ FDA 2014–2016 total diet study	Average consumers: 4.63 μg/day. Sources: Cereals and bread, leafy vegetables, potatoes, legumes and nuts, stem/root vegetables, and fruits contributed to 34%, 20%, 11%, 7% and 6% of total intake, respectively. High Cd foods: Spaghetti, bread, potatoes and potato chips contributed the most to total Cd intake, followed by lettuce, spinach, tomatoes, and beer. Lettuce was a main Cd source for whites and blacks. Tortillas and rice were main Cd sources for Hispanic Americans, and Asians plus other ethnicities. Cd concentration of raw leaf lettuce and iceberg lettuce were 0.066 and 0.051 mg/kg, respectively.	Average consumers: 1.7–5.3 μg/day. High consumers: 3.2–7.8 μg/day. Sources: Grains, beverages, vegetables, dairy, fruits, meat, and poultry plus fish contributed to 24.1%, 14.3%, 10.7%, 9.7%, 9.3% and 3.4% to total intake, respectively. High Pb foods: Chocolate syrup, liver, canned sweet potatoes, brownies, low-calorie buttermilk, salad dressing, raisins, English muffins, canned apricots, milk chocolate, candy bars, chocolate cake, chocolate chip cookies, wine and oat ring cereal with respective median levels of 14, 14, 14, 13, 13, 12, 10, 10, 9, 8, 8, 7 and 7 μg/kg.

A current tolerable Cd intake level established by FAO/WHO for the population of adults is 25 μg per kg body weight per month (58 μg per day for a 70-kg person) [41]. No tolerable Pb intake level has been identified after a previously established guideline was withdrawn in 2010 [41]. U.S. FDA interim safe intake level of Pb for the population of adults is 12.5 μg per day [42].

3.2.1. Estimated Cadmium Intake Levels in Various Populations

In a recent total diet study in China, the Cd intake among average consumers was 32.7 μg/day, with rice and vegetables being the main sources [89]. In Mongolia, potatoes were the main source of Cd, contributing 24% of the total Cd intake [89]. Nori, peanuts, squid, cuttlefish and mushrooms had relatively high Cd contents [90,91].

The Cd intake level among average consumers in South Korea was 12.6 μg/day [92]. Cereals and vegetables, beverages, fruits and nuts, and dairy products (milk included) were the main dietary sources. Cereals, oily seeds and fruits, and vegetables had relatively high Cd concentrations. A higher average Cd intake of 22 μg/day was reported in another Korean study ($n = 1245$), where Cd intake in gastric cancer cases was compared to noncancer controls [93]. An average amount of rice consumed by the control group was 587.3 g/day versus 610.9 g/day in gastric cancer cases. Rice was the major contributor (40.3%) to total Cd intake, followed by squid (11.8%), eel (11.0%), crab (8.6%), shellfish (3.6%), kimchi (Korean cabbage; 3.5%) and seaweed (3.5%).

The Cd intake levels among average and high consumers in Germany were 14.6 and 23.5 μg/day, respectively [94]. Cereals and vegetables were the main Cd sources, followed by beverages, fruits and nuts, and dairy products (milk included). Cereals, oily seeds and fruits, and vegetables had relatively high Cd contents [94].

The Cd intake among average consumers in Spain was 7.7 μg/day, with cereals and fish as the main sources, contributing to 38% and 29% of total Cd intake, respectively [95]. In another dietary study of 281 postmenopausal women in Spain, an average Cd intake was 30 (range, 20–41) μg/day [96]. These data illustrate that when the total diet study methodology is used, Cd intake from the diet showed a little variation and, in many cases, probably represented an underestimation of actual Cd intake.

The Cd intake among average consumers in the U.S. was 4.63 μg/day. Cereals and bread, leafy vegetables, potatoes, legumes and nuts, stem/root vegetables, and fruits contributed, respectively, to 34%, 20%, 11%, 7% and 6% of total intake [97]. Spaghetti, bread, potatoes and potato chips were the top three Cd sources, followed by lettuce, spinach, tomatoes, and beer. Lettuce was an important Cd source for whites and blacks. Tortillas and rice were the main Cd sources for Hispanic Americans, Asians and some other ethnicities. However, a higher dietary Cd intake of 10.9 μg/day was recorded in the U.S. Women's Health Initiative study [98]. The average Cd intake of 4.63 μg/day by adults in the U.S. was close to a median Cd intake of 5 μg/day reported for consumers in Northern Italy, where cereals, vegetables and sweets were the main Cd sources [99].

It is noteworthy that the average Cd intake in Sweden (10.6 μg/day), France (11.2 μg/day) and Belgium (9.8 μg/day) was higher in all of these countries than the average Cd intake in the U.S. of 4.63 μg/day [88,101,102]. For average consumers in France, bread and potato-based products contributed, respectively, to 35% and 26% of total Cd intake, while potatoes and wheat combined contributed to 40–50% of Cd intake among average consumers in Sweden. Likewise, cereal products and potatoes were the main sources, contributing more than 60% to total Cd intake among average consumers in Belgium [102]. For high consumers in Sweden, average Cd intake was 23 μg/day, with seafood (shellfish) and spinach being additional Cd sources [88]. For high consumers in France, Cd intake was 18.9 μg/day, with additional Cd coming from molluscs and crustaceans [101]. Cd contents in molluscs and crustaceans, offal, sweet and savoury biscuits and cereal bars, and chocolate in a French total diet study were 0.167, 0.053, 0.030, and 0.029 mg/kg, respectively.

In summary, the average Cd intake levels in China (32.7 μg/day), Korea (12.6 μg/day), Germany (14.6 μg/day), Spain (7.7 μg per day) and Sweden, France and Belgium (range, 9.81–11.2 μg/day) were all higher than the average Cd intake in the U.S (4.63 μg/day) [88,101,102]. For average consumers, staple foods were the main Cd sources. Seafood (shellfish), offal, spinach, lettuce and chocolate were additional sources of Cd among high consumers. These estimated Cd intake levels did not exceed a current FAO/WHO tolerable intake level of 58 μg/day [41]. However, evidence for adverse health effects has emerged from cross-sectional and longitudinal studies of populations from these countries, in which urinary and/or blood Cd levels were used to quantitate exposure levels (Section 5).

Thus, the utility of dietary intake estimates in health risk assessment is questionable. In another example, the total diet study undertaken in two areas of Japan affected by Cd pollution reported the median Cd intake levels in female farmers residing in the two areas as 47.8 and 55.7 μg/day [103]. These estimated Cd intake levels in Cd-polluted areas were lower than the FAO/WHO tolerable intake level, but adverse health effects were observed [103].

3.2.2. Estimated Lead Intake Levels in Various Populations

The Pb intake level among average consumers in China was 35.1 μg/day, with cereals, meats, vegetables, beverages and water as the main sources [89]. These food and beverage items together contributed to 73.26% of total Pb intake [89]. Kelp, nori, processed and preserved soybean, meat, and fungus products had relatively high Pb concentrations [90]. For the population of Jiangsu province, a higher mean Pb intake level of 73.9 μg/day was reported, with cereals and vegetables as the main sources, contributing to 57% of total Pb intake [91].

The Pb intake level among average consumers in South Korea was 9.8 μg/day [92]. High levels of Pb were found in a range of products, notably seaweed, shellfish and crustaceans, molluscs, fish, sugar and sugar products, and beverages (fruit juice, carbonated fruit juice, carbonated drinks, sports drinks and coffee).

The Pb intake levels among average and high consumers in Germany were 37.1 and 50.4 μg/day, respectively [100]. Beverages, vegetables, fruits and nuts and cereals were the main Pb sources. Foods with relatively high Pb concentrations were meat (offal included), fish (seafood), vegetables and cereals [100].

The Pb intake level among average consumers in Spain was 14.7 μg/day, with cereals as the main source at nearly half (49%) of total intake [95]. Sweeteners and condiments, vegetable oils, meat, and fish had relatively high Pb concentrations [95].

The Pb intake levels among average and high consumers in the U.S. were 1.7–5.3 and 3.2–7.8 μg/day, respectively [84]. Grains, beverages, vegetables, dairy products, fruits, meat, and poultry plus fish contributed to 24.1%, 14.3%, 10.7%, 9.7%, 9.3% and 3.4% of total intake, respectively. Foods with relatively high Pb concentrations were chocolate syrup, liver, canned sweet potatoes, brownies, low-calorie buttermilk, salad dressing, raisins, English muffins, canned apricots, milk chocolate, candy bars, chocolate cake, chocolate chip cookies, wine and oat ring cereal.

In summary, average Pb intake in China (35.1 μg/day) was close to the level of intake in Germany (37.1 μg/day). These Pb intake levels were higher than the intake figures estimated for average consumers in Spain (14.7 μg/day), Korea (9.8 μg/day) and the U.S. (1.7–5.3 μg/day). Pb intake from the diet was highest (50.4 μg/day) among high consumers in Germany. To date, a tolerable Pb intake level has not been identified after a tolerable intake level of 25 μg per kg body weight per week was withdrawn in 2010 [41]. An interim tolerable intake level for Pb of 12.5 μg per day has been proposed for the population of adults by the U.S. FDA [42,43]. Based on this interim safe-intake figure (12.5 μg/day), dietary Pb intake levels among average consumers in China, Germany and Spain could be considered as excessive and may pose a significant health risk.

3.3. *Absorption of Cadmium and Lead: An Overview*

As the body does not synthesize nor break down metals, transporter systems and pathways have evolved to acquire all required elements, notably calcium (Ca), zinc (Zn), manganese (Mn), copper (Cu), and iron (Fe), from exogenous sources [104]. These metal transporters and pathways also serve as routes of entry for toxic metals Cd and Pb in the diet [105–110]. Early work suggested that the iron (Fe^{2+}) transporter, divalent metal transporter1 (DMT1), was a likely route of entry for Cd and Pb [111,112]. Later, it was demonstrated that Pb entered enterocytes through a mechanism that was independent of DMT1 [113,114]. Additionally, although DMT1 has the same high affinity for Cd^{2+} as it does for Fe^{2+} [112], ferroportin 1 (FPN1) exports iron but not Cd [115]. Calbindin-D28k, a calcium-binding protein, may transport Cd to the basolateral membrane of enterocytes and may export Cd into the portal blood circulation [110,116].

Receptor-mediated endocytosis and transcytosis are the likely mechanisms for absorption of the Cd–metallothionein complex (CdMT) and the Cd–phytochelatin complex (CdPC) [117–119]. The specific metal transporters, carriers and receptors that have been implicated in the absorption of Cd and/or Pb include DMT1, a Zrt- and Irt-related protein (ZIP) of the zinc transporter family, the Ca^{2+}-selective channel TRPV6, and the human neutrophil gelatinase-associated lipocalin (hNGAL) receptor [110,120]. ZIP14 and TRPV6 are highly expressed by intestinal enterocytes [107–109,120].

3.4. The Kinetics of Cadmium and Lead in the Human Body

Figure 1 outlines exposure sources of Cd and Pb, their entry routes, tissue distribution, storage organs and targets of toxicity.

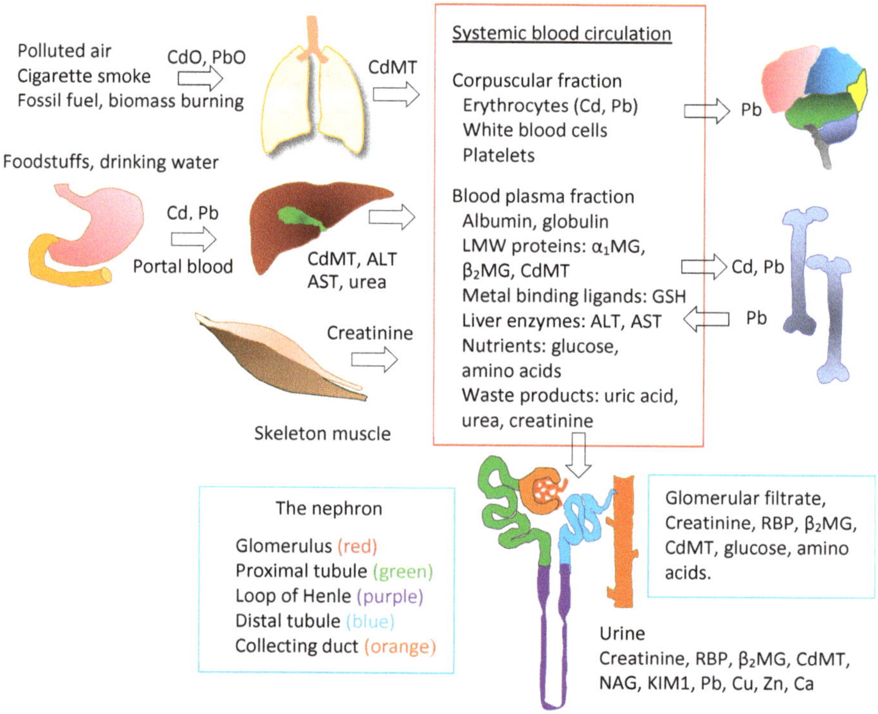

Figure 1. Entry routes, distribution, storage and urinary excretion of cadmium and lead.

Absorbed Cd and Pb are transported to the liver. Inhaled CdO and PbO are transported to the lungs. Cd induces the synthesis of MT in both liver and lung, and CdMT is formed. Hepatic and pulmonary CdMT are later released and contribute to $[CdMT]_b$. Pb does not induce MT in the liver or lung, and it binds presumably to GSH and other thiols in these organs. The fractions of absorbed Cd and Pb that are not taken up by the liver in the first pass then reach systemic circulation and are taken up by tissues and organs throughout the body, kidneys included. Pb is taken up mostly by bone and is later released, contributing to $[Pb]_b$. CdMT from all sources (liver, lung, intestine) passes glomerular membrane filtration, and the filtered CdMT is reabsorbed by proximal tubular cells. Small fractions of Cd and Pb in the body are excreted in urine. $[Cd]_u$ provides a useful indication of kidney injury and kidney burden. $[Pb]_u$ serves as a proxy for $[Pb]_p$.

Oxides of Cd and Pb in the air reach the lung, prompting an increase in the synthesis of MT, and CdMT is formed in situ [121]. Presumably, the induction of MT synthesis in the lung is attributable to Cd only because Pb is a weak inducer [122]. The pulmonary CdMT is later released into systemic circulation and redistributed to the kidneys [123,124]. Of note, while inhaled Cd increased pulmonary MT synthesis, a study in mice has shown that low-dose oral Cd did not induce pulmonary MT [125].

Cd and Pb in the diet are transported via the hepatic portal system to the liver, where Cd induces copiously the synthesis of MT, to which it becomes tightly bound as CdMT [126]. Pb does not induce MT synthesis in the liver. An increase in hepatic MT protein levels was a result of elevated plasma levels of interleukin 6 that followed Pb administration [127]. Of note, hepatic MT synthesis is intensified in rats given Pb plus Cd, although oral Pb alone does not affect the synthesis of MT in the liver [128]. Presumably, in hepatocytes, Pb initially forms complexes with GSH [24]. A small fraction of hepatic Cd and Pb is excreted in faeces via bile or may be reabsorbed and returned to the liver [129]. Hepatic CdMT is also continuously released into systemic circulation. This hepatic process contributes to $[Cd]_b$ and the redistribution of Cd (as CdMT) to kidneys long after exposure cessation. In this manner, the liver serves as a reservoir of Cd. The fraction of dietary Cd and Pb not taken up by hepatocytes in the first pass reaches systemic circulation and is taken up by tissues and organs throughout the body. Pb is preferentially taken up by bone, where it is stored and later released [130]. Thus, bone serves as a reservoir of Pb, and this organ contributes to $[Pb]_b$, as is discussed further in Section 4.2.

Through systemic circulation, CdMT and CdPC of dietary origin and intestinal and hepatic CdMT [126] all reach the kidneys, where they are filtered by glomeruli by virtue of their small molecular weights [8]. Once they pass the glomerular membrane into the tubular lumen, they are then subsequently reabsorbed by proximal tubular epithelial cells as these cells are equipped with protein internalization mechanisms [131–134]. Due to a lack of biologically active mechanisms to eliminate excess metals, nearly all reabsorbed Cd is retained in the kidneys.

In summary, ingested Cd is mostly reabsorbed and sequestered in kidneys [126,131–134], while ingested Pb is taken up and retained in bone [135]. Only a small fraction of Cd and Pb in the kidneys is excreted in urine (Section 3.4, Figure 2). An in-depth discussion on the source of excreted Cd is provided in Section 4.3.2. In effect, the kidney Cd content reflects cumulative lifetime exposure, while bone Pb is an indicator of Pb body burden.

3.5. Cadmium and Lead Accumulation in Kidneys and Urinary Excretion: Australian Experience

Figure 2 provides data on Cd and Pb levels in kidney cortex samples ($[Cd]_k$, $[Pb]_k$) from a subgroup of an Australian autopsy study ($n = 42$) [136,137]. The mean age, body mass index (BMI) and kidney weight were 38 years, 23.5 kg/m^2 and 267 g, respectively. Kidney weight relative to body weight showed a decrease in old age (Figure 2A). The means of $[Cd]_k$ and $[Pb]_k$ were 14.5 and 4.16 μg/g kidney cortex wet weight, respectively. Thus, the kidney cortex accumulated 3.5 times greater amounts of Cd than Pb on a weight basis and 6.4 times higher amounts of Cd than Pb on a molar basis (Figure 2B). In an analysis of Cd and Pb concentrations in urine samples ($[Cd]_u$, $[Pb]_u$) from 17–23 urinary bladders of subjects in this subgroup, $[Cd]_u$ increased linearly with age and $[Cd]_k$ (Figure 2C,D). Distinctly, $[Pb]_u$ did not correlate with age or $[Pb]_k$. The correlation between $[Cd]_u$, age and $[Cd]_k$ supports the use of $[Cd]_u$ as a kidney burden indicator. The mean $[Pb]_k$ of 4.16 μg/g wet weight observed in this Australian study was much higher than the median $[Pb]_k$ of 0.08 μg/g wet weight found in Swedish kidney transplant donors ($n = 109$, 24–70 years, median 51), but there was only a small difference in $[Cd]_k$ in Australian and Swedish studies (14.5 vs. 12.9 μg/g wet weight) [138].

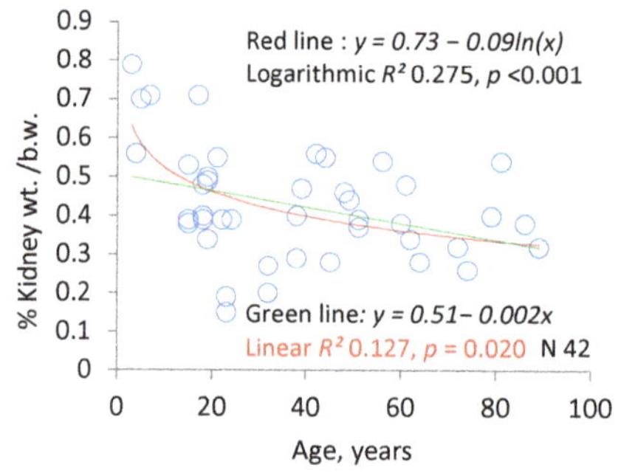

Parameters	Males N 30	Females N 12	All N 42
Age, years	34.9 ± 22.6	46.0 ± 27.4	38.0 ± 24.3
BMI, kg/m²	23.7 ± 5.75	22.8 ± 5.07	23.5 ± 5.52
Kidney wt., g	282 ± 97.4	230 ± 102	267 ± 100
% Kidney wt./b.w.	0.45 ± 0.14	0.38 ± 0.14	0.43 ± 0.14
Cd, μg/g wet wt.	13.8 ± 11.9	16.2 ± 16.5	14.5 ± 13.2
Pb, μg/g wet wt.	4.34 ± 9.66	3.66 ± 6.27	4.16 ± 8.80

Numbers are arithmetic means ± standard deviation

(B)

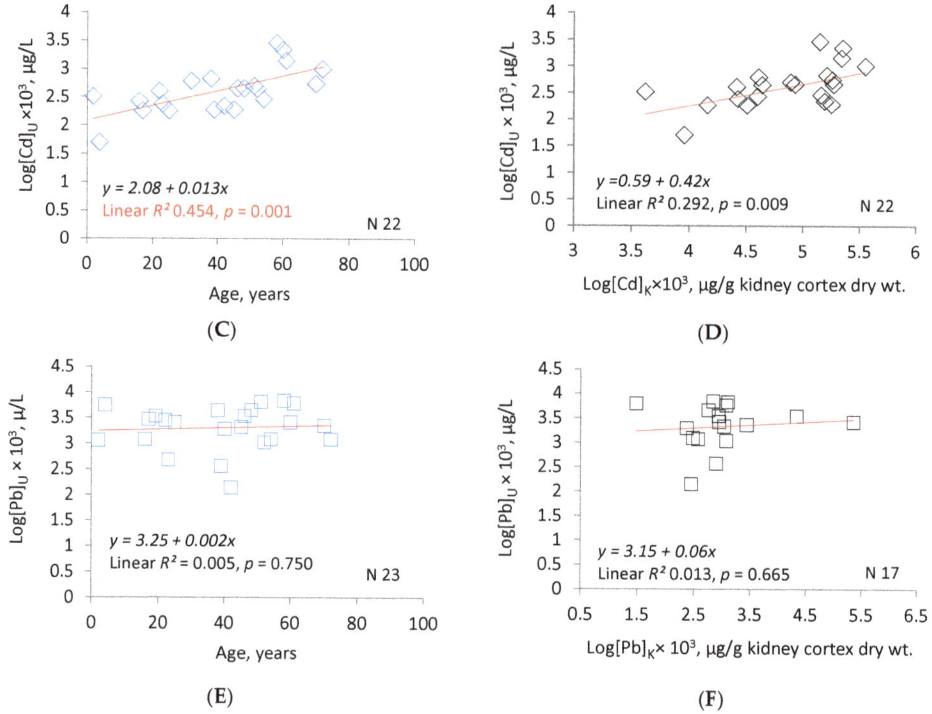

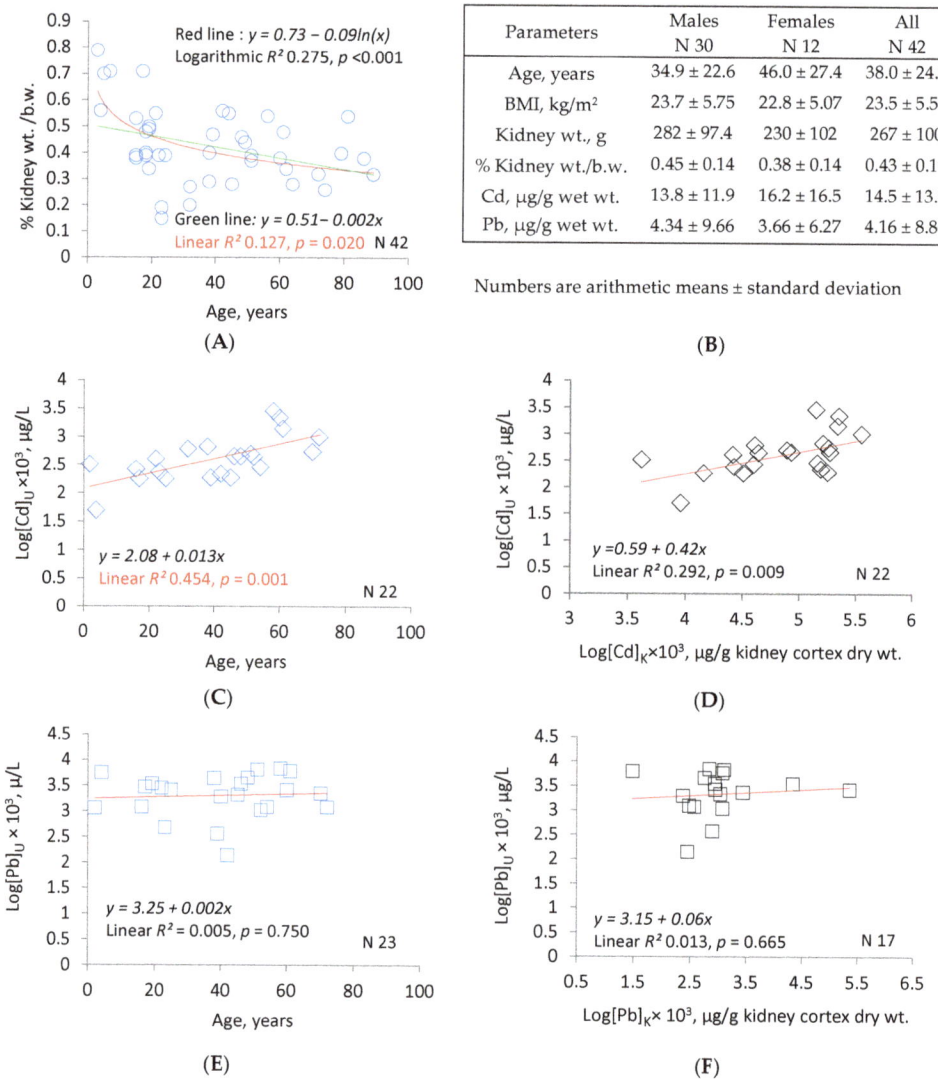

Figure 2. Cadmium and lead accumulation levels in kidneys and their levels in urine.

Figure 2A is a scatterplot that relates % kidney weight to body weight ratios to age in a subgroup of an Australian autopsy study (n = 42, mean age 38 years). Figure 2B provides data on age, BMI, kidney weight and Cd and Pb contents in kidney cortex ($[Cd]_k$, $[Pb]_k$). Figure 2C,D are scatterplots showing significant correlations between $[Cd]_u$ versus age and $[Cd]_u$ versus $[Cd]_k$, respectively. These correlations support the utility of $[Cd]_u$ in kidney burden assessment. Miniscule correlations between $[Pb]_u$ versus age and $[Pb]_u$ versus $[Pb]_k$ are indicated by scatter plots in Figure 2E,F, respectively.

4. Dosimetry and Nephrotoxicity Assessment

The dogma in health risk assessment states that for a given toxicant to pose a health risk, it must enter the body to reach its critical target of toxicity. The levels of a toxicant in body fluid and tissues and organs may serve as dosimetric matrices. In this section, we discuss the utility of urine, whole blood, blood plasma (serum), and erythrocytes in the assessment of Cd and Pb body burden. The manifestation of nephrotoxicities such as the leakage of intracellular proteins into the filtrate, a reduction in glomerular filtration rate, and impaired reabsorption of filtered proteins is discussed.

4.1. Cadmium Dosimetry

4.1.1. Blood Cadmium Versus Urinary Cadmium

In the studies examining decreases in $[Cd]_b$ and $[Cd]_u$ in groups of Cd-exposed Swedish workers after exposure had ceased, the estimated half-life values varied from 75 to 128 days for the fast component, representing $[Cd]_b$ [139,140]. For the slow component, representing Cd in tissues, the estimated half-life values varied from 7.4 to 16.0 years. A comparable half-life figure of 14 years (range, 9–28 years) was derived from a Japanese study [141]. In a separate analysis, the half-life of whole-body Cd in Japanese men with lower exposures ($[Cd]_u < 5$ µg/L) was 23.4 years, nearly two-fold longer than the half-life figure of 12.4 years, estimated for those with higher exposures [142]. A whole-body half-life of Cd over 45 years was estimated based on data from Swedish kidney transplant donors, who had much lower $[Cd]_u$, $[Cd]_b$ and $[Cd]_k$ than those in Japanese studies [143]. Collectively, these findings indicate that Cd is mostly retained in the body, particularly the kidneys, in low-level exposure situations, while there is a substantial loss of $[Cd]_k$ due to Cd-induced tubular injury in chronic high-exposure conditions [54].

The half-life of whole-body Cd falls in the same range as estimated half-life for Pb in bone (Section 4.2). Apparently, however, the half-life of blood Cd (between 75 and 128 days) is much longer than the 10-day half-life of blood Pb [144]. The estimated long half-life of $[Cd]_b$ could be due to continuing contribution to $[Cd]_b$ from tissues and organs, notably, the liver and lungs. To derive a half-life figure specific to exogenously derived Cd requires knowledge of contribution from the main endogenous sources, liver, lung and bone included, as depicted in Figure 1. Thus, at any given time, $[Cd]_b$ is considered to reflect recent exposure together with a continuing contribution from whole-body Cd, especially the liver and lungs.

Distinct from $[Cd]_b$, urinary excretion of Cd (E_{Cd}) is an indicator of cumulative lifelong exposure. E_{Cd} varies directly with $[Cd]_k$ (see Figure 2) and the determinants of $[Cd]_k$, such as age, gender, smoking, metalwork history and level of regional Cd pollution [8,136,145–148]. In a Swedish study, the highest Cd concentrations in copper smelter workers and the controls were seen in kidneys, followed by liver, lung and brain [148]. Of note, E_{Cd} showed stronger and more consistent associations with nephrotoxicity than $[Cd]_b$. E_{Cd} is discussed further in Section 4.3.2.

In an autopsy study in Poland, E_{Cd} of 1.7 µg/g creatinine corresponded to $[Cd]_k$ of 50 µg/g [145]. In another Swedish study, kidney transplant donors ($n = 109$) had a mean $[Cd]_k$ of 12.9 µg/g, and the "urine-to-kidney Cd ratio" of 1:60. Accordingly, E_{Cd} of 0.42 µg/g creatinine corresponded to $[Cd]_k$ of 25 µg/g wet kidney weight [146]. In another study of kidney transplant donors, the means for E_{Cd}, $[Cd]_b$, and $[Cd]_k$ in women were 0.34 µg/g creatinine, 0.54 µg/L and 17.1 µg/g kidney wet weight, respectively [147]. The corresponding figures in men were 0.23 µg/g creatinine, 0.46 µg/L and 12.5 µg/g, all of which were lower than in women [147].

4.1.2. Cadmium in Erythrocytes Versus Blood Plasma (Serum)

The vast majority of $[Cd]_b$ appears to be concentrated in the cytosol of red blood cells. The chloride/bicarbonate anion exchanger ([Cl−/HCO3−], AE1, SLC4A1), is the major Cd transporter responsible for its uptake [149–151]. High- and low-affinity "iron" transport mechanisms have also been suggested to mediate Cd uptake [152]. Of interest, these transport mechanisms are also responsible for Pb and Zn uptake by erythrocytes [152–154]. Although Cd is concentrated in red blood cells, the toxicity of Cd in these cells has not been examined. One potential toxic effect is that Cd causes erythrocytes to undergo suicidal death, known as eryptosis, the mechanism by which such injured cells are removed [155,156]. Enhanced eryptosis, seen in smokers, has been linked to oxidative stress and inflammation [157].

The Cd that remains in the plasma is bound to the amino acid histidine and proteins such as MT, pre-albumin, albumin, α_2-macroglobulin, and immunoglobulins G and A [126,158,159]. A range of low molecular weight thiols, including GSH, cysteine, cysteinylglycine, homocysteine, and γ-glutamylcysteine, are also possible carriers of Cd [160–162]. The total concentrations of these low molecular weight thiols are in the low µM range (12–20 µM), while albumin thiol is more abundant (~0.6 mM). As Cd in plasma is readily exchangeable with other metals in target tissues, $[Cd]_p$ is more relevant than $[Cd]_b$ (Cd in erythrocytes) to toxic injury in those tissues. This may explain the conflicting results when different indicators of exposure were used. For instance, an association was not observed between breast cancer risk and $[Cd]_b$ [163], while $[Cd]_u$ has been consistently associated with a significant increase in risk for cancer [164].

Presently, plasma/serum Cd is rarely used in health risk assessment. The true distribution of Cd in whole blood and serum (plasma) remains to be fully characterized. The relationship between $[Cd]_b$ and plasma Cd at varying exposure levels is not known, nor is there a way to predict plasma Cd from whole blood/erythrocyte Cd data that are abundantly available. Nonetheless, the utility of the serum Cd concentration has been demonstrated in the studies linking Cd to an increased risk of respiratory disease in a representative U.S. population. Serum Cd levels ≥ 0.73 µg/L were associated with a 2.5-fold increase in the risk of obstructive lung disease among participants in NHANES 2007–2010 [165], while serum Cd levels in the highest quartile were associated with a 2.8-fold increase in the risk of recurrent wheeze and asthma in NHANES 2007–2012 participants aged 20–79 years [166].

4.2. Lead Dosimetry

4.2.1. Blood Lead Versus Bone Lead

Blood Pb ($[Pb]_b$) constitutes less than 2% of the total body content of Pb. Ninety-nine percent of blood Pb is found in the cytosol of erythrocytes, while 1% or less is present in plasma [167–170]. However, $[Pb]_b$ is still the most frequently used marker of Pb exposure in epidemiologic studies because higher quantities are detectable by common analytical instruments compared with measurements of Pb in bone and urine. $[Pb]_b$ of 5 µg/dL is recommended as an actionable level or an excessive exposure level in infants and children, while $[Pb]_b$ of 20 µg/dL is adopted as an excessive exposure level in workplace settings [71].

At any given time, $[Pb]_b$ reflects recent intake plus the contribution from bone Pb (cumulative lifetime exposure). In children, the bone contribution is more than 90%, while the bone contribution to [Pb]b in adults ranges from 45% to 55% [171–173]. An estimated half-life of $[Pb]_b$ was 10 days (9.96 ± 3.92) in a study of Chinese children with Pb toxicity, in whom both bone Pb and $[Pb]_b$ were measured [144]. This estimated half-life of $[Pb]_b$ is much shorter than the previously estimated figures that ranged from 8–11 months to 2–3 years [174]. A half-life of as long as 2 years for $[Pb]_b$ was suggested in a study of the time required for $[Pb]_b$ to fall by 50% in Pb-exposed children undergoing chelation therapy [175]. The differences in $[Pb]_b$ half-life figures are due mostly to a correction for bone contribution in a recent study [144].

Bone Pb constitutes approximately 94% and 74% of the total body burden of this metal in adults and children, respectively [144,176–178]. The half-life of bone Pb varies from 10 to 20 years [179–182]. In a study of Pb accumulation in different types of bone from Swedish copper–lead smelter workers and controls, the highest Pb concentration was found in finger bone, followed in order by vertebrae, iliac crest and sternum [183]. Among soft tissues, Pb concentration was highest in the liver, followed by kidney, lung and brain [184]. Consistent with this study, an Australian study reported that liver contained Pb levels two times higher than kidney cortex: the mean hepatic and kidney cortex Pb levels were 0.19 and 0.09 µg/g wet tissue weight, respectively [137]. Bone Pb levels correlated with serum Pb levels in adults who were exposed to Pb in the workplace [185].

In environmental exposure scenarios, Pb in tibia showed stronger and more consistent associations with neurotoxicity than blood Pb. This supports bone Pb to be a better biomarker of cumulative dosimetry or the body burden than blood Pb [186–188]. In addition to the tibia, Pb in the patella was associated with declines in cognitive test scores in older persons [189]. In a prospective cohort study of men, chronic, low-level Pb exposure, assessed with bone Pb, has been linked to hypertension [190] and incident coronary heart disease [14]. The Western dietary patterns have also been linked to elevated bone and blood Pb levels in men [13,14].

4.2.2. Plasma (Serum) Lead Versus Urinary Lead

For the same reason as plasma Cd (see Section 4.1.2), $[Pb]_p$ is more relevant than $[Pb]_b$ to toxicity in tissues/organs. The superiority of plasma Pb has been demonstrated in an early study of Pb-exposed Japanese workers, in which the strength of correlations between $[Pb]_p$ and urinary indicators of adverse effect (the inhibition of heme biosynthesis), namely, urinary coproporphyrin and urinary delta-aminolevulinic acid (ALA), was stronger than the correlations of $[Pb]_b$ with these indicators [191]. Although only 1% of whole-blood Pb is in the plasma fraction, this percentage increases sharply in high-exposure conditions, a phenomenon that suggests the binding capacity of the erythrocytes has been exceeded. A linear relationship between $[Pb]_p$ and $[Pb]_b$ has been demonstrated using data from Pb-exposed workers [182,192]. Likewise, a linear relationship between $[Pb]_p$ and $[Pb]_b$ was observed in a study of U.S. women of child-bearing age [183].

Notably, however, the measurement of $[Pb]_p$ can be problematic because hemolysis causes a spurious increase in $[Pb]_p$. $[Pb]_u$ correlated more closely with $[Pb]_p$ than $[Pb]_b$ in a study of Pb-exposed workers in Japan [191]. $[Pb]_u$ may, thus, be used as a proxy for $[Pb]_p$. The utility of urine in monitoring Pb exposure has been illustrated in studies in Japan [193], Belgium [194], China [195], Thailand [12] and the U.S. [196]. In a Chinese study, workers in a lead–zinc mine had higher $[Pb]_u$, $[Cd]_u$ and urinary 8-hydroxydeoxyguanosine, an indicator of oxidative stress, compared with those who worked in a steel smelting plant [195].

In a Thai study, the 75th percentile level of $[Pb]_u$ was associated with a 2.3-fold increase in the risk of reduced eGFR [12]. This finding is reminiscent of studies relating E_{Cd} to eGFR (Section 4.3.2). In a follow-up study of 5316 participants in NHANES 1999–2010, $[Pb]_u$ levels > 1.26 µg/L were associated, respectively, with 1.79- and 6.60-fold increases in mortality from all causes and cancer [196].

4.3. *Assessment of Cadmium Nephrotoxicity*

As Figure 1 indicates, Cd enters the body from contaminated food, tobacco smoke, and polluted air. It is transported through the gut and lungs to the bloodstream, where it is bound primarily to albumin and taken up by red blood cells ([126], see Section 3.4). Most circulating Cd is eventually transferred to hepatocytes, which then synthesize the protein MT and store Cd in complexes of CdMT. As hepatocytes die, these complexes are released to the circulation, filtered by glomeruli, and reabsorbed primarily or entirely by proximal tubular cells [197,198]. After lysosomes within these cells degrade the complexes, Cd enters the cytoplasm, where it again induces the synthesis of MT, to which it is subsequently bound. Cd that remains free is believed to induce the release of copper (Cu), a transition metal, from MT; Cu then promotes the formation of reactive oxygen species, which inflict cellular injury [31,199]. The intensity of this injury is thought to be related to the concentration of free Cd in the cytoplasm [200,201]. As no mechanism exists for discharging Cd from intact tubular cells, the metal continues to accumulate in those cells as long as hepatocytes release CdMT to the bloodstream [202,203].

Commonly studied clinical expressions of tubular Cd toxicity include leakage of intracellular proteins into the filtrate, excretion of Cd itself, the estimated glomerular filtration rate (eGFR), and impaired reabsorption of small filtered proteins. Extreme toxicity also compromises reabsorption of filtered substances that are cotransported with sodium, including glucose, phosphate, urate, and amino acids. The resulting constellation of abnormalities, the so-called Fanconi syndrome, was once common in heavily contaminated regions of Japan [82]. As this syndrome is now a rare manifestation of Cd tubulopathy, it is not considered in this review.

4.3.1. Release of Intracellular Proteins into the Filtrate

After cellular injury, proteins synthesized in tubular cells may be released into the filtrate and detected in urine. In studies of Cd nephropathy, N-acetyl-β-D-glucosaminidase (NAG) and kidney injury molecule 1 (KIM1) have been assayed most frequently.

N-Acetyl-β-D-Glucosaminidase

NAG is present in lysosomes of proximal tubular cells. Mean normal rates of NAG excretion rise slightly with age [204]. The molecular weight of NAG, 150 kD, precludes glomerular filtration and, therefore, ensures that excreted NAG has emanated from tubules. The enzyme exists in two major isoforms, A and B. NAG-A is released by exocytosis into the filtrate at a stable rate that is unrelated to the cellular Cd content. NAG-B remains in lysosomes and enters the filtrate after cellular injury [204,205]. Its excretion is increased by Cd toxicity [205–207]. Reported measurements of NAG excretion have contributed significantly to our current synthesis of Cd nephropathy (see Section 4.3.2, Section 4.3.3, and Section 4.3.6).

Kidney Injury Molecule 1

KIM1 is a transmembrane glycoprotein that participates in the restoration of adhesion between regenerated proximal tubular cells. During this process, the ectodomain of KIM1 is released into the filtrate and excreted in urine. The protein is not detectable in the absence of injury [208].

KIM1 has been studied extensively in animals as a biomarker of Cd toxicity [209–211]. In rats treated with exogenous Cd, genetic expression and urinary excretion of KIM1 (E_{KIM1}) increased at 6 weeks; E_{Cd} and E_{NAG} rose 3 and 6 weeks later [209,210]. Apoptosis was sparsely evident at 6 weeks and more prevalent at 12 weeks; increased KIM1 excretion accompanied apoptosis but was also observed in the absence of apoptosis [211]. If rodent studies can be extrapolated to humans, E_{KIM1} identifies toxicity that has not yet led to cell death, and it is detectable before E_{Cd} rises. It appears to be the earliest appearing indicator of Cd tubulopathy.

At least four studies have examined the utility of E_{KIM1} in humans exposed to Cd. Pennemans and colleagues investigated a Belgian sample with chronic low-dose environmental exposure [212]. The geometric mean of Cd excretion in this group was 0.76 μg/g creatinine, which is approximately twice that reported in healthy populations and 15% of the conventional Cd threshold for tubular injury (5.24 μg/g creatinine) [41]. Pennemans and colleagues found that E_{KIM1} correlated with E_{Cd} even though the excretion of reabsorptive markers did not. A Thai group confirmed this correlation in a sample with higher E_{Cd} [213], but a Chinese report did not [214]. A second study from China showed that E_{KIM1} rose in a stepwise fashion with low-, middle-, and high-dose environmental exposure to Cd [58].

4.3.2. Excretion of Cadmium

Excreted Cd is either filtered and not reabsorbed or released from tubular cells into the filtrate [215]. Several lines of evidence support the second alternative. After inducing Cd nephropathy in rabbits, Nomiyama and Foulkes infused labelled CdMT at increasing rates to create a series of steady-state plasma concentrations of the complex. Although Cd poisoning had reduced the tubular maximum for CdMT, the excretion rates of total Cd greatly exceeded those accounted for by failure to reabsorb the label [216]. Most of the excreted Cd, therefore, emanated from the tubular cells.

In kidneys from rats intoxicated with Cd, Tanimoto and colleagues showed that E_{Cd} and numbers of apoptotic, sloughed cells in tubules rose in tandem [217]. In workers with occupational exposure to Cd, E_{Cd} correlated with the renal cortical content of the metal, as measured by neutron-capture gamma-ray analysis [218]. In human accident victims, the Cd content of renal tissue at autopsy correlated with the urine Cd concentration ([136]; Figure 2; see Section 4.1.1). In transplanted kidneys, the tissue Cd content correlated with the preoperative overnight E_{Cd} of living donors [140]. Three groups of investigators found that E_{Cd} varied directly with GFR, as though the number of intact nephrons had determined the rate of appearance in urine [219–221].

Reported correlations of E_{Cd} with E_{NAG} or E_{KIM1} provide additional evidence that urinary Cd emanates from tubular cells [205,212,214,222–226]. Importantly, these studies did not suggest that markers of cell injury began to rise at a threshold level of E_{Cd}; instead, the correlations extended in a linear fashion from normal to increased levels of E_{Cd} [205,222,225,226]. E_{KIM1}, the most sensitive indicator of Cd-induced toxicity, rose before E_{Cd} in animal studies [209,210].

Taken together, the foregoing observations suggest that Cd excretion does not result from a failure to reabsorb filtered Cd. It is more likely that Cd, NAG, and KIM1 emanate from the same source for the same reason. We infer that E_{Cd} is itself a marker of tubular cell injury.

4.3.3. Cadmium Toxicity and the Glomerular Filtration Rate (GFR)

A paradox emerges from the literature relating E_{Cd} to GFR. Three groups have reported that E_{Cd} rose with GFR in exposed populations [219–221], and three have stated that C_{cr} or eGFR declined steadily as E_{Cd} increased from modest levels [51,52,227–229]. To reconcile these observations, we speculate that in the progression of Cd nephropathy, cellular injury is evident before nephrons are lost; during that phase, E_{Cd} varies directly with the nephron number, which, in turn, varies directly with GFR. Cell death ensues as the burden of Cd rises; during this phase, Cd is released to filtrate at an increased rate even though nephrons are disappearing simultaneously. Estimated GFR falls as E_{Cd} continues to rise.

In Thai population samples, our group found inverse relationships between eGFR and E_{Cd} at all levels of environmental Cd exposure [52,54]. Moreover, investigators from multiple geographic regions documented a progressive decline in GFR despite mitigation or termination of occupational exposure [229–232]. This decline may have resulted from the continued transfer of CdMT from the liver to the kidneys [233], or it may have reflected continuous nephron destruction by a stable renal burden of the metal [234,235].

4.3.4. Impaired Reabsorption of Small Filterable Proteins

Small proteins are readily filtered by normal glomeruli and reabsorbed and degraded by proximal tubular cells. As reabsorption of such proteins is virtually complete, excretion rates above a cutoff value may be viewed as evidence of impaired reabsorptive capacity. The proteins most commonly studied for this purpose are β_2-microglobulin (β_2MG) and retinol-binding protein 4 (RBP4).

β2-Microglobulin

β_2MG is the light chain of class I major histocompatibility complexes and is, therefore, found on most nucleated cells. Its molecular weight is 11,000 Daltons. The rate at which β_2MG enters plasma ("influx") is relatively constant within and among healthy subjects, but it may rise in patients with chronic inflammatory conditions or hematologic malignancies [236].

β_2MG is eliminated exclusively by the kidneys. A modest fraction of the amount removed is taken up from peritubular capillaries [237], but most elimination results from glomerular filtration, proximal tubular reabsorption, and intracellular degradation. At least 90% of the circulating protein is ultrafilterable [238,239], and 99.9% of the filtered load is ordinarily reabsorbed. When the GFR is normal, the equilibrium between influx and renal processing establishes a plasma concentration ($[\beta_2MG]_p$) between 1.2 and 2.7 mg/L [236]. As GFR falls, the filtrate is presented to proximal tubules at a rate that is absolutely reduced but normal or increased per surviving nephron. $[\beta_2MG]_p$ rises secondarily, and equilibrium between the influx and the degradation of the protein is maintained [240–244].

In Cd research, it has been customary to declare that proximal tubular toxicity is present at $E_{\beta 2MG}$ > 300 μg/g creatinine [41]. At an arbitrary $E_{\beta 2MG}$ of 300 μg/d, E_{cr} of 1 g/d, GFR of 144 L/d (100 mL/min), and filterable $[\beta_2MG]_p$ of 2.0 mg/L, fractional excretion of β_2MG ($FE_{\beta 2MG}$) is 0.1% and fractional reabsorption ($FR_{\beta 2MG}$) is 99.9%. Doubling of $E_{\beta 2MG}$ to 600 μg/g creatinine, a clearly elevated value, entails an increase in $FE_{\beta 2MG}$ from 0.1% to 0.2% and a reduction in $FR_{\beta 2MG}$ to 99.8%. Miniscule Cd-induced reductions in $FR_{\beta 2MG}$, therefore, lead to substantial increments in $E_{\beta 2MG}$ [245].

The sensitivity of $E_{\beta 2MG}$ to slight reductions of $FR_{\beta 2MG}$ should not be interpreted as evidence that the underlying cellular injury is trivial. Values of E_{Cd} at which $E_{\beta 2MG}$ exceeds 300μg/g creatinine are at least 10 times higher than in normal populations [246,247]. If E_{Cd} itself is a marker of toxicity, then the customary cutoff value of $E_{\beta 2MG}$ is not a sensitive metric for detecting tubular injury. For pathophysiologic insight, $E_{\beta 2MG}$ is most logically related to the normal *maximal* reabsorptive capacity for the protein—i.e., the tubular maximum ($Tm_{\beta 2MG}$)—if such a Tm exists. Hall could not demonstrate one in dogs with an infusion of human β_2MG [237], but in rats, Gauthier documented a $Tm_{\beta 2MG}$ when $[\beta_2MG]_p$ was approximately four times the norm [238].

In theory, if a $Tm_{\beta 2MG}$ existed in humans, a decline in GFR might expose it. In this circumstance, surviving nephrons would be presented with a higher concentration of β_2MG in less total filtrate volume, and a normal rate of presentation to a reduced nephron mass could exceed a putative $Tm_{\beta 2MG}$. Multiple investigators have argued that this scenario occurs, but it is often possible that the disease lowering GFR has also lowered $Tm_{\beta 2MG}$ [241,244]. In patients with hepatorenal syndrome, in which the perfusion of normal kidneys is severely limited, a $Tm_{\beta 2MG}$ was not demonstrable despite extreme reductions in GFR and elevations in $[\beta_2MG]_p$ [243]. Similarly, in children with glomerular disease exclusively, on biopsy, $FE_{\beta 2MG}$ did not correlate with GFR [244].

If some humans can reabsorb all filtered β_2MG despite a low GFR and high $[\beta_2MG]_p$, then nephron loss is insufficient to explain excessive $E_{\beta 2MG}$ in patients with Cd nephropathy. It appears that Cd imposes a $Tm_{\beta 2MG}$ or reduces one that already exists, and increased $E_{\beta 2MG}$ indicates reduced β_2MG reabsorption per nephron at any GFR [248]. Once Cd has established a $Tm_{\beta 2MG}$, we expect $E_{\beta 2MG}$ to rise substantially as GFR falls. Multiple investigators have documented this phenomenon [53,232,249], but none have quantified the individual contributions of GFR and $Tm_{\beta 2MG}$ to excessive $E_{\beta 2MG}$.

Retinol-Binding Protein 4

RBP4, a small protein with molecular weight 21,000 Daltons, is synthesized in the liver. As its name implies, it binds to retinol (vitamin A) and transports the vitamin to tissues. Most RBP4 in plasma is bound to transthyretin (pre-albumin) in a complex that is too large to be filtered by normal glomeruli, but a minor fraction is unbound and readily filtered [239,250]. The total plasma concentration of RBP4 ($[RBP]_p$) is normally 40–60 μg/mL [251].

As is the case with β_2MG, over 99.9% of filtered RBP is normally reabsorbed. Urinary excretion (E_{RBP}) increases markedly in tubulointerstitial disease, and it also rises substantially as GFR falls [233,252]. We are unable to ascertain whether nephron loss per se raises free $[RBP]_p$ to a threshold at which the reabsorptive capacity of surviving nephrons is exceeded. Bernard and colleagues reported a threshold $[RBP]_p$ of 25 mg/L at which $[RBP]_u$ rose acutely, but all of the patients with CKD had tubulopathies [253]. Mason and colleagues described a similar finding at high rates of Cd excretion, but we presume that their subjects had sustained Cd-induced tubular injury [233].

RBP4 differs in some respects from β_2MG. β_2MG is a positive acute-phase reactant (APR), and its plasma concentration rises in association with inflammation. RBP4 is a negative APR, and its concentration falls with inflammation [250]. Whereas β_2MG is unstable at $pH < 5.5$, RBP4 is stable at any physiologic urine pH. Because of this attribute, some have argued that RBP4 should be the reabsorptive marker of choice in studies of Cd tubulopathy [253].

4.3.5. Normalization of Excretion Rates to Creatinine Excretion or Creatinine Clearance

The kidney is the final repository of assimilated Cd and the principal site of persistent toxicity [254]. To study that toxicity, it is reasonable to quantify excretion rates of relevant substances (abbreviated E_x for a given substance x). In practice, however, urine aliquots are more conveniently obtained than timed collections, and concentrations of x ($[x]_u$) are measured instead of E_x. To nullify the effect of urine volume on these concentrations, $[x]_u$ is usually normalized to the urine creatinine concentration ($[cr]_u$) because volume affects $[x]_u$ and $[cr]_u$ proportionately.

This practice may lead to erroneous conclusions. As E_x and E_{cr} are biologically unrelated, each excretion rate is influenced by at least one variable that does not affect the other. E_{cr} is determined primarily by muscle mass [255], which has no relationship to E_x; consequently, in a physically diverse population, normalization of a given $[x]_u$ to $[cr]_u$ alters $[x]_u/[cr]_u$—in theory, by as much as fourfold—for a reason unrelated to E_x [256]. Conversely, if substance x emanates from tubular cells, E_x varies directly with the number of cells and the intracellular concentration of x, neither of which is related to E_{cr}. If nephron mass is normal, E_x may rise as a consequence of cellular injury; if Cd destroys nephrons, E_x may fall. As E_{cr} does not change importantly in either circumstance, $[x]_u/[cr]_u$ may overstate tubular injury per nephron when GFR is normal and understate it when GFR is reduced [221,229].

To circumvent these issues, we recently introduced the practice of normalizing E_x to creatinine clearance (C_{cr}), a surrogate for GFR, in studies of Cd nephrotoxicity [52,54]. C_{cr} is the excretion rate divided by the plasma concentration of creatinine; if V_u is the urine flow rate, $C_{cr} = [cr]_u V_u/[cr]_p$ and $E_x/C_{cr} = [x]_u V_u/([cr]_u V_u/[cr]_p)$, which simplifies to $[x]_u[cr]_p/[cr]_u$. Whereas the unit of $[x]_u/[cr]_u$ is mass of x per mass of creatinine, the unit of E_x/C_{cr} is mass of x excreted *per volume of filtrate*. Since C_{cr} varies directly with the number of nephrons, E_x/C_{cr} also depicts excretion of x per intact nephron. As the formula for E_x/C_{cr} includes the ratio $[x]_u/[cr]_u$, E_x/C_{cr}, like $[x]_u/[cr]_u$, is unaffected by urine volume; since $[cr]_p$ rises with E_{cr} at a given C_{cr}, E_x/C_{cr} is also unaffected by muscle mass. Most importantly, if substance x is released by tubular cells into urine, E_x/C_{cr} prevents overstatement of injury per nephron at normal GFR and understatement at reduced GFR.

4.3.6. A Pathophysiologic Synopsis of Cadmium Nephropathy

We recently published an analysis of cross-sectional data from Thai subjects living in areas of low, moderate, and high intensity of environmental Cd exposure. The patients were clinically well and were not hemodynamically predisposed to reductions in GFR [54]. In each subset and in the entire sample, we examined linear and quadratic regressions of eGFR on E_{Cd}/C_{cr} and E_{NAG}/C_{cr}, regressions of E_{NAG}/C_{cr} on E_{Cd}/C_{cr}, and regressions of $E_{\beta 2MG}$ on E_{Cd}/C_{cr} and E_{NAG}/C_{cr}. All regressions were statistically significant except those of $E_{\beta 2MG}/C_{cr}$ on E_{Cd}/C_{cr} and E_{NAG}/C_{cr} in the low-exposure subset. In general, effect size (standardized β) and coefficients of determination (R^2) rose with exposure intensity. A minority of subjects was found to have eGFR < 60 mL/min/1.73 m^2; in the absence of renal hypoperfusion, which would have been accompanied by disqualifying signs and symptoms, the only plausible explanation for subnormal glomerular filtration was a reduction in the number of intact nephrons. "Nephron loss" is a widely used term to describe this state [257].

Our goals in the analysis of these data were to explain the correlation of E_{Cd}/C_{cr} with E_{NAG}/C_{cr}, identify the source of excreted Cd, and elucidate the inverse relationship of eGFR to E_{Cd}/C_{cr} and E_{NAG}/C_{cr}. Although we recognized that tubular injury might interfere with reabsorption of filtered CdMT, we doubted that *this interference* would lead to a statistically significant relationship of E_{NAG}/C_{cr} to E_{Cd}/C_{cr}. As multiple lines of evidence suggested that excreted Cd, like NAG, emanates from proximal tubular cells (see Section 4.3.2), we reasoned that a common origin of the two substances would account for the relationship between E_{NAG} and E_{Cd}.

Whereas we consider both E_{Cd}/C_{cr} and E_{NAG}/C_{cr} to be parameters of cellular injury at the time of testing, eGFR reflects progressive nephron loss due to continuous accrual of Cd in proximal tubules. To explain why eGFR varied inversely with E_{Cd}/C_{cr} and E_{NAG}/C_{cr} despite these temporal differences, we argued that all three parameters were either current or historical functions of the same intracellular Cd content. We concluded that Cd-induced injury had led to tubular cell death and a reduction of GFR. Relationships of eGFR to E_{Cd}/C_{cr} and E_{NAG}/C_{cr} suggested that the severity of cellular injury had determined the extent of nephron loss.

In the literature on Cd toxicity, we occasionally encounter the concept that a reduction of GFR implies injury to glomeruli by the metal. Ample evidence suggests that this concept is both erroneous and unnecessary. CKD is a common sequela of ischemic acute tubular necrosis and numerous acute and chronic tubulointerstitial (TI) diseases that do not affect glomeruli [257–262]. Moreover, primary glomerular disease also leads to TI inflammation and fibrosis, presumably because reabsorbed, inappropriately filtered proteins are toxic to tubular cells [263]. Whether glomeruli or tubules are injured initially, the extent of TI fibrosis is the histologic finding that correlates best with GFR in CKD [264,265]. Possible filtration-reducing effects of TI fibrosis include the destruction of post-glomerular peritubular capillaries, amputation of glomeruli from tubules, and obstruction of nephrons with cellular debris [257,266].

We have not found English-language reports relating histopathology to GFR in asymptomatic humans exposed to Cd. However, in 61 autopsied subjects with itai-itai disease (IID), a syndrome of painful osteomalacia and proximal tubular dysfunction associated with severe Cd toxicity, Baba and colleagues showed that the most extreme osteomalacia was associated with the most advanced renal shrinkage [267]. In autopsies of 15 patients with IID, Yasuda and colleagues found that low kidney weight correlated with loss of tubules on microscopy; severely afflicted kidneys showed interstitial fibrosis and widespread atrophy of tubular epithelium [268]. Although reduced kidney weight and disrupted cortical architecture suggest that GFRs were reduced in these studies, neither Baba nor Yasuda provided relevant quantitative information. In contrast, Saito and colleagues performed extensive renal function studies (but no histopathology) in 13 patients with IID; endogenous creatinine clearance, a surrogate for GFR, was reduced in 12 [269]. Nogawa and associates measured serum creatinine concentrations in 4 of 5 patients with severe skeletal manifestations of IID, and the concentrations were substantially increased in each case [270]. Yasuda mentions that numerous Japanese patients with IID required chronic dialysis [268]; this choice of treatment suggests that extreme Cd toxicity reduced the GFR to levels that could not sustain life.

4.3.7. Assessment of Cadmium Nephrotoxicity: Summary

Cd is a cumulative toxin to proximal tubular cells. Ample evidence suggests that the metal inflicts injury by promoting the creation of reactive oxygen species. The injury commences at a low intracellular concentration of Cd and intensifies as the concentration rises. Excretion of KIM1 is the first identifiable manifestation of toxicity, and NAG and Cd are subsequently released from injured or apoptotic cells. Inflammation and fibrosis follow, nephrons are lost, and GFR falls. After significant proximal tubular injury has occurred, reabsorption of small filtered proteins decreases and excretion of these proteins exceeds the normal limit. Once a $Tm_{\beta 2MG}$ is established, $E_{\beta 2MG}$ rises rapidly as GFR falls.

E_{NAG} and E_{KIM1} correlate with E_{Cd}. This observation and many others suggest that Cd excretion results from the cellular release of the metal rather than filtration without reabsorption. If this conclusion is accepted, then increased E_{Cd} is itself a manifestation of Cd toxicity, and the concept of a threshold E_{Cd} at which $E_{\beta 2MG}$ becomes excessive loses its pathophysiologic relevance. In subjects with low environmental exposure to Cd, eGFR is statistically related to E_{Cd}/C_{cr} when $E_{\beta 2MG}/C_{cr}$ is not, and the relationship grows stronger as exposure increases. Markers of cellular injury at the time of testing, e.g., E_{NAG}/C_{cr} and E_{Cd}/C_{cr}, correlate with eGFR, an indicator of historical injury, because all three parameters are determined by the intracellular concentration of Cd. Tubular injury inflicted by Cd is sufficient to explain reductions in GFR and progression of CKD.

5. Environmental Exposure to Cd and Pb, Toxic Kidney Burden, CKD, and Other Common Ailments

Environmental exposures are estimated to account for 70–90% of the risk of acquiring chronic ailments such as diabetes type 2, CKD and cancer [271,272]. The kidney is particularly at risk of injury from long-term use of therapeutic drugs and chronic exposure to environmental toxicants, especially when they are present in the diet [273–275]. The increased risk of kidney injury is attributed to its large blood flow (20–25% of cardiac output) and exposure to high solute concentrations as the primary glomerular filtrate is concentrated [276]. In the following sections, we discuss cross-sectional studies that suggest that Cd and Pb are synergistic CKD risk factors and longitudinal studies that implicate combined Cd and Pb exposure in enhanced mortality risk.

5.1. The Increased Risk of CKD Associated with Cadmium and Lead Exposure

CKD afflicts 8% to 16% of the world population. Diabetes and hypertension are the most common risk factors universally, while obesity is an additional risk factor, especially in industrialized countries [272–279]. CKD is a cause of morbidity and mortality as it is an important predictor of end-stage kidney disease (ESKD), stroke and cardiovascular disease (CVD) [280–285]. CKD is characterized by albuminuria (a urinary albumin to creatinine ratio, uACR, above 30 μg/g) and/or a decrease of GFR to ≤60 mL/min/1.73 m^2 that persists for at least three months [48–50].

GFR is considered the best indicator of overall kidney function because it reflects the number of functioning nephrons at any given time [50]. In practice, the GFR is estimated from equations, notably, the Chronic Kidney Disease Epidemiology Collaboration (CKD-EPI) equations [47–49], and is reported as eGFR. The CKD-EPI equations, which have been validated using inulin clearance, are considered as the most accurate approximation of GFR [286]. CKD in its early stage is asymptomatic, and CKD staging is vital to evaluate nephron loss. Accordingly, CKD stages 1, 2, 3a, 3b, 4, and 5 correspond to eGFR of 90–119, 60–89, 45–59, 30–44, 15–29, and <15 mL/min/1.73 m^2, respectively [48,287]. For simplicity, a low eGFR refers to an eGFR of <60 mL/min/1.73 m^2, and albuminuria refers to uACRs above 30 μg/g.

5.1.1. U.S. Population

An increment of $[Pb]_b$ to 10 μg/dL was associated with a decrease in creatinine clearance of 10.4 mL/min in an early study of U.S. men participating in the Normative Aging Study between 1988 and 1991 [288]. Subsequently, an increased risk of CKD was associated with Pb and Cd exposures in participants of various NHANES cycles. In NHANES 1999–2006, adults with $[Cd]_u$ levels ≥ 1 μg/L had 1.48- and 1.41-fold increases in the risk of low eGFR and albuminuria [44], while those with $[Cd]_b$ ≥0.6 μg/L had 1.53-, 1.92-, and 2.91-fold increases in the risk of low eGFR, albuminuria and low eGFR plus albuminuria, respectively [289]. In addition, $[Pb]_b$ ≥ 2.4 μg/dL, which is 12% of the exposure limit in occupational exposure settings of 20 μg/dL, was associated with a 1.56-fold increase in the risk of low eGFR [289]. Of interest, the risk of CKD was increased further when subjects were exposed to both metals: the odds ratios for low eGFR, albuminuria, low eGFR plus albuminuria rose to 1.98, 2.34, and 4.10 in participants who had both $[Cd]_b$ and $[Pb]_b$ in the highest quartiles, compared with those who had $[Cd]_b$ and $[Pb]_b$ in the lowest quartiles [289]. Likewise, in adults enrolled in NHANES 2007–2012, $[Cd]_b$ > 0.61 μg/L was associated, respectively, with 1.80- and 1.60-fold higher risk of having low eGFR and albuminuria, compared with $[Cd]_b$ ≤ 0.11 μg/L [45]. A pronounced effect of Cd on eGFR was seen in women who had diabetes and/or hypertension. On average, women with diabetes, hypertension and $[Cd]_b$ in the highest quartile (0.61−9.3 μg/L) had 4.9 mL/min/1.73 m^2 lower eGFR than nondiabetic, normotensive women who had the lowest $[Cd]_b$ (0.11−0.21 μg/L) [46]. In those women with hypertension and the highest $[Cd]_b$ quartile, the mean eGFR was 5.77 mL/min/1.73 m^2 lower than the normotensive with the same lowest $[Cd]_b$ quartile [46].

In another analysis of data from adult participants in NHANES 2011–2012, $[Cd]_b$ > 0.53 μg/L was associated with 2.21- and 2.04-fold increases in the risk of low eGFR and albuminuria, respectively. $[Cd]_u$ as low as 0.22 μg/L was associated with higher urinary albumin excretion, compared with $[Cd]_u$ < 0.126 μg/L, but neither Pb nor Hg was associated with elevated albumin excretion [290].

5.1.2. Swedish Population

In a study of Swedish women, 53–64 years of age, $[Cd]_u$ ≥ 0.6 μg/g creatinine was associated with a significant increase in tubular injury and decrease in eGFR [227]. In a longitudinal study (n = 4341), $[Pb]_b$ ≥ 3.3 μg/dL was associated with a 1.49-fold increase in the incidence of CKD, and the mean eGFR of subjects with this range of $[Pb]_b$ fell by 24 mL/min/1.73 m^2 during a 16-year follow-up period [291]. In a prospective, nested case–control study, 118 cohort participants developed ESKD during a 7-year period [292]. The mean values for erythrocyte Cd and Pb of these cases were 1.3 and 7.6 μg/dL, respectively. After adjusting for potential confounders, including Cd and Hg, smoking, body mass index, diabetes, and hypertension, only erythrocyte Pb was associated with an increase in the risk of developing ESKD [292].

5.1.3. Thai Population

Even though the environmental exposure of the general population in Thailand to Cd and Pb is low [293], a Bangkok study has shown that even a urinary Cd excretion rate (E_{Cd}) as low as 0.38 μg/L (0.44 μg/g creatinine) was associated with a decrease in eGFR [12]. The risk of a decrease in eGFR was 2.9-fold higher in those who had E_{Cd} in the highest quartile. Likewise, in those with $[Pb]_u$ in the highest quartile, the risk of eGFR decrease was 2.3-fold higher than those in the lowest quartile of $[Pb]_u$ [12]. Of note, a positive association between eGFR levels and serum ferritin in men suggested a protective effect of adequate body iron status. Women may be more predisposed to absorption of ingested Cd and Pb because of their lower levels of body iron stores [12].

In a Cd-polluted region of Thailand, more than half (66%) of the residents had elevated Cd body burdens, reflected by $E_{Cd} \geq 2$ μg/g creatinine, and the prevalence of CKD was 16.1% [294]. In a 5-year follow up study, a further decrease in eGFR was observed in residents who had high Cd exposure ($E_{Cd} \geq 5$ μg/g creatinine) [229]. These findings suggest that nephron loss associated with high Cd exposure and increasing kidney dysfunction continues even when the consumption of Cd-contaminated rice is reduced [229]. Other studies have reported an even greater effect of Cd on eGFR in women who had hypertension [51,52], as has been noted in the U.S. population study [46].

5.1.4. Chinese Population

In a Chinese population study (n = 8429), intake levels of dietary Cd were inversely associated with eGFR, and the risk of CKD rose with Cd intake levels in a dose-dependent manner: Cd intake levels of 23.2, 29.6 and 36.9 μg/day were associated with 1.73-, 2.93- and 4.05-fold increments of CKD risk, compared with a Cd intake level of 16.7 μg/day [15]. $[Pb]_b$ of 10 μg/dL was associated with tubular injury in Chinese men who were exposed to Pb in the workplace [295]. In a coexposure analysis of residents in Cd-polluted and control areas in China [296], the risk of tubular injury, as assessed with $[NAG]_u$, was highest in subjects who had $[Cd]_b \geq 2$ μg/L and $[Pb]_b \geq 10$ μg/dL, while the risk of a decrease in eGFR was highest in those with $E_{Cd} \geq 3$ μg/g creatinine and $E_{Pb} \geq 10$ μg/g creatinine.

5.1.5. Korean and Belgian Populations

The prevalence of CKD in a representative Korean population (n = 1797) was 7.1% and the population means for $[Pb]_b$, $[Hg]_b$ and $[Cd]_b$ were 2.37, 4.35 and 1.17 μg/L, respectively [297]. Elevated $[Cd]_b$ levels were associated with 1.52- and 1.92-fold increases in the risk of CKD in those with diabetes and hypertension, respectively. Neither $[Pb]_b$ nor $[Hg]_b$ showed such a relationship [297]. Supporting Cd as a risk factor for CKD is another study of 2992 Koreans, 20–65 years of age; $[Cd]_b > 1.74$ μg/L was associated with a 1.97-fold increase in odds for CKD in women [298]. In a study of a subset of participants (n = 2005, aged ≥20 years) in a nationwide survey (n = 8641), Cd exposure was again found to be an important risk factor for CKD in Korea: $[Cd]_b$ levels in the highest quartile (mean, 2.08 μg/L) were associated with a 1.93-fold increase in the risk of CKD [283]. In contrast, $[Pb]_b$ levels in the highest quartile (mean, 4.13 μg/dl) were not associated with a significant increase in CKD risk in this subset analysis [299].

Intriguingly, although Pb exposure levels in Korea did not seem to affect CKD risk, evidence that Pb coexposure may enhance Cd toxicity in kidneys has emerged from another Korean population study (n = 1953, aged 18–83 years) in which $[Pb]_b$ and $[Cd]_u$ both correlated positively with $[\beta_2MG]_u$, a marker of tubular dysfunction [300]. However, the correlation between $[Cd]_b$ and $[\beta_2MG]_u$ was strengthened in those who had $[Pb]_b$ above the median of 2.20 μg/dL. Similar to Korean findings, a study of Belgian metallurgic refinery workers suggested that there is a Cd–Pb interaction [301]. The associations between $[Cd]_u$, $[NAG]_u$ and $[RBP]_u$ were only seen in workers who had high levels of $[Pb]_b$ (≥21.9 μg/dL), corresponding to the 75th percentile or higher. In addition, the associations between $[Cd]_b$, $[NAG]_u$ and [intestinal alkaline phosphatase]$_u$ only became statistically significant in workers who had $[Pb]_b \geq 21.9$ μg/dL [285]. This Cd–Pb interaction was seen although blood Pb in Belgian workers of 21.9 μg/dL was 6-fold higher than the 90th percentile blood Pb level of 3.66 μg/dL in a Korean study [300]. Of note, $[Pb]_b$ of ~20 μg/dL did not exceed the exposure limit for neurotoxicity in adults of 25 μg/dL [71]. Further epidemiologic research is required to examine the mechanisms underlying the interaction of Cd and Pb in chronic Cd and Pb exposure conditions.

5.2. Environmental Exposures and Mortality from All Causes

In the previous section, exposures to Cd and Pb have been identified as risk factors for CKD across populations. In this section, we summarize the observations across populations that demonstrated the overall impact of chronic lifelong exposure to Cd and Pb on life prognosis and risks of death from CVD and cancer.

5.2.1. Cadmium and Mortality in the U.S.

Temporal trend analysis indicated a 29% reduction in environmental Cd exposure among a representative cohort of men in the U.S. over an 18-year follow-up period (1988–2006) during which the mean E_{Cd} fell from 0.58 to 0.41 μg/g creatinine [302]. A reduction in environmental Cd exposure in women over the same 18-year period was statistically insignificant.

Cd exposure was associated with heart disease in cross-sectional studies [303–305]. Cd exposure was also an independent risk factor for ischemic stroke in another cross-sectional study ($n = 2540$), with a mean and a 75th percentile E_{Cd} of 0.42 and 0.68 μg/g creatinine, respectively [306]. These associations may account for the increased mortality from CVD seen in various follow-up studies of NHANES participants. In a follow-up study of participants in NHANES 1988–2006, $[Cd]_b$ was linked to an increase in death from CVD, especially in women [302]. E_{Cd} of ≥0.37 to ≥0.65 μg/g creatinine was linked to increased risk of death from heart disease among participants in NHANES 1999–2008 [307,308].

A 4.29-fold increase in death from malignant disease was seen among participants from NHANES (1988–1994) who had $E_{Cd} > 0.48$ μg/g creatinine [309]. In men only, a 2-fold increase in E_{Cd} was respectively associated with 28%, 55%, 21%, and 36% increases in death from all causes, cancer, CVD, and coronary heart disease, after adjustment for potential confounders, including cigarette smoking [309]. E_{Cd} of ≥0.37 to ≥0.65 μg/g creatinine was linked to increased risk of breast cancer among women participating in NHANES 1999–2008 [307,308].

In other follow-up studies of NHANES 1988–1994 participants, a two-fold increase in E_{Cd} was associated with 26% and 21% increases in cancer mortality in men and women, respectively [310]. The mortality from lung cancer in men was increased by 3.22-fold, while the mortality from liver-related nonmalignant disease was increased by 3.42-fold in participants who had E_{Cd} of ≥0.58 to ≥0.65 μg/g creatinine [310,311].

Among the ≥65 years of age participants of NHANES 1999–2004, $[Cd]_b$ levels > 0.6 μg/L were associated with a 3.83-fold increase in the risk of the mortality from Alzheimer's disease [312]. In another publication based on the data from the same NHANES cycle showed that elevated urinary Cd levels were associated with a 58% increase in the risk of death from Alzheimer's disease in the 60–85 years age group [313].

5.2.2. Cadmium and Mortality in Sweden and Australia

In a Swedish cohort study, the overall mortality was increased by 2.06-fold in women who had $[Cd]_b \geq 0.69$ μg/L compared with those with $[Cd]_b \leq 0.18$ μg/L [314]. In this Swedish study on women, the median, 25th and 75th percentile levels of $[Cd]_b$ were 0.28, 0.18 and 0.51 μg/L, respectively [314].

In a follow-up study of women in Western Australia ($n = 1359$), there was 2.7-fold higher $[Cd]_u$ in those with atherosclerotic vascular disease. This $[Cd]_u$ was associated with a 36% increase in the risk of dying from heart failure and a 17% increase in the risk of having a heart failure event [299]. Hence, a reduction in survival was observed even though the kidney burden of Cd among the study women was low: the median, 25th and 75th percentile levels of $[Cd]_u$ were 0.18, 0.09 and 0.32 µg/L, respectively [315].

5.2.3. Cadmium and Mortality in Japan

A dose–response relationship between mortality risk and elevated body burden of Cd was seen in men who were residents of nonpolluted areas of Japan: the mortality risk from all causes was increased by 35% and 64% in men who had E_{Cd} 1.96–3.22 and ≥3.23 µg/g creatinine, respectively [316]. In women from the same nonpolluted areas, a 49% increase in mortality from all causes was associated with $E_{Cd} \geq 4.66$ µg/g creatinine. A 6% increase risk of death from cancer at any site was also seen only in women. There was a 13% increase in mortality from pancreatic cancer for every 1 µg/g creatinine increment of E_{Cd} [317].

In a region of Japan with Cd pollution, all-cause mortality increased by 1.57-and 2.40-fold in men and women with proteinuria and glycosuria, attributable to their elevated Cd exposure [318]. An increase in deaths from ischemic heart disease and incidences of diabetes and kidney disease was observed [302]. A 1.49-fold increase in deaths from cancer in any site was observed, especially in women with evidence of Cd-related kidney pathologies [319]. The increase in the risk of dying from a specific cancer type was 3.85, 7.71 and 10.1 for cancer of the uterus, kidney and kidney plus urinary tract [319]. The median $[Cd]_u$ in women and men with proteinuria and glycosuria was 8.3 µg/L and 10 µg/L, respectively. Paradoxically, in men, the risk of lung cancer and the risk of dying from cancer were reduced by 47% and 21%, respectively [319].

5.2.4. Lead and Mortality in the U.S., Korea and China

In a follow-up study of a subset of participants in NHANES 1988–1994, there was a 48% increase in cancer mortality risk in those with $[Pb]_b \geq 5$ µg/dL [320]. In another follow-up of participants in the same cycle, $[Pb]_b$ 1.0–6.7 µg/dL was associated with 1.37-, 1.70- and 2.08-fold increases in death from all causes, CVD, and ischemic heart disease [321]. In the NHANES 1999–2010 follow-up study ($n = 5316$), exposure to low levels of Pb, reflected by $[Pb]_u > 1.26$ µg/dL, may increase the risk of deaths from all causes and cancer by 1.79- and 6.60-fold, respectively [196]. A 44% increase in CVD mortality was observed for every 10-fold increase in hematocrit-corrected $[Pb]_b$ in a follow-up of participants, aged ≥40 years, in NHANES 1999–2010 ($n = 18{,}602$) [322].

In a cohort study of lead-exposed workers of South Korea ($n = 81{,}067$), $[Pb]_b$ 10–20 µg/dL was associated with 36% and 93% increases in the risk of death from all causes in men and women, respectively [323]. The mortality risk from bronchial and lung cancer rose by 10.45- and 12.68-fold in female workers with $[Pb]_b$ of 10–20 µg/dL. In male workers, the same $[Pb]_b$ range of 10–20 µg/dL was associated with hospital admission for ischemic heart disease, cerebrovascular disease, angina pectoris and cerebral infarction [324].

A 25% increase in deaths from all causes was recorded in a follow-up study of a Chinese population ($n = 2832$) with the median Pb intake level of 101.9 µg/day [16]. Compared with Pb intake levels in Quartile 1 (67 µg/day), Pb intake levels in Quartile 3 (111.4 µg/day) and Quartile 4 (147 µg/day) were associated with 1.52- and 3-fold increases in cancer mortality, respectively [16].

Table 2 summarizes exposure levels reflected by blood concentrations, urinary excretion, and dietary intake estimates of Cd and Pb that have been associated with nephrotoxicity, enhanced risks for CKD, and mortality in various populations that include the U.S., Sweden, Australia, Japan, China, Thailand, Belgium, and Korea.

Table 2. Toxic exposure levels of cadmium and lead observed in various populations.

Countries	Exposure Levels and Estimates of Disease and Mortality Risks
U.S. [44–46,289]	$[Cd]_u \geq 1$ µg/L, $[Cd]_b \geq 0.6$ µg/L, $[Pb]_b \geq 2.4$ µg/dL and $[Cd]_b \geq 0.6$ plus $[Pb]_b \geq 2.4$ µg/dL were associated with 1.48-, 1.32-,1.56- and 2.34-fold increment in CKD risk, respectively. $[Cd]_b$ of >0.53 to >0.61 µg/L were associated with 1.80- to 2.2-fold increases in CKD risk.
U.S. [302,308–313,319–321]	E_{Cd} of ≥0.37 to ≥0.65 µg/g creatinine were associated with increased mortality from heart disease. E_{Cd} of >0.48 and ≥0.58 µg/g creatinine were linked to 4.29-fold and 3.22-fold increments in cancer mortality and lung cancer mortality in men, respectively. $[Cd]_b > 0.6$ µg/L was linked to a 3.83-fold increase in mortality from Alzheimer's disease. $[Pb]_b \geq 5$ µg/dL was linked to a 1.48-fold increment of cancer mortality$[Pb]_b$ 1.0–6.7 µg/dL were linked to 1.37-, 1.70- and 2.08-fold increments of morality from all causes and cardiovascular and ischaemic heart diseases. $[Pb]_u$ levels >1.26 µg/L were linked to 1.79- and 6.60-fold increments of mortality from all causes and cancer, respectively.
Sweden [291,292,314]	$[Pb]_b \geq 3.3$ µg/dL was associated with a 1.49-fold rise of incidence of CKD and erythrocyte Pb was associated with developing ESKD. $[Cd]_b \geq 0.69$ µg/L was linked to a 2.06-fold increase in mortality from all causes.
Australia [315]	A 2.7-fold higher $[Cd]_u$ were linked to a 36% increase in mortality from heart failure and a 17% increase in the risk of having a heart failure event.
Japan [316–319]	E_{Cd} of ≥3.23 and ≥4.66 µg/g creatinine were linked to increased mortality by 64%, and 49% in men and women, respectively. The mortality from pancreatic cancer in women rose by 13% for every 1 µg/g creatinine increase in E_{Cd}. In women with signs of Cd-related kidney pathologies, there were 3.85-, 7.71- and 10.1-fold increases in mortality from cancer of the uterus, kidney, and kidney plus urinary tract, respectively.
China [15,16]	Cd intake levels of 23.2, 29.6 and 36.9 µg/day were associated with 1.73-, 2.93- and 4.05-fold increments of CKD risk, For every 30 µg/day intake of Pb, all-cause mortality rose by 25%. Pb intake levels of 111.4 and 147 µg/day were linked to 1.52- and 3-fold increases in cancer mortality.
Thailand [53]	$E_{\beta 2MG}$ of 100–299, 300–999 and ≥1000 µg/g creatinine were associated with 4.66-, 6.16-, and 11.47-fold increases in CKD risk, compared with $E_{\beta 2MG} < 100$ µg/g creatinine. An inverse association of $E_{\beta 2}$MG with eGFR was seen only in those with eGFR below 60 mL/min/1.73 m^2, indicative of nephron loss. $E_{\beta 2MG}$ did not show an association with eGFR in those with normal eGFR.
Belgium [301]	Associations of $[Cd]_u$ with $[NAG]_u$ and $[RBP]_u$ were seen in workers who had $[Pb]_b \geq 21.9$ µg/dL, corresponding to the 75th percentile or higher.
Korea [300]	A correlation between $[Cd]_b$ and $[\beta_2MG]_u$ was strengthened in those who had $[Pb]_b$ above the median of 2.20 µg/dL.

$[x]_u$ = urinary concentration of x; $[x]_b$ = blood concentration of x; CKD = chronic kidney disease; ESKD = end stage kidney disease; E_{Cd} = excretion rate of Cd; β_2MG = β_2-microglobulin; $E_{\beta 2MG}$ = excretion rate of β_2MG; NAG = N-acetyl-β-D-glucosaminidase. CKD is defined as estimated glomerular filtration rate < 60 mL/min/1.73 m^2. $E_{\beta 2MG} \geq 300$ µg/g creatinine was the conventional cutoff value to define an adverse effect of excessive intake of Cd [41].

6. Summary and Conclusions

Dietary assessment by the total diet study method shows that both Cd and Pb are present in virtually all foodstuffs. Foods which are frequently consumed in large quantities, such as cereals, rice, potatoes and vegetables, contribute the most to the total intake of these toxic metals. Seafood (shellfish), offal, spinach, lettuce and chocolate are Cd sources among high consumers of these foods. Beverage, chocolate syrup, raisins, fish, meats (offal included), preserved soybean, and fungus products are sources of Pb for high consumers of these products. Cd intake levels of 23.2, 29.6 and 36.9 µg/day were associated with 1.73-, 2.93- and 4.05-fold increments of CKD risk, compared with the 16.7 µg/day intake rate. A Cd intake level of 23.2 µg/day is 40% of the FAO/WHO current tolerable intake level. Pb intake levels of 111.4 and 147 µg/day were associated with 1.52- and 3-fold increases in cancer mortality, compared with the 67 µg/day intake rate. A Pb intake level of 111.4 µg/day exceeds the FDA interim safe intake rate of 12.5 µg/day.

Historically, the health risk assessment of Cd has relied on $E_{\beta 2MG}$. This practice follows the FAO/WHO guidelines in which $E_{\beta 2MG} \geq 300$ µg/g creatinine were cutoff values to define the level of health concern (nephrotoxicity). However, multiple lines of evidence discussed in this review indicate that the established cutoff value of $E_{\beta 2MG}$ is not a sensitive indicator of tubular cell toxicity. KIM1 is the first identifiable marker of Cd-induced injury, and in our opinion, any elevation of E_{Cd} also signifies such injury. Estimated GFR is a function of intact nephron mass and is universally employed for diagnosis and staging of CKD. Health risk assessment of Cd should be based on the dose–response relationship between E_{Cd} and GFR.

The variable effect of low-level environmental exposure to Cd and Pb on GFR has caused some controversy. Consequently, governments worldwide have not established the necessary regulations to protect their populations. To improve comparability of guidelines among populations, normalization of $[Cd]_u$ to C_{cr} is proposed to nullify urine flow rate as a confounder, circumvent the effect of muscle mass on $[cr]_u$, and facilitate the expression of relevant excretion rates as functions of intact nephron mass.

Risk assessment of Cd is conventionally based on the urinary Cd threshold limit of 5.24 μg/g creatinine, which was the mean E_{Cd} at which $E_{\beta 2MG}$ exceeded 300 μg/g creatinine. However, a $[Cd]_u$ level as low as 1 μg/L (E_{Cd} ~0.5 μg/g creatinine) is associated with a significant increase in the risk of CKD and mortality from cardiovascular disease and cancer. As Cd and Pb exposure is highly prevalent, even a small increase in disease risk can result in a large number of people affected by a disease that is preventable. Environmental exposure to low-level Pb ($[Pb]_b$ 1.0–6.7 μg/dL) is associated with mortality from cardiovascular disease and ischemic heart disease. $[Pb]_u$ levels > 1.26 μg/L are associated with increased mortality from cancer.

Given the continuing rise in the incidence of CKD worldwide and the escalating treatment costs associated with dialysis and/or kidney transplants needed for survival, developing strategies to prevent CKD is of global importance. Furthermore, Cd and Pb are associated with cardiovascular morbidity and reduced life expectancy, independently of CKD. Prevention of Cd- and Pb-related ailments and mortality requires minimization of their environmental contamination. Accordingly, public measures to reduce environmental pollution and the food-chain transfer of Cd and Pb are vital, as are risk reduction measures through setting a maximally permissible concentration of Cd and Pb in staple foods to the lowest achievable levels.

Author Contributions: S.S., G.C.G., D.A.V. and K.R.P. conceptualized the review. S.S. prepared an outline and an initial draft with G.C.G., and D.A.V. provided logical data interpretation. K.R.P. wrote the section on the assessment of nephrotoxicity. G.C.G., D.A.V. and K.R.P. reviewed and edited the draft manuscript. All authors have read and agreed to the published version of the manuscript.

Funding: This research received no external funding.

Acknowledgments: This work was partially supported with the resources of the Kidney Disease Research Centre, The University of Queensland Faculty of Medicine and Translational Research Institute. Additionally, this work was supported by the Stratton Veteran Affairs Medical Center, Albany, NY, USA, and was made possible by resources and facilities at that institution. Opinions expressed in this paper are those of the authors and do not represent the official position of the United States Department of Veterans' Affairs.

Conflicts of Interest: The authors have no potential conflict of interest to declare.

Abbreviations

Ca	Calcium
Cd	Cadmium
Cu	Copper
Pb	Lead
Zn	Zn
MT	Metallothionein
PC	Phytochelatin
CdMT	Cadmium-metallothionein complex
CdPC	Cadmium-phytochelatin complex
GSH	Glutathione
δ-ALAD	Delta-aminolevulinic acid dehydratase
δ-ALA	Delta-aminolevulinic acid
AST	Aspartate aminotransferase

ALT	Alanine aminotransferase
β_2MG	Beta$_2$-microglobulin
KIM1	Kidney injury molecule 1
NAG	N-acetyl-β-D-glucosaminidase
RBP	Retinol-binding protein
GFR	Glomerular filtration rate, units of volume/time
eGFR	Estimated glomerular filtration rate, units of mL/min/1.73 m^2
CKD-EPI	Chronic kidney disease epidemiology collaboration
JECFA	The Joint Expert Committee on Food Additives and Contaminants of the Food and Agriculture Organization and the World Health Organization of the United Nations
PTWI	Provisional tolerable weekly intake
TMI	Tolerable monthly intake
TDS	Total diet study
$[x]_u$	Urinary concentration of x.
$[x]_p$	Plasma concentration of x.
$[x]_b$	Blood concentration of x.
$[x]_k$	Kidney content of x.
C_{cr}	Creatinine clearance, units of volume/time
V_u	Urine flow rate, units of volume/time
E_x/C_{cr}	Excretion rate of x per volume of filtrate, units of mass/volume, where x = Cd, NAG, or β_2MG
$FE_{\beta 2MG}$	Fractional excretion of β_2MG, %
$FR_{\beta 2MG}$	Fractional reabsorption of β_2MG, %

References

1. Satarug, S.; Vesey, D.A.; Gobe, G.C. Health risk assessment of dietary cadmium intake: Do current guidelines indicate how much is safe? *Environ. Health Perspect.* **2017**, *125*, 284–288. [CrossRef]
2. Satarug, S.; Vesey, D.A.; Gobe, G.C. Current health risk assessment practice for dietary cadmium: Data from different countries. *Food Chem. Toxicol.* **2017**, *106*, 430–445. [CrossRef] [PubMed]
3. Shefa, S.T.; Héroux, P. Both physiology and epidemiology support zero tolerable blood lead levels. *Toxicol. Lett.* **2017**, *280*, 232–237. [CrossRef] [PubMed]
4. Daley, G.M.; Pretorius, C.J.; Ungerer, J.P. Lead toxicity: An Australian perspective. *Clin. Biochem. Rev.* **2018**, *39*, 61–98. [PubMed]
5. World Health Organization (WHO). Preventing Disease through Healthy Environments: Ten Chemicals of Major Public Health Concern; Public Environment WHO: Geneva, Switzerland. Available online: https://www.who.int/ipcs/features/10chemicals_en.pdf?ua=1 (accessed on 12 August 2020).
6. Satarug, S.; Haswell-Elkins, M.R.; Moore, M.R. Safe levels of cadmium intake to prevent renal toxicity in human subjects. *Br. J. Nutr.* **2000**, *84*, 791–802. [CrossRef] [PubMed]
7. Satarug, S.; Baker, J.R.; Urbenjapol, S.; Haswell-Elkins, M.; Reilly, P.E.; Williams, D.J.; Moore, M.R. A global perspective on cadmium pollution and toxicity in non-occupationally exposed population. *Toxicol. Lett.* **2003**, *137*, 65–83. [CrossRef]
8. Satarug, S. Dietary cadmium intake and its effects on kidneys. *Toxics* **2018**, *6*, 15. [CrossRef]
9. Satarug, S. Long-term exposure to cadmium in food and cigarette smoke, liver effects and hepatocellular carcinoma. *Curr. Drug Metab.* **2012**, *13*, 257–271. [CrossRef]
10. Satarug, S.; Moore, M.R. Emerging roles of cadmium and heme oxygenase in type-2 diabetes and cancer susceptibility. *Tohoku J. Exp. Med.* **2012**, *228*, 267–288. [CrossRef]
11. Gibb, H.J.; Barchowsky, A.; Bellinger, D.; Bolger, P.M.; Carrington, C.; Havelaar, A.H.; Oberoi, S.; Zang, Y.; O'Leary, K.; Devleesschauwer, B. Estimates of the 2015 global and regional disease burden from four foodborne metals-arsenic, cadmium, lead and methylmercury. *Environ. Res.* **2019**, *174*, 188–194. [CrossRef]
12. Satarug, S.; Gobe, G.C.; Ujjin, P.; Vesey, D.A. A comparison of the nephrotoxicity of low doses of cadmium and lead. *Toxics* **2020**, *8*, 18. [CrossRef] [PubMed]
13. Wang, X.; Ding, N.; Tucker, K.L.; Weisskopf, M.G.; Sparrow, D.; Hu, H.; Park, S.K. A Western diet pattern is associated with higher concentrations of blood and bone lead among middle-aged and elderly men. *J. Nutr.* **2017**, *147*, 1374–1383. [CrossRef] [PubMed]

14. Ding, N.; Wang, X.; Tucker, K.L.; Weisskopf, M.G.; Sparrow, D.; Hu, H.; Park, S.K. Dietary patterns, bone lead and incident coronary heart disease among middle-aged to elderly men. *Environ. Res.* **2019**, *168*, 222–229. [CrossRef] [PubMed]
15. Shi, Z.; Taylor, A.W.; Riley., M.; Byles., J.; Liu, J.; Noakes, M. Association between dietary patterns, cadmium intake and chronic kidney disease among adults. *Clin. Nutr.* **2018**, *37*, 276–284. [CrossRef]
16. Shi, Z.; Zhen, S.; Orsini, N.; Zhou, Y.; Zhou, Y.; Liu, J.; Taylor, A.W. Association between dietary lead intake and 10-year mortality among Chinese adults. *Environ. Sci. Pollut. Res.* **2017**, *24*, 12273–12280. [CrossRef]
17. Gobe, G.; Crane, D. Mitochondria, reactive oxygen species and cadmium toxicity in the kidney. *Toxicol. Lett.* **2010**, *198*, 49–55. [CrossRef]
18. Nair, A.R.; Lee, W.K.; Smeets, K.; Swennen, Q.; Sanchez, A.; Thévenod, F.; Cuypers, A. Glutathione and mitochondria determine acute defense responses and adaptive processes in cadmium-induced oxidative stress and toxicity of the kidney. *Arch. Toxicol.* **2015**, *89*, 2273–2289. [CrossRef]
19. Matović, V.; Buha, A.; Đukić-Ćosić, D.; Bulat, Z. Insight into the oxidative stress induced by lead and/or cadmium in blood, liver and kidneys. *Food Chem. Toxicol.* **2015**, *78*, 130–140. [CrossRef]
20. Satarug, S.; Vesey, D.A.; Gobe, G.C. Kidney cadmium toxicity, diabetes and high blood pressure: The perfect storm. *Tohoku J. Exp. Med.* **2017**, *241*, 65–87. [CrossRef]
21. Garza-Lombó, C.; Posadas, Y.; Quintanar, L.; Gonsebatt, M.E.; Franco, R. Neurotoxicity linked to dysfunctional metal ion homeostasis and xenobiotic metal exposure: Redox signaling and oxidative stress. *Antioxid. Redox Signal.* **2018**, *28*, 1669–1703. [CrossRef]
22. Valko, M.; Jomova, K.; Rhodes, C.J.; Kuča, K.; Musílek, K. Redox- and non-redox-metal-induced formation of free radicals and their role in human disease. *Arch. Toxicol.* **2016**, *90*, 1–37. [CrossRef] [PubMed]
23. Moulis, J.M.; Bourguinon, J.; Catty, P. Chapter 23 Cadmium. In *RSC Metallobiology Series No. 2, Binding, Transport. and Storage of Metal. Ions in Biological Cells*; Wolfgang, M., Anthony, W., Eds.; The Royal Society of Chemistry: London, UK, 2014; pp. 695–746.
24. Cangelosi, V.; Pecoraro, V. Chapter 28 Lead. In *RSC Metallobiology Series No. 2, Binding, Transport. and Storage of Metal. Ions in Biological Cells*; Wolfgang, M., Anthony, W., Eds.; The Royal Society of Chemistry: London, UK, 2014; pp. 843–882.
25. Sanders, T.; Liu, Y.; Buchner, V.; Tchounwou, P.B. Neurotoxic effects and biomarkers of lead exposure: A review. *Rev. Environ. Health* **2009**, *24*, 15–45. [CrossRef] [PubMed]
26. Carpenter, M.C.; Shami Shah, A.; DeSilva, S.; Gleaton, A.; Su, A.; Goundie, B.; Croteau, M.L.; Stevenson, M.J.; Wilcox, D.E.; Austin, R.N. Thermodynamics of Pb(ii) and Zn(ii) binding to MT-3, a neurologically important metallothionein. *Metallomics* **2016**, *8*, 605–617. [CrossRef] [PubMed]
27. Satarug, S.; Baker, J.R.; Reilly, P.E.; Esumi, H.; Moore, M.R. Evidence for a synergistic interaction between cadmium and endotoxin toxicity and for nitric oxide and cadmium displacement of metals in the kidney. *Nitric Oxide* **2000**, *4*, 431–440. [CrossRef]
28. Satarug, S.; Baker, J.R.; Reilly, P.E.; Moore, M.R.; Williams, D.J. Changes in zinc and copper homeostasis in human livers and kidneys associated with exposure to environmental cadmium. *Hum. Exp. Toxicol.* **2001**, *20*, 205–213. [CrossRef]
29. Satarug, S.; Nishijo, M.; Ujjin, P.; Moore, M.R. Chronic exposure to low-level cadmium induced zinc-copper dysregulation. *J. Trace Elem. Med. Biol.* **2018**, *46*, 32–38. [CrossRef]
30. Prozialeck, W.C.; Lamar, P.C.; Edwards, J.R. Effects of sub-chronic Cd exposure on levels of copper, selenium, zinc, iron and other essential metals in rat renal cortex. *Toxicol. Rep.* **2016**, *3*, 740–746. [CrossRef]
31. Thevenod, F. Nephrotoxicity and the proximal tubule. Insights from cadmium. *Nephron Physiol.* **2003**, *93*, 87–93. [CrossRef]
32. Moulis, J.M. Cellular mechanisms of cadmium toxicity related to the homeostasis of essential metals. *Biometals* **2010**, *23*, 877–896. [CrossRef]
33. Nzengue, Y.; Candéias, S.M.; Sauvaigo, S.; Douki, T.; Favier, A.; Rachidi, W.; Guiraud, P. The toxicity redox mechanisms of cadmium alone or together with copper and zinc homeostasis alteration: Its redox biomarkers. *J. Trace Elem. Med. Biol.* **2011**, *25*, 171–180. [CrossRef]
34. Nzengue, Y.; Steiman, R.; Rachidi, W.; Favier, A.; Guiraud, P. Oxidative stress induced by cadmium in the C6 cell line: Role of copper and zinc. *Biol. Trace Elem. Res.* **2012**, *146*, 410–419. [CrossRef] [PubMed]

35. Eom, S.Y.; Yim, D.H.; Huang, M.; Park, C.H.; Kim, G.B.; Yu, S.D.; Choi, B.S.; Park, J.D.; Kim, Y.D.; Kim, H. Copper-zinc imbalance induces kidney tubule damage and oxidative stress in a population exposed to chronic environmental cadmium. *Int. Arch. Occup. Environ. Health* **2020**, *93*, 337–344. [CrossRef] [PubMed]
36. Rubino, F.M. Toxicity of glutathione-binding metals: A review of targets and mechanisms. *Toxics* **2015**, *3*, 20–62. [CrossRef] [PubMed]
37. Phillips, J.D. Heme biosynthesis and the porphyrias. *Mol. Genet. Metab.* **2019**, *128*, 164–177. [CrossRef] [PubMed]
38. Tobwala, S.; Wang, H.-J.; Carey, J.W.; Banks, W.A.; Ercal, N. Effects of lead and cadmium on brain endothelial cell survival, monolayer permeability, and crucial oxidative stress markers in an in vitro model of the blood-brain barrier. *Toxics* **2014**, *2*, 258–275. [CrossRef]
39. Wang, W.; Duan, B.; Xu, H.; Xu, L.; Xu, T.L. Calcium-permeable acid-sensing ion channel is a molecular target of the neurotoxic metal ion lead. *J. Biol. Chem.* **2006**, *281*, 2497–2505. [CrossRef] [PubMed]
40. FAO/WHO. *Evaluation of Certain Food Additives and Contaminants (Forty-First Report of the Joint FAO/WHO Expert Committee on Food Additives)*; WHO Technical Report Series No. 837; World Health Organization: Geneva, Switzerland, 1993.
41. Food and Agriculture Organization of the United Nations (FAO); World Health Organization (WHO). Summary and Conclusions. In Proceedings of the Joint FAO/WHO Expert Committee on Food Additives Seventy-Third Meeting, Geneva, Switzerland, 8–17 June 2010; Available online: http://www.who.int/foodsafety/publications/chem/summary73.pdf (accessed on 12 August 2020).
42. Flannery, B.M.; Dolan, L.C.; Hoffman-Pennesi, D.; Gavelek, A.; Jones, O.E.; Kanwal, R.; Wolpert, B.; Gensheimer, K.; Dennis, S.; Fitzpatrick, S.U.S. Food and Drug Administration's interim reference levels for dietary lead exposure in children and women of childbearing age. *Regul. Toxicol. Pharmacol.* **2020**, *110*, 104516. [CrossRef]
43. Dolan, L.C.; Flannery, B.M.; Hoffman-Pennesi, D.; Gavelek, A.; Jones, O.E.; Kanwal, R.; Wolpert, B.; Gensheimer, K.; Dennis, S.; Fitzpatrick, S. A review of the evidence to support interim reference level for dietary lead exposure in adults. *Regul. Toxicol. Pharmacol.* **2020**, *111*, 104579. [CrossRef] [PubMed]
44. Ferraro, P.M.; Costanzi, S.; Naticchia, A.; Sturniolo, A.; Gambaro, G. Low level exposure to cadmium increases the risk of chronic kidney disease: Analysis of the NHANES 1999–2006. *BMC Public Health* **2010**, *10*, 304. [CrossRef]
45. Lin, Y.S.; Ho, W.C.; Caffrey, J.L.; Sonawane, B. Low serum zinc is associated with elevated risk of cadmium nephrotoxicity. *Environ. Res.* **2014**, *134*, 33–38. [CrossRef]
46. Madrigal, J.M.; Ricardo, A.C.; Persky, V.; Turyk, M. Associations between blood cadmium concentration and kidney function in the U.S. population: Impact of sex, diabetes and hypertension. *Environ. Res.* **2018**, *169*, 180–188. [CrossRef] [PubMed]
47. Crinnion, W.J. The CDC fourth national report on human exposure to environmental chemicals: What it tells us about our toxic burden and how it assists environmental medicine physicians. *Altern. Med. Rev.* **2010**, *15*, 101–108. [PubMed]
48. Levey, A.S.; Stevens, L.A.; Schmid, C.H.; Zhang, Y.; Castro, A.F., III; Feldman, H.I.; Kusek, J.W.; Eggers, P.; Van Lente, F.; Greene, T.; et al. A new equation to estimate glomerular filtration rate. *Ann. Intern. Med.* **2009**, *150*, 604–612. [CrossRef] [PubMed]
49. Levey, A.S.; Inker, L.A.; Coresh, J. GFR estimation: From physiology to public health. *Am. J. Kidney Dis.* **2014**, *63*, 820–834. [CrossRef] [PubMed]
50. Levey, A.S.; Becker, C.; Inker, L.A. Glomerular filtration rate and albuminuria for detection and staging of acute and chronic kidney disease in adults: A systematic review. *JAMA* **2015**, *313*, 837–846. [CrossRef] [PubMed]
51. Satarug, S.; Ruangyuttikarn, W.; Nishijo, M.; Ruiz, P. Urinary cadmium threshold to prevent kidney disease development. *Toxics* **2018**, *6*, 26.
52. Satarug, S.; Boonprasert, K.; Gobe, G.C.; Ruenweerayut, R.; Johnson, D.W.; Na-Bangchang, K.; Vesey, D.A. Chronic exposure to cadmium is associated with a marked reduction in glomerular filtration rate. *Clin. Kidney J.* **2018**, *12*, 468–475. [CrossRef]
53. Satarug, S.; Vesey, D.A.; Nishijo, M.; Ruangyuttikarnm, W.; Gobe, G.C. The inverse association of glomerular function and urinary β_2-MG excretion and its implications for cadmium health risk assessment. *Environ. Res.* **2019**, *173*, 40–47. [CrossRef]

54. Satarug, S.; Vesey, D.A.; Ruangyuttikarn, W.; Nishijo, M.; Gobe, G.C.; Phelps, K.R. The source and pathophysiologic significance of excreted cadmium. *Toxics* **2019**, *7*, 55. [CrossRef]
55. Järup, L. Hazards of heavy metal contamination. *Br. Med. Bull.* **2003**, *68*, 167–182. [CrossRef]
56. Wu, S.; Deng, F.; Hao, Y.; Shima, M.; Wang, X.; Zheng, C.; Wei, H.; Lv, H.; Lu, X.; Huang, J.; et al. Chemical constituents of fine particulate air pollution and pulmonary function in healthy adults: The Healthy Volunteer Natural Relocation study. *J. Hazard. Mater.* **2013**, *260*, 183–191. [CrossRef] [PubMed]
57. Jung, M.S.; Kim, J.Y.; Lee, H.S.; Lee, C.G.; Song, H.S. Air pollution and urinary N-acetyl-β-glucosaminidase levels in residents living near a cement plant. *Ann. Occup. Environ. Med.* **2016**, *28*, 52. [CrossRef] [PubMed]
58. Jin, Y.; Lu, Y.; Li, Y.; Zhao, H.; Wang, X.; Shen, Y.; Kuang, X. Correlation between environmental low-dose cadmium exposure and early kidney damage: A comparative study in an industrial zone vs. a living quarter in Shanghai, China. *Environ.Toxicol. Pharmacol.* **2020**, *79*, 103381. [CrossRef] [PubMed]
59. Repić, A.; Bulat, P.; Antonijević, B.; Antunović, M.; Džudović, J.; Buha, A.; Bulat, Z. The influence of smoking habits on cadmium and lead blood levels in the Serbian adult people. *Environ. Sci. Pollut. Res. Int.* **2020**, *27*, 751–760. [CrossRef]
60. Dumkova, J.; Vrlikova, L.; Vecera, Z.; Putnova, B.; Docekal, B.; Mikuska, P.; Fictum, P.; Hampl, A.; Buchtova, M. Inhaled cadmium oxide nanoparticles: Their in vivo fate and effect on target organs. *Int. J. Mol. Sci.* **2016**, *17*, 874. [CrossRef]
61. Dumková, J.; Smutná, T.; Vrlíková, L.; Le Coustumer, P.; Večeřa, Z.; Dočekal, B.; Mikuška, P.; Čapka, L.; Fictum, P.; Hampl, A.; et al. Sub-chronic inhalation of lead oxide nanoparticles revealed their broad distribution and tissue-specific subcellular localization in target organs. *Part. Fibre Toxicol.* **2017**, *14*, 55. [CrossRef]
62. Tulinska, J.; Masanova, V.; Liskova, A.; Mikusova, M.L.; Rollerova, E.; Krivosikova, Z.; Stefikova, K.; Uhnakova, I.; Ursinyova, M.; Babickova, J.; et al. Six-week inhalation of CdO nanoparticles in mice: The effects on immune response, oxidative stress, antioxidative defense, fibrotic response, and bones. *Food Chem. Toxicol.* **2020**, *136*, 110954. [CrossRef]
63. Sutunkova, M.P.; Solovyeva, S.N.; Chernyshov, I.N.; Klinova, S.V.; Gurvich, V.B.; Shur, V.Y.; Shishkina, E.V.; Zubarev, I.V.; Privalova, L.I.; Katsnelson, B.A. Manifestation of systemic toxicity in rats after a short-time inhalation of lead oxide nanoparticles. *Int. J. Mol. Sci.* **2020**, *21*, 690. [CrossRef]
64. Zahran, S.; McElmurry, S.P.; Sadler, R.C. Four phases of the Flint qater crisis: Evidence from blood lead levels in children. *Environ. Res.* **2017**, *157*, 160–172. [CrossRef]
65. Roy, S.; Tang, M.; Edwards, M.A. Lead release to potable water during the Flint, Michigan water crisis as revealed by routine biosolids monitoring data. *Water Res.* **2019**, *160*, 475–483. [CrossRef]
66. Bandara, J.M.; Wijewardena, H.V.; Liyanege, J.; Upul, M.A.; Bandara, J.M. Chronic renal failure in Sri Lanka caused by elevated dietary cadmium: Trojan horse of the green revolution. *Toxicol. Lett.* **2010**, *198*, 33–39. [CrossRef] [PubMed]
67. Kader, M.; Lamb, D.T.; Mahbub, K.R.; Megharaj, M.; Naidu, R. Predicting plant uptake and toxicity of lead (Pb) in long-term contaminated soils from derived transfer functions. *Environ. Sci. Pollut. Res. Int.* **2016**, *23*, 15460–15470. [CrossRef] [PubMed]
68. Lamb, D.T.; Kader, M.; Ming, H.; Wang, L.; Abbasi, S.; Megharaj, M.; Naidu, R. Predicting plant uptake of cadmium: Validated with long-term contaminated soils. *Ecotoxicology* **2016**, *25*, 1563–1574. [CrossRef] [PubMed]
69. Wilkinson, J.M.; Hill, J.; Phillips, C.J. The accumulation of potentially-toxic metals by grazing ruminants. *Proc. Nutr. Soc.* **2003**, *62*, 267–277. [CrossRef]
70. Bischoff, K.; Hillebrandt, J.; Erb, H.N.; Thompson, B.; Johns, S. Comparison of blood and tissue lead concentrations from cattle with known lead exposure. *Food Addit. Contam. Part A Chem. Anal. Control. Expo. Risk Assess.* **2016**, *33*, 1563–1569. [CrossRef]
71. Centers for Disease Control and Prevention. CDC Response to Advisory Committee on Childhood Lead Poisoning Prevention Recommendations in "Low Level Lead Exposure Harms Children: A Renewed Call of Primary Prevention". 2012. Available online: http://www.cdc.gov/nceh/lead/ACCLPP/CDC_Response_Lead_Exposure_Recs.pdf (accessed on 12 August 2020).
72. Feng, C.X.; Cao., J.; Bendell, L. Exploring spatial and temporal variations of cadmium concentrations in pacific oysters from British Columbia. *Biometrics* **2011**, *67*, 1142–1152. [CrossRef]

73. Losasso, C.; Bille, L.; Patuzzi, I.; Lorenzetto, M.; Binato, G.; Pozza, M.D.; Ferrè, N.; Ricci, N. Possible influence of natural events on heavy metals exposure from shellfish consumption: A case study in the north-east of Italy. *Front. Public Health* **2015**, *3*, 21. [CrossRef]
74. Guéguen, M.; Amiard, J.-C.; Arnich, N.; Badot, P.-M.; Claisse, D.; Guérin, T.; Vernoux, J.-P. Shellfish and residual chemical contaminants: Hazards, monitoring, and health risk assessment along French coasts. *Rev. Environ. Contam. Toxicol.* **2011**, *213*, 55–111.
75. Burioli, E.A.V.; Squadrone, S.; Stella, C.; Foglini, C.; Abete, M.C.; Prearo, M. Trace element occurrence in the Pacific oyster Crassostrea gigas from coastal marine ecosystems in Italy. *Chemosphere* **2017**, *187*, 248–260. [CrossRef]
76. Renieri, E.A.; Alegakis, A.K.; Kiriakakis, M.; Vinceti, M.; Ozcagli, E.; Wilks, M.F.; Tsatsakis, A.M. Cd, Pb and Hg biomonitoring in fish of the Mediterranean region and risk estimations on fish consumption. *Toxics* **2014**, *2*, 417–442. [CrossRef]
77. Cobbett, C.S. Phytochelatins and their roles in heavy metal detoxification. *Plant. Physiol.* **2000**, *123*, 825–832. [CrossRef] [PubMed]
78. Cobbett, C.; Goldsbrough, P. Phytochelatins and metallothioneins: Roles in heavy metal detoxification and homeostasis. *Annu. Rev. Plant Biol.* **2002**, *53*, 159–182. [CrossRef] [PubMed]
79. Pivato, M.; Fabrega-Prats, M.; Masi, A. Low-molecular-weight thiols in plants: Functional and analytical implications. *Arch. Biochem. Biophys.* **2014**, *560*, 83–99. [CrossRef] [PubMed]
80. Klaassen, C.D.; Liu, J.; Diwan, B.A. Metallothionein protection of cadmium toxicity. *Toxicol. Appl. Pharmacol.* **2009**, *238*, 215–220. [CrossRef]
81. Scott, S.R.; Smith, K.E.; Dahman, C.; Gorski, P.R.; Adams, S.V.; Shafer, M.M. Cd isotope fractionation during tobacco combustion produces isotopic variation outside the range measured in dietary sources. *Sci. Total Environ.* **2019**, *688*, 600–608. [CrossRef]
82. Aoshima, K. Epidemiology and tubular dysfunction in the inhabitants of a cadmium-polluted area in the Jinzu River basin in Toyama Prefecture. *Tohoku J. Exp. Med.* **1987**, *152*, 151–172. [CrossRef]
83. Spungen, J.H. Children's exposures to lead and cadmium: FDA total diet study 2014–2016. *Food Addit. Contam. Part A Chem. Anal. Control. Expo. Risk Assess.* **2019**, *36*, 893–903. [CrossRef]
84. Gavelek, A.; Spungen, J.; Hoffman-Pennesi, D.; Flannery, B.; Dolan, L.; Dennis, S.; Fitzpatrick, S. Lead exposures in older children (males and females 7–17 years), women of childbearing age (females 16–49 years) and adults (males and females 18+ years): FDA total diet study 2014-16. *Food Addit. Contam. Part A Chem. Anal. Control. Expo. Risk Assess.* **2020**, *37*, 104–109. [CrossRef]
85. European Food Safety Agency (EFSA). Statement on tolerable weekly intake for cadmium. *EFSA J.* **2011**, *9*, 1975.
86. European Food Safety Agency (EFSA). Cadmium dietary exposure in the European population. *EFSA J.* **2012**, *10*, 2551. [CrossRef]
87. Callan, A.; Hinwood, A.; Devine, A. Metals in commonly eaten groceries in Western Australia: A market basket survey and dietary assessment. *Food Addit. Contam. Part A Chem. Anal. Control. Expo. Risk Assess.* **2014**, *31*, 1968–1981. [CrossRef] [PubMed]
88. Sand, S.; Becker, W. Assessment of dietary cadmium exposure in Sweden and population health concern including scenario analysis. *Food Chem. Toxicol.* **2012**, *50*, 536–544. [CrossRef] [PubMed]
89. Wei, J.; Gao, J.; Cen, K. Levels of eight heavy metals and health risk assessment considering food consumption by China's residents based on the 5th China total diet study. *Sci. Total Environ.* **2019**, *689*, 1141–1148. [CrossRef] [PubMed]
90. Xiao, G.; Liu, Y.; Dong, K.F.; Lu, J. Regional characteristics of cadmium intake in adult residents from the 4th and 5th Chinese total diet study. *Environ. Sci. Pollut. Res. Int.* **2020**, *27*, 3850–3857. [CrossRef]
91. Jin, Y.; Liu, P.; Sun, J.; Wang, C.; Min, J.; Zhang, Y.; Wang, S.; Wu, Y. Dietary exposure and risk assessment to lead of the population of Jiangsu province, China. Food Addit. *Contam. Part A Chem. Anal. Control. Expo. Risk Assess.* **2014**, *31*, 1187–1195.
92. Lim, J.A.; Kwon, H.J.; Ha, M.; Kim, H.; Oh, S.Y.; Kim, J.S.; Lee, S.A.; Park, J.D.; Hong, Y.S.; Sohn, S.J.; et al. Korean research project on the integrated exposure assessment of hazardous substances for food safety. *Environ. Health Toxicol.* **2015**, *30*, e2015004. [CrossRef]

93. Kim, H.; Lee, J.; Woo, H.D.; Kim, D.W.; Choi, I.J.; Kim, Y.I.; Kim, J. Association between dietary cadmium intake and early gastric cancer risk in a Korean population: A case-control study. *Eur. J. Nutr.* **2019**, *58*, 3255–3266. [CrossRef]
94. Schwarz, M.A.; Lindtner, O.; Blume, K.; Heinemeyer, G.; Schneider, K. Cadmium exposure from food: The German LExUKon project. *Food Addit. Contam. Part A Chem. Anal. Control. Expo. Risk Assess.* **2014**, *31*, 1038–1051. [CrossRef]
95. Marín, S.; Pardo, O.; Báguena, R.; Font, G.; Yusà, V. Dietary exposure to trace elements and health risk assessment in the region of Valencia, Spain: A total diet study. *Food Addit. Contam. Part A Chem. Anal. Control. Expo. Risk Assess.* **2017**, *34*, 228–240. [CrossRef]
96. Puerto-Parejo, L.M.; Aliaga, I.; Canal-Macias, M.L.; Leal-Hernandez, O.; Roncero-Martín, R.; Rico-Martín, S.; Moran, J.M. Evaluation of the dietary intake of cadmium, lead and mercury and its relationship with bone health among postmenopausal women in Spain. *Int. J. Environ. Res. Public Health* **2017**, *14*, 564. [CrossRef]
97. Kim, K.; Melough, M.M.; Vance, T.M.; Noh, H.; Koo, S.I.; Chun, O.K. Dietary cadmium intake and sources in the US. *Nutrients* **2018**, *11*, 2. [CrossRef] [PubMed]
98. Adams, S.V.; Quraishi, S.M.; Shafer, M.M.; Passarelli, M.N.; Freney, E.P.; Chlebowski, R.T.; Luo, J.; Meliker, J.R.; Mu, L.; Neuhouser, M.L.; et al. Dietary cadmium exposure and risk of breast, endometrial, and ovarian cancer in the Women's Health Initiative. *Environ. Health Perspect.* **2014**, *122*, 594–600. [CrossRef] [PubMed]
99. Filippini, T.; Cilloni, S.; Malavolti, M.; Violi, F.; Malagoli, C.; Tesauro, M.; Bottecchi, I.; Ferrari, A.; Vescovi, L.; Vinceti, M. Dietary intake of cadmium, chromium, copper, manganese, selenium and zinc in a Northern Italy community. *J. Trace Elem. Med. Biol.* **2018**, *50*, 508–517. [CrossRef] [PubMed]
100. Schneider, K.; Schwarz, M.A.; Lindtner, O.; Blume, K.; Heinemeyer, G. Lead exposure from food: The German LExUKon. *Food Addit. Contam. Part A Chem. Anal. Control. Expo. Risk Assess.* **2014**, *31*, 1052–1063. [CrossRef]
101. Arnich, N.; Sirot, V.; Rivière, G.; Jean, J.; Noël, L.; Guérin, T.; Leblanc, J.-C. Dietary exposure to trace elements and health risk assessment in the 2nd French Total Diet Study. *Food Chem. Toxicol.* **2012**, *50*, 2432–2449. [CrossRef]
102. Vromman, V.; Waegeneers, N.; Cornelis, C.; De Boosere, I.; Van Holderbeke, M.; Vinkx, C.; Smolders, E.; Huyghebaert, A.; Pussemier, L. Dietary cadmium intake by the Belgian adult population. *Food Addit. Contam. Part A Chem. Anal. Control. Expo. Risk Assess.* **2010**, *27*, 1665–1673. [CrossRef]
103. Horiguchi, H.; Oguma, E.; Sasaki, S.; Miyamoto, K.; Hosoi, Y.; Ono, A.; Kayama, F. Exposure assessment of cadmium in female farmers in cadmium-polluted areas in Northern Japan. *Toxics* **2020**, *8*, 44. [CrossRef]
104. Nishito, Y.; Kambe, T. Absorption mechanisms of iron, copper, and zinc: An overview. *J. Nutr. Sci. Vitaminol.* **2018**, *64*, 1–7. [CrossRef]
105. Vesey, D.A. Transport pathways for cadmium in the intestine and kidney proximal tubule: Focus on the interaction with essential metals. *Toxicol. Lett.* **2010**, *198*, 13–19. [CrossRef]
106. Thévenod, F.; Lee, W.-K.; Garrick, M.D. Iron and cadmium entry into renal mitochondria: Physiological and toxicological implications. *Front. Cell Develop. Biol.* **2020**, *8*, 848. [CrossRef]
107. Kovacs, G.; Danko, T.; Bergeron, M.J.; Balazs, B.; Suzuki, Y.; Zsembery, A.; Hediger, M.A. Heavy metal cations permeate the TRPV6 epithelial cation channel. *Cell Calcium.* **2011**, *49*, 43–55. [CrossRef] [PubMed]
108. Kovacs, G.; Montalbetti, N.; Franz, M.C.; Graeter, S.; Simonin, A.; Hediger, M.A. Human TRPV5 and TRPV6: Key players in cadmium and zinc toxicity. *Cell Calcium.* **2013**, *54*, 276–286. [CrossRef] [PubMed]
109. Fujishiro, H.; Hamao, S.; Tanaka, R.; Kambe, T.; Himeno, S. Concentration-dependent roles of DMT1 and ZIP14 in cadmium absorption in Caco-2 cells. *J. Toxicol. Sci.* **2017**, *42*, 559–567. [CrossRef] [PubMed]
110. Thevenod, F.; Fels, J.; Lee, W.-K.; Zarbock, R. Channels, transporters and receptors for cadmium and cadmium complexes in eukaryotic cells: Myths and facts. *Biometals* **2019**, *32*, 469–489. [CrossRef]
111. Mackenzie, B.; Takanaga, H.; Hubert, N.; Rolfs, A.; Hediger, M.A. Functional properties of multiple isoforms of human divalent metal-ion transporter 1 (DMT1). *Biochem. J.* **2007**, *403*, 59–69. [CrossRef]
112. Illing, A.C.; Shawki, A.; Cunningham, C.L.; Mackenzie, B. Substrate profile and metal-ion selectivity of human divalent metal-ion transporter-1. *J. Biol. Chem.* **2012**, *287*, 30485–30496. [CrossRef]
113. Bannon, D.I.; Abounader, R.; Lees, P.S.; Bressler, J.P. Effect of DMT1 knockdown on iron, cadmium, and lead uptake in Caco-2 cells. *Am. J. Physiol. Cell Physiol.* **2003**, *284*, C44–C50. [CrossRef]
114. Aduayom, I.; Jumarie, C. Reciprocal inhibition of Cd and Pb sulfocomplexes for uptake in Caco-2 cells. *J. Biochem. Mol. Toxicol.* **2005**, *19*, 256–265. [CrossRef]

115. Mitchell, C.J.; Shawki, A.; Ganz, T.; Nemeth, E.; Mackenzie, B. Functional properties of human ferroportin, a cellular iron exporter reactive also with cobalt and zinc. *Am. J. Physiol. Cell Physiol.* **2014**, *306*, C450–C459. [CrossRef]
116. Jeon, H.-K.; Jin, H.-S.; Lee, D.-H.; Choi, W.-S.; Moon, C.-K.; Oh, Y.J.; Lee, T.H. Proteome analysis associated with cadmium adaptation in U937 cells: Identification of calbindin-D28k as a secondary cadmium-responsive protein that confers resistance to cadmium-induced apoptosis. *J. Biol. Chem.* **2004**, *279*, 31575–31583. [CrossRef]
117. Fujita, Y.; ElBelbasi, H.I.; Min, K.-S.; Onosaka, S.; Okada, Y.; Matsumoto, Y.; Mutoh, N.; Tanaka, K. Fate of cadmium bound to phytochelatin in rats. *Res. Commun. Chem. Pathol. Pharmacol.* **1993**, *82*, 357–365. [PubMed]
118. Langelueddecke, C.; Roussa, E.; Fenton, R.A.; Thévenod, F. Expression and function of the lipocalin-2 (24p3/NGAL) receptor in rodent and human intestinal epithelia. *PLoS ONE* **2013**, *8*, e71586. [CrossRef] [PubMed]
119. Langelueddecke, C.; Lee, W.-K.; Thevenod, F. Differential transcytosis and toxicity of the hNGAL receptor ligands cadmium-metallothionein and cadmium-phytochelatin in colon-like Caco-2 cells: Implications for cadmium toxicity. *Toxicol. Lett.* **2014**, *226*, 228–235. [CrossRef] [PubMed]
120. Jorge-Nebert, L.F.; Gálvez-Peralta, M.; Figueroa, J.L.; Somarathna, M.; Hojyo, S.; Fukada, T.; Nebert, D.W. Comparing gene expression during cadmium uptake and distribution: Untreated versus oral Cd-treated wild-type and ZIP14 knockout mice. *Toxicol. Sci.* **2015**, *143*, 26–35. [CrossRef]
121. McKenna, I.M.; Gordon, T.; Chen, L.C.; Anver, M.R.; Waalkes, M.P. Expression of metallothionein protein in the lungs of Wistar rats and C57 and DBA mice exposed to cadmium oxide fumes. *Toxicol. Appl. Pharmacol.* **1998**, *153*, 169–178. [CrossRef]
122. Takeda, K.; Fujita, H.; Shibahara, S. Differential control of the metal-mediated activation of the human heme oxygenase-1 and metallothionein IIA genes. *Biochem. Biophys. Res. Commun.* **1995**, *207*, 160–167. [CrossRef]
123. Hart, B.A. Cellular and biochemical response of the rat lung to repeated inhalation of cadmium. *Toxicol. Appl. Pharmacol.* **1986**, *82*, 281–291. [CrossRef]
124. Hart, B.A.; Gong, Q.; Eneman, J.D. Pulmonary metallothionein expression in rats following single and repeated exposure to cadmium aerosols. *Toxicology* **1996**, *112*, 205–218. [CrossRef]
125. Chandler, J.D.; Wongtrakool, C.; Banton, S.A.; Li, S.; Orr, M.L.; Barr, D.B.; Neujahr, D.C.; Sutliff, R.L.; Go, Y.M.; Jones, D.P. Low-dose oral cadmium increases airway reactivity and lung neuronal gene expression in mice. *Physiol. Rep.* **2016**, *4*, e12821. [CrossRef]
126. Sabolić, I.; Breljak, D.; Skarica, M.; Herak-Kramberger, C.M. Role of metallothionein in cadmium traffic and toxicity in kidneys and other mammalian organs. *Biometals* **2010**, *23*, 897–926. [CrossRef]
127. Yu, J.; Fujishiro, H.; Miyataka, H.; Oyama, T.M.; Hasegawa, T.; Seko, Y.; Miura, N.; Himeno, S. Dichotomous effects of lead acetate on the expression of metallothionein in the liver and kidney of mice. *Biol. Pharm. Bull.* **2009**, *32*, 1037–1042. [PubMed]
128. Dai, S.; Yin, Z.; Yuan, G.; Lu, H.; Jia, R.; Xu, J.; Song, X.; Li, L.; Shu, Y.; Liang, X.; et al. Quantification of metallothionein on the liver and kidney of rats by subchronic lead and cadmium in combination. *Environ. Toxicol. Pharmacol.* **2013**, *36*, 1207–1216. [CrossRef] [PubMed]
129. Kikuchi, Y.; Nomiyama, T.; Kumagai, N.; Dekio, F.; Uemura, T.; Takebayashi, T.; Nishiwaki, Y.; Matsumoto, Y.; Sano, Y.; Hosoda, K.; et al. Uptake of cadmium in meals from the digestive tract of young non-smoking Japanese female volunteers. *J. Occup. Health* **2003**, *45*, 43–52. [CrossRef] [PubMed]
130. Wang, X.; Kim, D.; Tucker, K.L.; Weisskopf, M.G.; Sparrow, D.; Hu, H.; Park, S.K. Effect of dietary sodium and potassium on the mobilization of bone lead among middle-aged and older men: The Veterans Affairs Normative Aging Study. *Nutrients* **2019**, *11*, 2750.
131. Nielsen, R.; Christensen, E.I.; Birn, H. Megalin and cubilin in proximal tubule protein reabsorption: From experimental models to human disease. *Kidney Int.* **2016**, *89*, 58–67.
132. Onodera, A.; Tani, M.; Michigami, T.; Yamagata, M.; Min, K.S.; Tanaka, K.; Nakanishi, T.; Kimura, T.; Itoh, N. Role of megalin and the soluble form of its ligand RAP in Cd-metallothionein endocytosis and Cd-metallothionein-induced nephrotoxicity in vivo. *Toxicol. Lett.* **2012**, *212*, 91–96.
133. Langelueddecke, C.; Roussa, E.; Fenton, R.A.; Wolff, N.A.; Lee, W.K.; Thévenod, F. Lipocalin-2 (24p3/neutrophil gelatinase-associated lipocalin (NGAL)) receptor is expressed in distal nephron and mediates protein endocytosis. *J. Biol. Chem.* **2012**, *287*, 159–169.

134. Fels, J.; Scharner, B.; Zarbock, R.; Zavala Guevara, I.P.; Lee, W.K.; Barbier, O.C.; Thévenod, F. Cadmium complexed with β2-microglubulin, albumin and lipocalin-2 rather than metallothionein cause megalin:cubilin dependent toxicity of the renal proximal tubule. *Int. J. Mol. Sci.* **2019**, *20*, 2379.
135. Nascimento, C.R.B.; Risso, W.E.; Martinez, C.B.D.R. Lead accumulation and metallothionein content in female rats of different ages and generations after daily intake of Pb-contaminated food. *Environ. Toxicol. Pharmacol.* **2016**, *48*, 272–277.
136. Satarug, S.; Baker, J.R.; Reilly, P.E.; Moore, M.R.; Williams, D.J. Cadmium levels in the lung, liver, kidney cortex, and urine samples from Australians without occupational exposure to metals. *Arch. Environ. Health* **2002**, *57*, 69–77.
137. Baker, J.R.; Edwards, R.J.; Lasker, J.M.; Moore, M.R.; Satarug, S. Renal and hepatic accumulation of cadmium and lead in the expression of CYP4F2 and CYP2E1. *Toxicol. Lett.* **2005**, *159*, 182–191. [PubMed]
138. Barregard, L.; Fabricius-Lagging, E.; Lundh, T.; Mölne, J.; Wallin, M.; Olausson, M.; Modigh, C.; Sallstenm, G. Cadmium, mercury, and lead in kidney cortex of living kidney donors: Impact of different exposure sources. *Environ. Res.* **2010**, *110*, 47–54. [PubMed]
139. Järup, L.; Rogenfelt, A.; Elinder, C.G.; Nogawa, K.; Kjellström, T. Biological half-time of cadmium in the blood of workers after cessation of exposure. *Scand. J. Work Environ. Health* **1983**, *9*, 327–331. [PubMed]
140. Börjesson, J.; Bellander, T.; Järup, L.; Elinder, C.G.; Mattsson, S. In vivo analysis of cadmium in battery workers versus measurements of blood, urine, and workplace air. *Occup. Environ. Med.* **1997**, *54*, 424–531.
141. Suwazono, Y.; Kido, T.; Nakagawa, H.; Nishijo, M.; Honda, R.; Kobayashi, E.; Dochi, M.; Nogawa, K. Biological half-life of cadmium in the urine of inhabitants after cessation of cadmium exposure. *Biomarkers* **2009**, *14*, 77–81. [CrossRef]
142. Ishizaki, M.; Suwazono, Y.; Kido, T.; Nishijo, M.; Honda, R.; Kobayashi, E.; Nogawa, K.; Nakagawa, H. Estimation of biological half-life of urinary cadmium in inhabitants after cessation of environmental cadmium pollution using a mixed linear model. *Food Addit. Contam. Part A Chem. Anal. Control. Expo. Risk Assess.* **2015**, *32*, 1273–1276.
143. Fransson, M.N.; Barregard, L.; Sallsten, G.; Akerstrom, M.; Johanson, G. Physiologically-based toxicokinetic model for cadmium using Markov-chain Monte Carlo analysis of concentrations in blood, urine, and kidney cortex from living kidney donors. *Toxicol. Sci.* **2014**, *141*, 365–376.
144. Specht, A.J.; Lin, Y.; Weisskopf, M.; Yan, C.; Hu, H.; Xu, J.; Nie, L.H. XRF-measured bone lead (Pb) as a biomarker for Pb exposure and toxicity among children diagnosed with Pb poisoning. *Biomarkers* **2016**, *21*, 347–352.
145. Orlowski, C.; Piotrowski, J.K.; Subdys, J.K.; Gross, A. Urinary cadmium as indicator of renal cadmium in humans: An autopsy study. *Hum. Exp. Toxicol.* **1998**, *17*, 302–306.
146. Akerstrom, M.; Barregard, L.; Lundh, T.; Sallsten, G. The relationship between cadmium in kidney and cadmium in urine and blood in an environmentally exposed population. *Toxicol. Appl. Pharmacol.* **2013**, *268*, 286–293.
147. Wallin, M.; Sallsten, G.; Lundh, T.; Barregard, L. Low-level cadmium exposure and effects on kidney function. *Occup. Environ. Med.* **2014**, *71*, 848–854. [CrossRef] [PubMed]
148. Gerhardsson, L.; Englyst, V.; Lundström, N.G.; Sandberg, S.; Nordberg, G. Cadmium, copper and zinc in tissues of deceased copper smelter workers. *J. Trace Elem. Med. Biol.* **2002**, *16*, 261–266. [CrossRef]
149. Lou, M.; Garay, R.; Alda., J.O. Cadmium uptake through the anion exchanger in human red blood cells. *J. Physiol.* **1991**, *443*, 123–136. [CrossRef] [PubMed]
150. Wu, F.; Satchwell, T.J.; Toye, A.M. Anion exchanger 1 in red blood cells and kidney: Band 3's in a pod. *Biochem. Cell Biol.* **2011**, *89*, 106–114. [PubMed]
151. Parker, M.D.; Boron, W.F. The divergence, actions, roles, and relatives of sodium-coupled bicarbonate transporters. *Physiol. Rev.* **2013**, *93*, 803–959. [CrossRef]
152. Savigni, D.L.; Morgan, E.H. Transport mechanisms for iron and other transition metals in rat and rabbit erythroid cells. *J. Physiol.* **1998**, *508*, 837–850. [CrossRef] [PubMed]
153. Simons, T.J. The role of anion transport in the passive movement of lead across the human red cell membrane. *J. Physiol.* **1986**, *378*, 287–312. [CrossRef]
154. Simons, T.J. Lead transport and binding by human erythrocytes in vitro. *Pflugers Arch.* **1993**, *423*, 307–313. [CrossRef]

155. Lang, F.; Abed, M.; Lang, E.; Föller, M. Oxidative stress and suicidal erythrocyte death. *Antioxid. Redox Signal.* **2014**, *21*, 138–153. [CrossRef]
156. Lang, E.; Lang, F. Mechanisms and pathophysiological significance of eryptosis, the suicidal erythrocyte death. *Semin. Cell Dev. Biol.* **2015**, *39*, 35–42. [CrossRef]
157. Attanzio, A.; Frazzitta, A.; Vasto, S.; Tesoriere, L.; Pintaudi, A.M.; Livrea, M.A.; Cilla, A.; Allegra, M. Increased eryptosis in smokers is associated with the antioxidant status and C-reactive protein levels. *Toxicology* **2019**, *411*, 43–48. [CrossRef] [PubMed]
158. Scott, B.J.; Bradwell, A.R. Identification of the serum binding proteins for iron, zinc, cadmium, nickel, and calcium. *Clin. Chem.* **1983**, *29*, 629–633. [CrossRef] [PubMed]
159. Horn, N.M.; Thomas, A.L. Interactions between the histidine stimulation of cadmium and zinc influx into human erythrocytes. *J. Physiol.* **1996**, *496*, 711–718. [CrossRef] [PubMed]
160. Turell, L.; Radi, R.; Alvarez, B. The thiol pool in human plasma: The central contribution of albumin to redox processes. *Free Radic. Biol. Med.* **2013**, *65*, 244–253. [CrossRef] [PubMed]
161. Morris, T.T.; Keir, J.L.; Boshart, S.J.; Lobanov, V.P.; Ruhland, A.M.; Bahl, N.; Gailer, J. Mobilization of Cd from human serum albumin by small molecular weight thiols. *J. Chromatogr. B Anal. Technol. Biomed. Life Sci.* **2014**, *958*, 16–21. [CrossRef] [PubMed]
162. Sagmeister, P.; Gibson, M.A.; McDade, K.H.; Gailer, J. Physiologically relevant plasma d,l-homocysteine concentrations mobilize Cd from human serum albumin. *J. Chromatogr. B Anal. Technol. Biomed. Life Sci.* **2016**, *1027*, 181–186. [CrossRef] [PubMed]
163. Gaudet, M.M.; Deubler, E.L.; Kelly, R.S.; Diver, W.R.; Teras, L.R.; Hodge, J.M.; Levine, K.E.; Haines, L.G.; Lundh, T.; Lenner, P.; et al. Blood levels of cadmium and lead in relation to breast cancer risk in three prospective cohorts. *Int. J. Cancer* **2019**, *144*, 1010–1016. [CrossRef] [PubMed]
164. Lin, J.; Zhang, F.; Lei, Y. Dietary intake and urinary level of cadmium and breast cancer risk: A meta-analysis. *Cancer Epidemiol.* **2016**, *42*, 101–107. [CrossRef]
165. Rokadia, H.K.; Agarwal, S. Serum heavy metals and obstructive lung disease: Results from the National Health and Nutrition Examination Survey. *Chest* **2013**, *143*, 388–397. [CrossRef]
166. Yang, G.; Sun, T.; Han, Y.Y.; Rosser, F.; Forno, E.; Chen, W.; Celedón, J.C. Serum cadmium and lead, current wheeze, and lung function in a nationwide study of adults in the United States. *J. Allergy Clin. Immunol. Pract.* **2019**, *7*, 2653–2660.e3. [CrossRef]
167. Bergdahl, I.A.; Schütz, A.; Gerhardsson, L.; Jensen, A.; Skerfving, S. Lead concentrations in human plasma, urine and whole blood. *Scand. J. Work Environ. Health* **1997**, *23*, 359–363. [CrossRef] [PubMed]
168. Manton, W.I.; Rothenberg, S.J.; Manalo, M. The lead content of blood serum. *Environ. Res.* **2001**, *86*, 263–273. [CrossRef] [PubMed]
169. Smith, D.; Hernandez-Avila, M.; Téllez-Rojo, M.M.; Mercado, A.; Hu, H. The relationship between lead in plasma and whole blood in women. *Environ. Health Perspect.* **2002**, *110*, 263–268. [CrossRef]
170. Barbosa, F., Jr.; Tanus-Santos, J.E.; Gerlach, R.F.; Parsons, P.J. A critical review of biomarkers used for monitoring human exposure to lead: Advantages, limitations, and future needs. *Environ. Health Perspect.* **2005**, *113*, 1669–1674. [CrossRef]
171. Gulson, B.L.; Mizon, K.J.; Korsch, M.J.; Horwarth, D.; Phillips, A.; Hall, J. Impact on blood lead in children and adults following relocation from their source of exposure and contribution of skeletal tissue to blood lead. *Bull. Environ. Contam. Toxicol.* **1996**, *56*, 543–550.
172. Gulson, B.L.; Mahaffey, K.R.; Mizon, K.F.; Korsch, M.J.; Cameron, M.A.; Vimpani, G. Contribution of tissue lead to bone lead in adult female subjects based on stable lead-isotope methods. *J. Lab. Clin. Med.* **1995**, *125*, 703–712. [PubMed]
173. Gwiazda, R.; Campbell, C.; Smith, D. A noninvasive isotopic approach to estimate the bone lead contribution to blood in children: Implications for assessing the efficacy of lead abatement. *Environ. Health Perspect.* **2005**, *113*, 104–110. [CrossRef] [PubMed]
174. Manton, W.I.; Angle, C.R.; Stanek, K.L.; Reese, Y.R.; Kuehnemann, T.J. Acquisition and retention of lead by young children. *Environ. Res.* **2000**, *82*, 60–80. [CrossRef]
175. Roberts, J.R.; Reigart., J.R.; Ebeling., M.; Hulsey, T.C. Time required for blood lead levels to decline in nonchelated children. *Clin. Toxicol.* **2001**, *39*, 153–160. [CrossRef]
176. Landrigan, P.J.; Todd, A.C. Direct measurement of lead in bone-a promising biomarker. *JAMA* **1994**, *271*, 239–240. [CrossRef]

177. O'Flaherty, E.J. Physiologically based models for bone-seeking elements V: Lead absorption and disposition in childhood. *Toxicol. Appl. Pharmacol.* **1995**, *131*, 297–308. [CrossRef] [PubMed]
178. Hu, H.; Rabinowitz, M.; Smith., D. Bone lead as a biological marker in epidemiologic studies of chronic toxicity: Conceptual paradigms. *Environ. Health Perspect.* **1998**, *106*, 1–8. [CrossRef]
179. Nilsson, U.; Attewell, R.; Christoffersson, J.O.; Schütz, A.; Ahlgren, L.; Skerfving, S.; Mattsson, S. Kinetics of lead in bone and blood after end of occupational exposure. *Pharmacol. Toxicol.* **1991**, *68*, 477–484. [CrossRef] [PubMed]
180. Price, J.; Grudzinski, A.W.; Craswell, P.W.; Thomas, B.J. Repeated bone lead levels in Queensland, Australia—Previously a high lead environment. *Arch. Environ. Health* **1992**, *47*, 256–262. [CrossRef] [PubMed]
181. Brito, J.A.; McNeill, F.E.; Stronach, I.; Webber, C.E.; Wells, S.; Richard, N.; Chettle, D.R. Longitudinal changes in bone lead concentration: Implications for modelling of human bone lead metabolism. *J. Environ. Monit.* **2001**, *3*, 343–351. [CrossRef] [PubMed]
182. Wilker, E.; Korrick, S.; Nie, L.H.; Sparrow, D.; Vokonas, P.; Coull, B.; Wright, R.O.; Schwartz., J.; Hu, H. Longitudinal changes in bone lead levels: The VA normative aging study. *J. Occup. Environ. Med.* **2011**, *53*, 850–855. [CrossRef] [PubMed]
183. Gerhardsson, L.; Akantis, A.; Lundström, N.G.; Nordberg, G.F.; Schütz, A.; Skerfving, S. Lead concentrations in cortical and trabecular bones in deceased smelter workers. *J. Trace Elem. Med. Biol.* **2005**, *19*, 209–215. [CrossRef] [PubMed]
184. Gerhardsson, L.; Englyst, V.; Lundström, N.G.; Nordberg, G.; Sandberg, S.; Steinvall, F. Lead in tissues of deceased lead smelter workers. *J. Trace Elem. Med. Biol.* **1995**, *9*, 136–143. [CrossRef]
185. Hernandez-Avila, M.; Smith, D.; Meneses, F.; Sanin, L.H.; Hu, H. The influence of bone and blood lead on plasma lead levels in environmentally exposed adults. *Environ. Health Perspect.* **1998**, *106*, 473–477. [CrossRef]
186. Hu, H.; Shih, R.; Rothenberg, S.; Schwartz, B.S. The epidemiology of lead toxicity in adults: Measuring dose and consideration of other methodologic issues. *Environ. Health Perspect.* **2007**, *115*, 455–462. [CrossRef]
187. Shih, R.A.; Hu, H.; Weisskopf, M.G.; Schwartz, B.S. Cumulative lead dose and cognitive function in adults: A review of studies that measured both blood lead and bone lead. *Environ. Health Perspect.* **2007**, *115*, 483–492. [CrossRef] [PubMed]
188. Farooqui, Z.; Bakulski, K.M.; Power, M.C.; Weisskopf, M.G.; Sparrow, D.; Spiro, A., III; Vokonas, P.S.; Nie, L.H.; Hu, H.; Park, S.K. Associations of cumulative Pb exposure and longitudinal changes in mini-mental status exam scores, global cognition and domains of cognition: The VA normative aging study. *Environ. Res.* **2017**, *152*, 102–108. [CrossRef] [PubMed]
189. Wright, R.O.; Tsaih, S.W.; Schwartz, J.; Spiro, A., III; McDonald, K.; Weiss, S.T.; Hu, H. Lead exposure biomarkers and mini-mental status exam scores in older men. *Epidemiology* **2003**, *14*, 713–718. [CrossRef] [PubMed]
190. Zheutlin, A.R.; Hu, H.; Weisskopf, M.G.; Sparrow, D.; Vokonas, P.S.; Park, S.K. Low-level cumulative lead and resistant hypertension: A prospective study of men participating in the Veterans Affairs normative aging study. *J. Am. Heart Assoc.* **2018**, *7*, e010014. [CrossRef] [PubMed]
191. Hirata, M.; Yoshida, T.; Miyajima, K.; Kosaka, H.; Tabuchi, T. Correlation between lead in plasma and other indicators of lead exposure among lead-exposed workers. *Int. Arch. Occup. Environ. Health* **1995**, *68*, 58–63. [CrossRef] [PubMed]
192. Schütz, A.; Olsson, M.; Jensen, A.; Gerhardsson, L.; Börjesson, J.; Mattsson, S.; Skerfving, S. Lead in finger bone, whole blood, plasma and urine in lead-smelter workers: Extended exposure range. *Int. Arch. Occup. Environ. Health* **2005**, *78*, 35–43. [CrossRef] [PubMed]
193. Fukui, Y.; Miki, M.; Ukai, H.; Okamoto, S.; Takada, S.; Higashikawa, K.; Ikeda, M. Urinary lead as a possible surrogate of blood lead among workers occupationally exposed to lead. *Int. Arch. Occup. Environ. Health* **1999**, *72*, 516–520. [CrossRef]
194. Bai, Y.; Laenen, A.; Haufroid, V.; Nawrot, T.S.; Nemery, B. Urinary lead in relation to combustion-derived air pollution in urban environments. A longitudinal study of an international panel. *Environ. Int.* **2019**, *125*, 75–81. [CrossRef]
195. Wang, X.; Jin, P.; Zhou, Q.; Liu, S.; Wang, F.; Xi, S. Metal biomonitoring and comparative assessment in urine of workers in lead-zinc and steel-iron mining and smelting. *Biol. Trace Elem. Res.* **2019**, *189*, 1–9. [CrossRef]

196. Li, S.; Wang, J.; Zhang, B.; Liu, Y.; Lu, T.; Shi, Y.; Shan, G.; Dong, L. Urinary lead concentration is an independent predictor of cancer mortality in the U.S. general population. *Front. Oncol.* **2018**, *8*, 242. [CrossRef]
197. Dudley, R.E.; Gammal, L.M.; Klaassen, C.D. Cadmium-induced hepatic and renal injury in chronically exposed rats: Likely role of hepatic cadmium-metallothionein in nephrotoxicity. *Toxicol. Appl. Pharmacol.* **1985**, *77*, 414–426. [CrossRef]
198. Chan, H.M.; Zhu, L.F.; Zhong, R.; Grant, D.; Goyer, R.A.; Cherian, M.G. Nephrotoxicity in rats following liver transplantation from cadmium-exposed rats. *Toxicol. Appl. Pharmacol.* **1993**, *123*, 89–96. [CrossRef] [PubMed]
199. Shaikh, Z.A.; Vu, T.T.; Zaman, K. Oxidative stress as a mechanism of chronic cadmium-induced hepatoxicity and renal toxicity and protection by antioxidants. *Toxicol. Appl. Pharmacol.* **1999**, *154*, 256–263. [CrossRef] [PubMed]
200. Goyer, R.A.; Miller, C.R.; Zhu, S.-Y.; Victery, W. Non-metallothionein-bound cadmium in the pathogenesis of cadmium nephrotoxicity in the rat. *Toxicol. Appl. Pharmacol.* **1989**, *101*, 232–244. [CrossRef]
201. Liu, Y.; Liu, J.; Habeebu, S.S.M.; Klaasen, C.D. Metallothionein protects against the nephrotoxicity produced by chronic CdMT exposure. *Toxicol. Sci.* **1999**, *50*, 221–227. [CrossRef] [PubMed]
202. Vestergaard, P.; Shaikh, Z.A. The nephrotoxicity of intravenously administered cadmium-metallothionein: Effect of dose, mode of administration, and preexisting renal cadmium burden. *Toxicol. Appl. Pharmacol.* **1994**, *126*, 240–247. [CrossRef] [PubMed]
203. Min, K.S.; Onosaka, S.; Tanaka, K. Renal accumulation of cadmium and nephropathy following long-term administration of cadmium-metallothionein. *Toxicol. Appl. Pharmacol.* **1996**, *141*, 102–109. [CrossRef]
204. Price, R.G. The role of NAG (N-acetyl-β-D-glucosaminidase) in the diagnosis of kidney disease including the monitoring of nephrotoxicity. *Clin. Nephrol.* **1992**, *38*, S14–S19.
205. Bernard, A.; Thielemans, N.; Roels, H.; Lauwerys, R. Association between NAG-B and cadmium in urine with no evidence of a threshold. *Occup. Environ. Med.* **1995**, *52*, 177–180. [CrossRef]
206. Jin, T.; Nordberg, G.; Wu, X.; Kong, Q.; Wang, Z.; Zhuang, F.; Cai, S. Urinary N-acetyl-beta-D-glucosaminidase isoenzymes as biomarker of renal dysfunction caused by cadmium in a general population. *Environ. Res.* **1999**, *81*, 167–173. [CrossRef]
207. Tassi, C.; Abbritti, G.; Mancuso, F.; Morucci, P.; Feligioni, L.; Muzi, G. Activity and isoenzyme profile of N-acetyl-beta-D-glucosaminidase in urine from workers exposed to cadmium. *Clin. Chim. Acta* **2000**, *299*, 55–64. [CrossRef]
208. Prozialeck, W.C.; Edwards, J.R. Early biomarkers of cadmium exposure and nephrotoxicity. *Biometals* **2010**, *23*, 793–809. [CrossRef] [PubMed]
209. Prozialeck, W.C.; Vaidya, V.S.; Liu, J.; Waalkes, M.P.; Edwards, J.R.; Lamar, P.C.; Bernard, A.M.; Dumont, X.; Bonventre, J.V. Kidney injury molecule-1 is an early biomarker of cadmium nephrotoxicity. *Kidney Int.* **2007**, *72*, 985–993. [CrossRef]
210. Prozialeck, W.C.; Edwards, J.R.; Vaidya, V.S.; Bonventre, J.V. Preclinical evaluation of novel urinary biomarkers of cadmium nephrotoxicity. *Toxicol. Appl. Pharmacol.* **2009**, *238*, 301–305. [CrossRef] [PubMed]
211. Prozialeck, W.C.; Edwards, J.R.; Lamar, P.C.; Liu, J.; Vaidya, V.S.; Bonventre, J.V. Expression of kidney injury molecule-1 (Kim-1) in relation to necrosis and apoptosis during the early stages of Cd-induced proximal tubular injury. *Toxicol. Appl. Pharmacol.* **2009**, *238*, 306–314. [CrossRef]
212. Pennemans, V.; De Winter, L.M.; Munters, E.; Nawrot, T.S.; Van Kerhove, E.; Rigo, J.-M.; Reynders, C.; Dewitte, H.; Carleer, R.; Penders, J.; et al. The association between urinary kidney injury molecule 1 and urinary cadmium in elderly during long-term, low-dose cadmium exposure: A pilot study. *Environ. Health* **2011**, *10*, 77. [CrossRef]
213. Ruangyuttikarn, W.; Panyamoon, A.; Nambunmee, K.; Honda, R.; Swaddiwudhipong, W.; Nishijo, M. Use of the kidney injury molecule-1 as a biomarker for early detection of renal tubular dysfunction in a population chronically exposed to cadmium in the environment. *Springerplus* **2013**, *2*, 533. [CrossRef]
214. Zhang, Y.; Wang, P.; Liang, X.; Chuen, S.; Tan, J.; Wang, J.; Huang, Q.; Huang, R.; Li, Z.; Chen, W.; et al. Associations between urinary excretion of cadmium and renal biomarkers in nonsmoking females: A cross-sectional study in rural areas of South China. *Int. J. Environ. Res. Public Health* **2015**, *12*, 11988–12001. [CrossRef]
215. Chaumont, A.; Voisin, C.; Deumer, G.; Haufroid, V.; Annesi-Maesano, I.; Roels, H.; Thijs, L.; Staessen, J.; Bernard, A. Associations of urinary cadmium with age and urinary proteins: Further evidence of physiological

variations unrelated to metal accumulation and toxicity. *Environ. Health Perspect.* **2013**, *121*, 1047–1053. [CrossRef]
216. Nomiyama, K.; Foulkes, E.C. Reabsorption of filtered cadmium-metallothionein in the rabbit kidney. *Proc. Soc. Exp. Biol. Med.* **1977**, *156*, 97–99. [CrossRef]
217. Tanimoto, A.; Hamada, T.; Koide, O. Cell death and regeneration of renal proximal tubular cells in rats with subchronic cadmium intoxication. *Toxicol. Pathol.* **1993**, *21*, 341–352. [CrossRef] [PubMed]
218. Roels, H.A.; Lauwerys, R.R.; Buchyet, J.-P.; Bernard, A.; Chettle, D.R.; Harvey, T.C.; Al-Haddad, I.K. In vivo measurement of liver and kidney cadmium in workers exposed to this metal: Its significance with respect to cadmium in blood and urine. *Environ. Res.* **1981**, *26*, 217–240. [CrossRef]
219. Weaver, V.M.; Kim, N.-S.; Jaar, B.G.; Schwartz, B.S.; Parsons, P.J.; Steuerwald, A.J.; Todd, A.C.; Simon, D.; Lee, B.-K. Associations of low-level urine cadmium with kidney function in lead workers. *Occup. Environ. Med.* **2011**, *68*, 250–256. [CrossRef] [PubMed]
220. Buser, M.C.; Ingber, S.Z.; Raines, N.; Fowler, D.A.; Scinicariello, F. Urinary and blood cadmium and lead and kidney function: NHANES 2007–2012. *Int. J. Hyg. Environ. Health* **2016**, *219*, 261–267. [CrossRef]
221. Jin, R.; Zhu, X.; Shrubsole, M.J.; Yu, C.; Xia, Z.; Dai, Q. Associations of renal function with urinary excretion of metals: Evidence from NHANES 2003–2012. *Environ. Int.* **2018**, *121*, 1355–1362. [CrossRef]
222. Kawada, T.; Koyama, H.; Suzuki, S. Cadmium, NAG activity, and β2-microglobulin in the urine of cadmium pigment workers. *Br. J. Ind. Med.* **1989**, *46*, 52–55.
223. Kawada, T.; Shinmyo, R.R.; Suzuki, S. Urinary cadmium and N-acetyl-β-D-glucosaminidase excretion of inhabitants living in a cadmium-polluted area. *Int. Arch. Occup. Environ. Health* **1992**, *63*, 541–546. [CrossRef]
224. Koyama, H.; Satoh, H.; Suzuki, S.; Tohyama, C. Increased cadmium excretion and its relationship to urinary N-acetyl-β-D-glucosaminidase activity in smokers. *Arch. Toxicol.* **1992**, *66*, 598–601. [CrossRef]
225. Thomas, L.D.; Hodgson, S.; Nieuwenhuijsen, M.; Jarup, L. Early kidney damage in a population exposed to cadmium and other heavy metals. *Environ. Health Perspect.* **2009**, *117*, 181–184. [CrossRef]
226. Wang, D.; Sun, H.; Wu, Y.; Zhou, Z.; Ding, Z.; Chen, X.; Xu, Y. Tubular and glomerular kidney effects in the Chinese general population with low environmental cadmium exposure. *Chemosphere* **2016**, *147*, 3–8. [CrossRef]
227. Akesson, A.; Lundh, T.; Vahter, M.; Bjellerup, P.; Lidfeldt, J.; Nerbrand, C.; Samsioe, G.; Strömberg, U.; Skerfving, S. Tubular and glomerular kidney effects in Swedish women with low environmental cadmium exposure. *Environ. Health Perspect.* **2005**, *113*, 1627–1631. [CrossRef] [PubMed]
228. Eom, S.-Y.; Seo, M.-N.; Lee, Y.-S.; Park, K.-S.; Hong, Y.-S.; Sohn, S.-J.; Kim, Y.-D.; Choi, B.-S.; Lim, J.-A.; Kwon, H.-J.; et al. Low-level environmental cadmium exposure induces kidney tubule damage in the general population of Korean adults. *Arch. Environ. Contam. Toxicol.* **2017**, *73*, 401–409. [CrossRef] [PubMed]
229. Swaddiwudhipong, W.; Limpatanachote, P.; Mahasakpan, P.; Krintratun, S.; Punta, B.; Funkhiew, T. Progress in cadmium-related health effects in persons with high environmental exposure in northwestern Thailand: A five-year follow-up. *Environ. Res.* **2012**, *112*, 194–198. [CrossRef] [PubMed]
230. Piscator, M. Long-term observations on tubular and glomerular function in cadmium-exposed persons. *Environ. Health Perspect.* **1984**, *54*, 175–179. [CrossRef] [PubMed]
231. Roels, H.A.; Lauwerys, R.R.; Buchyet, J.P.; Bernard, A.M.; Vos, A.; Oversteyns, M. Health significance of cadmium induced renal dysfunction: A five year follow up. *Br. J. Ind. Med.* **1989**, *46*, 755–764. [CrossRef] [PubMed]
232. Jarup, L.; Persson, B.; Elinder, C.G. Decreased glomerular filtration rate in solderers exposed to cadmium. *Occup. Environ. Med.* **1995**, *52*, 818–822. [CrossRef] [PubMed]
233. Mason, H.J.; Davison, A.G.; Wright, A.L.; Guthrie, C.J.G.; Fayers, P.M.; Venables, K.M.; Smith, N.J.; Chettle, D.R.; Franklin, D.M.; Scott, M.C.; et al. Relations between liver cadmium, cumulative exposure, and renal function in cadmium alloy workers. *Br. J. Ind. Med.* **1988**, *45*, 793–802. [CrossRef] [PubMed]
234. Satarug, S.; Moore, M.R. Adverse health effects of chronic exposure to low-level cadmium in foodstuffs and cigarette smoke. *Environ. Health Perspect.* **2004**, *112*, 1099–1103. [CrossRef] [PubMed]
235. Schnaper, H.W. The tubulointerstitial pathophysiology of progressive kidney disease. *Adv. Chronic Kidney Dis.* **2017**, *24*, 107–116. [CrossRef]
236. Schardijn, G.H.C.; Statius van Eps, L.W. β_2-microglobulin: Its significance in the evaluation of renal function. *Kidney Int.* **1987**, *32*, 635–641. [CrossRef]

237. Hall, P.W., III; Chung-Park, M.; Vacca, C.V.; London, M.; Crowley, A.Q. The renal handling of beta$_2$-microglobulin in the dog. *Kidney Int.* **1982**, *22*, 156–161. [CrossRef] [PubMed]
238. Gauthier, C.; Nguyen-Simonnet, H.; Vincent, C.; Revillard, J.-P.; Pellet, M.V. Renal tubular absorption of β2-microglobulin. *Kidney Int.* **1984**, *26*, 170–175. [CrossRef] [PubMed]
239. Norden, A.G.W.; Lapsley, M.; Lee, P.J.; Pusey, C.D.; Scheinman, S.J.; Tam, F.W.K.; Thakker, R.V.; Unwin, R.J.; Wrong, O. Glomerular protein sieving and implications for renal failure in Fanconi syndrome. *Kidney Int.* **2001**, *60*, 1885–1892. [CrossRef] [PubMed]
240. Wibell, L.; Evrin, P.-E.; Berggard, J. Serum β$_2$-microglobulin in renal disease. *Nephron* **1973**, *10*, 320–331. [CrossRef]
241. Wibell, L.B. Studies on β2-microglobulin in patients and normal subjects. *Acta Clin. Belg.* **1976**, *31*, 14–26.
242. Wibell, L. The serum level and urinary excretion of β2-microglobulin in health and renal disease. *Pathol. Biol. (Paris)* **1978**, *26*, 295–301.
243. Hall, P.W., III; Ricanati, E.S. Renal handling of β2-microglobulin in renal disorders with special reference to hepatorenal syndrome. *Nephron* **1981**, *27*, 62–66. [CrossRef]
244. Portman, R.J.; Kissane, J.M.; Robson, A.M. Use of β2-microglobulin to diagnose tubulo-interstitial renal lesions in children. *Kidney Int.* **1986**, *30*, 91–98. [CrossRef]
245. Bernard, A. Renal dysfunction induced by cadmium: Biomarkers of critical effects. *Biometals* **2004**, *17*, 519–523. [CrossRef]
246. Nogawa, K.; Kobayashi, E.; Honda, R. A study of the relationship between cadmium concentrations in urine and renal effects of cadmium. *Environ. Health Perspect.* **1979**, *28*, 161–168. [CrossRef]
247. Ikeda, M.; Ezaki, T.; Moriguchi, J.; Fukui, Y.; Ukai, H.; Okamoto, S.; Sakurai, H. The threshold cadmium level that causes a substantial increase in β2-microglobulin in urine of general populations. *Tohoku J. Exp. Med.* **2005**, *205*, 247–261. [CrossRef] [PubMed]
248. Peterson, P.A.; Evrin, P.-E.; Berggard, I. Differentiation of glomerular, tubular, and normal proteinuria: Determinations of urinary excretion of β2-microglobulin, albumin, and total protein. *J. Clin. Investig.* **1969**, *48*, 1189–1198. [CrossRef] [PubMed]
249. Elinder, C.G.; Edling, C.; Lindberg, E.; Agedal, B.K.; Vesterberg, A. Assessment of renal function in workers previously exposed to cadmium. *Br. J. Ind. Med.* **1985**, *42*, 754–760. [CrossRef]
250. Norden, A.G.W.; Lapsley, M.; Unwin, R.J. Urine retinol-binding protein 4: A functional biomarker of the proximal renal tubule. *Adv. Clin. Chem.* **2014**, *63*, 85–122. [PubMed]
251. Blaner, W.S. Retinol-binding protein: The serum transport protein for vitamin A. *Endocri. Rev.* **1989**, *10*, 308–316. [CrossRef]
252. Pallet, N.; Chauvet, S.; Chasse, J.-F.; Vincent, M.; Avilloach, P.; Levi, C.; Meas-Yedid, V.; Olivo-Marin, J.-C.; Nga-Matsogo, D.; Beaune, P.; et al. Urinary retinol binding protein is a marker of the extent of interstitial kidney fibrosis. *PLoS ONE* **2014**, *9*, e84708. [CrossRef]
253. Bernard, A.; Vyskocyl, A.; Mahieu, P.; Lauwerys, R. Effect of renal insufficiency on the concentration of free retinol-binding protein in urine and serum. *Clin. Chim. Acta* **1988**, *171*, 85–94. [CrossRef]
254. Jarup, L.; Akesson, A. Current status of cadmium as an environmental health problem. *Toxicol. Appl. Pharmacol.* **2009**, *238*, 201–208. [CrossRef]
255. Heymsfield, S.B.; Arteaga, C.; McManus, C.; Smith, J.; Moffitt, S. Measurement of muscle mass in humans: Validity of the 24-hour urinary creatinine method. *Am. J. Clin. Nutr.* **1983**, *37*, 478–494. [CrossRef]
256. Jenny-Burri, J.; Haldimann, M.; Bruschweiler, B.J.; Bochuyd, M.; Burnier, M.; Paccaud, F.; Dudler, V. Cadmium body burden of the Swiss population. *Food Addit. Contam. Part A Chem. Anal. Control. Expo. Risk Assess.* **2015**, *32*, 1265–1272. [CrossRef]
257. Chevalier, R.L.; Forbes, M.S. Generation and evolution of atubular glomeruli in the progression of renal disorders. *J. Am. Soc. Nephrol.* **2008**, *19*, 197–206. [CrossRef]
258. Ferenbach, D.A.; Bonventre, J.V. Acute kidney injury and chronic kidney disease: From the laboratory to the clinic. *Nephrol. Ther.* **2016**, *12* (Suppl. 1), S41–S48. [CrossRef]
259. Zammouri, A.; Barbouch, S.; Najjar, M.; Aoudia, R.; Jaziri, F.; Kaaroud, H.; Hedri, H.; Abderrahim, E.; Goucha, R.; Hamida, F.B.; et al. Tubulointerstitial nephritis due to sarcoidosis: Clinical, laboratory, and histological features and outcome in a cohort of 24 patients. *Saudi J. Kidney Dis. Transpl.* **2019**, *30*, 1276–1284. [CrossRef]

260. Goules, A.; Geetha, D.; Arend, L.J.; Baer, A.N. Renal involvement in primary Sjogren's syndrome: Natural history and treatment outcome. *Clin. Exp. Rheumatol.* **2019**, *37* (Suppl. 118), S123–S132.
261. Jasiek, M.; Karras, A.; Le Guern, V.; Krastinova, E.; Mesbah, R.; Faguer, S.; Jourde-Chiche, N.; Fauchais, A.-L.; Chiche, L.; Dernis, E.; et al. A multicentre study of 95 biopsy-proven cases of renal disease in primary Sjogren's syndrome. *Rheumatology* **2017**, *56*, 362–370. [CrossRef] [PubMed]
262. Kelly, C.J.; Neilson, E.G. Tubulointerstitial diseases. In *Brenner & Rector's The Kidney*, 10th ed.; Taal, M.W., Chertow, G.M., Marsden, P.A., Skorecki, K., Alan, S.L., Brenner, B.M., Eds.; Elsevier: Philadelphia, PA, USA, 2011; pp. 1209–1230.
263. Nath, K.A. Tubulointerstitial changes as a major determinant in the progression of renal damage. *Am. J. Kidney Dis.* **1992**, *20*, 1–17. [CrossRef]
264. Risdon, R.A.; Sloper, J.C.; De Wardener, H.E. Relationship between renal function and histological changes found in renal-biopsy specimens from patients with persistent glomerular nephritis. *Lancet* **1968**, *292*, 363–366. [CrossRef]
265. Schainuck, L.I.; Striker, G.E.; Cutler, R.E.; Benditt, E.P. Structural-functional correlations in renal disease: Part II: The correlations. *Human Pathol.* **1970**, *1*, 631–641. [CrossRef]
266. Bohle, A.; von Gise, H.; Mackensen-Haen, S.; Stark-Jakob, B. The obliteration of the postglomerular capillaries and its influence upon the function of both glomeruli and tubuli. Functional interpretation of morphologic findings. *Klin. Wochenschr.* **1981**, *59*, 1043–1051. [CrossRef]
267. Baba, H.; Tsuneyama, K.; Kumada, T.; Aoshima, K.; Imura, J. Histopathological analysis for osteomalacia and tubulopathy in itai-itai disease. *J. Toxicol. Sci.* **2014**, *39*, 91–96. [CrossRef]
268. Yasuda, M.; Miwa, A.; Kitagawa, M. Morphometric studies of renal lesions in itai-itai disease: Chronic cadmium nephropathy. *Nephron* **1995**, *69*, 14–19. [CrossRef] [PubMed]
269. Saito, H.; Shioji, R.; Hurukawa, Y.; Nagai, K.; Arikawa, T. Cadmium-induced proximal tubular dysfunction in a cadmium-polluted area. *Contrib. Nephrol.* **1977**, *6*, 1–12. [PubMed]
270. Nogawa, K.; Ishizaki, A.; Fukushima, M.; Shibata, I.; Hagino, N. Studies on the women with acquired Fanconi syndrome observed in the Ichi River basin polluted by cadmium. *Environ. Res.* **1975**, *10*, 280–307. [CrossRef]
271. Rappaport, S.M.; Smith, M.T. Environment and disease risks. *Science* **2010**, *330*, 460–461. [CrossRef]
272. Lee, J.; Oh, S.; Kang, H.; Kim, S.; Lee, G.; Li, L.; Kim, C.T.; An, J.N.; Oh, Y.K.; Lim, C.S.; et al. Environment-wide association study of CKD. *Clin. J. Am. Soc. Nephrol.* **2020**, *15*, 766–775. [CrossRef]
273. Soderland, P.; Lovekar, S.; Weiner, D.E.; Brooks, D.R.; Kaufman, J.S. Chronic kidney disease associated with environmental toxins and exposures. *Adv. Chronic Kidney Dis.* **2010**, *17*, 254–264. [CrossRef]
274. Chevalier, R.L. The proximal tubule is the primary target of injury and progression of kidney disease: Role of the glomerulotubular junction. *Am. J. Physiol. Renal. Physiol.* **2016**, *311*, F145–F161. [CrossRef]
275. Crowley, S.D.; Coffman, T.M. The inextricable role of the kidney in hypertension. *J. Clin. Investig.* **2014**, *124*, 2341–2347.
276. Nakhoul, N.; Batuman, V. Role of proximal tubules in the pathogenesis of kidney disease. *Contrib. Nephrol.* **2011**, *169*, 37–50.
277. De Nicola, L.; Zoccali, C. Chronic kidney disease prevalence in the general population: Heterogeneity and concerns. *Nephrol. Dial. Transplant.* **2016**, *31*, 331–335. [CrossRef]
278. Glassock, R.J.; David, G.; Warnock, D.G.; Delanaye, P. The global burden of chronic kidney disease: Estimates, variability and pitfalls. *Nat. Rev. Nephrol.* **2017**, *13*, 104–114. [CrossRef] [PubMed]
279. Chen, T.K.; Knicely, D.H.; Grams, M.E. Chronic kidney disease diagnosis and management: A review. *JAMA* **2019**, *322*, 1294–1304. [CrossRef] [PubMed]
280. Lees, J.S.; Welsh, C.E.; Celis-Morales, C.A.; Mackay, D.; Lewsey, J.; Gray, S.R.; Lyall, D.M.; Cleland, J.G.; Gill, J.M.R.; Jhund, P.S.; et al. Glomerular filtration rate by differing measures, albuminuria and prediction of cardiovascular disease, mortality and end-stage kidney disease. *Nat. Med.* **2019**, *25*, 1753–1760. [CrossRef] [PubMed]
281. Sarnak, M.J.; Amann, K.; Bangalore, S.; Cavalcante, J.L.; Charytan, D.M.; Craig, J.C.; Gill, J.S.; Hlatky, M.A.; Jardine, A.G.; Landmesser, U.; et al. Chronic kidney disease and coronary artery disease: JACC state-of-the-art review. *J. Am. Coll. Cardiol.* **2019**, *74*, 1823–1838. [CrossRef] [PubMed]
282. Liu, Y.; Lv, P.; Jin, H.; Cui, W.; Niu, C.; Zhao, M.; Fan, C.; Teng, Y.; Pan, B.; Peng, Q.; et al. Association between low estimated glomerular filtration rate and risk of cerebral small-vessel diseases: A meta-analysis. *J. Stroke Cerebrovasc. Dis.* **2016**, *25*, 710–716. [CrossRef] [PubMed]

283. Kelly, D.M.; Rothwell, P.M. Does chronic kidney disease predict stroke risk independent of blood pressure? A systematic review and meta-regression. *Stroke* **2019**, *50*, 3085–3092. [CrossRef] [PubMed]
284. Akoudad, S.; Sedaghat, S.; Hofman, A.; Koudstaal, P.J.; van der Lugt, A.; Ikram, M.A.; Vernooij, M.W. Kidney function and cerebral small vessel disease in the general population. *Int. J. Stroke* **2015**, *10*, 603–608. [CrossRef] [PubMed]
285. Sedaghat, S.; Ding, J.; Eiriksdottir, G.; van Buchem, M.A.; Sigurdsson, S.; Ikram, M.A.; Meirelles, O.; Gudnason, V.; Levey, A.S.; Launer, L.J. The AGES-Reykjavik study suggests that change in kidney measures is associated with subclinical brain pathology in older community-dwelling persons. *Kidney Int.* **2018**, *94*, 608–615. [CrossRef]
286. White, C.A.; Allen, C.M.; Akbari, A.; Collier, C.P.; Holland, D.C.; Day, A.G.; Knoll, G.A. Comparison of the new and traditional CKD-EPI GFR estimation equations with urinary inulin clearance: A study of equation performance. *Clin. Chim. Acta* **2019**, *488*, 189–195. [CrossRef]
287. George, C.; Mogueo, A.; Okpechi, I.; Echouffo-Tcheugui, J.B.; Kengne, A.P. Chronic kidney disease in low-income to middle-income countries: The case for increased screening. *BMJ Glob. Health* **2017**, *2*, e000256. [CrossRef]
288. Payton, M.; Hu, H.; Sparrow, D.; Weiss, S.T. Low-level lead exposure and renal function in the Normative Aging Study. *Am. J. Epidemiol.* **1994**, *140*, 821–829. [CrossRef] [PubMed]
289. Navas-Acien, A.; Tellez-Plaza, M.; Guallar, E.; Muntner, P.; Silbergeld, E.; Jaar, B.; Weaver, V. Blood cadmium and lead and chronic kidney disease in US adults: A joint analysis. *Am. J. Epidemiol.* **2009**, *170*, 1156–1164. [CrossRef] [PubMed]
290. Zhu, X.J.; Wang, J.J.; Mao, J.H.; Shu, Q.; Du, L.Z. Relationships between cadmium, lead and mercury levels and albuminuria: Results from the National Health and Nutrition Examination Survey Database 2009−2012. *Am. J. Epidemiol.* **2019**, *188*, 1281–1287. [CrossRef] [PubMed]
291. Harari, F.; Sallsten, G.; Christensson, A.; Petkovic, M.; Hedblad, B.; Forsgard, N.; Melander, O.; Nilsson, P.M.; Borné, Y.; Engström, G.; et al. Blood lead levels and decreased kidney function in a population-based cohort. *Am. J. Kidney Dis.* **2018**, *72*, 381–389. [CrossRef] [PubMed]
292. Sommar, J.N.; Svensson, M.K.; Björ, B.M.; Elmståhl, S.I.; Hallmans, G.; Lundh, T.; Schön, S.M.; Skerfving, S.; Bergdahl, I.A. End-stage renal disease and low level exposure to lead, cadmium and mercury; a population-based, prospective nested case-referent study in Sweden. *Environ. Health* **2013**, *12*, 9. [CrossRef] [PubMed]
293. Satarug, S.; Swaddiwudhipong, W.; Ruangyuttikarn, W.; Nishijo, M.; Ruiz, P. Modeling cadmium exposures in low- and high-exposure areas in Thailand. *Environ. Health Perspect.* **2013**, *121*, 531–536. [CrossRef] [PubMed]
294. Swaddiwudhipong, W.; Nguntra, P.; Kaewnate, Y.; Mahasakpan, P.; Limpatanachote, P.; Aunjai, T.; Jeekeeree, W.; Punta, B.; Funkhiew, T.; Phopueng, I. Human health effects from cadmium exposure: Comparison between persons living in cadmium-contaminated and non-contaminated areas in northwestern Thailand. *Southeast Asian J. Trop. Med. Public Health* **2015**, *46*, 133–142.
295. Sun, Y.; Sun, D.; Zhou, Z.; Zhu, G.; Lei, L.; Zhang, H.; Chang, X.; Jin, T. Estimation of benchmark dose for bone damage and renal dysfunction in a Chinese male population occupationally exposed to lead. *Ann. Occup. Hyg.* **2008**, *52*, 527–533.
296. Chen, X.; Zhu, G.; Wang, Z.; Zhou, H.; He, P.; Liu, Y.; Jin, T. The association between lead and cadmium co-exposure and renal dysfunction. *Ecotoxicol. Environ. Saf.* **2019**, *173*, 429–435. [CrossRef]
297. Kim, N.H.; Hyun, Y.Y.; Lee, K.B.; Chang, Y.; Ryu, S.; Oh, K.H.; Ahn, C. Environmental heavy metal exposure and chronic kidney disease in the general population. *J. Korean Med. Sci.* **2015**, *30*, 272–277. [CrossRef]
298. Myong, J.P.; Kim, H.R.; Baker, D.; Choi, B. Blood cadmium and moderate-to-severe glomerular dysfunction in Korean adults: Analysis of KNHANES 2005−2008 data. *Int. Arch. Occup. Environ. Health* **2012**, *85*, 885–893. [CrossRef] [PubMed]
299. Chung, S.; Chung, J.H.; Kim, S.J.; Koh, E.S.; Yoon, H.E.; Park, C.W.; Chang, Y.S.; Shin, S.J. Blood lead and cadmium levels and renal function in Korean adults. *Clin. Exp. Nephrol.* **2014**, *18*, 726–734. [CrossRef]
300. Lim, H.; Lim, J.A.; Choi, J.H.; Kwon, H.J.; Ha, M.; Kim, H.; Park, J.D. Associations of low environmental exposure to multiple metals with renal tubular impairment in Korean adults. *Toxicol. Res.* **2016**, *32*, 57–64. [CrossRef]

301. Hambach, R.; Lison, D.; D'Haese, P.C.; Weyler, J.; De Graef, E.; De Schryver, A.; Lamberts, L.V.; van Sprundel, M. Co-exposure to lead increases the renal response to low levels of cadmium in metallurgy workers. *Toxicol. Lett.* **2013**, *222*, 233–238. [CrossRef] [PubMed]
302. Ferraro, P.M.; Sturniolo, A.; Naticchia, A.; D'Alonzo, S.; Gambaro, G. Temporal trend of cadmium exposure in the United States population suggests gender specificities. *Intern. Med. J.* **2012**, *42*, 691–697. [CrossRef] [PubMed]
303. Agarwal, S.; Zaman, T.; Tuzcu, E.M.; Kapadia, S.R. Heavy metals and cardiovascular disease: Results from the National Health and Nutrition Examination Survey (NHANES) 1999–2006. *Angiology* **2011**, *62*, 422–429. [CrossRef]
304. Hecht, E.M.; Arheart, K.L.; Lee, D.J.; Hennekens, C.H.; Hlaing, W.M. Interrelation of cadmium, smoking, and cardiovascular disease (from the National Health and Nutrition Examination Survey). *Am. J. Cardiol.* **2016**, *118*, 204–209. [CrossRef]
305. Hecht, E.M.; Arheart, K.L.; Lee, D.J.; Hennekens, C.H.; Hlaing, W.M. Interrelationships of cadmium, smoking, and angina in the National Health and Nutrition Examination Survey, a cross-sectional study. *Cardiology* **2018**, *141*, 177–182. [CrossRef]
306. Chen, C.; Xun, P.; Tsinovoi, C.; McClure, L.A.; Brockman, J.; MacDonald, L.; Cushman, M.; Cai, J.; Kamendulis, L.; Mackey, J.; et al. Urinary cadmium concentration and the risk of ischemic stroke. *Neurology* **2018**, *91*, e382–e391. [CrossRef]
307. Gallagher, C.M.; Chen, J.J.; Kovach, J.S. Environmental cadmium and breast cancer risk. *Aging (Albany NY)* **2010**, *2*, 804–814. [CrossRef]
308. Tellez-Plaza, M.; Navas-Acien, A.; Menke, A.; Crainiceanu, C.M.; Pastor-Barriuso, R.; Guallar, E. Cadmium exposure and all-cause and cardiovascular mortality in the U.S. general population. *Environ. Health Perspect.* **2012**, *120*, 1017–1022. [CrossRef]
309. Menke, A.; Muntner, P.; Silbergeld, E.K.; Platz, E.A.; Guallar, E. Cadmium levels in urine and mortality among U.S. adults. *Environ. Health Perspect.* **2009**, *117*, 190–196. [CrossRef] [PubMed]
310. Adams, S.V.; Passarelli, M.N.; Newcomb, P.A. Cadmium exposure and cancer mortality in the Third National Health and Nutrition Examination Survey cohort. *Occup. Environ. Med.* **2012**, *69*, 153–156. [CrossRef] [PubMed]
311. Hyder, O.; Chung, M.; Cosgrove, D.; Herman, J.M.; Li, Z.; Firoozmand, A.; Gurakar, A.; Koteish, A.; Pawlik, T.M. Cadmium exposure and liver disease among US adults. *J. Gastrointest. Surg.* **2013**, *17*, 1265–1273. [CrossRef] [PubMed]
312. Min, J.Y.; Min, K.B. Blood cadmium levels and Alzheimer's disease mortality risk in older US adults. *Environ. Health* **2016**, *15*, 69. [CrossRef]
313. Peng, Q.; Bakulski, K.M.; Nan, B.; Park, S.K. Cadmium and Alzheimer's disease mortality in U.S. adults: Updated evidence with a urinary biomarker and extended follow-up time. *Environ. Res.* **2017**, *157*, 44–51. [CrossRef]
314. Moberg, L.; Nilsson, P.M.; Samsioe, G.; Sallsten, G.; Barregard, L.; Engström, G.; Borgfeldt, C. Increased blood cadmium levels were not associated with increased fracture risk but with increased total mortality in women: The Malmö Diet and Cancer Study. *Osteoporos Int.* **2017**, *28*, 2401–2408. [CrossRef]
315. Deering, K.E.; Callan, A.C.; Prince, R.L.; Lim, W.H.; Thompson, P.L.; Lewis, J.R.; Hinwood, A.L.; Devine, A. Low-level cadmium exposure and cardiovascular outcomes in elderly Australian women: A cohort study. *Int. J. Hyg. Environ. Health* **2018**, *221*, 347–354. [CrossRef]
316. Suwazono, Y.; Nogawa, K.; Morikawa, Y.; Nishijo, M.; Kobayashi, E.; Kido, T.; Nakagawa, H.; Nogawa, K. All-cause mortality increased by environmental cadmium exposure in the Japanese general population in cadmium non-polluted areas. *J. Appl. Toxicol.* **2015**, *35*, 817–823. [CrossRef]
317. Watanabe, Y.; Nogawa, K.; Nishijo, M.; Sakurai, M.; Ishizaki, M.; Morikawa, Y.; Kido, T.; Nakagawa, H.; Suwazono, Y. Relationship between cancer mortality and environmental cadmium exposure in the general Japanese population in cadmium non-polluted areas. *Int. J. Hyg. Environ. Health* **2020**, *223*, 65–70. [CrossRef]
318. Maruzeni, S.; Nishijo, M.; Nakamura, K.; Morikawa, Y.; Sakurai, M.; Nakashima, M.; Kido, T.; Okamoto, R.; Nogawa, K.; Suwazono, Y.; et al. Mortality and causes of deaths of inhabitants with renal dysfunction induced by cadmium exposure of the polluted Jinzu River basin, Toyama, Japan; a 26-year follow-up. *Environ. Health* **2014**, *13*, 18. [CrossRef] [PubMed]

319. Nishijo, M.; Nakagawa, H.; Suwazono, Y.; Nogawa, K.; Sakurai, M.; Ishizaki, M.; Kido, T. Cancer mortality in residents of the cadmium-polluted Jinzu River basin in Toyama, Japan. *Toxics* **2018**, *6*, 23. [CrossRef] [PubMed]
320. van Bemmel, D.M.; Li, Y.; McLean, J.; Chang, M.H.; Dowling, N.F.; Graubard, B.; Rajaraman, P. Blood lead levels, ALAD gene polymorphisms, and mortality. *Epidemiology* **2011**, *22*, 273–278. [CrossRef] [PubMed]
321. Lanphear, B.P.; Rauch, S.; Auinger, P.; Allen, R.W.; Hornung, R.W. Low-level lead exposure and mortality in US adults: A population-based cohort study. *Lancet Public Health* **2018**, *3*, e177–e184. [CrossRef]
322. Aoki, Y.; Brody, D.J.; Flegal, K.M. Blood lead and other metal biomarkers as risk factors for cardiovascular disease mortality. *Medicine* **2016**, *95*, e2223. [CrossRef]
323. Kim, M.G.; Ryoo, J.H.; Chang, S.J.; Kim, C.B.; Park, J.K.; Koh, S.B.; Ahn, Y.S. Blood lead levels and cause-specific mortality of inorganic lead-exposed workers in South Korea. *PLoS ONE* **2015**, *10*, e0140360. [CrossRef]
324. Min, Y.S.; Ahn, Y.S. The association between blood lead levels and cardiovascular diseases among lead-exposed male workers. *Scand. J. Work Environ. Health* **2017**, *43*, 385–390. [CrossRef]

toxics

MDPI

Review

Effects of Cadmium, Lead, and Mercury on the Structure and Function of Reproductive Organs

Peter Massányi [1,2,*], Martin Massányi [3], Roberto Madeddu [4], Robert Stawarz [2] and Norbert Lukáč [1]

1 Department of Animal Physiology, Slovak University of Agriculture in Nitra, Tr. A. Hlinku 2, SK 94976 Nitra, Slovakia; norbert.lukac@uniag.sk
2 Institute of Biology, Pedagogical University of Kraków, ul. Podchorążych 2, 30-084 Kraków, Poland; robert.stawarz@gmail.com
3 Department of Animal Husbandry, Slovak University of Agriculture in Nitra, Tr. A. Hlinku 2, SK 94976 Nitra, Slovakia; martinmassanyi@yahoo.com
4 Department of Biomedical Sciences-Histology, University of Sassari, Viale San Pietro 43/B, 07100 Sassari, Italy; rmadeddu@uniss.it
* Correspondence: peter.massanyi@uniag.sk; Tel.: +421-37-641-4284

Received: 21 August 2020; Accepted: 23 October 2020; Published: 29 October 2020

Abstract: Reproductive organs are essential not only for the life of an individual but also for the survival and development of the species. The response of reproductive organs to toxic substances differs from that of other target organs, and they may serve as an ideal "barometer" for the deleterious effects of environmental pollution on animal and human health. The incidence of infertility, cancers, and associated maladies has increased in the last fifty years or more, while various anthropogenic activities have released into the environment numerous toxic substances, including cadmium, lead, and mercury. Data from epidemiological studies suggested that environmental exposure to cadmium, lead, and mercury may have produced reproductive and developmental toxicity. The present review focused on experimental studies using rats, mice, avian, and rabbits to demonstrate unambiguously effects of cadmium, lead, or mercury on the structure and function of reproductive organs. In addition, relevant human studies are discussed. The experimental studies reviewed have indicated that the testis and ovary are particularly sensitive to cadmium, lead, and mercury because these organs are distinguished by an intense cellular activity, where vital processes of spermatogenesis, oogenesis, and folliculogenesis occur. In ovaries, manifestation of toxicity induced by cadmium, lead, or mercury included decreased follicular growth, occurrence of follicular atresia, degeneration of the corpus luteum, and alterations in cycle. In testes, toxic effects following exposure to cadmium, lead, or mercury included alterations of seminiferous tubules, testicular stroma, and decrease of spermatozoa count, motility and viability, and aberrant spermatozoa morphology.

Keywords: toxic metals; cadmium; lead; mercury; reproduction; testicular and ovarian structure

1. Introduction

Reproduction is an important biological trait to produce new individual organisms and is fundamental for the life of an individual as well as the survival and development of the species [1]. The reproductive system controls the morphological development and physiological differences between males and females as well as influences the behavior of the organism. Environmental and occupational exposure to toxic elements produces various alterations to the biological system, and infertility is one of the global public health concerns as it affects 15% of couples of reproductive age. The toxic mechanisms are described as ion mimicry, disruption of cell signaling pathways, oxidative stress, altered gene expression, epigenetic regulation of gene expression, apoptosis, disruption of the testis–blood barrier, inflammation, and endocrine disruption [2].

Industrial development and agricultural activities have resulted in varying degrees of environmental pollution and reorganization of toxic elements in the food chain [3]. Many elements have been described as highly toxic, while others are essential to living systems. Subfertility and sterility are male reproductive disorders and are interesting in relation to the environment. Adverse trends in male reproductive health are related to environmental impact and have attracted increased attention recently. Declining spermatozoa counts and an increase in reproductive disorders in some areas have been reported during the past 50 years. Because of the relatively short time period in which this has occurred, a crucial role of the environment compared to genetic factors is suggested. Alteration in male reproductive system function may serve as a very sensitive marker of environmental hazards, and the effects can clearly affect reproductive function. The best-reported risk factors related to male reproductive function have included physical exposure and chemical exposure. The doses and exposures demonstrate relatively well the impact of toxic elements at low levels of exposure to the male reproductive structure and function.

Impaired reproductive function is often related to environmental exposure to toxic substances, including toxic metals, namely cadmium, lead, and mercury to which most populations are exposed. These metals are listed by the World Health Organization (WHO) as toxicants of major public health concern (https://www.who.int/ipcs/assessment/public_health/chemicals_phc/en/). Accordingly, we sought to review evidence for reproductive toxicity induced by cadmium, lead, and mercury focusing on changes in the structure and function of male and female reproductive organs of various animal species. Some of these aspects have been covered in published reports [4–9]. It was conceivable that male and female reproductive toxicity should be best described by various and new perspectives with respect to dose-dependent effects of environmental exposure on the spermatozoa and ova/follicles [10–15]. In addition, we discussed evidence from epidemiological studies that linked impaired reproductive function to cadmium, lead, and mercury to which most people are exposed through their diet [3].

2. Cadmium (Cd)

Cadmium is an environmental contaminant from industrial processes and agricultural activities [9,16–19]. Food is the main source of cadmium exposure for the non-smoking general population [18–20]. Cadmium absorption from food in humans is relatively low (3–5%), and it is efficiently reabsorbed in kidneys, with a long biological half-life estimated from 10 to 30 years [21–27]. In relation to male infertility, cadmium is ranked as a highly toxic element [28,29].

2.1. *Toxicity of Cadmium in Female Reproductive Organs*

The effects of cadmium on the structure and function of ovaries were first reported in 1959 [30]. A significant study was published, a couple of years later, to describe the effect of a subcutaneous injection of cadmium salts on the ovaries of adult rats in persistent estrus [31].

In one of our early experimental works, cadmium was administered to 32 adult mice of the ICR Institute of Cancer Research (ICR) strain in two single doses (0.25 and 0.5 mg $CdCl_2$, per kg bw, via i.p. route), and a particularly high cadmium concentration was found in ovaries 48 h after cadmium administration [32]. Similarly, high cadmium accumulation in reproductive organs was observed in an experiment with rabbits [33].

In ovaries of rabbits, a decreased relative volume of growing follicles and increased stroma were found following cadmium administration (i.p. and p.o.) [34,35]. The number of atretic follicles was also significantly elevated by cadmium. The undulation of external nuclear membrane and dilatation of perinuclear cistern and endoplasmic reticulum were the most frequently observed ultrastructural alterations of granulosa, luteal, stroma, and endothelial cells [36]. In all types of cells studied, altered mitochondrial structures were evident [37]. In a later study, the effect of cadmium on the ovarian structure in Japanese quails was studied [38]. A reduction in relative volume of primary follicles was seen in cadmium-treated groups [32]. In addition, the number of follicles undergoing atresia increased as did the number of atretic primary follicles and atretic growing follicles in cadmium-treated groups [38].

In another study, exposed rats had a significantly higher ovarian weight and a higher number of antral and atretic follicles, compared with controls [33]. The effects of cadmium on ovarian follicles were related to changes in gonadotropin hormones and decreases in follicular stimulating hormone (FSH) and luteinizing hormone (LH). A significant formation of oxidative stress in ovarian of Cd-exposed rats was evident from increased levels of the lipid peroxidation product, malondialdehyde (MDA) in combination with decreased levels of an antioxidant enzyme, catalase [39].

In adult female Wistar rats exposed to cadmium, a statistically significant prolongation of the cycle was noted [40]. This effect was observed not only by the estrus phase but also by the diestrus phase. At the highest dose of cadmium (4.5 mg/kg bw), diestrus was extended, whereas proestrus was shortened although no significant increase in the duration of the cycle length was observed. Histopathological alterations in the ovaries of the cadmium-exposed rats were degeneration of the corpus luteum and damaged and fewer oocytes [40].

Cadmium decreases antioxidants and increases the concentrations of MDA and hydrogen peroxide (H_2O_2) in ovaries of rats [41]. Histopathological analysis of the ovaries indicates a significant decrease in follicle number [41]. Ovaries of the cadmium-exposed rats showed a decrease in the number of follicles, with a distorted Graafian follicle.

Cadmium also affects the maturation of follicles, degradation of the corpus luteum and the arrangement of follicles and corpus luteum and increases the number of atresia follicles [42]. In an analysis of ovary morphology, visualized by the expression of the granulosa-cell-specific factor (AMH), there were no differences in the follicle number in each stage (primordial, primary, secondary, and antral follicles) in cadmium-exposed groups [43]. The number of TUNEL-positive cells in the ovaries of cadmium-exposed groups did not differ from controls as did the levels of SOD and MDA in the ovaries [44].

An age-specific effect of cadmium in women was evident from a study using anti-Mullerian hormone (AMH) that is secreted by granulosa cells of antral follicles as an indicator of ovarian function [44]. An inverse association between cadmium and AMH was seen only in women aged between 30 and 35 years. Therefore, it is concluded that environmental exposure to cadmium may alter the AMH level and ovarian function depending on age [44].

Exposure to moderate and high doses of cadmium (i.p.; 1 mg/kg for 5 days/week for 6 weeks) affects steroid synthesis in reproductive organs in female rats [45]. A low-dose cadmium exposure has potent estrogen- and androgen-like activities as cadmium directly binds to estrogen and androgen receptors [46]. Cadmium, like estradiol, can cause rapid activation of ERK1/2 and AKT [47]. However, the exact mechanisms explaining cadmium as an endocrine disruptor remain to be investigated.

The toxicity of cadmium on female reproduction was studied in birds (50-day-old Hy-Line white hens, fed with two doses containing 140 and 210 mg/kg $CdCl_2$ for 20, 40 and 60 days), and increased MDA, nitric oxide (NO) and the activity of nitric oxide synthase (NOS) in the ovary were noted [48]. In addition, the levels of glutathione peroxidase (GPx) and SOD activity decreased in experimental groups. The number of apoptotic cells in the ovary increased in the cadmium-exposed groups, and extensive damage was observed in the ovary [49].

Table 1 summarizes the most significant changes in the ovary due to cadmium exposure.

A few studies have examined effects of cadmium on the structure and function of the oviduct. The highest relative volume of epithelium was seen in the oviduct after long-term Cd administration [36]. Histological analysis reports edematization of the oviduct tissue, which is related to the disintegration of the capillary wall. Further analysis describes dilatation of perinuclear cistern, enlarged intercellular spaces and alterations in cell junctions. Mainly after a long-term cadmium administration, nuclear chromatin disintegration was present [36]. The effects of cadmium on embryo transport through the oviduct were studied in the rat after administration of 2.5, 5, 10 mg/kg $CdCl_2$ on day 1 of pregnancy. Cadmium accumulated in oviducts in dose- and time-dependent manners [49]. Our previous studies reported similarly high concentrations of cadmium in the oviduct [50,51].

Table 1. Alteration in ovaries induced by cadmium.

Administration/Dose/Species/Form	Changes	References
Per os 5 mg/kg; 6 weeks, daily; 6 weeks Sprague Dawley rats $CdCl_2$	- Higher number of antral and atretic follicles	Ruslee et al., 2020 [39]
Single i.p. 1.5 mg/kg; killed after 48 h **Per os** 1.0 mg/kg/day; 5 months Rabbits $CdCl_2$	- Decrease in the relative volume of growing follicles; - Increased number of atretic follicles	Massanyi et al., 2020 [37]
Per os (gavage) 0.09–4.5 mg/kg, 90 days Rat (Wistar) $CdCl_2$	- Prolongation of the cycle length - Degeneration of the corpus luteum - Damaged and fewer oocytes	Nasiadek et al., 2019 [40]
Per os 5 mg/kg; 14 day Rat (Wistar) $CdCl_2$	- Decrease in follicle number	Nna et al., 2017 [41]
Per os 50, 100 and 150 ppm (in water); 50 days Swiss albino mice $CdCl_2$	- Increased numbers of atretic follicles - Decreased number of follicles in different stages of maturation - Disorganization, edema and decreased number of yellow bodies	Lubo-Palma et al., 2006 [52]

i.p.—intraperitoneal administration.

Effects of a single subcutaneous injection (1.5 mg/100 g bw) of cadmium chloride were studied in the oviduct of Indian koel (*Eudynamys scolopacea*). The stromal tissue showed hyperemia and profuse hemorrhage, leading to some cellular destruction. A marked degeneration was noticed in the lamina propria of magnum [53].

A large population-based cohort study of Swedish postmenopausal women described an association between dietary cadmium intake and endometrial cancer and showed potential estrogenic effects [54]. The average estimated cadmium intake was 15 μg/day and 378 cases of endometroid adenocarcinoma were found in a 16-year follow-up. It is noteworthy that an average cadmium intake level among Swedish women of 15 μg/day was 25.8% of an established safe intake level of 58 μg/day for a 70-kg person (0.83 μg/kg bw per week) [18].

Increased incidence of hormone-related cancers and diseases in Western populations may reflect that cadmium has estrogen-like activity in vivo [55]. Environmental contaminants that mimic the effects of estrogen have been linked to the disruption of the reproductive systems of wild animals [55].

A morphological study during the estrus stage reported that cadmium administered orally (0.09, 0.9, 1.8, and 4.5 mg/kg bw) for 90 days caused increased thickness of the epithelial layer. However, in high doses, cadmium induces atrophy of endometrium [55]. Authors also conclude that high-dose cadmium does not induce estradiol-like hyperplasia of endometrium but results in endometrial edema [55].

In the rabbit uterus, a significant adverse effect of cadmium exposure was reflected by the relative volume of glandular epithelium [36]. The increase of stroma was a sign of uterus edematization caused by damage in the wall of blood vessels and subsequent diapedesis [36].

In a study examining myometrial responsiveness, cadmium exposure increased both absolute tension and mean integral tension in female rats exposed to 3, 10, and 30 ppm of cadmium in drinking water for 28 days [56]. Cadmium accumulated in the myometrium of rats and altered response to oxytocin, histamine, calcium chloride, and phenylephrine. These effects were differentially mediated depending on the levels of exposure, possibly through voltage-dependent calcium channel and Ca^{2+}-mimicking pathways [57]. In another study, female BALB/c mice were exposed to 200 ppm cadmium in drinking water for either 30 or 60 days. Cadmium exposure resulted in significant decreases in endometrial thickness, number of glands in estrus-phase uteri and endometrial eosinophilia. Cadmium exposure also increased the number of mast cells. The apoptotic index increased with time in both experimental cadmium-exposed groups, while the proliferation index decreased. Authors conclude that 60-day Cd exposure increased apoptosis in the endometrium, which may affect the receptivity of the uterus for implantation [58].

Cadmium contents in uterine cancer and uterine myoma were studied, and a correlation was observed between tissue cadmium contents and age [59]. An analysis of cadmium content of collected samples of uterine myomas, uterine cancer, and non-lesion uterine tissues from the same women, aged 32–79 showed that cadmium content of myoma was lower than non-lesion tissue [60].

2.2. Toxicity of Cadmium in Male Reproductive Organs

For cadmium as a toxic element, people and animals are exposed to it through contaminated food and the environment. It has been reported that cadmium causes damage to the male testis in animals as well as humans. Cadmium was stated to induce alterations of seminiferous tubules, Sertoli cells, blood–testis barrier, and the loss of spermatozoa. Cadmium alters Leydig cell development and function and induces Leydig cell tumors. Furthermore, cadmium disrupts the vascular system of the testis. As an inducer of reactive oxygen species, cadmium possibly causes DNA damage and subsequently leads to male subfertility/infertility [61].

In a study with two experimental groups exposed to cadmium via injection: acute exposure to $CdCl_2$ 3 mg/kg for 5 days, and chronic exposure to $CdCl_2$ 1 mg/kg for 30 days. In acute exposure conditions, part of seminiferous tubes swelled and the arrangement of spermatogenic cells was mildly disordered [62]. In a chronic exposure conditions, the layers of seminiferous tubes were irregular, and there was loss of spermatogenic cells and a dramatic increase of spermatozoa in tubules [63].

In rats receiving subcutaneous injections of $CdCl_2$ (3 mg/kg bw) once a week for four weeks, cadmium induced biochemical alterations in testicular tissues such as increase in MDA and decrease in antioxidant markers SOD, catalase (CAT), and glutathione (GSH) and functional markers such as alkaline phosphatase (ALP) and lactate dehydrogenase (LDH) [63]. Microscopic changes were manifested as desquamation of basal lamina, shrunken tubules, generalized germ cell depletion with multinucleated giant cells, degenerating Leydig cells, vascular congestion, interstitial edema, and a significant reduction in spermatodynamic count [63].

Tubular damage (vacuolization of the seminiferous epithelium, germ cell detachment and seminiferous tubule degeneration) was seen in the Swiss adult male mice received $CdCl_2$ (1.5 mg/kg i.p., 30 mg/kg oral single dose, and 4.28 mg/kg oral fractional dose for 7 consecutive days) [63]. Authors observed also seminiferous epithelium degeneration, death of germ cells and Leydig cell damages, which were evident in both groups of mice receiving cadmium via i.p. and oral routes. Of note, the damages were more intense in the oral route than i.p. route [64]. In another experiment, the reduction in the diameter of seminiferous tubules was also found [65].

In a study aimed at the mechanisms of cadmium-induced reproductive toxicity in a male mouse model, results demonstrated that the severity of testes injury increased with cadmium concentrations [66]. In low doses, cadmium decreased the thickness of the testicular seminiferous tubule walls, with less apparent swirling contours, and no obvious changes in the appearance of testicular stromal cells were detected. In moderate doses, cadmium caused the thinning of germinal epithelium, sporadic bleeding in the testicular stroma, cells with aberrant swirling contours and decreased spermatogenesis. In high doses, cadmium caused severe thinning of germinal epithelium, seminiferous tubules with aberrant morphology, markedly low level of normal spermatogenesis, and apparent abnormalities of the testicular stroma [66].

In subchronic exposure conditions using rats, structural changes in testis and epididymis were observed together with the increases in testis and epididymis weights 90 days after peroral administration of cadmium at 30 mg/L of drinking water [67]. Testicular damage seen included a significant thickening of seminiferous epithelium, cellular degeneration, and necrosis [60]. Desquamation of immature germ cells resulted in a significant increment of intraepithelial spaces and reduction of tubular volume [67].

Table 2 summarizes the most significant changes in testes due to cadmium exposure.

Table 2. Alteration in testes induced by cadmium.

Administration/Dose/Species/Form	Changes	References
i.p. 2.5 mg/kg; 35 days Kunming mice $CdCl_2$	- Decreased number of spermatogenic tubules - Decreased cell level in the spermatogenic tubules - Disordered spermatogenic cells	Han et al., 2020 [67]
i.p. 3 mg/kg; 5 days and 1 mg/kg for 30 days BALB/c mice $CdCl_2$	- Alterations in spermatogenic cells arrangement - Irregular layers of seminiferous tubes - Loss of spermatogenic cells and spermatozoa	Liu et al., 2020 [60]
Per os 5 mg/kg, 30 days Rats (Wistar) $CdCl_2$	- Decreased spermatozoa count, motility and viability; altered spermatozoa morphology - Atrophy of the seminiferous tubules - Disrupted testicular architecture	Olaniyi et al., 2020 [68]
Per os 2, 4, 8 mg/kg, 8 days Mice (Institute of Cancer Research male specific pathogen-free) $CdCl_2$	- Thin germinal epithelium, seminiferous tubules with aberrant morphology - Markedly low level of normal spermatogenesis - Abnormalities of the testicular stroma	Ren et al., 2019 [65]
i.p. single dose, 2.25 mg/kg, 48 h **Per os** 1.0 mg Cd/kg, 5 months Rabbit $CdCl_2$	- Significant decrease in germinal epithelium volume and increase in stroma volume - Various injury of the seminiferous epithelium - Alterations in the basal membrane structure	Toman et al., 2002 [69]

i.p.—intraperitoneal administration.

Activation of the Erk/MAPK signaling pathway has been proposed as a driver for cadmium-induced prostate cancer. In an in vitro study using non-malignant human normal prostate epithelial cells and PWR1E cell line, chronic exposure to cadmium caused a significant increase in cell proliferation in conjunction with a reduction in apoptosis [69]. An increase in phosphorylation of the Erk1/2 and Mek1/2 was observed in Cd-RWPE1 and Cd-PWR1E cells compared to parental cells, thereby confirming that Cd-exposure induces activation of the Erk/MAPK pathway. It is concluded that Erk/MAPK signaling may be involved in malignant transformation of normal prostate cells by cadmium [70].

Chronic cadmium exposure causes also defective autophagy in prostate epithelial cells, leading to a malignant phenotype transformation [71]. Authors suggest also that chronic exposure to cadmium induces endoplasmic reticulum (ER) stress, which triggers the phosphorylation of stress transducers, and results in defective autophagy in RWPE-1 cells following exposure to cadmium [68].

3. Lead (Pb)

Lead is used in lead acid batteries, coloring agents, paints, smelters, and printing presses and is metallically alloyed as shielding material. It is a toxic metal affecting various organs and developing fetus [72,73]. Acute lead poisoning occurs in humans exposed to high doses, and its chronic exposure can become fatal when lead builds up in the body gradually via continuous exposures to small amounts [74]. It affects almost all organs of the human body and causes physical and mental impairments. Lead remains a noteworthy cause of environmental, occupational, public, and animal health problems [75–79].

3.1. Toxicity of Lead in Female Reproductive Organs

In 1960, a paper describing alteration in the ovary of the rhesus monkey with chronic lead intoxication was published [80], and authors stated that it has long been known that women exposed to lead show disturbances in menstruation, such as amenorrhea, dysmenorrhea, and menorrhagia. Later, results of an experiment with rats (control vs. treated with 5 μg or 100 μg for 30 days) indicated irregularity of the estrus cycle, while the group treated with higher concentrations had persistent vaginal estrus after a period of normal estrus, and the development of ovarian follicular cysts with a reduction in the number of corpora lutea was noted [81].

Lead exposure affects female reproduction mainly by impairing menstruation, reducing fertility potential, delaying conception time and altering hormonal production and circulation, affecting pregnancy and its outcome [82]. Reported effects of lead include infertility, miscarriage, early membrane rupture, preeclampsia, pregnancy hypertension, and preterm birth [83]. A review of studies from China described the possible links between low-level lead exposure and adverse effects on the reproductive system. Effects manifested mainly as high prevalence rates of menstrual disturbance, spontaneous abortion, and threatened abortion in exposed females [84].

Lead exposure is associated with hormonal imbalance causing reproductive impairment, and the accumulation of lead affects many endocrine glands [85]. It affects the hypothalamic–pituitary axis, causing blunted thyroid-stimulating hormone, growth hormone, and follicle-stimulating hormone (FSH)/luteinizing hormone (LH) responses to thyrotropin-releasing hormone, growth hormone–releasing hormone and gonadotropin-releasing hormone stimulation.

A study was done on female workers with a mean age of 32 years employed in a storage battery with a lead exposure period of 7.4 years (1–17 years). The incidence of polymenorrhea, prolonged and abnormal menstruations, and hypermenorrhea was significantly increased in the lead-exposed group, and the incidence of spontaneous abortions was also reported. Authors concluded that the occupational lead exposure results in impairment of the reproductive functions [86].

In a study of 259 healthy women, aged 18–44 years, the amplitude of estradiol showed a tendency to decrease with increasing lead exposure [87]. Thus, environmental exposure to lead experienced by healthy premenopausal women may produce modest changes in reproductive hormone levels [88].

Increment of serum FSH levels with increasing blood lead levels was observed in a study of women, aged 35–60 years [89]. Such increase of serum FSH levels with blood lead levels was seen in postmenopausal women, women with both ovaries removed and premenopausal women [89]. These data suggest that lead may act directly or indirectly to increase ovarian concentrations of FSH and LH [90].

High blood lead levels were associated with a delay in the onset of puberty, after adjustment for possible confounders [89]. Blood lead levels (≥5 μg/dL) were associated with lower levels of maturation at 9 years of age, and slower progression of pubic hair and breast development [91]. Gender differences in the effects of prenatal and postnatal lead exposure on pubertal development have been noted [90]. Accumulating evidence suggests that chronic exposure to low levels of environmental lead may have the following effects in females: menstruation cycles, offspring development, the intellectual ability, offspring weight, and hormonal production [91].

Effects of lead accumulation in the ovary and damage to folliculogenesis were seen in mice exposed to lead as $PbNO_3$ via intraperitoneal (i.p.) injection at 10 mg/kg/day for 15 days or 10 mg/kg/week for 15 weeks [92]. Dysfunction of folliculogenesis, expressed as decreased primordial follicles and an increase of atretic antral follicles was observed [88]. No significant difference in antral follicles was found. The percentages of primordial follicles were significantly lower than in controls (39.7 ± 3.5% vs. 50.7 ± 3.2%), while the percentages of growing follicles (44.7 ± 4.5% vs. 35.0 ± 5.3%) and atretic follicles (17.2 ± 2.4% vs. 4.6 ± 0.8%) were significantly higher compared to control ovaries. In lead-exposed mice, more oocytes had resumed meiosis in the follicles compared to controls. The ovaries from lead-exposed mice contained atretic antral follicles, with detached granulosa cells, pyknotic nuclei in the granulosa wall, and a hypertrophic theca layer.

Another study observed the effects of lead acetate on the histomorphology of the ovary in an animal model—mice of BALBc strain [93]. Animals were given lead acetate at a dose of 30 mg/kg per day for two months. The primary follicular count decreased significantly in the lead-exposed group. In general, the authors also reported that the morphology of the ovary was affected after exposure to lead acetate. Thus, lead clearly interferes with the development of growing follicles [94].

In a study of adult female rats with an oral chronic dose of 60 mg/kg for 90 days, the effect on the reproductive functions was noted [94]. Histological studies of ovaries showed atresia in all the stages of folliculogenesis, supportive of the poor fertility observations. Authors described various stages of follicles undergoing atresia, mainly antrum-formed Graafian follicles with complete detachment of granulosa cells from theca [94].

Histological changes in the ovaries were investigated using Wistar female rats exposed to lead acetate in drinking water in concentration between 0.050 and 0.150 mg/L for 12 months [95]. Such long-term exposure to lead resulted in a statistically significant increase of lead concentrations in ovaries (+42.13% to 9.4-fold increment). In low-dose exposure conditions, some areas with optical empty spaces were present in ovaries with diffuse edemas and ovarian follicle denudation. In high-dose exposure conditions, the most noticeable alterations—edemas and necrosis of the ovarian follicles were observed.

One study compared lead contents of malignant epithelial ovarian cancers ($n = 20$), borderline ovarian tumors ($n = 15$), and non-neoplastic ovarian tissues ($n = 20$) [96]. Lead contents were significantly higher in malignant tissues than controls. Lead contents of papillary and capsular samples of the borderline tumors were also higher than normal ovarian tissues. Thus, accumulation of lead in ovarian tissue showed associations with borderline and malignant proliferation of the surface epithelium [96].

An inverse association was observed between the amount of lead in follicular fluid from a single follicle and in vitro oocyte fertilization outcomes [97]. Later, a higher level of lead was found in the follicular fluid of the women from Taranto compared to the control group. It is concluded that chronic exposure to heavy metals, lead in particular, may decrease the production of estradiol and the number of retrieved mature oocytes [98]. A significantly higher lead concentration was also reported in the polycystic ovary syndrome (PCOS) group compared to the control [99].

Table 3 summarizes the most significant changes in ovaries due to lead exposure.

Table 3. Alteration in ovaries induced by lead.

Administration/Dose/Species/Form	Changes	References
Per os 1.5 mg/kg daily; 21 days Wistar rat Lead acetate	- Follicular edema - Ovarian follicle necrosis	Uchewa and Ezugworie, 2019 [100]
Per os (drinking water) 0.050–0.150 mg/L; 12 months Wistar female rats Lead acetate	- Areas with optical empty spaces - Diffuse edemas and ovarian follicle denudation - Necrosis of the ovarian follicles	Dumitrescu et al., 2015 [95]
Per os (gavage) 30 mg/kg/day; two months mice BALBc Lead acetate	- Decreased primary follicular count - Interference with the development of growing follicles in the ovary	Waseem et al., 2014 [93]
Per os 60 mg/kg; 90 days rats (Disease-free albino rats) Not specified	- Irregular estrous cycle; drop of fertility rate - Atresia in all the stages of folliculogenesis	Dhir and Dhand, 2010 [94]
i.p. acute 10 mg/kg; 15 days; chronic 10 mg/kg; 15 weeks Mice, C57 Bl × CBA $Pb(NO_3)$	- Dysfunction of folliculogenesis - The deceased amount of primordial follicles - Increase in atretic antral follicles	Taupeau et al., 2001 [92]

i.p.—intraperitoneal administration.

An in vitro study of porcine ovarian granulosa cells, low doses of lead (0.063 mg/mL and 0.046 mg/mL) inhibited IGF-I release from ovarian granulosa cells [101]. The authors concluded that lead can affect the pathway of proliferation and apoptosis of porcine ovarian granulosa cells through intracellular substances such as cyclin B1 and caspase 3 [96]. In another in vitro study (with lead acetate), effects of lead on total antioxidant status (TAS) and activity of SOD in ovarian granulosa cells were observed [102]. Further research demonstrated that lead causes a significant reduction in gonadotropin binding, which altered the steroidogenic enzyme activity of granulosa cells [103–106].

The reported effects of lead acetate (10 mg/kg) on uterus histomorphology include lead-induced inflammatory alterations, which were characterized by narrowing of the uterine lumen; atrophy of the endometrium; vacuolar degeneration in endometrial epithelial cells; damaged and decreased number of endometrial glands; and increased filtration of inflammatory cells [105]. In a previously described experiment [95], the levels of lead in uterus with oviduct were also significantly increased in the experimental groups. At the same level of lead exposure, necrosis of the uterine glands in the uterus and fallopian tubes was detected [95].

3.2. Toxicity of Lead in Male Reproductive Organs

Several pathways might be involved in lead-induced impairments of male reproductive health [83,84,105]. Lead reduces male fertility by decreasing spermatozoa quality. The blood–testis barrier can protect testicular tissue from direct exposure to high blood lead concentrations. Furthermore, it has been stated that environmental and occupational exposure to lead may adversely affect the hypothalamic–pituitary–testicular axis, impairing spermatogenesis. Dysfunction at the reproductive axis, mainly testosterone suppression, is most susceptible and irreversible during pubertal development. Lead poisoning also affects the process of spermatogenesis and spermatozoa function. Generation of excessive reactive oxygen species due to lead exposure potentially affects spermatozoa viability, motility, DNA fragmentation, and chemotaxis for spermatozoa–oocyte fusion, all of which can contribute to deterring fertilization [106].

Several reports indicate that lead has toxic effects on male reproduction through libido decline, spermatogenesis, semen quality, and hormonal production and regulation. It has been generally concluded that exposure to low-to-moderate levels of environmental lead affects certain reproductive parameters [107]. Blood lead levels >40 μg/dL have been linked to impaired male reproductive function, possibly by reducing spermatozoa count, volume, and density or by changing spermatozoa motility and morphology [108]. Total spermatozoa count decreases as blood lead increases, and the concentrations of lead in semen show an inverse association with total spermatozoa count, ejaculate volume, and serum testosterone [109]. No significant association was seen between blood lead levels and spermatozoa concentrations [109]. A significant decrease in spermatozoa motility and an increase in testosterone level were seen in patients with a blood lead concentration of ≥20 μg/dL [110].

Various signs of damage in the testicular architecture were noted in adult male Kunming mice (8 weeks old) receiving lead (lead acetate, 100 mg/kg) for 3 weeks [111]. The seminiferous tubules showed disorganization, and tubules were shrunken and distorted with complete absences of the spermatogenesis process. Histological evaluation was further confirmed by the Johnson score, which was lower in the lead-exposed group compared to control [111].

Another study described the effects of lead on the hypothalamic–pituitary–testicular axis, steroidogenesis, spermatozoa parameters, and testicular antioxidant enzyme activity of male Wistar rats after an administration of lead acetate [112]. In this study, adult male Wistar rats received lead (10 mg/kg) had decreased serum luteinizing hormone (LH) and testosterone levels; testicular 17β-hydroxysteroid dehydrogenase (HSD) activity; androgen receptor expression; spermatozoa motility, viability and counts; catalase activity (CAT); and SOD when compared with controls. Abnormal spermatozoa morphology and MDA increased significantly in the lead experimental group [112].

Administration of lead acetate (orally, 20 mg/kg bw, 10 days) to adult rats induced oxidative stress via attenuation of LH, total testosterone, and follicle-stimulating hormone levels in serum [113].

The testes of animals in experimental groups showed an increase in ROS levels, lipid peroxide levels, and lysosomal enzyme activity. The testicular tissue showed clear degeneration with loss of spermatogenic series related to lead administration [114].

The results of another study showed non-significant changes in the absolute and relative weights of epididymis and testes in the lead-exposed group compared with the control, but significant increases were recorded in the spermatozoa analysis and luteinizing hormone, as was a decrease in follicle-stimulating hormone (FSH) [115]. A 25% decrease in testicular CAT activities in the lead-exposed group was detected. The histopathological analysis of testes treated with lead showed edema, hydrocele, and inflamed tunica albuginea [115].

A significant decrease in the weights of testes and epididymis compared to the control group was noted in a study of male albino rats receiving lead acetate (20 mg/kg, orally) for 56 successive days [116]. Decreases in epididymal spermatozoa concentration, motility and viability were also observed. Histopathological analysis showed marked testicular lesions as disorganization and complete hyalinization, tubular blockage with sloughed germinal epithelium and germinal epithelium hypocellularity. The spermatogenesis score showed a significant reduction. Bax antigen staining showed higher intensity in testes of the lead-exposed group [107]. In addition, in lead-exposed rats, strong staining intensity of caspase-3 antigen in Sertoli cells and the resident germ cells was found. Lead induced a significant increase in testicular MDA and NO compared to the control as well as a significant reduction in testicular SOD and GSH [114].

Wistar rats exposed to lead acetate in drinking water for 45 days showed a significant reduction in testis weight, spermatozoa count, testosterone levels, and antioxidant enzymes levels. Testicular histological sections in lead-exposed animals were devoid of germ cells and maturation arrest with the formation of giant primary spermatocytes [116].

Table 4 summarizes the most significant changes in testes due to lead exposure.

Table 4. Alteration in testes induced by lead.

Administration/Dose/Species/Form	Changes	References
Per os 100 mg/kg; 3 weeks Kunming mice Lead acetate	- Disorganization of seminiferous tubules - Complete absences of the spermatogenesis	Elsheikh et al., 2020 [111]
Per os 20 mg/kg; daily for 10 days Albino rats Lead acetate	- Degeneration of testicular tissue with loss of spermatogenic series - Elevation of ROS level, lipid peroxide levels and lysosomal enzyme activity	Kelainy et al., 2019 [113]
Per os 50 g of lead acetate dissolved in 12 mL of 1N HCl; 4 weeks Albino Wistar rats Lead acetate	- Edema, hydrocele and inflamed tunica albuginea	Ezejiofor and Orisakwe, 2019 [114]
Per os 20 mg/kg, 56 days Albino rats Lead acetate	- Significant decrease in the weights of testes - Marked testicular lesions of seminiferous tubules - Disorganization seminiferous tubules, complete hyalinization, tubular blockage, sloughed germinal epithelium, and germinal epithelium hypocellularity - Decreased spermatogenesis score	Hassan et al., 2019 [116]
Per os Wistar rats 0.15%; 45 days Lead acetate	- Significant reduction in testis weight, spermatozoa count, testosterone levels and, antioxidant enzymes levels - Devoid of germ cells and maturation arrest; formation of giant primary spermatocytes	Santhoshkumar and Asha Devi, 2019 [117]

In our previous study, we observed the dilatation of blood capillaries in the interstitium, undulation of basal membrane, and occurrence of empty spaces in the seminiferous epithelium in testes of rats that received lead ($PbNO_3$) in single intraperitoneal doses (12.5–50 mg/kg) [37]. There was also an increased incidence of apoptosis in the spermatogenetic cells. Further morphometric analysis confirmed significant differences between control and treated groups in evaluated parameters. The number of cell nuclei was decreased in lead-treated groups consistent with the occurrence of empty spaces and higher apoptosis incidence in the germinal epithelium [37,118].

The relationship between semen quality and the concentrations of lead in seminal plasma of various species have been reported in our previous studies [119–124]. It has been reported that environmental lead affects semen quality and spermatozoa chromatin considering lead in seminal fluid, spermatozoa and blood as exposure biomarkers in urban men (9.3 μg/dL blood lead). Authors report that 44% of subjects showed decreases in spermatozoa quality, concentration, motility, morphology, and viability that were associated negatively with lead concentration in seminal plasma [121]. Seminal lead concentrations showed inverse associations with spermatozoa concentration, motility, and percentage of abnormal spermatozoa [125]. Authors concluded that exposure to lead (5.29–7.25 μg/dL) affects semen quality [126]. Similarly, blood plasma lead concentrations were reported to be significantly higher in azospermic and oligospermic men compared to normospermic men [127].

4. Mercury (Hg)

Mercury exists as elemental, inorganic, and organic forms [128]. Human exposure to mercury occurs mostly through seafood or sashimi consumption, and also to a lesser extent through dental amalgams, broken thermometers, fluorescent light bulbs, button cell batteries, and skin-lightening creams [129,130]. Mercury exposure is related to its concentrations in the environment [131–133] and various food products [134–140]. Possible health impacts have been reported [141].

In an analysis of data from the U.S. National Health and Nutrition Examination Survey (NHANES) 2011–2012 (n = 7920), the overall population mean for whole blood total mercury (THg) was 0.70 μg/L [142]. In a comparative study, 3.8% of seafood consumers had whole blood THg higher than 5.8 μg/L, while 9.4% of them had whole blood THg higher than 3.4 μg/L [143]. In addition, seafood consumers had higher geometric mean for whole blood THg (0.89 μg/L) than non-seafood consumers (0.31 μg/L) [143]. Fish/seafood was found to be likely sources of mercury exposure among seafood consumers, whereas wine, rice, vegetables, vegetable oil, or liquor were dietary sources of mercury exposure among non-seafood consumers [142]. Intriguingly, a 2.57-fold increase in risk of infertility was seen among women enrolled in NHANES 2013–2016 who had high levels of whole blood THg (>5.278 μg/L) [143].

4.1. *Toxicity of Mercury in Female Reproductive Organs*

Studies related to the reproductive toxicity of mercury were first reported many years ago [144]. Later studies developed the knowledge of mercury effects on female reproductive organs [145,146]. There are few studies reporting the effect of mercury in animal and human female reproductive organs.

In females, mercury can accumulate in ovaries and can cause changes in reproductive behavior, infertility and ovarian failure [147,148]. Studies using experimental animals have shown that increased doses of mercury inflate the potential number of reproductive disorders (i.e., infertility, stillbirth, congenital malformations, and spontaneous abortion) [149].

Evidence from human and animal studies suggests that mercury may adversely affect reproductive function. Increased mercury levels have been linked to infertility or subfertility. Infertile subjects with unclear reasons for infertility had higher mercury concentrations in hair, blood, and urine than fertile subjects. Mercury exposure has been associated with increased incidence of menstrual and hormonal disorders as well as increased rates of adverse reproductive outcomes [150]. Increased exposure to mercury was seen among subjects with polycystic ovary syndrome (PCOS) in a case-control study of 84 patients with PCOS and 70 healthy volunteers [151]. In females, mercury has been shown to have an inhibitory effect on the release of luteinizing hormone (LH) and follicle-stimulating hormone (FSH) from the anterior pituitary [152,153]. This can tip the levels of estrogen and progesterone, causing painful or irregular menstruation, tipped uterus, premature menopause, and often different ovarian dysfunctions. Mercury exposure has been associated with multiple menstrual disorders such as shortening or prolonging of menstrual cycles, abnormal bleeding, or pain [153].

Female mice exposed to 0.25–1.00 mg/kg/day (gavage) of methylmercury showed reduced fertility and survival indices in experimental groups although the exposure did not affect their litter size. Notably, authors stated that microscopic lesions were randomly distributed among the control and experimental groups, and the severity, as well as the distribution, was not consistent with methylmercury-induced toxicity [154].

A positive relationship was observed between the accumulation of mercury in ovaries and the follicular atresia rate in laying hens (40-week-old Hy-Line Brown) fed with four experimental diets containing graded levels of mercury (0.280, 3.325, 9.415, and 27.240 mg/kg) [155]. Progesterone levels significantly decreased in all mercury treatment groups. On the other hand, FSH and LH levels showed inverse correlations with mercury doses. The activities of catalase, superoxide dismutase, glutathione reductase, and glutathione content significantly decreased in experimental groups [155].

Exposure concentration-related effects of mercury vapor were evaluated in rats exposed to 0, 1, 2, or 4 mg/m^3 Hg degrees vapor for 2 h/day for 11 consecutive days. Slightly prolonged estrous cycles were detected in groups with higher mercury exposure. A lengthening of the cycle was detected, and morphological changes were observed in the corpora lutea after exposure for 6 days. Authors concluded that exposure to mercury vapor alters the estrous cycle but has no significant effect on ovulation, implantation, or maintenance of first pregnancy [156]. Another study confirms the effect of mercury vapor (HgO) inhalation on rat ovary structure and function. Ovaries exposed to mercury had various histo-morphometric alterations. A reduction of the total number of primordial, primary, and Graaf follicles was detected. The average mean volume of ovary, medulla and cortex, corpus luteum and Graaf follicles was decreased in the mercury-exposed group. There was also a significant increase in the total volume of the atretic follicles [156].

In an experiment (daily s.c. dose; 1 mg of $HgCl_2$), it was reported that, in the ovary, more mercury was concentrated in the corpora lutea than in the follicles and interstitium. Moreover, when hamsters were given a total of 3 or 4 mg of $HgCl_2$ during the first cycle, 60% of the animals did not ovulate by day 1 of the third cycle [157].

Mercury-exposed rats exhibited irregular estrous cycles and abnormal duration spent in the different phases of the estrous cycle. Mercury-exposed rats (i.m.) spent less time in the proestrus phase compared with control. Authors observed significantly lower ovarian weight in mercury-exposed rats than in control, and ovaries displayed irregular ovarian follicular development. Ovaries had a reduced ovarian antral follicles number and an increase in the number of atretic ovarian follicles (approx. 57%). On the other hand, experimental rats showed an increase in the number of ovarian cystic follicles. No significant changes were observed in the number of primordial, primary, and preantral ovarian follicles and corpus luteum (CL). An increase in the O_2- levels was also observed in mercury-exposed rats [158].

A statistically significant increase in pre- and early post-implantation fetal losses was confirmed in female BALB/c mice treated with a single intraperitoneal injection (2.5–7.5 mg methyl mercury chloride per kg body weight) [159].

It has been reported that that mercury chloride (1.5 mg/kg bw) damages the ovary function and reduces the number of superovulation oocytes in vitro. Results also show that mercury inhibits the extruding of the first polar body and affects the quality and viability of mouse oocyte. Authors also indicate that mercury could affect the meiotic maturation of mouse oocyte, obviously block the IVF and injure or reduce mice's reproductive capacity [160].

Table 5 summarizes the most significant changes in ovaries due to mercury exposure.

In an in vitro study of porcine ovarian granulosa, the effect of mercury on secretion activity of progesterone and insulin-like growth factor-I (IGF-I) was analyzed. Results show that progesterone release by granulosa cells was significantly inhibited, while IGF-I release was not affected. An increasing trend of apoptosis of granulosa cells was confirmed. Results of this study also confirm a direct effect of mercury on the release of steroid hormone progesterone as well as interference of mercury in the pathways of steroidogenesis and apoptosis [161]. Other data confirm that mercury administration has a dose-dependent association with the hormonal release by porcine ovarian granulosa cells [162].

Another study analyzed skin-lightening creams, which are used by women in particular in an attempt to whiten their skin, and men and older people use these creams to remove age spots or other pigmentation disorders [148]. The authors found the presence of high mercury levels in skin-lightening cream. The mercury content in the ovary tissues increased with the frequency of cream applications and was highest in the ovaries of mice treated twice a day with Fair & Lovely and once a day with Rose. Data indicate that dermal exposure to mercury can result in significant accumulation in ovaries of mice following skin-lightening cream application [148].

Table 5. Alteration in ovaries induced by mercury.

Administration/Species/Form	Changes	References
i.m. 4.6 μg/kg + subsequent dose 0.07 μg/kg; 30 days Wistar rats Mercuric chloride	- Irregular estrous cycles - Abnormal duration spent in the different phases of the estrous cycle - Reduced number of ovarian antral follicles number - Increase in the number of atretic ovarian follicles - Increase of lipid deposition	Merlo et al., 2019 [158]
inhalation 1–4 mg/m^3 Hg°; 11 days Sprague–Dawley rats Hg° vapor	- Necropsy of corpora lutea at estrus or metestrus - Immature corpora lutea - Prolonged estrous cycles	Davis et al., 2001 [153]
s.c. 1 mg per day; each day of the 4-day cycle, Golden hamsters Mercuric chloride	- Retarded follicular development and morphologically prolonged corpora lutea	Lamperti et al., 1973 [163]
s.c. 1–4 mg Golden hamster Mercuric chloride	- Higher mercury concentration in the corpora lutea than the follicles of the interstitium - Absent ovulation by Day 1 of the third cycle - Atretic follicles in the primary and secondary stages	Lamperti and Printz, 1974 [157]

i.m.—intramuscular administration; s.c.—subcutaneous administration.

Effects of mercury on oviducts are studied mostly in female birds as the oviduct is important for egg development. A significant eggshell thinning and deformation and inhibited egg production have been noted in domestic fowls receiving methyl mercury—5 mg daily for 6 consecutive days and 1 mg daily for 50 consecutive days [164]. In an in vitro analysis, mercury added to a homogenate of eggshell gland mucosa significantly stimulated the synthesis of prostaglandin F2-alpha (PGF2-α) and prostaglandin E2 (PGE2). Authors conclude that this effect is related to a direct inhibitory effect of mercury on calcium uptake from the gastrointestinal tract and/or to mobilization of medullary bone [164].

The ultrastructure of the surface epithelium of the oviduct of ducks has been reported. Pekin ducks were fed with different doses of methylmercury (0.5; 5.0; 15.0 ppm) for 12 weeks [165]. The primary and secondary folds of magnum and the shell gland regions were densely populated with ciliated cells. In the medium-exposure group, areas of ciliary loss were observed. In the group with the highest mercury exposure, ciliary loss was more extensive and disruption of the apex of cells was also detected. Transmission electron microscopy (TEM) showed degeneration of cytoplasmic organelles—severely damaged ciliated cells, loss of ciliary extensions, and formation of compound cilia [165].

Subcutaneous injection of female hamsters with 6.2–8.2 mg of mercury per kilogram body weight led to a disruption of estrus 1–4 days after treatment [166]. Normal uterine hypertrophy and follicular maturation inhibition, morphological prolongation of corpora lutea, and alteration of progesterone concentrations were noted [167].

Effects of mercury on myometrial activity were examined using Wistar rats receiving 5, 50, and 500 μg/L mercuric chloride in drinking water for 28 days [168]. A significant increase in the receptor-dependent (PGF2α-induced) and receptor-independent ($CaCl_2$-induced and high K+-depolarizing solution-induced) myometrial contraction was observed in rats that received the lowest mercury. Authors concluded that mercury at a low dose produced a detrimental effect on myometrial activity by altering calcium entry into the smooth muscle and/or the release of calcium from intracellular stores [167]. These authors also confirmed that mercury ($HgCl_2$) produced a concentration-dependent uterotonic effect. This study shows that mercury evidently interacts with muscarinic receptors and activates calcium signaling cascades involving calcium channels, Rho-kinase, protein kinase-C, and phospholipase-C pathways to exert an uterotonic effect in rats [169].

Animals exposed to mercury showed uterus inflammatory cells in the endometrium and myometrium [170]. The uterine endometrial area was decreased compared to control, while the myometrium area showed no difference between the groups [170].

In another human study, elevated mercury concentrations were observed in the hyperplasia tissue samples from pre-menopausal women, aged less than 50 years, who had different endometrial pathologies: typical endometrial hyperplasia, endometrial cancer and normal endometrial tissues [169].

4.2. *Toxicity of Mercury in Male Reproductive Organs*

Negative effects of mercury on reproductive traits in male rats include impairment of spermatogenesis, decrease in spermatozoa motility, and increase in pathological changes [171–177].

Testicular toxicity of mercury chloride ($HgCl_2$) in adult male Wistar rats was reported [174]. In the mercury-exposed group (40 mg/kg bw; $HgCl_2$; orally daily; 28 days), histological profiles of the testes showed a derangement of the cytoarchitecture and deterioration of spermatozoa quality. The weights of testes and the gonadosomatic indexes were significantly lower in the mercury-treated group compared to the control. In the mercury-exposed group, degeneration of the spermatogenic cells of the germinal epithelium, occlusion of the lumen of seminiferous tubules, hypertrophy of seminiferous tubules, and irregular vacuolized basement membrane were found. After 28 days of administration, a significant decrease in mean spermatozoa motility and spermatozoa count was detected in the mercury-exposed group [174]. Similar changes in testes were also confirmed after peroral mercury administration. Authors found a decline in spermatozoa, disorganization and degeneration of some spermatogenic cells and vacuolated areas within the seminiferous tubules in the mercury experimental group [175].

Necrosis, disintegration of spermatocytes from basement membrane, undulation of basal membrane and severe edema in interstitial tissue of testis were observed in male Wistar rats exposed to mercury (mercuric chloride; 1 mg/kg bw per day; per os–gavage; 4 weeks) [176]. However, it is noteworthy that no histological changes were observed in the testes, neither in Leydig cells nor in seminiferous tubules in Wistar rats receiving tap water containing methylmercury [177].

An effect of a very low dose of mercury (4 ppm) on possible induction of testicular damage was examined also in mice. Mercury (drinking water; CD-1 male mice; 4 ppm $HgCl_2$; 12 weeks) significantly reduced the epididymal spermatozoa number. Histological study showed that mercury caused degenerative lesions in the testes [178]. Authors also report that mercury exposure leads to disruption of spermiation as disintegration and necrosis of spermatocytes were detected.

A significant decrease in the total volume of testes, diameters of seminiferous tubules, and total volume of seminiferous tubules was observed in rats exposed to mercury vapor at 1 mg/m^{-3} per day in a chamber for six weeks [179]. A significant decrease was also detected in the numbers of Sertoli cells, spermatogonia, spermatocytes, and spermatids. The spermatogenic cells were degenerated, and seminiferous tubules were atrophied [179].

In another study, testicular atrophy was induced by mercuric chloride [180]. The formation of a fibrotic histopathological structure of mature active seminiferous tubules was seen in the testes of rats exposed to mercury via s.c. injection (5 mg/kg mercury chloride; 5 days). The mercury experimental group also showed a decreased number of spermatocytes [180]. Table 6 summarizes the most significant changes in testes due to mercury exposure.

Table 6. Alteration in testes induced by mercury.

Administration/Species/Form	Changes	References
Per os (gastric gavage) 40 mg/kg; once a day; 28 consecutive days Wistar rats Mercuric chloride	- Degeneration of the spermatogenic cells of the germinal epithelium - Occlusion of the lumen of seminiferous tubules - Hypertrophy of seminiferous tubules - Irregular vacuolized basement membrane	Adelakun et al., 2020 [174]
s.c. 5 mg/kg; 5 days Wistar rats Mercury chloride	- Formation of fibrotic histopathological structure of mature active seminiferous tubules - Decreased number of spermatocytes	Fadda et al., 2020 [180]
i.p. 1.23 mg/kg; 7 days Sprague Dawley rats Mercuric chloride	- Severe edema in the interstitium - Necrotic and degenerative changes - Thinned tubular wall - Severe levels of TNF-α and COX-2 expressions in the intertubular areas	Kandemir et al., 2020 [179]
Per os 0.4 mg/kg; 28 days Wistar rats Mercuric chloride	- Decline in spermatozoa - Disorganization and degeneration of spermatogenic cells - Vacuolated area within the seminiferous tubules	Almeer et al., 2020 [181]
i.p. (single) 5–20 mg/kg Rats Mercuric chloride	- Undulation of basal membrane - Dilatation of blood vessels in interstitium - Occurrence of empty spaces in germinal epithelium - Decreased relative volume of germinal epithelium, increased relative volume of interstitium - Increased apoptosis - Decreased number of nuclei in germinal epithelium	Massányi et al., 2007 [182]

s.c.—subcutaneous administration; i.p.—intraperitoneal administration.

One study aimed to assess the effects and underlying mechanisms of chronic exposure to low levels of mercury (Wistar rats; $HgCl_2$; i.m.; 1st dose 4.6 μg/kg and subsequent doses 0.07 μg/kg per day; 60 days) [177]. Administration of mercury decreased spermatozoa production, count, and motility and increased head and tail morphologic abnormalities. Within head phenotypes, more banana head and total head abnormalities were observed. For tail morphology, more bent tail and total tail abnormalities were detected. In the spermatozoa, motility-decreased type A spermatozoa accompanied by increases in type C spermatozoa (immotile) in mercury-treated rats were observed [178]. In a subsequent paper, authors proved the correlation between sperm pathologies and enhanced oxidative stress in reproductive organs. The authors concluded that chronic exposure to low mercury doses impairs spermatozoa quality and adversely affects male reproductive functions, which may be due to enhanced oxidative stress [183].

In rats, mice, hamsters, and guinea pigs exposed to mercury in the form of mercuric chloride intraperitoneally (1, 2 or 5 mg/kg; 1 month), testicular degeneration and cellular deformation of the seminiferous tubules and Leydig cells were found at the highest dosage. On the other hand, a lower dose of mercury resulted only in testicular degeneration in hamsters and partially in rats and mice with no effects in guinea pigs [184,185].

A reproductive alteration due to mercury was also reported in male Sprague Dawley rats (1.23 mg/kg/bw, 7 days). Authors confirm edema in the interstitial areas, necrosis of spermatogonia, degeneration, edema in intertubular areas, severe thinning of the tubular wall, and a higher percentage of dead spermatozoa in semen [183].

Furthermore, an effect mercury on the motility and structural integrity of rabbit spermatozoa has been demonstrated using an in vitro cell-culture study (5.0–83.3 μg $HgCl_2$/mL) [184]. Decreased spermatozoa motility in mercury-exposed cultures was found. Detailed analysis showed a decrease in spermatozoa distance and velocity parameters, straightness, linearity, wobble amplitude of lateral head displacement, and beat cross frequency of spermatozoa. In mercury-exposed cultures, a positive reaction proved alteration in the anterial part of the head (acrosome), connection part (connection piece), and mitochondrial segment [185].

5. Conclusions and Future Directions

The signs of toxicity of cadmium, lead, and mercury in reproductive organs appear to be strikingly similar when each is administered individually. In ovaries, the most significant changes are decreased follicular growth, increased number of atretic follicles, degeneration of the corpus luteum, and prolonged and/or irregular cycle. In testes, the most significant changes include disorganization of seminiferous tubules; alterations in spermatogenic cell arrangement; alterations in the basal membrane structure; abnormalities of the testicular stroma; decreased spermatozoa count, motility, and viability; and altered spermatozoa morphology. These are signs of adverse effects of cadmium, lead, and mercury on the architecture of reproductive organs, which are both dose- and time-dependent. In general, toxic effects of various substances in reproductive organs occur at low concentrations. Because toxic mechanisms of each individual metal have been established, future research should be aimed to elucidate molecular mechanism(s) of action of these metals in combinations to mimic human co-exposure situations. In addition, toxicity preventive strategies and the synergistic or antagonistic interactions during the simultaneous presence of more than one of these three metals should be examined in future research.

Author Contributions: Conceptualization, P.M., M.M., R.M., R.S., N.L.; methodology, P.M., M.M.; writing—original draft preparation, P.M., M.M., R.M., R.S., N.L.; review and editing, P.M., R.M.; supervision, P.M., R.S., N.L. All authors have read and agreed to the published version of the manuscript.

Funding: This work was supported by projects of the Scientific Grant Agency of the Ministry of Education, Science, Research and Sport of the Slovak Republic (project 1/0539/18); The Slovak Research and Development Agency (project APVV-15-0543) and Cultural and Educational Agency of the Ministry of Education, Science, Research and Sport of the Slovak Republic (project KEGA 010/SPU-4/2018). Authors prepared this review in relation to their activities in the International Society for Research on Cadmium and Trace Element Toxicity (P.M., R.M., N.L.) and CeRA research team at SUA in Nitra (P.M., N.L.).

Acknowledgments: This work was supported by projects VEGA 1/0539/18, APVV-15-0543 and KEGA 010/SPU-4/2018.

Conflicts of Interest: The authors declare no conflict of interest.

Abbreviations

Cd	Cadmium
Pb	Lead
Hg	Mercury
17β-HSD	17β-hydroxysteroid dehydrogenase
ALP	Alkaline phosphatase
AMH	Anti-Mullerian hormone
CAT	Catalase
CL	Corpus luteum
ERK1/2	Extracellular signal-regulated kinases 1 and 2
FSH	Follicular stimulating hormone
GPx	Glutathione peroxidase
IGF-I	Insulin-like growth factor 1
LDH	Lactate dehydrogenase
LH	Luteinizing hormone
MAPK	Mitogen-activated protein kinases
MDA	Malondialdehyde
NO	Nitric oxide
NOS	Nitric oxide synthase
PCOS	Polycystic ovary syndrome
PGF2-α	Prostaglandin F2-alpha
PGE2	Prostaglandin E2
ROS	Reactive oxygen species
RWPE1, PWR1E	Non-malignant prostate epithelial cells
SOD	Superoxide dismutase
TAS	Total antioxidant status
TEM	Transmission electron microscopy
WHO	World Health Organization

References

1. Roychoudhury, S.; Massányi, P. *Introduction to Male Reproduction and Toxicity*; Slovak University of Agriculture in Nitra: Nitra, Slovakia, 2014; p. 30.
2. Lukáč, N.; Massányi, P.; Kročková, J.; Nad', P.; Slamečka, J.; Ondruška, L.; Formicki, G.; Trandžík, J. Relationship between trace element concentrations and spermatozoa quality in rabbit semen. *Slovak J. Anim. Sci.* **2009**, *42*, 46–50.
3. Satarug, S.; Gobe, G.C.; Vesey, D.A.; Phelps, K.R. Cadmium and lead exposure, nephrotoxicity, and mortality. *Toxics* **2020**, *8*, 86. [CrossRef]
4. Anyanwu, B.O.; Orisakwe, O.E. Current mechanistic perspectives on male reproductive toxicity induced by heavy metals. *J. Environ. Sci. Health Part C Toxicol. Carcinog.* **2020**, *38*, 204–244. [CrossRef] [PubMed]
5. Reis, M.M.S.; Moreira, A.C.; Sousa, M.; Mathur, P.P.; Oliveira, P.F.; Alves, M.G. Sertoli cell as a model in male reproductive toxicology: Advantages and disadvantages. *J. Appl. Toxicol.* **2015**, *35*, 870–883. [CrossRef] [PubMed]
6. Rzymski, P.; Tomczyk, K.; Rzymski, P.; Poniedziałek, B.; Opala, T.; Wilczak, M. Impact of heavy metals on the female reproductive system. *Ann. Agric. Environ. Med.* **2015**, *22*, 259–264. [CrossRef] [PubMed]
7. Qiao, Z.; Dai, J.-B.; Wang, Z.-X. The hazardous effects of tobacco smoking on male fertility. *Asian J. Androl.* **2015**, *17*, 954–960. [CrossRef] [PubMed]
8. Zeng, X.; Xu, X.; Boezen, H.M.; Huo, X. Children with health impairments by heavy metals in an e-waste recycling area. *Chemosphere* **2016**, *148*, 408–415. [CrossRef]

9. Ramos-Treviño, J.; Bassol-Mayagoitia, S.; Hernández-Ibarra, J.A.; Ruiz-Flores, P.; Nava-Hernández, M.P. Toxic effect of cadmium, lead, and arsenic on the Sertoli cell: Mechanisms of damage involved. *DNA Cell Biol.* **2018**, *37*, 600–608. [CrossRef]
10. Bonde, J.P. Male reproductive organs are at risk from environmental hazards. *Asian J. Androl.* **2010**, *12*, 152–156. [CrossRef]
11. Bonde, J.P.E.; Ernst, E.; Jensen, T.K.; Hjollund, N.H.I.; Kolstad, H.A.; Scheike, T.H.; Giwercman, A.; Skakkebæk, N.E.; Henriksen, T.B.; Olsen, J. Relation between semen quality and fertility: A population-based study of 430 first-pregnancy planners. *Lancet* **1998**, *352*, 1172–1177. [CrossRef]
12. Kolesárová, A.; Capcarová, M.; Roychoudhury, S. *Metal Induced Ovarian Signaling*; Slovak University of Agriculture in Nitra: Nitra, Slovakia, 2010; p. 135. ISBN 978-80-552-0456-7.
13. Massányi, P.; Cigánková, V.; Fabiš, M.; Kováčik, J.; Massányiová, K.; Toman, R. *Reproductive Toxicology (in Slovak)*; Slovak University of Agriculture in Nitra: Nitra, Slovakia, 1999; p. 144.
14. Massányi, P.; Bárdos, L.; Roychoudhury, S.; Stawarz, R. Foreword. *J. Environ. Sci. Health A Toxic Hazard Subst. Environ. Eng.* **2012**, *47*, 1201. [CrossRef]
15. Meeker, J.D.; Rossano, M.G.; Protas, B.; Diamond, M.P.; Puscheck, E.; Daly, D.; Paneth, N.; Wirth, J.J. Cadmium, Lead, and Other Metals in Relation to Semen Quality: Human Evidence for Molybdenum as a Male Reproductive Toxicant. *Environ. Health Perspect.* **2008**, *116*, 1473–1479. [CrossRef] [PubMed]
16. Satarug, S.; Garrett, S.H.; Sens, M.A.; Sens, D.A. Cadmium, Environmental Exposure, and Health Outcomes. *Environ. Health Perspect.* **2010**, *118*, 182–190. [CrossRef] [PubMed]
17. Sall, M.L.; Diaw, A.K.D.; Gningue-Sall, D.; Aaron, S.E.; Aaron, J.-J. Toxic heavy metals: Impact on the environment and human health, and treatment with conducting organic polymers, a review. *Environ. Sci. Pollut. Res. Int.* **2020**, *27*, 29927–29942. [CrossRef] [PubMed]
18. Satarug, S. Dietary Cadmium intake and its effects on kidneys. *Toxics* **2018**, *6*, 15. [CrossRef]
19. Janicka, M.; Binkowski, Ł.J.; Błaszczyk, M.; Paluch, J.; Wojtaś, W.; Massanyi, P.; Stawarz, R. Cadmium, lead and mercury concentrations and their influence on morphological parameters in blood donors from different age groups from southern Poland. *J. Trace Elem. Med. Biol.* **2015**, *29*, 342–346. [CrossRef]
20. Capcarová, M.; Harangozó, L.; Árvay, J.; Tóth, T.; Gabríny, L.; Binkowski, Ł.J.; Palšová, L.; Skalická, M.; de la Luz Garcia Pardo, M.; Stawarz, R.; et al. Essential and xenobiotic elements in cottage cheese from the Slovak market with a consumer risk assessment. *J. Environ. Sci. Health Part B* **2020**, *55*, 677–686. [CrossRef]
21. Schwarz, P.; Lukáčová, A.; Formicki, G.; Massányi, P.; Golian, J.; Kiss, Z. Heavy metals in Slovakian meat and milk samples. *Hungarian Vet. J.* **2013**, *135*, 565–571.
22. Stawarz, R.; Formicki, G.; Massanyi, P. Daily fluctuations and distribution of xenobiotics, nutritional and biogenic elements in human milk in Southern Poland. *J. Environ. Sci. Health Part A* **2007**, *42*, 1169–1175. [CrossRef]
23. Satarug, S.; Gobe, G.C.; Ujjin, P.; Vesey, D. A Comparison of the Nephrotoxicity of Low Doses of Cadmium and Lead. *Toxics* **2020**, *8*, 18. [CrossRef]
24. Satarug, S.; Boonprasert, K.; Gobe, G.C.; Ruenweerayut, R.; Johnson, D.W.; Na-Bangchang, K.; Vesey, D. Chronic exposure to cadmium is associated with a marked reduction in glomerular filtration rate. *Clin. Kidney J.* **2018**, *12*, 468–475. [CrossRef] [PubMed]
25. Genchi, G.; Sinicropi, M.S.; Lauria, G.; Carocci, A.; Catalano, A. The Effects of Cadmium Toxicity. *Int. J. Environ. Res. Public Health* **2020**, *17*, 3782. [CrossRef] [PubMed]
26. Gašparík, J.; Binkowski, Ł.J.; Jahnátek, A.; Šmehýl, P.; Dobiaš, M.; Lukac, N.; Błaszczyk, M.; Semla, M.; Massanyi, P. Levels of Metals in Kidney, Liver, and Muscle Tissue and their Influence on the Fitness for the Consumption of Wild Boar from Western Slovakia. *Biol. Trace Elem. Res.* **2017**, *177*, 258–266. [CrossRef] [PubMed]
27. Kramárová, M.; Massanyi, P.; Slamecka, J.; Tataruch, F.; Jancová, A.; Gasparik, J.; Fabis, M.; Kovacik, J.; Toman, R.; Galová, J.; et al. Distribution of Cadmium and Lead in Liver and Kidney of Some Wild Animals in Slovakia. *J. Environ. Sci. Health Part A Toxic Hazard Subst. Environ. Eng.* **2005**, *40*, 593–600. [CrossRef]
28. Zhu, Q.; Li, X.; Ge, R.-S. Toxicological Effects of Cadmium on Mammalian Testis. *Front. Genet.* **2020**, *11*, 527. [CrossRef]
29. Jenardhanan, P.; Panneerselvam, M.; Mathur, P.P. Effect of environmental contaminants on spermatogenesis. *Semin. Cell Dev. Biol.* **2016**, *59*, 126–140. [CrossRef]

30. Kar, A.B.; Das, R.P.; Karkun, J.N. Ovarian changes in prepuberal rats after treatment with cadmium chloride. *Acta Biol. Med. Ger.* **1959**, *3*, 372–399.
31. Pařízek, J.; Ošťádalová, I.; Benes, I.; Pitha, J. The effect of a subcutaneous injection of cadmium salts on the ovaries of adult rats in persistent oestrus. *J. Reprod. Fertil.* **1968**, *17*, 559. [CrossRef]
32. Massanyi, P.; Bárdos, L.; Oppel, K.; Hluchý, S.; Kovácik, J.; Csicsai, G.; Toman, R. Distribution of cadmium in selected organs of mice: Effects of cadmium on organ contents of retinoids and beta-carotene. *Acta Physiol. Hung.* **1999**, *86*, 99–104.
33. Massanyi, P.; Toman, R.; Valent, M.; Cupka, P. Evaluation of selected parameters of a metabolic profile and levels of cadmium in reproductive organs of rabbits after an experimental administration. *Acta Physiol. Hung.* **1995**, *83*, 267–273.
34. Massányi, P.; Uhrín, V. Histological changes in the ovaries of rabbits after an administration of cadmium. *Reprod. Dom. Anim.* **1996**, *31*, 4–5, 629–632.
35. Massanyi, P.; Uhrín, V.; Valent, M. Correlation relationship between cadmium accumulation and histological structures of ovary and uterus in rabbits. *J. Environ. Sci. Health Part A Environ. Sci. Eng. Toxicol.* **1997**, *32*, 1621–1635. [CrossRef]
36. Massanyi, P.; Lukac, N.; Uhrin, V.; Toman, R.; Pivko, J.; Rafay, J.; Forgács, Z.; Somosy, Z. Female reproductive toxicology of cadmium. *Acta Biol. Hung.* **2007**, *58*, 287–299. [CrossRef] [PubMed]
37. Massanyi, P.; Lukac, N.; Massanyi, M.; Stawarz, R.; Formicki, G.; Danko, J. Effects of Xenobiotics on Animal Reproduction in Vivo: Microscopical Examination. *Microsc. Microanal.* **2020**, *26*, 63. [CrossRef]
38. Naď, P.; Massanyi, P.; Skalicka, M.; Koréneková, B.; Cigankova, V.; Almášiová, V. The effect of cadmium in combination with zinc and selenium on ovarian structure in Japanese quails. *J. Environ. Sci. Health Part A* **2007**, *42*, 2017–2022. [CrossRef]
39. Ruslee, S.S.; Zaid, S.S.M.; Bakrin, I.H.; Goh, Y.M.; Mustapha, N.M. Protective effect of Tualang honey against cadmium-induced morphological abnormalities and oxidative stress in the ovary of rats. *BMC Complement. Med. Ther.* **2020**, *20*, 1–11. [CrossRef]
40. Nasiadek, M.; Danilewicz, M.; Klimczak, M.; Stragierowicz, J.; Kilanowicz, A. Subchronic Exposure to Cadmium Causes Persistent Changes in the Reproductive System in Female Wistar Rats. *Oxidative Med. Cell. Longev.* **2019**, *2019*, 6490820. [CrossRef]
41. Nna, V.U.; Usman, U.Z.; Ofutet, E.O.; Owu, D.U. Quercetin exerts preventive, ameliorative and prophylactic effects on cadmium chloride—Induced oxidative stress in the uterus and ovaries of female Wistar rats. *Food Chem. Toxicol.* **2017**, *102*, 143–155. [CrossRef]
42. Wang, Y.; Wang, X.; Wang, Y.; Fan, R.; Qiu, C.; Zhong, S.; Wei, L.; Luo, D. Effect of Cadmium on Cellular Ultrastructure in Mouse Ovary. *Ultrastruct. Pathol.* **2015**, *39*, 324–328. [CrossRef]
43. Zhang, T.; Gao, X.; Luo, X.; Li, L.; Ma, M.; Zhu, Y.; Zhao, L.; Li, R. The effects of long-term exposure to low doses of cadmium on the health of the next generation of mice. *Chem. Interact.* **2019**, *312*, 108792. [CrossRef]
44. Lee, Y.M.; Chung, H.W.; Jeong, K.; Sung, Y.-A.; Lee, H.; Ye, S.; Ha, E. Association between cadmium and anti-Mullerian hormone in premenopausal women at particular ages. *Ann. Occup. Environ. Med.* **2018**, *30*, 44. [CrossRef] [PubMed]
45. Zhang, W.; Pang, F.; Huang, Y.; Yan, P.; Lin, W. Cadmium exerts toxic effects on ovarian steroid hormone release in rats. *Toxicol. Lett.* **2008**, *182*, 18–23. [CrossRef] [PubMed]
46. Takiguchi, M.; Yoshihara, S. New aspects of cadmium as endocrine disruptor. *Environ. Sci. Int. J. Environ. Physiol. Toxicol.* **2006**, *13*, 107–116.
47. Chen, L.; Liu, L.; Huang, S. Cadmium activates the mitogen-activated protein kinase (MAPK) pathway via induction of reactive oxygen species and inhibition of protein phosphatases 2A and 5. *Free Radic. Biol. Med.* **2008**, *45*, 1035–1044. [CrossRef] [PubMed]
48. Yang, S.; Zhang, Z.; He, J.; Li, J.; Zhang, J.; Xing, H.; Xu, S. Ovarian toxicity induced by dietary cadmium in hen. *Biol. Trace Elem. Res.* **2012**, *148*, 53–60. [CrossRef] [PubMed]
49. Paksy, K.; Varga, B.; Náray, M.; Olajos, F.; Folly, G. Altered ovarian progesterone secretion induced by cadmium fails to interfere with embryo transport in the oviduct of the rat. *Reprod. Toxicol.* **1992**, *6*, 77–83. [CrossRef]
50. Massányi, P.; Toman, R.; Najmik, F. Concentrations of cadmium in ovary, oviductus, uterus, testis and tunica albuginea of testis in cattle. *J. Environ. Sci. Health A Toxic Hazard Subst. Environ. Eng.* **1995**, *30*, 1685–1692.

51. Massányi, P.; Najmik, F.; Renon, P. Concentrazione del cadmio in organi riproduttivi di bovino. *Arch. Vet. Ital.* **1995**, *46*, 62–66.
52. Lubo-Palma, A.; Nava-Leal, C.; Villasmil, V. Efectos del cadmio sobre el parénquima ovarico en ratones albinos suizos [Effects of cadmium on the ovarian parenchyma in Swiss albino mice]. *Investig. Clin.* **2006**, *47*, 219–231.
53. Sarkar, A.K.; Maitra, S.K.; Midya, T. Histological, histochemical and biochemical effects of cadmium chloride in female koel (*Eudynamys scolopacea*). *Acta Histochem.* **1976**, *57*, 205–211. [CrossRef]
54. Åkesson, A.; Julin, B.; Wolk, A.; Locke, J.A.; Guns, E.S.; Lubik, A.A.; Adomat, H.; Hendy, S.C.; Wood, C.A.; Ettinger, S.L.; et al. Long-term Dietary Cadmium Intake and Postmenopausal Endometrial Cancer Incidence: A Population-Based Prospective Cohort Study. *Cancer Res.* **2008**, *68*, 6435–6441. [CrossRef]
55. Johnson, M.D.; Kenney, N.; Stoica, A.; Hilakivi-Clarke, L.; Singh, B.; Chepko, G.; Clarke, R.; Sholler, P.F.; Lirio, A.A.; Foss, C.; et al. Cadmium mimics the in vivo effects of estrogen in the uterus and mammary gland. *Nat. Med.* **2003**, *9*, 1081–1084. [CrossRef] [PubMed]
56. Nasiadek, M.; Danilewicz, M.; Sitarek, K.; Świątkowska, E.; Daragó, A.; Stragierowicz, J.; Kilanowicz, A. The effect of repeated cadmium oral exposure on the level of sex hormones, estrous cyclicity, and endometrium morphometry in female rats. *Environ. Sci. Pollut. Res. Int.* **2018**, *25*, 28025–28038. [CrossRef] [PubMed]
57. Saroj, V.K.; Nakade, U.P.; Sharma, A.; Choudhury, S.; Hajare, S.W.; Garg, S.K. Dose-Dependent Differential Effects of In Vivo Exposure of Cadmium on Myometrial Activity in Rats: Involvement of VDCC and Ca2+-Mimicking Pathways. *Biol. Trace Elem. Res.* **2017**, *181*, 272–280. [CrossRef] [PubMed]
58. Sapmaz-Metin, M.; Topcu-Tarladacalisir, Y.; Kurt-Omurlu, I.; Weller, B.K.; Unsal-Atan, S. A morphological study of uterine alterations in mice due to exposure to cadmium. *Biotech. Histochem.* **2017**, *92*, 264–273. [CrossRef]
59. Nasiadek, M.; Krawczyk, T.; Sapota, A. Tissue levels of cadmium and trace elements in patients with myoma and uterine cancer. *Hum. Exp. Toxicol.* **2005**, *24*, 623–630. [CrossRef]
60. Liu, D.; Wan, J.; Liu, Z.; Zhao, Z.; Zhang, G.; Leng, Y. Determination of cadmium induced acute and chronic reproductive toxicity with Raman spectroscopy. *Lasers Med. Sci.* **2020**, 1–8. [CrossRef]
61. Rajendar, B.; Bharavi, K.; Rao, G.S.; Kishore, P.V.S.; Kumar, P.R.; Kumar, C.S.V.S.; Kumar, D.S. Protective effect of alpha-tocopheral on biochemical and histological alterations induced by cadmium in rat testes. *Indian J. Physiol. Pharmacol.* **2012**, *55*, 213–220.
62. Mouro, V.G.S.; Martins, A.L.P.; Silva, J.; Menezes, T.P.; Gomes, M.L.M.; Oliveira, J.A.; De Melo, F.C.S.A.; Da Matta, S.L.P. Subacute Testicular Toxicity to Cadmium Exposure Intraperitoneally and Orally. *Oxidative Med. Cell. Longev.* **2019**, *2019*, 3429635. [CrossRef]
63. Mouro, V.G.S.; Siman, V.A.; Da Silva, J.; Dias, F.C.R.; Damasceno, E.M.; Cupertino, M.D.C.; De Melo, F.C.S.A.; Da Matta, S.L.P. Cadmium-Induced Testicular Toxicity in Mice: Subacute and Subchronic Route-Dependent Effects. *Biol. Trace Elem. Res.* **2019**, *193*, 466–482. [CrossRef]
64. Momeni, H.R.; Eskandari, N. Curcumin protects the testis against cadmium-induced histopathological damages and oxidative stress in mice. *Hum. Exp. Toxicol.* **2020**, *39*, 653–661. [CrossRef] [PubMed]
65. Ren, Y.; Shao, W.; Zuo, L.; Zhao, W.; Qin, H.; Hua, Y.; Lu, D.; Mi, C.; Zeng, S.; Zu, L. Mechanism of cadmium poisoning on testicular injury in mice. *Oncol. Lett.* **2019**, *18*, 1035–1042. [CrossRef] [PubMed]
66. Adamkovičová, M.; Toman, R.; Cabaj, M.; Massanyi, P.; Martiniaková, M.; Omelka, R.; Krajcovicova, V.; Duranova, H. Effects of Subchronic Exposure to Cadmium and Diazinon on Testis and Epididymis in Rats. *Sci. World J.* **2014**, *2014*, 632581. [CrossRef]
67. Han, C.; Zhu, Y.; Yang, Z.; Fu, S.; Zhang, W.; Liu, C. Protective effect of Polygonatum sibiricum against cadmium-induced testicular injury in mice through inhibiting oxidative stress and mitochondria-mediated apoptosis. *J. Ethnopharmacol.* **2020**, *261*, 113060. [CrossRef] [PubMed]
68. Olaniyi, K.S.; Amusa, O.A.; Oniyide, A.A.; Ajadi, I.O.; Akinnagbe, N.T.; Babatunde, S.S. Protective role of glutamine against cadmium-induced testicular dysfunction in Wistar rats: Involvement of G6PD activity. *Life Sci.* **2020**, *242*, 117250. [CrossRef]
69. Toman, R.; Massányi, P.; Uhrín, V. Changes in the testis and epididymis of rabbits after an intraperitoneal and peroral administration of cadmium. *Trace Elem. Electrol.* **2002**, *19*, 114–117.
70. Dasgupta, P.; Kulkarni, P.; Bhat, N.S.; Majid, S.; Shiina, M.; Shahryari, V.; Yamamura, S.; Tanaka, Y.; Gupta, R.K.; Dahiya, R.; et al. Activation of the Erk/MAPK signaling pathway is a driver for cadmium induced prostate cancer. *Toxicol. Appl. Pharmacol.* **2020**, *401*, 115102. [CrossRef]

71. Kolluru, V.; Tyagi, A.; Chandrasekaran, B.; Ankem, M.; Damodaran, C. Induction of endoplasmic reticulum stress might be responsible for defective autophagy in cadmium-induced prostate carcinogenesis. *Toxicol. Appl. Pharmacol.* **2019**, *373*, 62–68. [CrossRef]
72. Zhang, Y.; Wang, B.; Cheng, Q.; Li, X.; Li, Z. Removal of Toxic Heavy Metal Ions (Pb, Cr, Cu, Ni, Zn, Co, Hg, and Cd) from Waste Batteries or Lithium Cells Using Nanosized Metal Oxides: A Review. *J. Nanosci. Nanotechnol.* **2020**, *20*, 7231–7254. [CrossRef]
73. Kabamba, M.; Tuakuila, J. Toxic metal (Cd, Hg, Mn, Pb) partition in the maternal/foetal unit: A systematic mini—Review of recent epidemiological studies. *Toxicol. Lett.* **2020**, *332*, 20–26. [CrossRef]
74. Nkwunonwo, U.; Odika, P.O.; Onyia, N.I. A Review of the Health Implications of Heavy Metals in Food Chain in Nigeria. *Sci. World J.* **2020**, *2020*, 6594109. [CrossRef]
75. Okereafor, U.; Makhatha, M.E.; Mekuto, L.; Uche-Okereafor, N.; Sebola, T.; Mavumengwana, V. Toxic Metal Implications on Agricultural Soils, Plants, Animals, Aquatic life and Human Health. *Int. J. Environ. Res. Public Health* **2020**, *17*, 2204. [CrossRef] [PubMed]
76. Charkiewicz, A.E.; Backstrand, J.R. Lead Toxicity and Pollution in Poland. *Int. J. Environ. Res. Public Health* **2020**, *17*, 4385. [CrossRef]
77. Kumar, A.; M.M.S., C.-P.; Chaturvedi, A.K.; Shabnam, A.A.; Subrahmanyam, G.; Mondal, R.; Gupta, D.K.; Malyan, S.K.; Kumar, S.S.; Khan, S.A.; et al. Lead Toxicity: Health Hazards, Influence on Food Chain, and Sustainable Remediation Approaches. *Int. J. Environ. Res. Public Health* **2020**, *17*, 2179. [CrossRef]
78. Binkowski, Ł.J.; Błaszczyk, M.; Przystupińska, A.; Ożgo, M.; Massanyi, P. Metal concentrations in archaeological and contemporary mussel shells (Unionidae): Reconstruction of past environmental conditions and the present state. *Chemosphere* **2019**, *228*, 756–761. [CrossRef] [PubMed]
79. Massanyi, P.; Stawarz, R.; Halo, M.; Formicki, G.; Lukac, N.; Cupka, P.; Schwarcz, P.; Kovacik, A.; Tušimová, E.; Kováčik, J. Blood concentration of copper, cadmium, zinc and lead in horses and its relation to hematological and biochemical parameters. *J. Environ. Sci. Health Part A* **2014**, *49*, 973–979. [CrossRef] [PubMed]
80. Eck, G.J.V.-V.; Meigs, J.W. Changes in the Ovary of the Rhesus Monkey After Chronic Lead Intoxication. *Fertil. Steril.* **1960**, *11*, 223–234. [CrossRef]
81. Hilderbrand, D.C.; Der, R.; Griffin, W.T.; Fahim, M.S. Effect of lead acetate on reproduction. *Am. J. Obstet. Gynecol.* **1973**, *115*, 1058–1065. [CrossRef]
82. Kumar, S. Occupational and Environmental Exposure to Lead and Reproductive Health Impairment: An Overview. *Indian J. Occup. Environ. Med.* **2018**, *22*, 128–137. [PubMed]
83. Winder, C. Lead, reproduction and development. *NeuroToxicology* **1993**, *14*, 303–317.
84. Xuezhi, J.; Youxin, L.; Yilan, W. Studies of lead exposure on reproductive system: A review of work in China. *Biomed. Environ. Sci.* **1992**, *5*, 266–275. [PubMed]
85. Doumouchtsis, K.K.; Doumouchtsis, S.K.; Doumouchtsis, E.K.; Perrea, D.N. The effect of lead intoxication on endocrine functions. *J. Endocrinol. Investig.* **2009**, *32*, 175–183. [CrossRef]
86. Tang, N.; Zhu, Z.Q. Adverse reproductive effects in female workers of lead battery plants. *Int. J. Occup. Med. Environ. Health* **2003**, *16*, 359–361. [PubMed]
87. Pollack, A.Z.; Schisterman, E.F.; Goldman, L.R.; Mumford, S.L.; Albert, P.S.; Jones, R.L.; Wactawski-Wende, J. Cadmium, Lead, and Mercury in Relation to Reproductive Hormones and Anovulation in Premenopausal Women. *Environ. Health Perspect.* **2011**, *119*, 1156–1161. [CrossRef] [PubMed]
88. Krieg, E.F., Jr.; Feng, H.A. The relationships between blood lead levels and serum follicle stimulating hormone and luteinizing hormone in the National Health and Nutrition Examination Survey 1999–2002. *Reprod. Toxicol.* **2011**, *32*, 277–285. [CrossRef]
89. Naicker, N.; Norris, S.A.; Mathee, A.; Becker, P.; Richter, L. Lead exposure is associated with a delay in the onset of puberty in South African adolescent females: Findings from the Birth to Twenty cohort. *Sci. Total. Environ.* **2010**, *408*, 4949–4954. [CrossRef] [PubMed]
90. Nkomo, P.; Richter, L.M.; Kagura, J.; Mathee, A.; Naicker, N.; Norris, S.A. Environmental lead exposure and pubertal trajectory classes in South African adolescent males and females. *Sci. Total. Environ.* **2018**, 1437–1445. [CrossRef] [PubMed]
91. De Queiroz, E.K.R.; Waissmann, W. Occupational exposure and effects on the male reproductive system. *Cadernos de Saúde Pública* **2006**, *22*, 485–493. [CrossRef]
92. Taupeau, C.; Poupon, J.; Nomé, F.; Lefèvre, B. Lead accumulation in the mouse ovary after treatment-induced follicular atresia. *Reprod. Toxicol.* **2001**, *15*, 385–391. [CrossRef]

93. Waseem, N.; Butt, S.A.; Hamid, S. Amelioration of lead induced changes in ovary of mice, by garlic extract. *J. Pak. Med. Assoc.* **2014**, *64*, 798–801.
94. Dhir, V.; Dhand, P. Toxicological Approach in Chronic Exposure to Lead on Reproductive Functions in Female Rats (*Rattus norvegicus*). *Toxicol. Int. Former. Indian J. Toxicol.* **2010**, *17*, 1–7. [CrossRef]
95. Dumitrescu, E.; Chiurciu, V.; Muselin, F.; Popescu, R.; Brezovan, D.; Cristina, R.T. Effects of long-term exposure of female rats to low levels of lead: Ovary and uterus histological architecture changes. *Turk. J. Biol.* **2015**, *39*, 284–289. [CrossRef]
96. Canaz, E.; Kilinc, M.; Sayar, H.; Kiran, G.; Ozyurek, E. Lead, selenium and nickel concentrations in epithelial ovarian cancer, borderline ovarian tumor and healthy ovarian tissues. *J. Trace Elements Med. Biol.* **2017**, *43*, 217–223. [CrossRef]
97. Bloom, M.S.; Kim, K.; Kruger, P.C. Associations between toxic metals in follicular fluid and in vitro fertilization (IVF) outcomes. *J. Assist. Reprod. Genet.* **2012**, *29*, 1369–1379. [CrossRef] [PubMed]
98. Cavallini, A.; Lippolis, C.; Vacca, M.; Nardelli, C.; Castegna, A.; Arnesano, F.; Carella, N.; DePalo, R. The Effects of Chronic Lifelong Activation of the AHR Pathway by Industrial Chemical Pollutants on Female Human Reproduction. *PLoS ONE* **2016**, *11*, e0152181. [CrossRef] [PubMed]
99. Kirmizi, D.A.; Baser, E.; Turksoy, V.A.; Kara, M.; Yalvac, E.S.; Gocmen, A.Y. Are heavy metal eposure and trace element levels related to metabolic and endocrine poblems in polycystic ovary syndrome? *Biol. Trace Elem. Res.* **2020**. [CrossRef] [PubMed]
100. Uchewa, O.O.; Ezugworie, O.J.; Obinna, U.O.; Joseph, E.O. Countering the effects of lead as an environmental toxicant on the microanatomy of female reproductive system of adult wistar rats using aqueous extract of *Ficus vogelii*. *J. Trace Elem. Med. Biol.* **2019**, *52*, 192–198. [CrossRef] [PubMed]
101. Kolesarova, A.; Roychoudhury, S.; Slivkova, J.; Sirotkin, A.; Capcarová, M.; Massanyi, P. In vitro study on the effects of lead and mercury on porcine ovarian granulosa cells. *J. Environ. Sci. Health Part A* **2010**, *45*, 320–331. [CrossRef] [PubMed]
102. Capcarová, M.; Kolesarova, A.; Lukac, N.; Sirotkin, A.; Roychoudhury, S. Antioxidant status and selected biochemical parameters of porcine ovarian granulosa cells exposed to leadin vitro. *J. Environ. Sci. Health Part A* **2009**, *44*, 1617–1623. [CrossRef] [PubMed]
103. Nampoothiri, L.; Gupta, S. Simultaneous effect of lead and cadmium on granulosa cells: A cellular model for ovarian toxicity. *Reprod. Toxicol.* **2006**, *21*, 179–185. [CrossRef]
104. Albishtue, A.A.; Yimer, N.; Zakaria, Z.A.; Haron, A.W.; Babji, A.S.; Abubakar, A.A.; Baiee, F.H.; Almhanna, H.K.; Almhanawi, B.H. The role of edible bird's nest and mechanism of averting lead acetate toxicity effect on rat uterus. *Veter. World* **2019**, *12*, 1013–1021. [CrossRef] [PubMed]
105. Vigeh, M.; Smith, D.R.; Hsu, P.-C. How does lead induce male infertility? *Iran. J. Reprod. Med.* **2011**, *9*, 1–8. [PubMed]
106. Gandhi, J.; Hernandez, R.J.; Chen, A.; Smith, N.L.; Sheynkin, Y.R.; Joshi, G.; Khan, S.A. Impaired hypothalamic-pituitary-testicular axis activity, spermatogenesis, and sperm function promote infertility in males with lead poisoning. *Zygote* **2017**, *25*, 103–110. [CrossRef] [PubMed]
107. Pizent, A.; Tariba, B.; Živković, T. Reproductive Toxicity of Metals in Men. *Arch. Ind. Hyg. Toxicol.* **2012**, *63*, 35–46. [CrossRef]
108. Apostoli, P.; Kiss, P.; Porru, S.; Bonde, J.P.; Vanhoorne, M. Male reproductive toxicity of lead in animals and humans. ASCLEPIOS Study Group. *Occup. Environ. Med.* **1998**, *55*, 364–374. [CrossRef] [PubMed]
109. Alexander, B.H.; Checkoway, H.; Faustman, E.M.; van Netten, C.; Muller, C.H.; Ewers, T.G. Contrasting associations of blood and semen lead concentrations with semen quality among lead smelter workers. *Am. J. Ind. Med.* **1998**, *34*, 464–469. [CrossRef]
110. Hosni, H.; Selim, O.; Abbas, M.; Fathy, A. Semen quality and reproductive endocrinal function related to blood lead levels in infertile painters. *Andrologia* **2013**, *45*, 120–127. [CrossRef]
111. Elsheikh, N.A.H.; Omer, N.A.; Yi-Ru, W.; Mei-Qian, K.; Ilyas, A.; Abdurahim, Y.; Wang, G. Protective effect of betaine against lead-induced testicular toxicity in male mice. *Andrologia* **2020**, *52*, e13600. [CrossRef]
112. Oyeyemi, W.; Princely, A.C.; Oluwadamilare, A.A.; Oore-Oluwapo, D.O.; Blessing, A.O.; Alfred, E.F. Clomiphene citrate ameliorated lead acetate-induced reproductive toxicity in male Wistar rats. *JBRA Assist. Reprod.* **2019**, *23*, 336–343. [CrossRef]
113. Kelainy, E.G.; Laila, I.M.I.; Ibrahim, S.R. The effect of ferulic acid against lead-induced oxidative stress and DNA damage in kidney and testes of rats. *Environ. Sci. Pollut. Res. Int.* **2019**, *26*, 31675–31684. [CrossRef]

114. Ezejiofor, A.N.; Orisakwe, O.E. The protective effect of Costus afer Ker Gawl aqueous leaf extract on lead-induced reproductive changes in male albino Wistar rats. *JBRA Assist. Reprod.* **2019**, *23*, 215–224. [CrossRef]
115. Sudjarwo, S.A.; Sudjarwo, G.W.K. Protective effect of curcumin on lead acetate-induced testicular toxicity in Wistar rats. *Res. Pharm. Sci.* **2017**, *12*, 381–390. [CrossRef] [PubMed]
116. Hassan, E.; El-Neweshy, M.S.; Hassan, M.; Noreldin, A.E. Thymoquinone attenuates testicular and spermotoxicity following subchronic lead exposure in male rats: Possible mechanisms are involved. *Life Sci.* **2019**, *230*, 132–140. [CrossRef]
117. Santhoshkumar, R. Protective effect of Abutilon indicum against lead-induced reproductive toxicity in male Wistar rats. *J. Cell. Biochem.* **2019**, *120*, 11196–11205. [CrossRef]
118. Massanyi, P.; Lukac, N.; Makarevich, A.V.; Chrenek, P.; Forgacs, Z.; Zakrzewski, M.; Stawarz, R.; Toman, R.; Lazor, P.; Flesarova, S. Lead-induced alterations in rat kidneys and testesin vivo. *J. Environ. Sci. Health Part A* **2007**, *42*, 671–676. [CrossRef] [PubMed]
119. Błaszczyk, M.; Toporcerova, S.; Popelkova, M.; Semla, M.; Tvrda, E.; Lukac, N.; Massanyi, P.; Stawarz, R.; Binkowski, L. Semen metal profile, spermatozoa morphology and semen biochemical parameters in subfertile men with different lifestyle habits. *J. Elem.* **2019**, *24*, 603–614. [CrossRef]
120. Tvrdá, E.; Kňažická, Z.; Lukáčová, J.; Schneidgenová, M.; Goc, Z.; Greń, A.; Szabó, C.; Massányi, P.; Lukáč, N. The impact of lead and cadmium on selected motility, prooxidant and antioxidant parameters of bovine seminal plasma and spermatozoa. *J. Environ. Sci. Health Part A* **2013**, *48*, 1292–1300. [CrossRef]
121. Slivkova, J.; Popelkova, M.; Massanyi, P.; Toporcerová, S.; Stawarz, R.; Formicki, G.; Lukac, N.; Putała, A.; Guzik, M. Concentration of trace elements in human semen and relation to spermatozoa quality. *J. Environ. Sci. Health Part A* **2009**, *44*, 370–375. [CrossRef]
122. Massanyi, P.; Trandzik, J.; Nad, P.; Skalická, M.; Koréneková, B.; Lukac, N.; Fabis, M.; Toman, R. Seminal Concentration of Trace Elements in Fox and Relationships to Spermatozoa Quality. *J. Environ. Sci. Health Part A* **2005**, *40*, 1097–1105. [CrossRef]
123. Massányi, P.; Trandžík, J.; Nad', P. Concentration of copper, iron, zinc, cadmium, lead, and nickel in bull and ram semen and relation to the occurrence of pathological spermatozoa. *J. Environ. Sci. Health A Toxic Hazard Subst. Environ. Eng.* **2004**, *39*, 3005–3014. [CrossRef]
124. Massanyi, P.; Trandzík, J.; Nad, P.; Koréneková, B.; Skalická, M.; Toman, R.; Lukac, N.; Strapák, P.; Halo, M.; Turcan, J. Concentration of copper, iron, zinc, cadmium, lead, and nickel in boar semen and relation to the spermatozoa quality. *J. Environ. Sci. Health Part A* **2003**, *38*, 2643–2651. [CrossRef] [PubMed]
125. Hernández-Ochoa, I.; García-Vargas, G.; López-Carrillo, L.; Rubio-Andrade, M.; Morán-Martínez, J.; Cebrián, M.E.; Quintanilla-Vega, B. Low lead environmental exposure alters semen quality and sperm chromatin condensation in northern Mexico. *Reprod. Toxicol.* **2005**, *20*, 221–228. [CrossRef] [PubMed]
126. Pant, N.; Kumar, G.; Upadhyay, A.D.; Gupta, Y.K.; Chaturvedi, P.K. Correlation between lead and cadmium concentration and semen quality. *Andrologia* **2015**, *47*, 887–891. [CrossRef]
127. Famurewa, A.C.; Ugwuja, E.I. Association of Blood and Seminal Plasma Cadmium and Lead Levels With Semen Quality in Non-Occupationally Exposed Infertile Men in Abakaliki, South East Nigeria. *J. Fam. Reprod. Health* **2017**, *11*, 97–103.
128. U.S. EPA. Basic Information about Mercury 2019. Available online: https://www.epa.gov/mercury/basic-information-about-mercury (accessed on 15 August 2020).
129. Bank, M.S. *Mercury in the Environment: Pattern and Process*; Univ of California Press: Berkeley, CA, USA, 2012.
130. Ask, K.; Åkesson, A.; Berglund, M.; Vahter, M. Inorganic mercury and methylmercury in placentas of Swedish women. *Environ. Health Perspect.* **2002**, *110*, 523–526. [CrossRef] [PubMed]
131. Al-Saleh, I.; Shinwari, N.; Mashhour, A.; Mohamed, G.E.D.; Rabah, A. Heavy metals (lead, cadmium and mercury) in maternal, cord blood and placenta of healthy women. *Int. J. Hyg. Environ. Health* **2011**, *214*, 79–101. [CrossRef] [PubMed]
132. Gasparik, J.; Vladarova, D.; Capcarová, M.; Smehyl, P.; Slamecka, J.; Garaj, P.; Stawarz, R.; Massanyi, P. Concentration of lead, cadmium, mercury and arsenic in leg skeletal muscles of three species of wild birds. *J. Environ. Sci. Health Part A* **2010**, *45*, 818–823. [CrossRef] [PubMed]
133. Kolesarova, A.; Slamecka, J.; Jurcik, R.; Tataruch, F.; Lukac, N.; Kováčik, J.; Capcarová, M.; Valent, M.; Massanyi, P. Environmental levels of cadmium, lead and mercury in brown hares and their relation to blood metabolic parameters. *J. Environ. Sci. Health Part A* **2008**, *43*, 646–650. [CrossRef]

134. Massányi, P.; Tataruch, F.; Slamčeka, J.; Toman, R.; Jurík, R. Accumulation of lead, cadmium, and mercury in liver and kidney of the brown hare (*Lepus europaeus*) in relation to the season, age, and sex in the West Slovakian Lowland. *J. Environ. Sci. Health Part A* **2003**, *38*, 1299–1309. [CrossRef]
135. Capcarová, M.; Binkowski, L.J.; Stawarz, R.; Schwarczová, L.; Massányi, P. Levels of essential and xenobiotic elements and their relationships in milk available on the Slovak market with the estimation of consumer exposure. *Biol. Trace Elem. Res.* **2019**, *188*, 404–411. [CrossRef]
136. Semla, M.; Schwarcz, P.; Mezey, J.; Binkowski, Ł.J.; Błaszczyk, M.; Semla, M.; Greń, A.; Stawarz, R.; Massanyi, P. Biogenic and Risk Elements in Wines from the Slovak Market with the Estimation of Consumer Exposure. *Biol. Trace Elem. Res.* **2018**, *184*, 33–41. [CrossRef] [PubMed]
137. Árvay, J.; Tomáš, J.; Hauptvogl, M.; Massányi, P.; Harangozo, L'.; Tóth, T.; Stanovič, R.; Bryndzová, Š.; Bumbalová, M. Human exposure to heavy metals and possible public health risks via consumption of wild edible mushrooms from Slovak Paradise National Park, Slovakia. *J. Environ. Sci. Health Part B* **2015**, *50*, 833–843. [CrossRef] [PubMed]
138. Árvay, J.; Tomáš, J.; Hauptvogl, M.; Kopernická, M.; Kováčik, A.; Bajčan, D.; Massanyi, P. Contamination of wild-grown edible mushrooms by heavy metals in a former mercury-mining area. *J. Environ. Sci. Health Part B* **2014**, *49*, 815–827. [CrossRef] [PubMed]
139. Habán, M.; Habanova, M.; Otepka, P.; Lukac, N.; Massanyi, P. Concentration of heavy metals in various children's herbal tea types and their correlations. *J. Environ. Sci. Health Part B* **2008**, *43*, 533–538. [CrossRef]
140. Binkowski, Ł.J.; Rogoziński, P.; Roychoudhury, S.; Bruliński, K.; Kucharzewski, M.; Laciak, T.; Massanyi, P.; Stawarz, R. Accumulation of metals in cancerous and healthy tissues of patients with lung cancer in Southern Poland. *J. Environ. Sci. Health Part A* **2015**, *50*, 9–15. [CrossRef]
141. Mortensen, M.E.; Caudill, S.P.; Caldwell, K.L.; Ward, C.D.; Jones, R.L. Total and methyl mercury in whole blood measured for the first time in the U.S. population: NHANES 2011–2012. *Environ. Res.* **2014**, *134*, 257–264. [CrossRef]
142. Wells, E.M.; Kopylev, L.; Nachman, R.; Radke, E.G.; Segal, D. Seafood, wine, rice, vegetables, and other food items associated with mercury biomarkers among seafood and non-seafood consumers: NHANES 2011–2012. *J. Expo. Sci. Environ. Epidemiol.* **2020**, *30*, 504–514. [CrossRef]
143. Zhu, F.; Chen, C.; Zhang, Y.; Chen, S.; Huang, X.; Li, J.; Wang, Y.; Liu, X.; Deng, G.; Gao, J. Corrigendum to "Elevated blood mercury level has a non-linear association with infertility in U.S. women: Data from the NHANES 2013–2016" [Reprod. Toxicol. 91C (2020) 53–58]. *Reprod. Toxicol.* **2020**, *94*, 103. [CrossRef]
144. Colson, A. On the influence of mercury on the functions of the uterus. *Med. Chir. Rev.* **1829**, *10*, 471–472.
145. De Bellis, L. L'azione della formoguanamina e dei sali di mercurio sulla muscolatura liscia dell'utero isolato di coniglia [Action of formoguanamine and mercury salts on the smooth muscles of the isolated uterus of the rabbit]. *Boll. Soc. Ital. Biol. Sper.* **1952**, *28*, 48–50.
146. Baltrukiewicz, Z. Gromadzenie rteci w narzadach rodnych i płodach w róznych okresach ciazy po dozylnym podaniu neohydryny-Hg-203 [Accumulation of mercury in reproductive organs and fetuses in various periods of pregnancy after intravenous administration of neohydrin-Hg-203]. *Acta Physiol. Pol.* **1970**, *21*, 777–783. [PubMed]
147. Bjørklund, G.; Chirumbolo, S.; Dadar, M.; Pivina, L.; Lindh, U.; Butnariu, M.; Aaseth, J. Mercury exposure and its effects on fertility and pregnancy outcome. *Basic Clin. Pharmacol. Toxicol.* **2019**, *125*, 317–327. [CrossRef] [PubMed]
148. Al-Saleh, I.; Shinwari, N.; Al-Amodi, M. Accumulation of Mercury in Ovaries of Mice After the Application of Skin-lightening Creams. *Biol. Trace Elem. Res.* **2009**, *131*, 43–54. [CrossRef]
149. Schuurs, A. Reproductive toxicity of occupational mercury. A review of the literature. *J. Dent.* **1999**, *27*, 249–256. [CrossRef]
150. Henriques, M.C.; Loureiro, S.; Fardilha, M.; Herdeiro, M.T. Exposure to mercury and human reproductive health: A systematic review. *Reprod. Toxicol.* **2019**, *85*, 93–103. [CrossRef] [PubMed]
151. Lee, T.W.; Kim, D.H.; Ryu, J.Y. The effects of exposure to lead, cadmium and mercury on follicle-stimulating hormone levels in men and postmenopausal women: Data from the Second Korean National Environmental Health Survey (2012–2014). *Ann. Occup. Environ. Med.* **2019**, *31*, e21. [CrossRef]
152. Chen, Y.W.; Huang, C.F.; Tsai, K.S.; Yang, R.S.; Yen, C.C.; Yang, C.Y.; Lin-Shiau, S.Y.; Liu, S.H. Methylmercury Induces Pancreatic β-Cell Apoptosis and Dysfunction. *Chem. Res. Toxicol.* **2006**, *19*, 1080–1085. [CrossRef]

153. Davis, B.; Price, H.C.; O'Connor, R.W.; Fernando, R.; Rowland, A.S.; Morgan, D.L. Mercury vapor and female reproductive toxicity. *Toxicol. Sci.* **2001**, *59*, 291–296. [CrossRef]
154. Khan, A.T. Effects of inorganic mercury on reproductive performance of mice. *Food Chem. Toxicol.* **2004**, *42*, 571–577. [CrossRef]
155. Ma, Y.; Zhu, M.; Miao, L.; Zhang, X.; Dong, X.; Zou, X.T. Mercuric Chloride Induced Ovarian Oxidative Stress by Suppressing Nrf2-Keap1 Signal Pathway and its Downstream Genes in Laying Hens. *Biol. Trace Elem. Res.* **2018**, *185*, 185–196. [CrossRef]
156. Altunkaynak, B.Z.; Akgül, N.; Yahyazadeh, A.; Türkmen, A.P.; Unal, B. Effect of mercury vapor inhalation on rat ovary: Stereology and histopathology. *J. Obstet. Gynaecol. Res.* **2016**, *42*, 410–416. [CrossRef]
157. Lamperti, A.A.; Printz, R.H. Localization, Accumulation, and Toxic Effects of Mercuric Chloride on the Reproductive Axis of the Female Hamster. *Biol. Reprod.* **1974**, *11*, 180–186. [CrossRef]
158. Merlo, E.; Schereider, I.R.; Simões, M.R.; Vassallo, D.V.; Graceli, J.B. Mercury leads to features of polycystic ovary syndrome in rats. *Toxicol. Lett.* **2019**, *312*, 45–54. [CrossRef] [PubMed]
159. Verschaeve, L.; Leonard, A. Dominant lethal test in female mice treated with methyl mercury chloride. *Mutat. Res. Toxicol.* **1984**, *136*, 131–136. [CrossRef]
160. Shen, W.; Chen, Y.; Li, C.; Ji, Q. [Effect of mercury chloride on the reproductive function and visceral organ of female mouse]. *Wei Sheng Yan Jiu* **2000**, *29*, 75–77. [PubMed]
161. Roychoudhury, S.; Massanyi, P.; Slivkova, J.; Formicki, G.; Lukac, N.; Slamecka, J.; Slama, P.; Kolesarova, A. Effect of mercury on porcine ovarian granulosa cellsin vitro. *J. Environ. Sci. Health Part A* **2015**, *50*, 839–845. [CrossRef]
162. Kňažická, Z.; Lukáč, N.; Forgács, Z.; Tvrdá, E.; Lukáčová, J.; Slivková, J.; Binkowski, L.; Massányi, P. Effects of mercury on the steroidogenesis of human adrenocarcinoma (NCI-H295R) cell line. *J. Environ. Sci. Health Part A* **2013**, *48*, 348–353. [CrossRef] [PubMed]
163. Lamperti, A.A.; Printz, R.H. Effects of mercuric chloride on the reproductive cycle of the female hamster. *Biol. Reprod.* **1973**, *8*, 378–387. [CrossRef] [PubMed]
164. Lundholm, C. Effects of methyl mercury at different dose regimes on eggshell formation and some biochemical characteristics of the eggshell gland mucosa of the domestic fowl. *Comp. Biochem. Physiol. Part C Pharmacol. Toxicol. Endocrinol.* **1995**, *110*, 23–28. [CrossRef]
165. Balachandran, A.; Bhatnagar, M.K.; Geissinger, H.D. Scanning and transmission electron microscopic studies on the oviducts of Pekin ducks fed methyl mercury containing diets. *Scanning Electron Microsc.* **1985**, *1*, 311–322.
166. WHO. Elemental Mercury Andinorganic Mercury Compounds: Human Health Aspects. Available online: https://www.who.int/ipcs/publications/cicad/en/cicad50.pdf?ua=1 (accessed on 15 August 2020).
167. Koli, S.; Prakash, A.; Choudhury, S.; Mandil, R.; Garg, S.K. Mercury affects uterine myogenic activity even without producing any apparent toxicity in rats: Involvement of calcium-signaling cascades. *J. Trace Elem. Med. Biol.* **2020**, *57*, 40–47. [CrossRef] [PubMed]
168. Koli, S.; Prakash, A.; Choudhury, S.; Mandil, R.; Garg, S.K. Calcium Channels, Rho-Kinase, Protein Kinase-C, and Phospholipase-C Pathways Mediate Mercury Chloride-Induced Myometrial Contractions in Rats. *Biol. Trace Elem. Res.* **2019**, *187*, 418–424. [CrossRef] [PubMed]
169. Guyot, E.; Solovyova, Y.; Tomkiewicz, C.; Leblanc, A.; Pierre, S.; El Balkhi, S.; Le Frere-Belda, M.-A.; Lecuru, F.; Poupon, J.; Barouki, R.; et al. Determination of Heavy Metal Concentrations in Normal and Pathological Human Endometrial Biopsies and In Vitro Regulation of Gene Expression by Metals in the Ishikawa and Hec-1b Endometrial Cell Line. *PLoS ONE* **2015**, *10*, e0142590. [CrossRef]
170. Nakade, U.P.; Garg, S.K.; Sharma, A.; Choudhury, S.; Yadav, R.S.; Gupta, K.; Sood, N. Lead-induced adverse effects on the reproductive system of rats with particular reference to histopathological changes in uterus. *Indian J. Pharmacol.* **2015**, *47*, 22–26. [CrossRef]
171. Da Silva, D.A.F.; Teixeira, C.T.; Scarano, W.R.; Favareto, A.P.A.; Fernandez, C.D.; Grotto, D.; Barbosa, F.; Kempinas, W.D.G.; Barbosa, F. Effects of methylmercury on male reproductive functions in Wistar rats. *Reprod. Toxicol.* **2011**, *31*, 431–439. [CrossRef]
172. Boujbiha, M.A.M.; Hamden, K.; Guermazi, F.; Bouslama, A.; Omezzine, A.; El Feki, A. Impairment of Spermatogenesis in Rats by Mercuric Chloride: Involvement of Low 17β-Estradiol Level in Induction of Acute Oxidative Stress. *Biol. Trace Elem. Res.* **2011**, *142*, 598–610. [CrossRef]

173. Martinez, C.S.; Escobar, A.G.; Torres, J.G.D.; Brum, D.S.; Santos, F.W.; Alonso, M.J.; Salaices, M.; Vassallo, D.V.; Peçanha, F.M.; Leivas, F.G.; et al. Chronic Exposure to Low Doses of Mercury Impairs Sperm Quality and Induces Oxidative Stress in Rats. *J. Toxicol. Environ. Health Part A* **2014**, *77*, 143–154. [CrossRef]
174. Adelakun, S.; Ukwenya, V.O.; Akingbade, G.T.; Omotoso, O.D.; Aniah, J.A. Interventions of aqueous extract of Solanum melongena fruits (garden eggs) on mercury chloride induced testicular toxicity in adult male Wistar rats. *Biomed. J.* **2020**, *43*, 174–182. [CrossRef]
175. Almeer, R.S.; Albasher, G.; Kassab, R.B.; Ibrahim, S.R.; Alotibi, F.; Alarifi, S.; Ali, D.; Alkahtani, S.; Moneim, A.E.A. Ziziphus spina-christi leaf extract attenuates mercury chloride-induced testicular dysfunction in rats. *Environ. Sci. Pollut. Res.* **2020**, *27*, 3401–3412. [CrossRef]
176. Kalender, S.; Uzun, F.G.; Demir, F.; Uzunhisarcikli, M.; Aslanturk, A. Mercuric chloride-induced testicular toxicity in rats and the protective role of sodium selenite and vitamin E. *Food Chem. Toxicol.* **2013**, *55*, 456–462. [CrossRef]
177. Moussa, H.; Hachfi, L.; Trimèche, M.; Najjar, M.F.; Sakly, R. Accumulation of mercury and its effects on testicular functions in rats intoxicated orally by methylmercury. *Andrologia* **2010**, *43*, 23–27. [CrossRef]
178. Orisakwe, O.E.; Afonne, O.J.; Nwobodo, E.; Asomugha, L.; Dioka, C.E. Low-dose mercury induces testicular damage protected by zinc in mice. *Eur. J. Obstet. Gynecol. Reprod. Biol.* **2001**, *95*, 92–96. [CrossRef]
179. Altunkaynak, M.; Akgül, N.; Yahyazadeh, A.; Altunkaynak, B.; Türkmen, A.P.; Akgül, H.; Aksak, S.; Unal, B. A stereological and histopathological study of the effects of exposure of male rat testes to mercury vapor. *Biotech. Histochem.* **2015**, *90*, 529–534. [CrossRef] [PubMed]
180. Fadda, L.M.; Alhusaini, A.M.; Al-Qahtani, Q.H.; Ali, H.M.; Hasan, I.H. Role of α-tocopherol and Lactobacillus plantarum in the alleviation of mercuric chloride-induced testicular atrophy in rat's model: Implication of molecular mechanisms. *J. Biochem. Mol. Toxicol.* **2020**, *34*, e22481. [CrossRef]
181. Kandemir, F.M.; Caglayan, C.; Aksu, E.H.; Yıldırım, S.; Kucukler, S.; Gur, C.; Eser, G. Protective effect of rutin on mercuric chloride-induced reproductive damage in male rats. *Andrologia* **2020**, *52*, e13524. [CrossRef]
182. Massányi, P.; Lukáč, N.; Slivková, J.; Kováčik, J.; Makarevich, A.V.; Chrenek, P.; Toman, R.; Forgács, Z.; Somosy, Z.; Stawarz, R.; et al. Mercury-induced alterations in rat kidneys and testes in vivo. *J. Environ. Sci. Health Part A* **2007**, *42*, 865–870. [CrossRef] [PubMed]
183. Martinez, C.S.; Torres, J.G.D.; Peçanha, F.M.; Anselmo-Franci, J.A.; Vassallo, D.V.; Salaices, M.; Alonso, M.J.; Wiggers, G.A. 60-Day Chronic Exposure to Low Concentrations of $HgCl_2$ Impairs Sperm Quality: Hormonal Imbalance and Oxidative Stress as Potential Routes for Reproductive Dysfunction in Rats. *PLoS ONE* **2014**, *9*, e111202. [CrossRef]
184. Chowdhury, A.R.; Arora, U. Toxic effect of mercury on testes in different animal species. *Indian J. Physiol. Pharmacol.* **1982**, *26*, 246–249.
185. Slivková, J.; Massányi, P.; Pizzi, F.; Trandžík, J.; Roychoudhury, S.; Lukáč, N.; Danková, M.; Almášiová, V. In vitro toxicity of mercuric chloride on rabbit spermatozoa motility and cell membrane integrity. *J. Environ. Sci. Health Part A* **2010**, *45*, 767–774. [CrossRef]

toxics

MDPI

Review

Emerging Links between Cadmium Exposure and Insulin Resistance: Human, Animal, and Cell Study Data

Aleksandra Buha [1,*], Danijela Đukić-Ćosić [1], Marijana Ćurčić [1], Zorica Bulat [1], Biljana Antonijević [1], Jean-Marc Moulis [2,3], Marina Goumenou [4,5] and David Wallace [6]

1 Department of Toxicology "Akademik Danilo Soldatović", University of Belgrade-Faculty of Pharmacy, 11000 Belgrade, Serbia; danijela.djukic.cosic@pharmacy.bg.ac.rs (D.Đ.-Ć.); marijana.curcic@pharmacy.bg.ac.rs (M.Ć.); zorica.bulat@pharmacy.bg.ac.rs (Z.B.); biljana.antonijevic@pharmacy.bg.ac.rs (B.A.)
2 Alternative Energies and Atomic Energy Commission—Fundamental Research Division—Interdisciplinary Research Institute of Grenoble (CEA-IRIG), University of Grenoble Alpes, F-38000 Grenoble, France; jean-marc.moulis@cea.fr
3 Laboratory of Fundamental and Applied Bioenergetics (LBFA), University of Grenoble Alpes, Inserm U1055, F-38000 Grenoble, France
4 Centre of Toxicology and Forensic Sciences, Medicine School, University of Crete, 70013 Heraklion, Greece; marina.goumenou@gmail.com
5 General Chemical State Laboratory of Greek Republic, 71202 Heraklion, Greece
6 Department of Pharmacology & Toxicology, Oklahoma State University Center for Health Sciences, Tulsa, OK 74107, USA; david.wallace@okstate.edu
* Correspondence: aleksandra@pharmacy.bg.ac.rs

Received: 27 July 2020; Accepted: 18 August 2020; Published: 27 August 2020

Abstract: Recent research has helped clarify the role of cadmium (Cd) in various pathological states. We have demonstrated Cd involvement in pancreatic cancer, as well as the bioaccumulation of Cd in the pancreas. Bioaccumulation and increased toxicity suggest that Cd may also be involved in other pancreas-mediated diseases, like diabetes. Cd falls into the category of "hyperglycemic" metals, i.e., metals that increase blood glucose levels, which could be due to increased gluconeogenesis, damage to β-cells leading to reduced insulin production, or insulin resistance at target tissue resulting in a lack of glucose uptake. This review addresses the current evidence for the role of Cd, leading to insulin resistance from human, animal, and in vitro studies. Available data have shown that Cd may affect normal insulin function through multiple pathways. There is evidence that Cd exposure results in the perturbation of the enzymes and modulatory proteins involved in insulin signal transduction at the target tissue and mutations of the insulin receptor. Cd, through well-described mechanisms of oxidative stress, inflammation, and mitochondrial damage, may also alter insulin production in β-cells. More work is necessary to elucidate the mechanisms associated with Cd-mediated insulin resistance.

Keywords: cadmium; insulin; diabetes; hyperglycemia; hyperinsulinemia; lipogenic; β-cell toxicity

1. Introduction

Insulin-mediated glucose disposal widely varies in its sensitivity across populations [1], and depending on the level of compensatory hyperinsulinemia, resistance to insulin can or cannot be overcome. This insensitivity can lead to glucose intolerance, high-plasma triglyceride levels, low high-density lipoprotein cholesterol (HDL-C) concentrations, and hypertension [2]. If not overcome, it will lead to type 2 diabetes (T2D) development. Simultaneously, this collection of abnormalities has been linked with a significantly increased risk of cardiovascular diseases (CVD) [2].

The proposed association was formally established in the report of the adult treatment panel III of the National Cholesterol Educational Program. Formerly known as syndrome X, insulin resistance (IR) syndrome represents the insensitivity of the peripheral tissues (e.g., muscle, liver, adipose tissue) to the effects of insulin. IR is defined as a state wherein normal insulin concentrations evoke a less-than-normal biological response [3]. Although not a disease per se, it may be understood as a condition that increases the likelihood of developing a cluster of abnormalities, such as glucose intolerance, dyslipidemia, endothelial dysfunction, hemodynamic changes, increased testosterone secretion, and sleep-disordered breathing [4]. Additionally, it does not necessarily lead to, but instead increases the risk of clinical syndromes like CVD, essential hypertension, polycystic ovary syndrome, nonalcoholic fatty liver disease, and certain forms of cancers [2]. Metabolic syndrome (MS) is a collection of cardiometabolic risk factors. It is often characterized by IR that may provide a link between physical inactivity and MS development [5]. Most importantly, IR and impaired insulin secretion play a crucial role in the pathogenesis of T2D [6]. Although the potential causative connection has been shown for certain pollutants and IR development, the role of environmental chemicals in IR pathogenesis and the molecular mechanisms contributing to its development have not been fully elucidated yet [7].

Over fifty years ago, there was evidence suggesting that certain inorganic elements may alter glucose utilization in target tissues via sulfhydryl modification [8]. Since the 1970s, there has been a growing body of evidence that supports the involvement of these elements in various metabolic disorders associated with impaired β-cell function [9–12]. Several inorganic elements may influence the proper regulation of insulin/glucose homeostasis. They can be divided into two categories—hyperglycemic and hypoglycemic—based on their effects on insulin production or insulin action at target tissues [13]. The categorization of different elements is displayed in Table 1.

Table 1. Categorization of different elements as hyper- or hypoglycemic [13].

Hyperglycemic	Hypoglycemic
Arsenic	Zinc
Mercury	Vanadium
Iron	Chromium
Lead	Magnesium
Nickel	
Cadmium	

Our interest is focused on the actions of cadmium (Cd) and its ability to alter numerous cell and organ systems. This toxic metal is characterized by a high soil-to-plant transfer rate, which makes the dietary exposure to this metal inevitable and a matter of great public health concern [14,15]. Another important source of exposure of the general population to Cd is smoking, as shown by elevated Cd levels in the smokers' blood [16]. Once inside the organism, Cd has a long biological half-life, with estimates reaching 45 years for humans [17]. Whole-blood and urinary Cd concentrations are widely accepted markers of Cd exposure and accumulation [14,18]. Long-term exposure to Cd has been associated with various conditions, including various renal syndromes, osteoporosis and osteomalacia, CVD, and different types of cancer [14,15,19–25]. Its endocrine-disrupting properties have also been shown, suggesting its possible effects on estrogenic activity [26–29], alterations in semen and the testis [30–32], and a role in thyroid disorders [33–35]. The mode of toxic Cd actions in the organism have been extensively investigated, but still not entirely elucidated, mainly because they may change with the dose and the detailed health status of the exposed subjects. Recent reviews by Đukić-Ćosić et al. [36] and Wallace et al. [37] have summarized the most critical mechanisms of Cd toxicity: changes in gene expression and DNA repair, interference with autophagy and apoptosis pathways, oxidative stress induction, interaction with bioelements, and epigenetic modifications. These mechanisms underlie the possible role of Cd as a metabolic disruptor. Its direct pancreatotoxic actions are buttressed by the Cd's ability to accumulate in the pancreas, as shown in many human studies [22,38–40]. Similar results have been obtained in animal studies as well [41,42], with a dose-dependent accumulation pattern observed in rats [22]. In vitro studies have shown not only dose- but also a time-dependent accumulation of Cd in insulin-producing β-cells [43]. Furthermore, having in mind Cd's deleterious effects on the kidneys [14] and the role of kidneys in glucose homeostasis, which is accomplished through the processes of gluconeogenesis, glucose filtration, glucose reabsorption, and glucose consumption [44], it could be presumed that Cd's effects in the kidneys do contribute to IR development to a certain point. One of the first reports of Cd's ability to promote the development of diabetes appeared nearly four decades ago, when Merali and Singhal reported that neonatal exposure to Cd resulted in IR and diabetes development in rats [45]. The present review aims to provide an overview of the potential role of Cd exposure in IR collected in human, animal, and cell studies, focusing mainly on those conducted in the last two decades. Furthermore, the review will also briefly discuss the existence of a threshold for this effect.

2. Insulin Resistance and Cadmium: Human Studies

Human studies investigating the link between Cd exposure and IR are limited and have yielded somewhat conflicting data. The first association between Cd content, impaired fasting glucose (IFG), and diabetes was suggested by Schwartz et al. [46], who analyzed the data of the third National Health and Nutrition Examination Survey (NHANES III). This large, cross-sectional study revealed a significant, dose-dependent association between Cd urinary levels and IFG/diabetes prevalence, regardless of the source of Cd exposure. Another study analyzing NHANES participants for the years 2005 through 2010 aged ≥40 years revealed a complex, non-linear association between higher Cd levels and prediabetes state. Since this association varied across smoking groups and age, the authors suggested a complex relationship between Cd exposure, age, smoking habits, and prediabetes odds. Nevertheless, since no differences in the Homeostatic Model Assessment for IR (HOMA-IR) were observed across the exposure quintiles, the authors marked changes in IR as an unlikely cause of Cd effects on glucose levels [47]. The relationship between Cd exposure and T2D occurrence was confirmed in the study comparing the levels of Cd in various biological samples (blood, urine, and scalp hair) of patients having T2D (age range 31–60) with the levels in control subjects. Significantly higher levels of Cd were observed in scalp hair samples from patients compared to control individuals, along with a similar trend in observed values obtained from blood and urine samples [48]. Studies that followed tried to establish possible mechanisms of Cd in disturbing glucose metabolism. Pizzino et al. [49] investigated glycemic control, oxidative stress markers, and urinary Cd levels from 111 males (aged 12–14 years) living in polluted areas of Sicily and control age-matched population of 60 males living 28–45 km from the contaminated site. The results revealed altered glycemic control in adolescents that was associated with higher Cd levels. Altered glycemic control was demonstrated by the robust correlation between Cd and the homeostatic model assessment of HOMA-IR, along with markers of disturbed oxidative status. The authors identified oxidative stress disturbance to play a role in Cd-induced IR [49]. Apart from oxidative stress induction, Cd's ability to induce inflammation was also investigated. In a case-control, cross-sectional study, including 120 healthy controls and 105 systemic lupus erythematosus (SLE) patients, the relationship between various trace elements with SLE diagnosis, disease activity, and IR was assessed [50]. Serum levels of Cd were higher in patients with IR. Cd's ability to impair insulin sensitivity was connected to the positive association between Cd and the C-reactive protein (CRP). Namely, CRP as an inflammatory marker was shown to have a role in the development of diabetes [51].

Conflicting results from multiple studies have complicated the interpretation of Cd-mediated hyperglycemia. Jacquet et al. provided a comprehensive review of these conflicting reports in a 2016 review, where they categorized the effects as having "associations", "no association", or "potentiation" in diabetes [52]. Examples of this data variability is reflected in a study of Scandinavian Caucasian women, aged 64, which showed conflicting data with the previously mentioned studies [53]. Two thousand five hundred and ninety-five women were screened with oral glucose tolerance tests to identify subjects with T2D, impaired glucose tolerance (IGT), and normal glucose tolerance (NGT), and samples were randomly chosen from each group. Cd concentration was measured in blood and urine samples, while the HOMA-IR calculations assessed the acute insulin response. A follow-up examination was also performed. Both cross-sectional and prospective studies showed no association between Cd exposure and increased risk of T2D, impaired insulin secretion, or insulin sensitivity [53]. The discrepancies in these results with previously published data were explained by differences in the occurrence of T2D risk factors in investigated groups, such as age, obesity, smoking, lifestyle, and ethnic predispositions. Furthermore, all women studied were aged 64+, which does not inform on the behavior of other populations. Interestingly, however, Wu et al. [54], in their PRISMA-compliant systematic review and meta-analysis based on 11 cohort/cross-sectional studies included in the meta-analysis, determined that high Cd exposure may not be a risk factor for diabetes development. Moreover, Anetor et al. [55] found significantly lower Cd blood levels from diabetic patients when compared to controls. This conflicted finding was partly attributed to the observed higher Zn levels in the same group of patients and the relatively small sample size (65 participants). Indeed, Cd belongs to the same group of elements as zinc, and the number of common biological targets of the two metals abound [56–60]. The role of zinc in insulin regulation has been extensively examined [61–63]. Zinc associates with insulin in exocytosis granules, and a significant amount of zinc is subsequently released into the extracellular space. Zinc can act as an autocrine mediator, affecting the activity of surrounding β-cells [61]. Defects in the transporters, such as SLC30A (ZNT) for the Zn provision for insulin secretion or SLC39A (ZIP) for replenishment, result in reduced intracellular zinc and a reduction in functional insulin release [62]. Changes in functional insulin release and alterations in zinc homeostasis may thus combine to contribute to glucose intolerance and IR [63].

Swaddiwudhipong and associates conducted a series of studies in Cd-exposed adults from Mae Sot District, Tak Province, in northwestern Thailand. This region was contaminated by the Cd-rich waste of Zn mines, and the population was Cd-exposed by the consumption of rice and other crops irrigated by downstream water. No association between urinary Cd levels and an increase in diabetes prevalence and risk were found [64,65]. The follow-up examination conducted on 436 persons who had urinary Cd levels >5 μg/g creatinine revealed a significant increase in the prevalence of diabetes compared to baseline [66].

The question of the role of kidneys in Cd-induced IR has been raised earlier. The kidney is responsible for up to 20% of all glucose production, and these figures are even higher in diabetic conditions [44]. Moreover, IR represents an early metabolic alteration in chronic kidney disease (CKD) patients, with the skeletal muscle representing the primary site of IR [67]. On the other hand, a recent study in a group of 395 subjects from low- and high-Cd exposure areas demonstrated that glomerular filtration rate could be linked to Cd exposure and tubular toxicity [68]. This linkage was shown to act in both dose and toxicity severity-dependent manners. The association of Cd with CKD was recently highlighted in a review by Satarug [14], which addressed the connection between Cd dietary intake and its effects on kidneys. However, animal studies have shown that the Cd effect on fasting blood glucose elevation is evident before signs of renal dysfunction are overt [69]. It is, nevertheless, highly plausible that Cd acts synergistically with chronic hyperglycemia seen in diabetic nephropathy. For example, research on 65 participants, consisting of 45 T2D and 20 healthy individuals, revealed the association between higher Cd levels in the poor glycemic control group [55]. Thus, Cd should certainly be considered as the agent of high importance in the progression of diabetes-related kidney disease, and the toxic effects of Cd in the kidney certainly further contributes to the role of Cd in IR.

Studies conducted in human subjects have shown conflicting data on the role of Cd in IR development. The obtained results depend on many factors, and the actual prevalence of diabetes in the study population seems to have an important impact on them. Although questionable due to ethical reasons, prospective studies investigating the Cd levels, especially low-level exposure, before the presentation of pathologies/toxicity is warranted to establish the causality bases for this association.

3. Insulin Resistance and Cadmium: Animal Studies

For the last five decades, studies in animals have suggested that both acute and chronic Cd exposure can affect glucose metabolism and synthesis regulation, and alter insulin secretion [70,71]. Intraperitoneal administration of a single dose of Cd-acetate to mice (2.0–6.0 mg/kg body weight (b.w.) and rats (0.84 mg/kg b.w.) was shown to cause a significant increase of blood glucose [70,72]. In addition, feeding animals chow containing increasing amounts of Cd (0–200 ppm $CdCl_2$) for 30 days resulted in a significant dose-dependent elevation of blood glucose levels [73]. The ability of the pancreas to accumulate Cd has been demonstrated in multiple animal studies. Chronic oral administration of Cd for 60 days (100 mg/L) in rats resulted in the accumulation of the metal in the pancreas and a significant decrease in serum insulin levels, followed by a reduction in insulin gene expression [74]. Similar results were obtained after a single oral exposure to a high dose of Cd in rats, where the pancreas accumulated this toxic metal [22]. Studies directed at investigating the impact of environmentally relevant doses of Cd showed that Cd exhibited gender-specificity in glucose metabolism disruption, with females being more sensitive [75]. The same authors demonstrated that low-level maternal exposure to Cd influences glucose homeostasis in offspring and increases the risk of offspring developing T2D later in life [76].

Although different animal experiments indicate impaired glucose metabolism, insulin secretion, and tissue resistance to insulin, the exact mechanisms of these effects of Cd are still hardly known. Under physiological conditions, the maintenance of glucose homeostasis depends on a coordinated process of balancing circulating glucose levels and the release of insulin by the pancreatic β-cells. In the post-absorptive state, 75% of glucose uptake occurs in the insulin-independent tissues, mainly in the liver and brain tissue. In comparison, the remaining glucose uptake (25%) occurs in insulin-dependent tissues, as well as muscle and adipose tissue [77]. To some extent, β-cells can compensate hyperglycemic states by elevating the secretion of insulin at the expense of the likelihood of IR development in multiple peripheral tissues [78].

Based on the studies in animal models of Cd exposure, Cd can produce a direct effect on the pancreas and affect glucose transport in insulin-independent and insulin-dependent tissues. Numerous animal studies have demonstrated that Cd exposure influences glucose metabolism by directly affecting pancreas morphology and β-cell function, resulting in cellular damage. Furthermore, oxidative damage, as a known phenomenon important in diabetes development, may occur upon Cd accumulation [52].

A hyperglycemic state in animals involves the increased activity of the glycogenolysis pathway and stimulation of enzymes associated with the gluconeogenesis pathway [73]. Apart from the Cd effects on gluconeogenesis, Cd can influence insulin via different patterns. Lei et al. [74] demonstrated that subcutaneously administered cadmium (0.5, 1.0, and 2.0 mg/kg b.w.) decreased insulin gene expression in exposed rats. This investigation suggests that Cd can influence the biosynthesis of insulin but has no effects on its release. Additionally, the same study revealed pancreatic dysfunction occurring earlier than kidney dysfunction following Cd administration.

Apart from the direct Cd effect on pancreatic β-cells, exposure to this metal affects glucose transport in other tissues, all potential sites of Cd toxicity. In these tissues, insulin exhibits different effects: in skeletal muscle, it promotes glucose utilization and storage by increasing glucose transport and net glycogen synthesis; in the liver, it activates glycogen synthesis, increases lipogenic gene expression, and decreases gluconeogenic gene expression, whereas, in white adipocyte tissue (WAT), it suppresses lipolysis and increases glucose transport and lipogenesis [79,80]. Glucose uptake in different animal cell types is mediated by a family of intrinsic membrane proteins (products of the *GLUT/SCL2A* genes) that facilitate glucose transport through membranes. GLUT4, the insulin-responsive glucose transporter, is selectively produced in muscle and adipose cells, while GLUT2 occurs in hepatic cells [81,82].

Generally, in skeletal muscle, Cd-induced IR suppresses glucose utilization and storage by decreasing glucose transport and net glycogen synthesis [79,80]. One-month administration of $CdCl_2$ (50 mg/L) with drinking water in male rats resulted in a significant decrease in plasma insulin-like growth factor 1 (IGF-I) and insulin-like growth factor binding protein-3 (IGFBP-3) levels [83], factors known to be altered in IR. Insulin resistance in the muscle of rats chronically exposed to Cd has been associated with the reduction of glycogen synthesis. Studies with rodents exposed to Cd have shown decreased GLUT4 expression, which could partly explain the reduction in glycogen synthesis [79].

In the liver, insulin activates glycogen synthesis, increases lipogenic gene expression, and decreases gluconeogenic gene expression. Cadmium-induced IR in the liver leads to a significant increase in hepatic GLUT2, carbohydrate regulatory element-binding protein, glucokinase, and pyruvate kinase mRNA [84]. Zhang et al. [85] have demonstrated that animals exposed to Cd developed IR as the result of the activation of lipogenic proteins, leading to a significant increase in serum glucose and free fatty acids.

Finally, in adipose tissue, especially white adipocytes, insulin suppresses lipolysis and increases glucose transport and lipogenesis [80]. Thus, the adipose IR is the inability of insulin to activate adipose glucose transport, promote lipid uptake, and suppress lipolysis [86]. Several mechanisms were suggested to contribute to the adverse Cd effects on adipose tissue pathophysiology and subsequently increased IR. Han et al. [79] demonstrated that subacute administration of Cd (subcutaneously. 2 mg/kg daily for four days) produces impaired glucose tolerance (IGT) in rats, which was associated with a dose-dependent reduction in GLUT4 protein and GLUT4 mRNA levels in adipocytes. Furthermore, the IR state in adipose tissue favors lipolytic pathways, resulting in an elevation of free fatty acids (FFA), which additionally contributes to impaired insulin secretion when released in the plasma.

4. Insulin Resistance and Cadmium: Cellular Studies

4.1. Non-Pancreatic Cells

Many in vitro studies have used non-pancreatic cell lines, such as adipocytes or ovarian/granulosa cells, that are typically involved with insulin action or glucose utilization [87]. In adipocytes directly obtained from Wistar rats, exposure to 5 μM Cd increased the cellular metabolism of glucose, similar to zinc, but did not increase glucose uptake, which is the opposite of zinc's action [88]. The primary glucose transporter stimulated by insulin is GLUT4, and an early study suggests that Cd exposure decreases the activity of the GLUT1 transporter [89]. Exposure to Cd also reduces critical cellular mediators involved in the differentiation and normal function of adipocytes. Decreased leptin, adiponectin, and resistin alter cellular ability to normally process lipids, potentially leading to IR [90,91]. Proteins that interact with the motif cytosine–cytosine–adenosine–adenosine–thymidine (CCAAT) are referred to as "CCAAT-enhancer-binding proteins" and are a target of Cd action in adipocytes. There are six CCAAT-enhancer-binding proteins involved in normal adipogenesis, including β and δ, which are activated in early adipocyte differentiation, and α, which is upregulated in the later stages of adipogenesis. Early in adipogenesis, β and δ stimulate peroxisome proliferator–activator receptor-γ (PPARγ). Exposure to Cd has been shown to inhibit the production of both CCAAT-binding enhancer proteins and PPARγ, leading to IR and an increase in adipogenesis [91,92]. In adipocytes, exposure to Cd alters the cellular functions involved with lipid metabolism and IR development, leading to obesity or diabetes.

4.2. Pancreatic Cells

Of the various elements, arsenic is possibly the most studied with regard to its effects on pancreatic function and the subsequent development of diabetes. Directly comparing arsenic, manganese, and Cd actions, the reduction in glucose-stimulated insulin section after arsenic and manganese exposure appeared to be due to mitochondrial dysfunction. In contrast, the inhibitory effects observed following Cd exposure were due to a mitochondria-independent mechanism [9]. There is evidence that mitochondria can transport Cd via the calcium uniporter, resulting in interference of the K+/H+ exchanger [93]. Nearly forty years ago, a transport-specific deficiency was identified due to changes in Cd sensitivity encoded by the *SLC39A8* gene [94]. The transporter encoded by this gene is highly conserved across species and has been shown to encode a specific element cation transporter referred to as *ZIP8*. Examination of β-cell function after arsenic, manganese, and Cd exposure revealed a distinct pattern of miRNA expression changes unique to each element, suggesting that biochemical differences result in distinct responses. Exposure to inorganic arsenic gave rise to a significant 76% increase in miR-146a, while there was a 60% decrease in miR-195 expression following Cd exposure [95]. Since β-cells are excitable cells and involve cell depolarization, leading to insulin release, several studies have examined the effects of metal exposure on voltage-gated calcium channel function. In an early study, ex vivo, isolated, perfused rat pancreas demonstrated that the addition of Cd to the perfusion buffer reduced insulin release, possibly due to the blockade of calcium uptake, thus preventing β-cell depolarization [96]. Characterization of the calcium channels suggests that the L-type (long-lasting) calcium channel is the predominant channel on β-cells, and that Cd acts by preventing calcium uptake via L-type channels [97]. Voltage-dependent calcium uptake is dependent on β-cell depolarization via potassium channel activity. Cd-mediated effects on potassium channels appear negligible and are mediated by voltage-dependent calcium channel inhibition [98]. In addition to blocking calcium uptake, Cd itself can be transported into β-cells and accumulate within the cells. Interestingly, at relatively low concentrations (5 μM), in the absence of calcium applied for one hour, the non-stimulated insulin release from islets of obese–hyperglycemic mice increased, but not the glucose-stimulated one [99]. Changes in insulin release in the presence of 5 μM Cd appears to be independent of calcium involvement. Lower concentrations of Cd do not increase intracellular calcium, nor inositol 1,4,5-triphosphate (IP_3) [100]. When 1 h-applied Cd concentrations exceed approximately 160 μM, insulin release is inhibited [99]. One conclusion from earlier studies is that Cd acts like a "silent killer", being taken up into β-cells and accumulating with time. During the early stages, β-cells would function normally until the Cd detoxification systems are overcome. Cd content from normal, "non-diabetic" human β-cells is approximately 29 nmol/g protein, with significant variability between individuals; that is not high enough to impair normal pancreatic function, as indicated by the lack of diabetic symptomology [43]. Determining intracellular Cd concentration and correlating intracellular values to extracellular concentrations have been challenging. Mathematical modeling data obtained from intestinal cell lines suggests that an external concentration of 10 μM would lead to an intracellular Cd concentration of 5000 amol/cell [101]. Cd continuously accumulates over time, at concentrations that may not significantly alter cell viability or gene expression [43]. Changes in β-cell function at sub-lethal concentrations seem to involve mitochondrial adaptation. As Cd accumulates in β-cells to several hundred-fold over baseline concentrations, mitochondria begin to appear fragmented, with the fusion–fission state shifting towards fission [102]. Studies using the INS-1 human pancreatic β-cell line utilized Cd concentrations 10-fold below the threshold necessary for cell death. Concentrations of Cd that are subtoxic produced no effects on mitochondrial function that were assessed by the energy change and the synthesis of adenosine triphosphate (ATP). Yet there were no morphological changes, suggesting a mitochondrial adaptive response to low-level Cd. The authors concluded that if cellular Cd influx continues, impairment of this organelle may contribute to cellular dysfunction and decreased viability of β-cells [102].

Mitochondrial respiration (oxygen consumption) and energy state (adenosine triphosphate production) appear unchanged during this process, until the cells commit to the death pathways [93]. Disruptions of mitochondrial morphology and energy state are linked to the onset of apoptosis. The intracellular mechanisms associated with Cd-mediated apoptosis have not been completely elucidated. The intracellular apoptotic mechanisms usually co-exist with necrosis, with a proportion of each depending on the cadmium dose and other conditions [102]. Exposure to Cd has been shown to elevate oxidative stress in pancreatic cells [103]. Increases in oxidative stress are linked to increased levels of malondialdehyde, free cytochrome c, p53, extracellular-regulated kinases 1/2, p38-mitogen-activated kinase, and *c-jun* N-terminal kinase (JNK), but decreases in mitochondrial membrane potential and Bcl-2 have also been observed [104]. Of the changes observed following Cd exposure, the increase in JNK activity by increased oxidative stress has been postulated to be one trigger for apoptosis. Not only is the phosphorylation of JNK upregulated after just one hour of exposure to 10 μM Cd, the expression of CCAAT-enhancer binding protein homologous protein, CHOP, is significantly upregulated [105]. Mitogen-activated kinases are vital for the normal function of the cell through proliferation, differentiation, and apoptosis. CHOP has been linked as an apoptotic response to oxidative stress in the endoplasmic reticulum. Additionally, Cd-mediated effects have been demonstrated directly via activation of the extracellular, signal-regulated kinases (ERK1/2) [106,107]. In general, ERKs activate numerous downstream pathways and are involved in Cd-induced carcinogenesis [108,109]. Together, reported effects of Cd on β-cells provide different pathways for Cd-mediated responses, ultimately leading to apoptosis, cell death, and a lack of β-cell responsiveness to elevated glucose, leading to stimulated insulin release.

5. Insulin Resistance and Cadmium: Is There a Threshold?

Considering Cd-mediated IR, the critical question is as follows: is there is a threshold for this effect? As recently reviewed [110], uncertainties in the mechanisms of low-level metal toxicity for humans and the demonstration of the existence of a safe threshold remains a rather challenging issue in toxicology. The comparable issue of whether endocrine disruption (ED) occurs at a threshold value has been holding for years, and the scientific community still expresses controversial views. The Endocrine Disrupters Expert Advisory Group (ED EAG) of the European Commission published a report in 2013 [111] summarizing experts' opinions regarding the existence of ED thresholds of adversity and the possibility of estimating such thresholds from existing experimental data. Most experts expressed the view that a threshold is likely to exist, but it might be exceptionally low. The basis of this argument is that one molecule, bound to only one receptor, would not be enough to activate the cascade of events needed to lead to apical adversity. However, in the case of fetal development, a threshold might not exist, due to the immaturity of the endocrine system [112]. Furthermore, with regard to the possibility of non-monotonic dose-response curves (NMDRCs), the available assays and methodologies most probably are not adequate for estimating a threshold with sufficient accuracy and sensitivity [113]. Other experts have expressed the view that a threshold does not exist, as endogenous hormones are already present in the body, and only one molecule of a xenobiotic might be enough to overwhelm the homeostatic system [114,115]. Based on these arguments, the EDs' risk assessment in most cases in the European Union is based on a hazard-based (no-threshold) approach, although a different, case-by-case approach for the Registration, Evaluation, Authorisation and Restriction of Chemicals (REACH) regulation has been proposed [116]. Other countries, such as the United States, Canada, and Australia, have adopted a risk-based threshold approach to overcome the difficulties discussed previously [117,118].

The estimation of a threshold under which Cd does not precipitate IR (further than the theoretical discussion of existence or not of such a threshold) would necessitate the existence of appropriate validated assays. For the moment, the globally existing recognized and accepted testing approaches cover modalities related only to the estrogen, androgen, thyroid, and steroidogenesis (EATS) pathways, as described in the OECD's Conceptual Framework (CF) for Testing and Assessment of Endocrine Disrupters [119]. Assays designed explicitly for the IR are not available in clinical practice or the field of toxicology. However, we know that IR, at least as a syndrome, generates obesity, hypertension, high glucose, triglycerides, and an increased LDL/HDL ratio in the blood. These endpoints should be determined using validated assays, like the repeated dose 90-day study (OECD Test Guidelines (TG) 408) and chronic toxicity and carcinogenicity studies (OECD TGs 451, 452, and 453).

In a regulatory context, for setting an experimental threshold for Cd causing IR, the "no observed adverse effect level" (NOAEL) or, better, a benchmark dose (BMD) should be determined. To set a BMD, it should be defined (a) if adversity is considered only as the apical effect(s) or even earlier signs of effect, and (b) the exact values for the various endpoints and conditions that compose the IR as a syndrome. In relation to the apical adversity, as mentioned above, a practical approach could be to consider as such the combination of obesity, hypertension, high glucose, triglycerides, and increased LDL/HDL ratio in blood, as in clinical practice. In vivo experiments would be necessary, and consequently specific values that consider adverse effects should be set for animal studies (considering that an appropriate model exists). The available studies with rats and mice mentioned in the review of Tinkov et al. [84] have various shortcomings (such as very low duration, single dose used, use of engineered animals, and lack of adequate endpoints) to support the establishment of a NOAEL.

Additionally, the Cd mode of action or the related adverse outcome pathway should be elucidated, and adequate in vitro mechanistic assays should be developed and performed to prove causality. The exact cause(s) of IR is not yet known. Still, there are data supporting perturbations of the enzymes and modulatory proteins involved in insulin signal transduction. Oxidative stress, inflammation, insulin receptor mutations, endoplasmic reticulum stress, and mitochondrial dysfunction affecting the insulin-dependent cells of skeletal muscle and adipocytes have been put forward [120,121]. The study of which of the above mechanisms are the most sensitive to Cd and the possible existence of NMDRC through appropriate methodology are essential steps for substantiating the role of Cd in IR, and eventually proposing a scientifically robust and reliable threshold if any can be validated.

6. Conclusions and Remarks for Future

Even though evidence abounds suggesting the damaging role of Cd on glucose homeostasis, the debate continues over the importance of Cd toxicity in the increasing occurrence of diabetes. Conversations are ongoing about the preventive or curative measures that should be taken within the susceptible populations. Cd's biological harm has been documented at different levels, from cells to human populations. However, the ample literature on cadmium toxicity (more than 15,000 articles are referenced in PubMed) covers such a variety of experimental conditions and formats that it is difficult to draw convincing strong conclusions from the available data.

The main topic of the present review, namely IR, is no exception. Cd doses, origins of cells, and detailed information on the exposed populations are a few of the numerous variables that change and impair comparison between studies from different groups. At the time of writing this, we are still unable to propose a range of possible toxicity mechanisms, without knowing whether any level of exposure to environmental Cd can be accepted for human populations. Figure 1 briefly summarizes the role of Cd in impaired glucose metabolism in various organs.

Forthcoming studies should thus focus on the application of environmentally realistic doses in experimental studies since chronic low-level exposure of humans to Cd is seemingly inescapable. For its contribution to IR, parallel data would have to be obtained with optimized cellular models for each insulin target tissue. Meanwhile, cells and tissues involved in insulin turnover, secretion, and withdrawal would have to be similarly studied. The data at hand should now be enough to reach an international consensus on which concentration, (bio)chemical form, and duration of exposure should be implemented. In this process, negative results, i.e., a lack of observed effects as long as state-of-the-art methods are used, are as useful as positive ones. Since prospective population studies are precluded for obvious ethical reasons, and in the face of the skyrocketing diabetes development worldwide, it may be hoped that the above reductionist approach can define the most sensitive and useful markers of minute exposure for humans. This way, reliable monitoring of Cd-associated IR may be reached, and the degree of usefulness of preventive or corrective measures can be knowledgeably addressed.

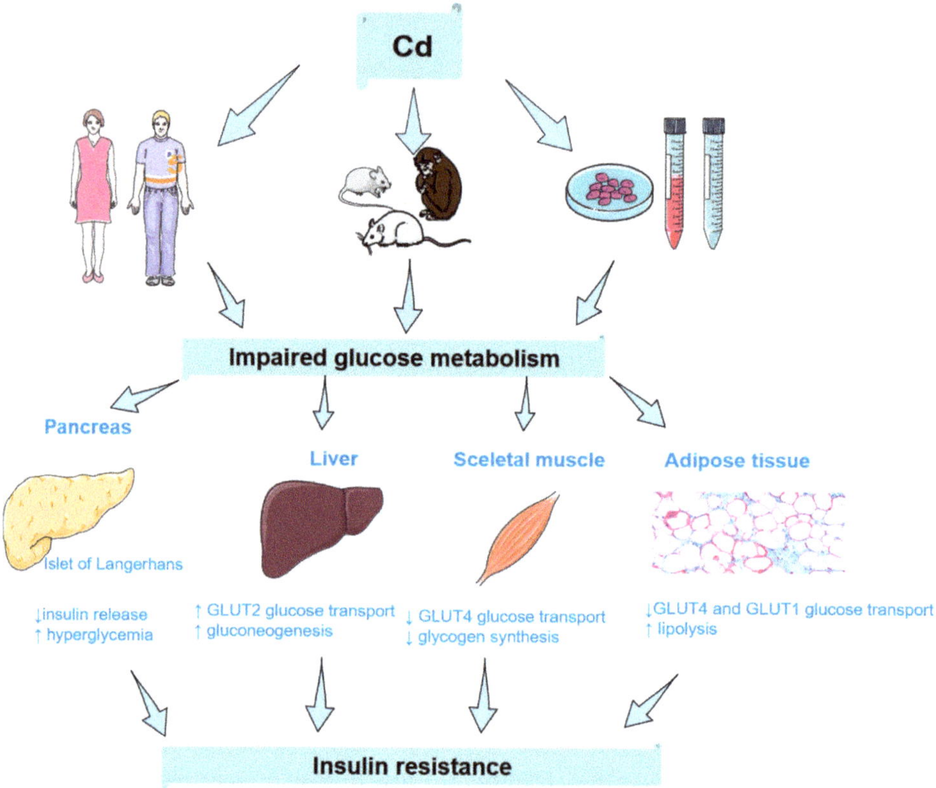

Figure 1. Cadmium's (Cd's) role in insulin resistance and glucose tolerance/impaired glucose metabolism in various organs: summary of the results obtained from human, animal, and cell studies. Insulin resistance appears first, followed by impairment of glucose metabolism. Cd's effects in the kidneys do contribute to IR development to a certain point. In the pancreas, Cd accumulates in insulin-producing β-cells, leading to a decrease of insulin release and an increase in blood glucose in blood. Besides the direct effect of Cd on the pancreas, this toxic metal affects glucose transport in insulin-independent (liver) and insulin-dependent tissues (skeletal muscle and adipose tissue).

Author Contributions: The role for each of the authors is as follows: conceptualization, A.B. and D.W.; investigation, M.Ć., M.G., Z.B., and B.A.; writing—original draft preparation, A.B., D.Đ.-Ć., J.-M.M., M.G., and D.W.; writing—review and editing, A.B., J.-M.M., Z.B., and D.W.; visualization, D.Đ.-Ć.; supervision, A.B., Z.B., and B.A., funding acquisition, A.B. All authors have read and agreed to the published version of the manuscript.

Funding: This work was supported by the Ministry of Education, Science and Technological Development, Republic of Serbia (No. 451-03-68/2020-14/200161; A.B., D.Đ.-Ć., M.Ć., Z.B., and B.A.). Oklahoma State University Center for Health Sciences Pilot/Seed Grant (1-54357; D.W.), and the French Agence Nationale de la Recherche (ANR-13-CESA-008-Cadmidia; J.-M.M.).

Conflicts of Interest: The authors declare no conflict of interest. No funding source had a role in the design of the study; in the writing of the manuscript, or in the decision to publish the results.

References

1. Yeni-Komshian, H.; Carantoni, M.; Abbasi, F.; Reaven, G.M. Relationship between several surrogate estimates of insulin resistance and quantification of insulin-mediated glucose disposal in 490 healthy nondiabetic volunteers. *Diabetes Care* **2000**, *23*, 171–175. [CrossRef]

2. Reaven, G. The metabolic syndrome or the insulin resistance syndrome? Different names, different concepts, and different goals. *Endocrinol. Metab. Clin. N. Am.* **2004**, *33*, 283–303. [CrossRef] [PubMed]
3. Ronald Kahn, C. Insulin resistance, insulin insensitivity, and insulin unresponsiveness: A necessary distinction. *Metabolism* **1978**, *27*, 1893–1902. [CrossRef]
4. Reaven, G.M. Role of insulin resistance in human disease. *Diabetes* **1988**, *37*, 1595–1607. [CrossRef] [PubMed]
5. Roberts, C.K.; Hevener, A.L.; Barnard, R.J. Metabolic syndrome and insulin resistance: Underlying causes and modification by exercise training. *Compr. Physiol.* **2013**, *3*, 1–58.
6. Lee, J.M.; Okumura, M.J.; Davis, M.M.; Herman, W.H.; Gurney, J.G. Prevalence and determinants of insulin resistance among U.S. adolescents: A population-based study. *Diabetes Care* **2006**, *29*, 2427–2432. [CrossRef]
7. Hectors, T.L.M.; Vanparys, C.; Van Gaal, L.F.; Jorens, P.G.; Covaci, A.; Blust, R. Insulin resistance and environmental pollutants: Experimental evidence and future perspectives. *Environ. Health Perspect.* **2013**, *121*, 1273–1281. [CrossRef]
8. Dixit, P.K.; Lazarow, A. Effects of metal ions and sulfhydryl inhibitors on glucose metabolism by adipose tissue. *Am. J. Physiol.* **1967**, *213*, 849–856. [CrossRef]
9. Dover, E.N.N.; Patel, N.Y.; Stýblo, M. Impact of in vitro heavy metal exposure on pancreatic β-cell function. *Toxicol. Lett.* **2018**, *299*, 137–144. [CrossRef]
10. Li, L.; Yang, X. The Essential Element Manganese, Oxidative Stress, and Metabolic Diseases: Links and Interactions. *Oxid. Med. Cell. Longev.* **2018**, *2018*, 1–11. [CrossRef]
11. Tripathi, D.; Mani, V.; Pal, R.P. Vanadium in Biosphere and Its Role in Biological Processes. *Biol. Trace Elem. Res.* **2018**, *186*, 52–67. [CrossRef] [PubMed]
12. Goldwaser, I.; Gefel, D.; Gershonov, E.; Fridkin, M.; Shechter, Y. Insulin-like effects of vanadium: Basic and clinical implications. *J. Inorg. Biochem.* **2000**, *80*, 21–25. [CrossRef]
13. González-Villalva, A.; Colín-Barenque, L.; Bizarro-Nevares, P.; Rojas-Lemus, M.; Rodríguez-Lara, V.; García-Pelaez, I.; Ustarroz-Cano, M.; López-Valdez, N.; Albarrán-Alonso, J.C.; Fortoul, T.I. Pollution by metals: Is there a relationship in glycemic control? *Environ. Toxicol. Pharmacol.* **2016**, *46*, 337–343. [CrossRef] [PubMed]
14. Satarug, S. Dietary Cadmium Intake and Its Effects on Kidneys. *Toxics* **2018**, *6*, 15. [CrossRef]
15. Satarug, S.; Vesey, D.A.; Gobe, G.C. Current health risk assessment practice for dietary cadmium: Data from different countries. *Food Chem. Toxicol.* **2017**, *106*, 430–445. [CrossRef]
16. Repić, A.; Bulat, P.; Antonijević, B.; Antunović, M.; Džudović, J.; Buha, A.; Bulat, Z. The influence of smoking habits on cadmium and lead blood levels in the Serbian adult people. *Environ. Sci. Pollut. Res.* **2020**, *27*, 751–760. [CrossRef]
17. Fransson, M.N.; Barregard, L.; Sallsten, G.; Akerstrom, M.; Johanson, G. Physiologically-based toxicokinetic model for cadmium using markov-chain monte carlo analysis of concentrations in blood, urine, and kidney cortex from living kidney donors. *Toxicol. Sci.* **2014**, *141*, 365–376. [CrossRef]
18. Nordberg, G.F.; Nogawa, K.; Nordberg, M.; Friberg, L.T. Cadmium. In *Handbook on the Toxicology of Metals*, 3rd ed.; Nordberg, G., Fowler, B., Nordberg, M., Nordberg, G., Fowler, L., Friberg, L., Eds.; Academic Press: Cambridge, MA, USA, 2007; pp. 445–486.
19. Satarug, S.; Garrett, S.H.; Sens, M.A.; Sens, D.A. Cadmium, Environmental Exposure, and Health Outcomes. *Environ. Health Perspect.* **2009**, *118*, 182–190. [CrossRef]
20. Mezynska, M.; Brzóska, M.M. Environmental exposure to cadmium—A risk for health of the general population in industrialized countries and preventive strategies. *Environ. Sci. Pollut. Res.* **2018**, *25*, 3211–3232. [CrossRef]
21. Buha, A.; Jugdaohsingh, R.; Matovic, V.; Bulat, Z.; Antonijevic, B.; Kerns, J.G.; Goodship, A.; Hart, A.; Powell, J.J. Bone mineral health is sensitively related to environmental cadmium exposure- experimental and human data. *Environ. Res.* **2019**, *176*, 108539. [CrossRef]
22. Djordjevic, V.R.; Wallace, D.R.; Schweitzer, A.; Boricic, N.; Knezevic, D.; Matic, S.; Grubor, N.; Kerkez, M.; Radenkovic, D.; Bulat, Z.; et al. Environmental cadmium exposure and pancreatic cancer: Evidence from case control, animal and in vitro studies. *Environ. Int.* **2019**, *128*, 353–361. [CrossRef] [PubMed]
23. Buha, A.; Wallace, D.; Matovic, V.; Schweitzer, A.; Oluic, B.; Micic, D.; Djordjevic, V. Cadmium Exposure as a Putative Risk Factor for the Development of Pancreatic Cancer: Three Different Lines of Evidence. *Biomed. Res. Int.* **2017**, *2017*, 1–8. [CrossRef] [PubMed]

24. Wallace, D.R.; Buha Djordjevic, A. Heavy metal and pesticide exposure: A mixture of potential toxicity and carcinogenicity. *Curr. Opin. Toxicol.* **2020**, *19*, 72–79. [CrossRef]
25. Browar, A.; Koufos, E.; Wei, Y.; Leavitt, L.; Prozialeck, W.; Edwards, J. Cadmium Exposure Disrupts Periodontal Bone in Experimental Animals: Implications for Periodontal Disease in Humans. *Toxics* **2018**, *6*, 32. [CrossRef]
26. Ronchetti, S.A.; Miler, E.A.; Duvilanski, B.H.; Cabilla, J.P. Cadmium Mimics Estrogen-Driven Cell Proliferation and Prolactin Secretion from Anterior Pituitary Cells. *PLoS ONE* **2013**, *8*, e81101. [CrossRef]
27. Silva, N.; Peiris-John, R.; Wickremasinghe, R.; Senanayake, H.; Sathiakumar, N. Cadmium a metalloestrogen: Are we convinced? *J. Appl. Toxicol.* **2012**, *32*, 318–332. [CrossRef]
28. Pollack, A.Z.; Schisterman, E.F.; Goldman, L.R.; Mumford, S.L.; Albert, P.S.; Jones, R.L.; Wactawski-Wende, J. Cadmium, lead, and mercury in relation to reproductive hormones and anovulation in premenopausal women. *Environ. Health Perspect.* **2011**, *119*, 1156–1161. [CrossRef]
29. Chen, X.; Zhu, G.; Jin, T. Effects of Cadmium Exposure on Age of Menarche and Menopause. *Toxics* **2017**, *6*, 6. [CrossRef]
30. Wang, Y.X.; Wang, P.; Feng, W.; Liu, C.; Yang, P.; Chen, Y.J.; Sun, L.; Sun, Y.; Yue, J.; Gu, L.J.; et al. Relationships between seminal plasma metals/metalloids and semen quality, sperm apoptosis and DNA integrity. *Environ. Pollut.* **2017**, *224*, 224–234. [CrossRef]
31. de Angelis, C.; Galdiero, M.; Pivonello, C.; Salzano, C.; Gianfrilli, D.; Piscitelli, P.; Lenzi, A.; Colao, A.; Pivonello, R. The environment and male reproduction: The effect of cadmium exposure on reproductive functions and its implication in fertility. *Reprod. Toxicol.* **2017**, *73*, 105–127. [CrossRef]
32. Tariba Lovaković, B. Cadmium, arsenic, and lead: Elements affecting male reproductive health. *Curr. Opin. Toxicol.* **2020**, *19*, 7–14. [CrossRef]
33. Buha, A.; Matovic, V.; Antonijevic, B.; Bulat, Z.; Curcic, M.; Renieri, E.A.; Tsatsakis, A.M.; Schweitzer, A.; Wallace, D. Overview of cadmium thyroid disrupting effects and mechanisms. *Int. J. Mol. Sci.* **2018**, *19*, 1501. [CrossRef] [PubMed]
34. Buha, A.; Antonijević, B.; Bulat, Z.; Jaćević, V.; Milovanović, V.; Matović, V. The impact of prolonged cadmium exposure and co-exposure with polychlorinated biphenyls on thyroid function in rats. *Toxicol. Lett.* **2013**, *221*, 83–90. [CrossRef] [PubMed]
35. Stojsavljević, A.; Rovčanin, B.; Krstić, Đ.; Jagodić, J.; Borković-Mitić, S.; Paunović, I.; Živaljević, V.; Mitić, B.; Gavrović-Jankulović, M.; Manojlović, D. Cadmium as main endocrine disruptor in papillary thyroid carcinoma and the significance of Cd/Se ratio for thyroid tissue pathophysiology. *J. Trace Elem. Med. Biol.* **2019**, *55*, 190–195. [CrossRef] [PubMed]
36. Đukić-Ćosić, D.; Baralić, K.; Javorac, D.; Djordjevic, A.B.; Bulat, Z. An overview of molecular mechanisms in cadmium toxicity. *Curr. Opin. Toxicol.* **2020**, *19*, 56–62. [CrossRef]
37. Wallace, D.R.; Taalab, Y.M.; Heinze, S.; Tariba Lovaković, B.; Pizent, A.; Renieri, E.; Tsatsakis, A.; Farooqi, A.A.; Javorac, D.; Andjelkovic, M.; et al. Toxic-Metal-Induced Alteration in miRNA Expression Profile as a Proposed Mechanism for Disease Development. *Cells* **2020**, *9*, 901. [CrossRef]
38. Amaral, A.F.S.; Porta, M.; Silverman, D.T.; Milne, R.L.; Kogevinas, M.; Rothman, N.; Cantor, K.P.; Jackson, B.P.; Pumarega, J.A.; López, T.; et al. Pancreatic cancer risk and levels of trace elements. *Gut* **2012**, *61*, 1583–1588. [CrossRef]
39. Luckett, B.G.; Su, L.J.; Rood, J.C.; Fontham, E.T.H. Cadmium Exposure and Pancreatic Cancer in South Louisiana. *J. Environ. Public Health* **2012**, *2012*, 1–11. [CrossRef]
40. Uetani, M.; Kobayashi, E.; Suwazono, Y.; Honda, R.; Nishijo, M.; Nakagawa, H.; Kido, T.; Nogawa, K. Tissue cadmium (Cd) concentrations of people living in a Cd polluted area. *Jpn. Biometals* **2006**, *19*, 521–525. [CrossRef]
41. Bashir, N.; Manoharan, V.; Miltonprabu, S. Grape seed proanthocyanidins protects against cadmium induced oxidative pancreatitis in rats by attenuating oxidative stress, inflammation and apoptosis via Nrf-2/HO-1 signaling. *J. Nutr. Biochem.* **2016**, *32*, 128–141. [CrossRef]
42. Bulat, Z.P.; Djukić-Ćosić, D.; Maličević, Ž.; Bulat, P.; Matović, V. Zinc or Magnesium Supplementation Modulates Cd Intoxication in Blood, Kidney, Spleen, and Bone of Rabbits. *Biol. Trace Elem. Res.* **2008**, *124*, 110–117. [CrossRef] [PubMed]

43. El Muayed, M.; Raja, M.R.; Zhang, X.; MacRenaris, K.W.; Bhatt, S.; Chen, X.; Urbanek, M.; O'Halloran, T.V.; Lowe, W.L., Jr. Accumulation of cadmium in insulin-producing β cells. *Islets* **2012**, *4*, 405–416. [CrossRef] [PubMed]
44. Mather, A.; Pollock, C. Glucose handling by the kidney. *Kidney Int.* **2011**, *79*, S1–S6. [CrossRef] [PubMed]
45. Merali, Z.; Singhal, R.L. Diabetogenic Effects of Chronic Oral Cadmium Administration To Neonatal Rats. *Br. J. Pharmacol.* **1980**, *69*, 151–157. [CrossRef]
46. Schwartz, G.G.; Il'Yasova, D.; Ivanova, A. Urinary cadmium, impaired fasting glucose, and diabetes in the NHANES III. *Diabetes Care* **2003**, *26*, 468–470. [CrossRef]
47. Wallia, A.; Allen, N.B.; Badon, S.; El Muayed, M. Association between urinary cadmium levels and prediabetes in the NHANES 2005–2010 population. *Int. J. Hyg. Environ. Health* **2014**, *217*, 854–860. [CrossRef]
48. Afridi, H.I.; Kazi, T.G.; Kazi, N.; Jamali, M.K.; Arain, M.B.; Jalbani, N.; Baig, J.A.; Sarfraz, R.A. Evaluation of status of toxic metals in biological samples of diabetes mellitus patients. *Diabetes Res. Clin. Pract.* **2008**, *80*, 280–288. [CrossRef]
49. Pizzino, G.; Irrera, N.; Bitto, A.; Pallio, G.; Mannino, F.; Arcoraci, V.; Aliquò, F.; Minutoli, L.; De Ponte, C.; D'Andrea, P.; et al. Cadmium-induced oxidative stress impairs glycemic control in adolescents. *Oxid. Med. Cell. Longev.* **2017**, *2017*, 1–6. [CrossRef]
50. Pedro, E.M.; da Rosa Franchi Santos, L.F.; Scavuzzi, B.M.; Iriyoda, T.M.V.; Peixe, T.S.; Lozovoy, M.A.B.; Reiche, E.M.V.; Dichi, I.; Simão, A.N.C.; Santos, M.J. Trace Elements Associated with Systemic Lupus Erythematosus and Insulin Resistance. *Biol. Trace Elem. Res.* **2019**, *191*, 34–44. [CrossRef]
51. Mugabo, Y.; Li, L.; Renier, G. The Connection Between C-Reactive Protein (CRP) and Diabetic Vasculopathy. Focus on Preclinical Findings. *Curr. Diabetes Rev.* **2010**, *6*, 27–34. [CrossRef]
52. Jacquet, A.; Ounnas, F.; Lénon, M.; Arnaud, J.; Demeilliers, C.; Moulis, J.-M. Chronic Exposure to Low-Level Cadmium in Diabetes: Role of Oxidative Stress and Comparison with Polychlorinated Biphenyls. *Curr. Drug Targets* **2016**, *17*, 1385–1413. [CrossRef] [PubMed]
53. Barregard, L.; Bergström, G.; Fagerberg, B. Cadmium exposure in relation to insulin production, insulin sensitivity and type 2 diabetes: A cross-sectional and prospective study in women. *Environ. Res.* **2013**, *121*, 104–109. [CrossRef] [PubMed]
54. Wu, M.; Song, J.; Zhu, C.; Wang, Y.; Yin, X.; Huang, G.; Zhao, K.; Zhu, J.; Duan, Z.; Su, L. Association between cadmium exposure and diabetes mellitus risk: A prisma-compliant systematic review and meta-analysis. *Oncotarget* **2017**, *8*, 113129–113141. [CrossRef] [PubMed]
55. Anetor, J.I.; Uche, C.Z.; Ayita, E.B.; Adedapo, S.K.; Adeleye, J.O.; Anetor, G.O.; Akinlade, S.K. Cadmium Level, Glycemic Control, and Indices of Renal Function in Treated Type II Diabetics: Implications for Polluted Environments. *Front. Public Heal.* **2016**, *4*, 114. [CrossRef]
56. Maret, W.; Moulis, J.-M. The Bioinorganic Chemistry of Cadmium in the Context of Its Toxicity. In *Cadmium: From Toxicity to Essentialit*; Sigel, A., Sigel, H., Sigel, R.K.O., Eds.; Springer: Dordrecht, The Netherland, 2013; pp. 1–29.
57. Moulis, J.M. Cellular mechanisms of cadmium toxicity related to the homeostasis of essential metals. *BioMetals* **2010**, *23*, 877–896. [CrossRef]
58. Matović, V.; Buha, A.; Bulat, Z.; Đukić-Ćosić, D. Cadmium Toxicity Revisited: Focus on Oxidative Stress Induction and Interactions with Zinc and Magnesium. *Arch. Ind. Hyg. Toxicol.* **2011**, *62*, 65–76. [CrossRef]
59. Bulat, Z.; Dukić-Ćosić, D.; Antonijević, B.; Buha, A.; Bulat, P.; Pavlović, Z.; Matović, V. Can zinc supplementation ameliorate cadmium-induced alterations in the bioelement content in rabbits? *Arh. Hig. Rada Toksikol.* **2017**, *68*, 38–45. [CrossRef]
60. Moulis, J.-M.; Bourguignon, J.; Catty, P. CHAPTER 23. cadmium. In *Metallobiology*; Maret, W., Wedd, A., Eds.; Royal Society of Chemistry: Cambridge, UK, 2014; pp. 695–746. ISBN 978-1-84973-599-5.
61. Li, Y.V. Zinc and insulin in pancreatic beta-cells. *Endocrine* **2014**, *45*, 178–189. [CrossRef]
62. Huang, L. Zinc and Its Transporters, Pancreatic β-Cells, and Insulin Metabolism. *Vitam. Horm.* **2014**, *95*, 365–390.
63. Cruz, K.J.C.; De Oliveira, A.R.S.; Morais, J.B.S.; Severo, J.S.; Mendes, P.M.V.; De Sousa Melo, S.R.; De Sousa, G.S.; Do Nascimento Marreiro, D. Zinc and insulin resistance: Biochemical and molecular aspects. *Biol. Trace Elem. Res.* **2018**, *186*, 407–412. [CrossRef]

64. Swaddiwudhipong, W.; Mahasakpan, P.; Limpatanachote, P.; Krintratun, S. Correlations of urinary cadmium with hypertension and diabetes in persons living in cadmium-contaminated villages in in northwestern Thailand: A population study. *Environ. Res.* **2010**, *110*, 612–616. [CrossRef] [PubMed]
65. Swaddiwudhipong, W.; Mahasakpan, P.; Funkhiew, T.; Limpatanachote, P. Changes in cadmium exposure among persons living in cadmium-contaminated areas in Northwestern Thailand: A five-year follow-up. *J. Med. Assoc. Thail.* **2010**, *93*, 1217–1222.
66. Swaddiwudhipong, W.; Limpatanachote, P.; Mahasakpan, P.; Krintratun, S.; Punta, B.; Funkhiew, T. Progress in cadmium-related health effects in persons with high environmental exposure in northwestern Thailand: A five-year follow-up. *Environ. Res.* **2012**, *112*, 194–198. [CrossRef] [PubMed]
67. Spoto, B.; Pisano, A.; Zoccali, C. Insulin resistance in chronic kidney disease: A systematic review. *Am. J. Physiol.-Ren. Physiol.* **2016**, *311*, F1087–F1108. [CrossRef]
68. Satarug, S.; Ruangyuttikarn, W.; Nishijo, M.; Ruiz, P. Urinary Cadmium Threshold to Prevent Kidney Disease Development. *Toxics* **2018**, *6*, 26. [CrossRef]
69. Edwards, J.R.; Prozialeck, W.C. Cadmium, diabetes and chronic kidney disease. *Toxicol. Appl. Pharmacol.* **2009**, *238*, 289–293. [CrossRef]
70. Ghafghazi, T.; Mennear, J.H. Effects of acute and subacute cadmium administration on carbohydrate metabolism in mice. *Toxicol. Appl. Pharmacol.* **1973**, *26*, 231–240. [CrossRef]
71. Ithakissios, D.S.; Ghafghazi, T.; Mennear, J.H.; Kessler, W.V. Effect of multiple doses of cadmium on glucose metabolism and insulin secretion in the rat. *Toxicol. Appl. Pharmacol.* **1975**, *31*, 143–149. [CrossRef]
72. Bell, R.R.; Early, J.L.; Nonavinakere, V.K.; Mallory, Z. Effect of cadmium on blood glucose level in the rat. *Toxicol. Lett.* **1990**, *54*, 199–205. [CrossRef]
73. Chapatwala, K.D.; Rajanna, E.; Desaiah, D. Cadmium Induced Changes in Gluconeogenic Enzymes in Rat Kidney and Liver. *Drug Chem. Toxicol.* **1980**, *3*, 407–420. [CrossRef]
74. Lei, L.J.; Jin, T.Y.; Zhou, Y.F. Insulin expression in rats exposed to cadmium. *Biomed. Environ. Sci.* **2007**, *20*, 295–301.
75. Jacquet, A.; Arnaud, J.; Hininger-Favier, I.; Hazane-Puch, F.; Couturier, K.; Lénon, M.; Lamarche, F.; Ounnas, F.; Fontaine, E.; Moulis, J.M.; et al. Impact of chronic and low cadmium exposure of rats: Sex specific disruption of glucose metabolism. *Chemosphere* **2018**, *207*, 764–773. [CrossRef] [PubMed]
76. Jacquet, A.; Barbeau, D.; Arnaud, J.; Hijazi, S.; Hazane-Puch, F.; Lamarche, F.; Quiclet, C.; Couturier, K.; Fontaine, E.; Moulis, J.M.; et al. Impact of maternal low-level cadmium exposure on glucose and lipid metabolism of the litter at different ages after weaning. *Chemosphere* **2019**, *219*, 109–121. [CrossRef] [PubMed]
77. DeFronzo, R.A. Pathogenesis of type 2 diabetes mellitus. *Med. Clin. N. Am.* **2004**, *88*, 787–835. [CrossRef] [PubMed]
78. Bertoluci, M.C.; Quadros, A.S.; Sarmento-Leite, R.; Schaan, B.D. Insulin resistance and triglyceride/HDLcindex are associated with coronary artery disease. *Diabetol. Metab. Syndr.* **2010**, *2*, 11. [CrossRef] [PubMed]
79. Han, J.C.; Park, S.Y.; Hah, B.G.; Choi, G.H.; Kim, Y.K.; Kwon, T.H.; Kim, E.K.; Lachaal, M.; Jung, C.Y.; Lee, W. Cadmium induces impaired glucose tolerance in rat by down-regulating GLUT4 expression in adipocytes. *Arch. Biochem. Biophys.* **2003**, *413*, 213–220. [CrossRef]
80. Petersen, M.C.; Shulman, G.I. Mechanisms of insulin action and insulin resistance. *Physiol. Rev.* **2018**, *98*, 2133–2223. [CrossRef]
81. Olson, A.L. Regulation of GLUT4 and Insulin-Dependent Glucose Flux. *ISRN Mol. Biol.* **2012**, *2012*, 1–12. [CrossRef]
82. Huang, S.; Czech, M.P. The GLUT4 Glucose Transporter. *Cell Metab.* **2007**, *5*, 237–252. [CrossRef]
83. Turgut, S.; Kaptanoğlu, B.; Turgut, G.; Emmungil, G.; Genç, O. Effects of cadmium and zinc on plasma levels of growth hormone, insulin-like growth factor I, and insulin-like growth factor-binding protein 3. *Biol. Trace Elem. Res.* **2005**, *108*, 197–204. [CrossRef]
84. Tinkov, A.A.; Filippini, T.; Ajsuvakova, O.P.; Aaseth, J.; Gluhcheva, Y.G.; Ivanova, J.M.; Bjørklund, G.; Skalnaya, M.G.; Gatiatulina, E.R.; Popova, E.V.; et al. The role of cadmium in obesity and diabetes. *Sci. Total Environ.* **2017**, *601–602*, 741–755. [CrossRef] [PubMed]
85. Zhang, S.; Jin, Y.; Zeng, Z.; Liu, Z.; Fu, Z. Subchronic Exposure of Mice to Cadmium Perturbs Their Hepatic Energy Metabolism and Gut Microbiome. *Chem. Res. Toxicol.* **2015**, *28*, 2000–2009. [CrossRef] [PubMed]
86. Czech, M.P. Mechanisms of insulin resistance related to white, beige, and brown adipocytes. *Mol. Metab.* **2020**, *34*, 27–42. [CrossRef] [PubMed]

87. Belani, M.; Purohit, N.; Pillai, P.; Gupta, S.; Gupta, S. Modulation of steroidogenic pathway in rat granulosa cells with subclinical Cd exposure and insulin resistance: An impact on female fertility. *Biomed. Res. Int.* **2014**, *2014*, 1–13. [CrossRef] [PubMed]
88. Yamamoto, A.; Wada, O.; Ono, T.; Ono, H.; Manabe, S.; Ishikawa, S. Cadmium-induced stimulation of lipogenesis from glucose in rat adipocytes. *Biochem. J.* **1984**, *219*, 979–984. [CrossRef]
89. Harrison, S.A.; Buxton, J.M.; Clancy, B.M.; Czech, M.P. Evidence that erythroid-type glucose transporter intrinsic activity is modulated by cadmium treatment of mouse 3T3-L1 cells. *J. Biol. Chem.* **1991**, *266*, 19438–19449.
90. Kawakami, T.; Nishiyama, K.; Kadota, Y.; Sato, M.; Inoue, M.; Suzuki, S. Cadmium modulates adipocyte functions in metallothionein-null mice. *Toxicol. Appl. Pharmacol.* **2013**, *272*, 625–636. [CrossRef]
91. Kawakami, T.; Sugimoto, H.; Furuichi, R.; Kadota, Y.; Inoue, M.; Setsu, K.; Suzuki, S.; Sato, M. Cadmium reduces adipocyte size and expression levels of adiponectin and Peg1/Mest in adipose tissue. *Toxicology* **2010**, *267*, 20–26. [CrossRef]
92. Lee, E.J.; Moon, J.Y.; Yoo, B.S. Cadmium inhibits the differentiation of 3T3-L1 preadipocyte through the C/EBPα and PPARγ pathways. *Drug Chem. Toxicol.* **2012**, *35*, 225–231. [CrossRef]
93. Lee, W.K.; Spielmann, M.; Bork, U.; Thévenod, F. Cd^{2+}-induced swelling-contraction dynamics in isolated kidney cortex mitochondria: Role of Ca^{2+} uniporter, K^+ cycling, and protonmotive force. *Am. J. Physiol.-Cell Physiol.* **2005**, *289*, 656–664. [CrossRef]
94. Nebert, D.W.; Liu, Z. SLC39A8 gene encoding a metal ion transporter: Discovery and bench to bedside. *Hum. Genom.* **2019**, *13*, 51. [CrossRef] [PubMed]
95. Beck, R.; Chandi, M.; Kanke, M.; Stýblo, M.; Sethupathy, P. Arsenic is more potent than cadmium or manganese in disrupting the INS-1 beta cell microRNA landscape. *Arch. Toxicol.* **2019**, *93*, 3099–3109. [CrossRef] [PubMed]
96. Ghagghazi, T.; Mennear, J.H. The inhibitory effect of cadmium on the secretory activity of the isolated perfused rat pancreas. *Toxicol. Appl. Pharmacol.* **1975**, *31*, 134–142. [CrossRef]
97. Plasman, P.O.; Hermann, M.; Herchuelz, A.; Lebrun, P. Sensitivity to Cd^{2+} but resistance to Ni^{2+} of Ca^{2+} inflow into rat pancreatic islets. *Am. J. Physiol.* **1990**, *258*, E529–E533. [CrossRef] [PubMed]
98. Jijakli, H.; Malaisse, W.J. Verapamil- and cadmium-resistant stimulation of calcium uptake and insulin release by D-glucose in depolarised pancreatic islets exposed to diazoxide. *Cell. Signal.* **1998**, *10*, 661–665. [CrossRef]
99. Nilsson, T.; Rorsman, F.; Berggren, P.O.; Hellman, B. Accumulation of cadmium in pancreatic beta cells is similar to that of calcium in being stimulated by both glucose and high potassium. *Biochim. Biophys. Acta* **1986**, *888*, 270–277. [CrossRef]
100. Nilsson, T.; Berggren, P.O.; Hellman, B. Cadmium-induced insulin release does not involve changes in intracellular handling of calcium. *BBA-Mol. Cell Res.* **1987**, *929*, 81–87. [CrossRef]
101. Gerasimenko, T.N.; Senyavina, N.V.; Anisimov, N.U.; Tonevitskaya, S.A. A Model of Cadmium Uptake and Transport in Caco-2 Cells. *Bull. Exp. Biol. Med.* **2016**, *161*, 187–192. [CrossRef]
102. Jacquet, A.; Cottet-Rousselle, C.; Arnaud, J.; Julien Saint Amand, K.; Ben Messaoud, R.; Lénon, M.; Demeilliers, C.; Moulis, J.M. Mitochondrial morphology and function of the pancreatic β-cells INS-1 model upon chronic exposure to sub-lethal cadmium doses. *Toxics* **2018**, *6*, 20. [CrossRef]
103. Wallace, D.; Spandidos, D.; Tsatsakis, A.; Schweitzer, A.; Djordjevic, V.; Djordjevic, A. Potential interaction of cadmium chloride with pancreatic mitochondria: Implications for pancreatic cancer. *Int. J. Mol. Med.* **2019**, *44*, 145–156. [CrossRef]
104. Chang, K.-C.C.; Hsu, C.-C.C.; Liu, S.-H.H.; Su, C.-C.C.; Yen, C.-C.C.; Lee, M.-J.J.; Chen, K.-L.L.; Ho, T.-J.J.; Hung, D.-Z.Z.; Wu, C.-C.C.; et al. Cadmium Induces Apoptosis in Pancreatic β-Cells through a Mitochondria-Dependent Pathway: The Role of Oxidative Stress-Mediated c-Jun N-Terminal Kinase Activation. *PLoS ONE* **2013**, *8*, e54374. [CrossRef] [PubMed]
105. Huang, C.C.; Kuo, C.Y.; Yang, C.Y.; Liu, J.M.; Hsu, R.J.; Lee, K.I.; Su, C.C.; Wu, C.C.; Lin, C.T.; Liu, S.H.; et al. Cadmium exposure induces pancreatic β-cell death via a Ca^{2+}-triggered JNK/CHOP-related apoptotic signaling pathway. *Toxicology* **2019**, *425*, 152252. [CrossRef] [PubMed]
106. Paniagua, L.; Diaz-Cueto, L.; Huerta-Reyes, M.; Arechavaleta-Velasco, F. Cadmium exposure induces interleukin-6 production via ROS-dependent activation of the ERK1/2 but independent of JNK signaling pathway in human placental JEG-3 trophoblast cells. *Reprod. Toxicol.* **2019**, *89*, 28–34. [CrossRef] [PubMed]

107. Ali, I.; Damdimopoulou, P.; Stenius, U.; Adamsson, A.; Mäkelä, S.I.; Åkesson, A.; Berglund, M.; Håkansson, H.; Halldin, K. Cadmium-induced effects on cellular signaling pathways in the liver of transgenic estrogen reporter mice. *Toxicol. Sci.* **2012**, *127*, 66–75. [CrossRef] [PubMed]
108. Dasgupta, P.; Kulkarni, P.; Bhat, N.S.; Majid, S.; Shiina, M.; Shahryari, V.; Yamamura, S.; Tanaka, Y.; Gupta, R.K.; Dahiya, R.; et al. Activation of the Erk/MAPK signaling pathway is a driver for cadmium induced prostate cancer. *Toxicol. Appl. Pharmacol.* **2020**, *401*, 115102. [CrossRef] [PubMed]
109. Ali, I.; Damdimopoulou, P.; Stenius, U.; Halldin, K. Cadmium at nanomolar concentrations activates Raf-MEK-ERK1/2 MAPKs signaling via EGFR in human cancer cell lines. *Chem. Biol. Interact.* **2015**, *231*, 44–52. [CrossRef]
110. Moulis, J.M.; Bulat, Z.; BuhaDjordjevic, A. Threshold in the toxicology of metals: Challenges and pitfalls of the concept. *Curr. Opin. Toxicol.* **2020**, *19*, 28–33. [CrossRef]
111. Munn, S.; Goumenou, M. Thresholds for endocrine disrupters and related uncertainties report of the endocrine disrupters expert advisory group. *JRC Sci. Policy Rep.* **2013**. [CrossRef]
112. Diamanti-Kandarakis, E.; Bourguignon, J.P.; Giudice, L.C.; Hauser, R.; Prins, G.S.; Soto, A.M.; Zoeller, R.T.; Gore, A.C. Endocrine-disrupting chemicals: An Endocrine Society scientific statement. *Endocr. Rev.* **2009**, *30*, 293–342. [CrossRef]
113. Vandenberg, L.N.; Colborn, T.; Hayes, T.B.; Heindel, J.J.; Jacobs, D.R.; Lee, D.H.; Shioda, T.; Soto, A.M.; vom Saal, F.S.; Welshons, W.V.; et al. Hormones and endocrine-disrupting chemicals: Low-dose effects and nonmonotonic dose responses. *Endocr. Rev.* **2012**, *33*, 378–455. [CrossRef]
114. Hass, U.; Christiansen, S.; Axelstad, M.; Boberg, J.; Andersson, A.; Skakkebæk, N.E.; Bay, K.; Holbech, H.; Kinnberg, K.L.; Bjerregaard, P. *Evaluation of 22 SIN List 2.0 Substances According to the Danish Proposal on Criteria for Endocrine Disrupters*; DTU Food: Copenhagen, Denmark, 2012.
115. Zoeller, R.T.; Vandenberg, L.N. Assessing dose-response relationships for endocrine disrupting chemicals (EDCs): A focus on non-monotonicity. *Environ. Heal. A Glob. Access Sci. Source* **2015**, *14*, 42. [CrossRef] [PubMed]
116. European Commission. Registration, Evaluation, Authorisation and Restriction of Chemicals (REACH). *Off. J. Eur. Union* **2006**, *49*, 396.
117. Brescia, S. Thresholds of adversity and their applicability to endocrine disrupting chemicals. *Crit. Rev. Toxicol.* **2020**, *50*, 213–218. [CrossRef] [PubMed]
118. Parrott, J.L.; Bjerregaard, P.; Brugger, K.E.; Gray, L.E.; Iguchi, T.; Kadlec, S.M.; Weltje, L.; Wheeler, J.R. Uncertainties in biological responses that influence hazard and risk approaches to the regulation of endocrine active substances. *Integr. Environ. Assess. Manag.* **2017**, *13*, 293–301. [CrossRef]
119. OCDE. OECD Conceptual Framework for Testing and Assessment of Endocrine Disrupters (as revised in 2012). *OECD Ser. Test. Assess.* **2012**, *8*, 1829.
120. Yaribeygi, H.; Farrokhi, F.R.; Butler, A.E.; Sahebkar, A. Insulin resistance: Review of the underlying molecular mechanisms. *J. Cell. Physiol.* **2019**, *234*, 8152–8161. [CrossRef]
121. Sesti, G. Pathophysiology of insulin resistance. *Best Pract. Res. Clin. Endocrinol. Metab.* **2006**, *20*, 665–679. [CrossRef]

toxics

MDPI

Article

Theoretical Modeling of Oral Glucose Tolerance Tests Guides the Interpretation of the Impact of Perinatal Cadmium Exposure on the Offspring's Glucose Homeostasis

Alexandre Rocca [1,2,*], Eric Fanchon [2,*] and Jean-Marc Moulis [3]

1 LJK, Grenoble INP, CNRS, Inria, Université Grenoble Alpes, 38000 Grenoble, France
2 TIMC-IMAG, UMR 5525, CNRS, Université Grenoble Alpes, 38041 Grenoble, France
3 Laboratory of Fundamental and Applied Bioenergetics (LBFA), CEA, Inserm U1005, Université Grenoble Alpes, 38000 Grenoble, France; jean-marc.moulis@cea.fr
* Correspondence: alexandre.rocca@univ-grenoble-alpes.fr (A.R.); eric.fanchon@univ-grenoble-alpes.fr (E.F.)

Received: 23 February 2020; Accepted: 6 April 2020; Published: 15 April 2020

Abstract: Oral glucose tolerance tests, in which the concentration of glucose is monitored in the circulation over 2 h after ingesting a bolus, probe diabetic or pre-diabetic conditions. The resulting glucose curves inform about glucose turnover, insulin production and sensitivity, and other parameters. However, extracting the relevant parameters from a single complex curve is not straightforward. We propose a simple modeling method recapitulating the most salient features of the role of insulin-secreting pancreatic β-cells and insulin sensitive tissues. This method implements four ordinary differential equations with ten parameters describing the time-dependence of glucose concentration, its removal rate, and the circulating and stored insulin concentrations. From the initial parameter set adjusted to a reference condition, fitting is done by minimizing a weighted least-square residual. In doing so, the sensitivity of β-cells to glucose was identified as the most likely impacted function at weaning for the progeny of rats that were lightly exposed to cadmium in the perigestational period. Later in life, after young rats received non-contaminated carbohydrate enriched food, differences are more subtle, but modeling agrees with long-lasting perturbation of glucose homeostasis.

Keywords: OGTT; minimal model; cadmium; glucose response mechanism

1. Introduction

The diagnostic and monitoring of diabetes mellitus rely on the experimental assessment of glucose homeostasis. Various tests and indices have been developed over time with the aim of identifying the sources of dysfunction among two main categories, deficient insulin secretion and insulin resistance. The former reflects the failure of β-cells in pancreatic islets of Langerhans to respond to increased glucose concentrations, whereas the latter corresponds to the increased inability of insulin-sensitive tissues, such as liver, muscles, and adipose tissue, to internalize glucose upon insulin stimulation together with deficient repression by insulin of hepatic glucose synthesis. Such conditions progressively develop in pre-diabetic states, and they are the hallmark of diabetes. However, discriminating between β-cells failure and insulin resistance is a challenge and involves invasive assays [1].

Among the environmental contributors to diabetes, particularly type 2 diabetes, exposure to the widespread metal cadmium has been regularly proposed. Epidemiological data promoted the idea at the beginning of the century [2], and, since then, conflicting results have bolstered debate on the issue [3–10] without reaching any clear consensus. The same statement applies to epidemiological studies considering the influence of the cadmium burden of the mother on the glucose homeostasis of both mother and child [11,12]. Besides, mechanistic investigations on the effects of cadmium on the function of the β-cells often focused on large, short-term, exposure (see [13,14] for the latest examples of such approaches) that bear little relevance to environmental conditions. Comparatively, very few studies investigated the relationship between low-level cadmium burden and impaired glucose homeostasis in relatively well defined conditions that can be implemented in the laboratory [15].

Among currently applied assays probing glucose homeostasis, oral glucose tolerance tests (OGTT) gather several advantages such as low-end staff and patient burden, integrated physiological behavior of the main contributors to glucose homeostasis, and clinically valuable information. In clinical practice, many parameters, such as 1-h or 2-h post-load glucose values that are extracted during OGTT, fasting glucose, or more indirect markers such as glycated haemoglobin, are considered in their ability to provide sensitive and cheap ways to diagnose dysglycemia and predict the development of diabetes. However, none gathers a consensus for application to all populations, or in the presence of the many confounding conditions [16]. By contrast, in research settings as with laboratory animals, the high information content of OGTT is more readily accessible since the kinetic data relative to blood glucose increase after the bolus and glucose disposal up to 2–3 h can be obtained.

The OGTT include a wealth of quantitative information that cannot always be extracted by mere examination of the curves presenting the variations of circulating glucose over time after a bolus, or even integration in the form of the area under the curve. We propose here a simple modeling and parameter analysis of such curves after cadmium exposure. The experimental data on which the present work is based were all reported before [17,18] for groups of rat pups exposed to low-level cadmium contamination through their mothers during gestation and lactation. All experimental details are available in these [17,18] and other [19] publications. In our hands [18], one of the frequently emphasized disadvantages of OGTT, namely its variability as compared to intravenous methods, has not been encountered as witnessed by the narrow spreading of measured values observed within experimental groups. This experimental advantage sets a strong basis for detailed analysis, which should allow us to focus on the variations of different parameters of glucose homeostasis obtained for these animals [18].

The purpose of the present study was to first build a simple kinetic model describing the evolution of the glucose concentration in the context of OGTT. Then, numerical simulations were run on previously obtained experimental results [17,18]. The process allowed us to test three groups of hypothesis via the sensitivity of the associated parameters as a function of cadmium exposure at three ages of pups post-weaning. These hypotheses were grouped as: (1) insulin sensitivity of glucose withdrawing tissues such as liver and muscles; (2) insulin turnover; and (3) insulin secretion by β-cells.

2. Materials and Methods

2.1. Summary of the Animal Study on Which Modeling Was Applied

The model built in the present study was applied to previously published data on pups born from cadmium-exposed dams [18]. The animal study was approved by the ethics committee (224_LBFA-U1055, 7 April 2015) affiliated to the animal facility (D3842110001) and agreed by the French Ministry of research (approval number 02397.02, 8 January 2018). A summary of the experimental protocol is shown in Figure 1. Shortly, dams were separated into three different groups and offered ad libitum doses of cadmium ($CdCl_2$) in drinking water adjusted to 0, 50, and 500 μg·(kg body mass)$^{-1}$·day^{-1} above the diet baseline [19]. The groups were reorganized post hoc as 'control', Cd1, and Cd2 according to the increasing Cd concentrations of the dam's kidneys [18]. This way, the OGTT measured for the respective pups are more representative of the cadmium exposure of the progeny via their mothers. The oral glucose tolerance tests (OGTT) measure, after overnight fasting, the evolution of plasma glucose concentration during the 2 h following force-feeding glucose intake at 2 mg per g of body mass. The tests were performed on the pups 21 days after birth, i.e., at weaning at Post-Natal Day 21 (PND21), at PND26, and at PND60. It has to be emphasized that the groups of pups were not exposed to different cadmium concentrations after weaning (>PND21) as they were all put on the same, not-intentionally cadmium-supplemented, diet. The population of the groups Control, Cd1 and Cd2 at the time points PND21, PND26, and PND60 are recalled in Table 1 to appreciate the statistical power of the studied data.

Table 1. Number of animals in the control, Cd1 and Cd2 groups at PND21, PND26, and PND60.

	PND21	PND26	PND60
Control	48	13	12
Cd1	38	18	17
Cd2	35	10	12

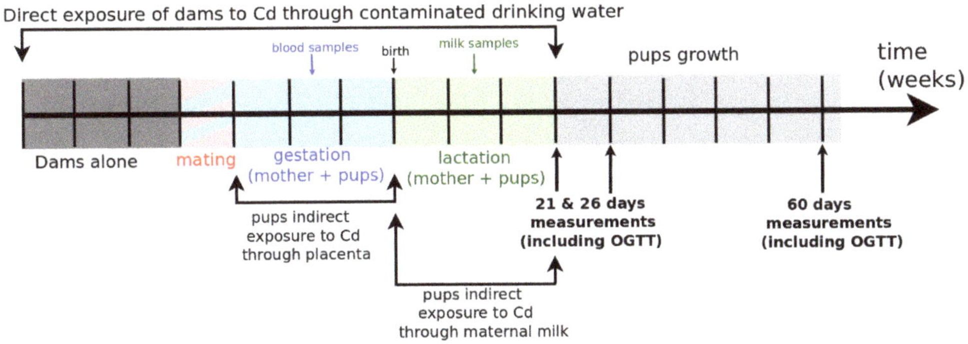

Figure 1. Protocol for indirect exposure of rat litters to cadmium through their mothers.

2.2. The Minimal Model (MINMOD)

As we plan in future work to apply formal or computationally expensive methods on our model, we built the simplest model possible while retaining important and meaningful variables for experimentalists, namely the plasma glucose concentration and the plasma insulin concentration. For this purpose, we used the minimal model (MINMOD) [20,21] as a starting point. The MINMOD model [21] is a small ODE model describing the evolution of glucose concentration after an initial intravenous injection of a glucose bolus.

$$\begin{aligned} \dot{G} &= -p_1(G(t) - G_b) - X(t)G(t) \\ \dot{X} &= -p_2X(t) + p_3(I(t) - I_b) \\ \dot{I} &= -n\,I(t) + \gamma\,(G(t) - h)\,t \end{aligned} \qquad (1)$$

The MINMOD model in Equation (1) has three variables: G is the glucose concentration in circulating blood, X is the rate of glucose withdrawal by muscles and adipocytes due to insulin, and I is the insulin concentration in circulating blood. This dynamic is modulated by seven parameters $p_1, p_2, p_3, n, \gamma, G_b, I_b$ and h. Parameters p_1 is a control rate on the glucose $G(t)$ to maintain the threshold concentration G_b in absence of insulin regulation and glucose intake. Parameter p_2 is the decrease rate of the variable glucose absorption rate $X(t)$. Parameter p_3 is the increase rate of $X(t)$, and is associated to the insulin threshold I_b. The parameters associated to insulin modeling in the MINMOD model are as follows: n is the degradation rate of insulin and γ is the long-term insulin production rate when glucose is above threshold h.

2.3. Glucose Tolerance Test Simulation Procedures

Numerical simulations were performed in JULIA using the DIFFERENTIALEQUATIONS library [22]. The process of fitting the parameter sets by minimizing Equation (5) for each dataset was performed manually. The code associated to these simulations can be found at https://github.com/roccaa/OGTT_Simulations.

3. Results

3.1. OGTT Modeling

In this approach, we first propose a model, which is adapted from the model MINMOD [21], to reproduce the OGTT results obtained in [17,18] from the protocol described in Figure 1. We refer to [23] for a review of glucose regulation models, and, together with [24–27], for a modeling of the OGTT in a more complex and exhaustive manner. Finally, we highlight the work [28] which contains a very detailed model of glucose response after a meal. The oral minimal model defined in [29] assembles three "minimal" models in order to build a quantitative minimal model of both glucose and insulin evolution in the context of OGTT. However, this model is still too complex for our simple purpose. The trade off of not using a model as detailed as [29] is that our conclusion will only be qualitative: the fitted models and parameters cannot be used for quantitative predictive purposes unlike those in [21,29].

The MINMOD model from [21] is not designed for OGTT, but for intravenous glucose tolerance tests (IvGTT). Therefore, we cannot consider that the plasma glucose is already at its maximal concentration at t = 0, as it is done for IvGTT studies.

Complex OGTT models such as [28] use compartmental modeling to represent the multiple stages of glucose distribution in the body, and to obtain the glucose rate of appearance in plasma after the meal. As a first approximation, we propose a simpler modeling using direct experimental results measuring the glucose rate of appearance after ingestion in rat, as follows. Following Wielinga et al. [30], we set the maximum of the rate of glucose appearance in the rat circulation ∼30 min after the meal (we consider that the time food spends in stomach is close to zero for the glucose solution). Similarly, the initial value of the rate of appearance was ∼70% of its maximum (see Figure 2). With this approximation, we eluded the steep increase of the glucose rate of appearance in the first few minutes of the experiments. This is justified as we focus on the simulation of the plasma glucose concentration with the first data point 10 min after glucose feeding. However, this implies imprecision with respect to the numerical variation of insulin between the fasting period and the peak of the insulin production. The curve of the glucose rate of appearance as a function of time was modeled by the continuous function $\mathrm{G_{RA}}(t)$:

$$\mathrm{G_{RA}}(t) = K\frac{1}{\sigma\sqrt{2\pi}}\mathrm{e}^{\frac{-(t-\mu)^2}{2\sigma^2}}, \tag{2}$$

where $\frac{1}{\sigma\sqrt{2\pi}}e^{\frac{-(t-\mu)^2}{2\sigma^2}}$ is a Gaussian function centred on μ. Fitting to the experimental curve in ([30], Figure 4), we chose $\mu = 30$ min that is the time of maximal appearance rate, and $\sigma = 35$ to obtain ∼70% of the maximum rate at $t = 0$. The value of the parameter K is determined by the actual quantity of glucose fed to the rats, such that all the glucose has to be absorbed over the $[0, +\infty[$ time interval. Let $\mathrm{m_{Glc}}$ be the mass of glucose fed to the rats (see Table 2 for the chosen rat body mass in the simulations at PND21, -26, and -60 with respect to the measurement in [17,18]) and V_{Blood} the rat blood volume (see Table 2) as given in [31]. Then, given an administrated concentration of glucose $\mathrm{m_{Glc}}/V_{Blood}$, the value of K (Table 2) is the solution of the following equation:

$$\int_0^{+\infty} K\frac{1}{\sigma\sqrt{2\pi}}\mathrm{e}^{\frac{-(t-\mu)^2}{2\sigma^2}}\,\mathrm{dt} = \frac{\mathrm{m_{Glc}}}{V_{Blood}}. \tag{3}$$

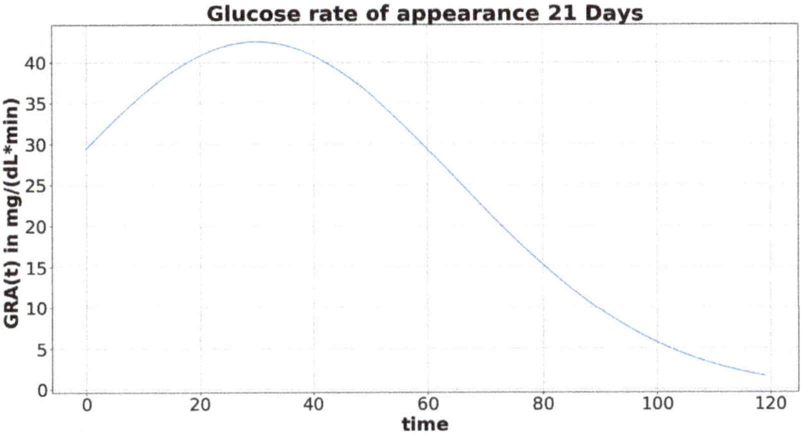

Figure 2. Approximation of the plasma glucose rate of appearance in 21-day-old rats (PND21).

Table 2. Values of body mass, blood volume, and parameter *K* at PND21, -26 and -60.

	PND21	PND26	PND60	Unit
Body mass	45	65	205	g
Blood volume	0.03	0.04	0.128	dL
K	3729	4040	3982	mg/(dL·min)

Upon secretagogue (here glucose) stimulation, insulin release by β-cells occurs in two overlapping phases [32]. The first phase, hereafter called 'fast', corresponds to the mobilization of granules belonging to the 'readily releasable pool' (RRP) by fusion to the plasma membrane and quasi-immediate excretion: it lasts for a few minutes. The second ('slow') phase lasts longer because it involves more complex phenomena such as trafficking to the surface of more deeply stored granules, and production and maturation of new insulin granules up to increased insulin transcription and synthesis to replenish the RRP. The duration of this second phase of the order of 1–2 h allows the organism to start responding to the insulin increase by the uptake of glucose in processing organs such as liver, muscles, and adipose tissues, and parallel insulin clearance by the liver. Measuring glucose clearance in the circulation over time thus integrates all these phenomena and probes the efficiency of insulin secretion by islets of Langerhans in response to glucose and the insulin sensitivity of glucose processing tissues. Of note, the first and second phases of insulin production cannot be distinguished in OGTT as delays in glucose levels in the circulation depend on intestinal absorption. The MINMOD model correctly simulates the slow phase of insulin production, but not the fast one outside of the IVGTT experimental context. To address this problem, we added a state variable representing the insulin already present and ready to be released in the blood circulation. Finally, the adapted MINMOD model is given by Equation (4).

$$\begin{aligned}
\dot{G} &= -p_1(G(t) - G_b) - r_{Cd}\,X(t)G(t) + G_{RA}(t) \\
\dot{X} &= -p_2X(t) + p_3(I(t) - I_b) \\
\dot{I} &= -n\,I(t) + \gamma\,(G(t) - h)\,t + p_4I_s(t) \\
\dot{I}_s &= -p_4I_s(t)
\end{aligned} \qquad (4)$$

We recall that, in the ODE system in Equation (4), G is the glucose concentration in circulating blood, X is the rate of glucose withdrawal by muscles and adipocytes due to insulin, I is the insulin concentration in circulating blood, and I_s is the insulin concentration stored in the β-cells and ready to be released. Here, we did not model the C-peptide concentration nor the liver production or absorption of glucose unlike in the more detailed model of [29].

The parameters $p_1, p_2, p_3, n, \gamma, G_b, I_b$, and h are original parameters of the MINMOD model. However, they were refitted in our experimental context. We refer to Section 2.2 for a more detailed introduction to the original MINMOD model. In addition to the parameters of the original MINMOD model, we added, for our purpose of modeling OGTT and cadmium impact, three additional parameters. The flux associated with glucose intake is modeled by $G_{RA}(t)$ in Equation (2). The efficiency of the rate of glucose withdrawal $X(t)$ is modeled by r_{Cd}. This parameter r_{Cd} was always taken equal to 1.0 in the simulations corresponding to the data of the control group. Finally, the parameter p_4 models the secretion rate of the readily releasable pool of insulin modeled by the variable $I_s(t)$.

The datasets were obtained from three groups of pups [18], namely control, Cd1, and Cd2 born from female rats with background, medium, and relatively high cadmium burden, respectively, still all corresponding to low exposure doses [18]. OGTT were performed on pups at weaning (21 days after birth, that is PND21), a few days later after shifting on a regular non contaminated chow (PND26), and pcorfive weeks later (PND60). To estimate the goodness of fit of a given simulation compared to the experimental data, we used the root of the weighted least squares error:

$$\varepsilon(\mathbf{k}) = \sqrt{\sum_i W_i(\mathbf{x}_{exp,i} - \mathbf{x}_{simu}(t_i, \mathbf{k}))^2}, \quad (5)$$

where $\mathbf{k}$ is a parameter set, $\mathbf{x}_{exp,i}$ are the mean values associated to an experimental dataset (see Table 1 for its corresponding population), and $\mathbf{x}_{simu}(t, \mathbf{k})$ its associated simulation of the OGTT. The weight W_i is determined by the equation:

$$W_i = \frac{1}{\nu_i^2(\sum_i \mathbf{x}_{exp,i}^2)},$$

where ν_i^2 are the variance to the mean associated to the ith data point.

It follows that, for a given parameter set $\mathbf{k}$, the lower the fitting error $\varepsilon(\mathbf{k})$, the better the fitting of the mean of the experimental data. When fitting the experimental results, this implies a bias in favor of the mean values of the data points as the error $\varepsilon(\mathbf{k})$ is 0 if the simulation goes through all mean points. Let us remark that the fitting error will decrease when the variances ν_i^2 increase: an experimental point is easier to fit when its experimental uncertainty increases. This adjustment allows giving more importance to the fitting of points which are experimentally in close positions as they will be the ones which really matter in the decrease of $\varepsilon(\mathbf{k})$. Here, the uncertainty on the experimental results not only comes from the precision of the measurements, but also, and mainly, from the individual variations within groups.

It is important to note that the error is *specific* to a dataset, and that errors associated to two different datasets cannot be compared. Only comparing the effect of two parameter sets to mean data points (and associated variances) corresponding to a given group (control, Cd1, or Cd2) at a given period (PND21, -26, or -60) makes sense. In Figure 3, we provide a schematic representation of our method to test the possible target of cadmium at PND21, PND26, and PND60, with respect to both our OGTT modeling and the experimental data.

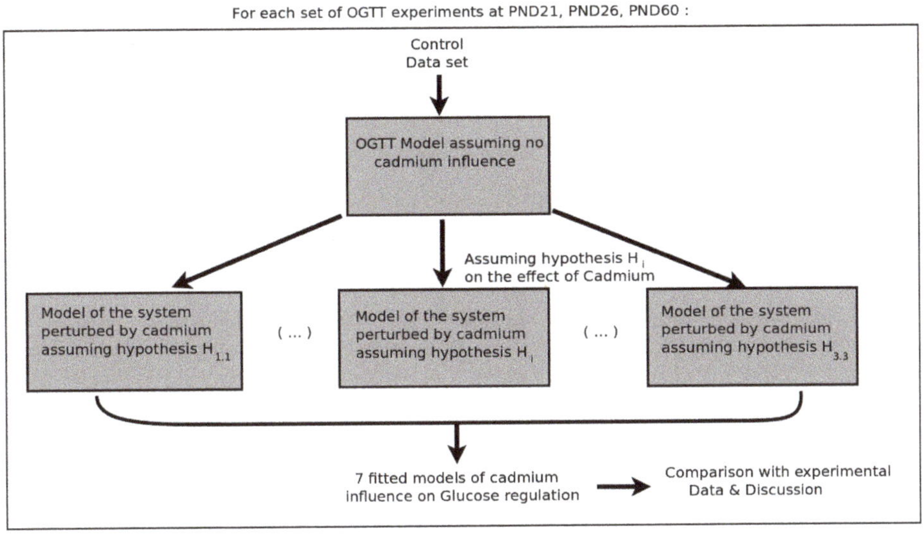

Figure 3. Modeling method to test hypotheses on the possible targets of cadmium. In the diagram, the index i spans hypotheses 1.1–3.3.

3.2. Parameter Analysis

The parameters were searched in the intervals proposed in [21], bloated by one order of magnitude, when possible. The initial value of the concentration of readily releasable insulin was fitted for the control group at PND21 and kept the same for the other experiments. The initial concentration of fasting glucose and insulin in plasma were taken from [18]. We chose to take $X(0) = 0$ as initial condition of the withdrawal rate of glucose: this implies a lack of regulation effect at t = 0. To relax the parameter search, when fitting the parameters to the datasets corresponding to groups Cd1 and Cd2, we only considered a few hypotheses on the evolution of the parameters, starting from the ones fitting the control group, by only altering one parameter at a time.

We considered the following hypotheses for the possible effects of cadmium of plasma glucose regulation:

Hypothesis 1. *Modification of the sensitivity of insulin sensitive tissues.*

- ***Hypothesis 1.1:*** r_{Cd} *varies: this shows the effect of cadmium on the glucose removal by the tissues. If* $r_{Cd} < 1$*, then the system has developed insulin resistance.*
- ***Hypothesis 1.2:*** p_3 *varies: this represents the effect of insulin on the rate of glucose withdrawal from the circulation.*
- ***Hypothesis 1.3:*** p_2 *varies: this affects the decrease rate of* $X(t)$*, which is the glucose withdrawal rate.*

Hypothesis 2. *n varies: this models an effect on insulin degradation.*

Hypothesis 3. *Modification of the insulin release rate.*

- ***Hypothesis 3.1:*** γ *varies: this models an evolution of the insulin release rate, in response to glucose, in the slow phase of insulin production.*
- ***Hypothesis 3.2:*** p_4 *varies: this models the stored insulin release rate.*
- ***Hypothesis 3.3:*** *h varies: this affects the glucose response threshold.*

The hypotheses on the effect of cadmium on the regulation of circulating glucose were tested in the following manner. We first looked for a starting parameter set $\mathbf{k}_{ctrl}$ minimizing Equation (5) for the experimental results of the control group. Then, for experimental results of group Cd1 (respectively Cd2), we first took a hypothesis H_i and we refitted a parameter set $\mathbf{k}_{H_i}$ by varying only one parameter at a time as defined above; the values of the other parameters were taken equal to the ones in the $\mathbf{k}_{ctrl}$ parameter set.

3.2.1. Results at PND21 (Weaning)

For 21-day-old pups at weaning, the goodness of fit for each hypothesis and associated to group Cd1 dataset are shown in Table 3. Considering the initial conditions from Table 4, the associated best parameter sets are given in Table 5. The simulation corresponding to the best parameter fits are shown in Figure 4. It should be reminded here that the experimental points reported in Figure 4 showed significant differences between the animal groups for the areas under the arbitrary drawn curves (AUC) in previously published data [17,18]. Here, the goodness of fit associated to the control group dataset is 0.00311 (Table 6). The best fits for group Cd1 are obtained considering Hypothesis 3.1, i.e., decreased response of β-cells to glucose in the slow phase of insulin production. For the experiment associated to group Cd2 at PND21, the best fit is also obtained for Hypothesis 3.1 and yields a goodness of 0.00433: it shows a continuous decrease of γ as a function of increased cadmium burden of the dams (Table 5).

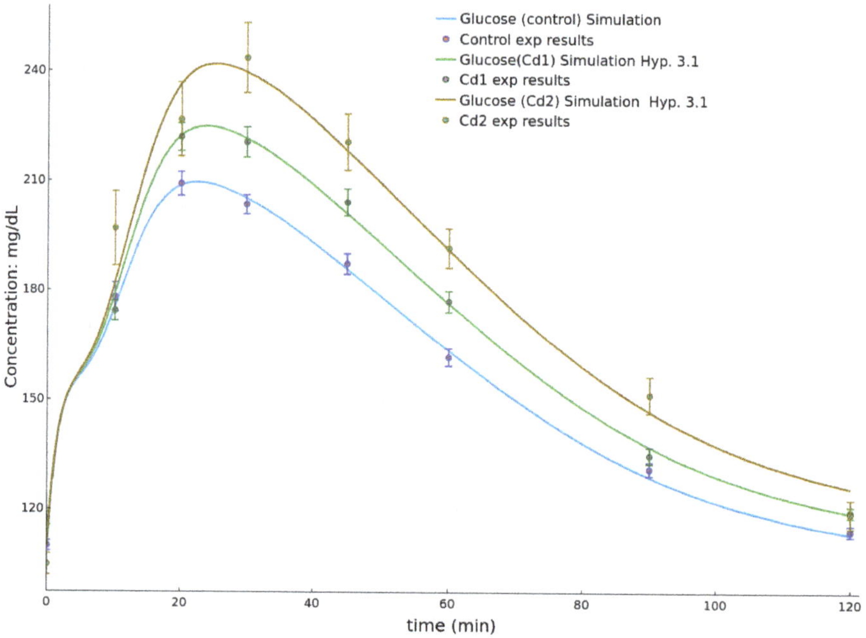

Figure 4. Simulations of the OGTT at PND21 for the control group, Cd1 and Cd2 groups.

Table 3. Goodness of fit from Equation (5) of each hypothesis applied to the Cd1 and Cd2 datasets at PND21. The symbol – denotes a value no better than the control parameter set.

Hypothesis	Cd1	Cd2
No Hyp.	0.0188	0.0144
Hyp 1.1	0.0144	0.00820
Hyp 1.2	0.0144	0.00821
Hyp 1.3	0.0140	0.00789
Hyp 2	0.0145	0.00852
Hyp 3.1	0.00566	0.00433
Hyp 3.2	–	0.0137
Hyp 3.3	0.0102	0.00740

Table 4. Initial condition determined for the control group at PND21. These initial conditions are conserved for groups Cd1 and Cd2. Note that 1 U = 0.0347 mg of insulin.

Variable	Value	Unit
G(0)	110.0	mg/dL
X(0)	0.0	min^{-1}
I(0)	16.0	nU/dL
$I_s(0)$	5950.0	nU/dL

Table 5. Parameters values fitted for the control group as well as groups Cd1 and Cd2 at PND21 (considering Hypothesis 3.1 for both groups).

Parameters	Ctrl	Cd1	Cd2	Unit
p_1	0.01	–	–	min^{-1}
G_b	100.0	–	–	mg/dL
p_2	0.56	–	–	min^{-1}
p_3	0.0155	–	–	$(dL/nU)min^{-2}$
I_b	10.0	–	–	nU/dL
n	10.53	–	–	min^{-1}
γ	0.0310	0.0258	0.0215	$(nU/dL)min^{-2}$
h	85.0	–	–	mg/dL
p_4	0.033	–	–	min^{-1}
r_{Cd}	1.0	–	–	N.U.

Table 6. Goodness of fit from Equation (5) for each dataset of the control group at PND21, -26 and -60.

Control Groups	Goodness of Fit
PND21	0.00311
PND26	0.00315
PND60	0.00251

3.2.2. Results at PND26

Concerning the experiments at PND26, after weaning at PND21 the pups shifted from a milk-based, i.e., lipid-dominated, diet to conventional rodent chow which is rich in carbohydrates. This change of diet induces important changes in the regulation mechanism: this translates into considerable changes of the parameter set fitting the control group dataset. In addition, the three groups of young animals were no longer differently exposed to cadmium after weaning, and the AUC as previously reported [18] did not show any statistically significant difference.

The initial conditions at PND26 are given in Table 7. The goodness of fit for each hypothesis on groups Cd1 and Cd2 are given in Table 8. The associated best parameters sets are given in Table 9. The simulation associated to the best fits are shown in Figure 5. The goodness of fit associated to the control group dataset is 0.00315 (see Table 6). We note that, unlike at PND21, there is no clear hypothesis that appears more likely than the others. Indeed, for group Cd1, although Hypothesis 2 yielded the best results, there is only a small difference with Hypotheses 1.1–1.3: thus, the present data cannot discriminate between changes of the insulin sensitivity of muscle and adipose tissue or of the insulin degradation rate.

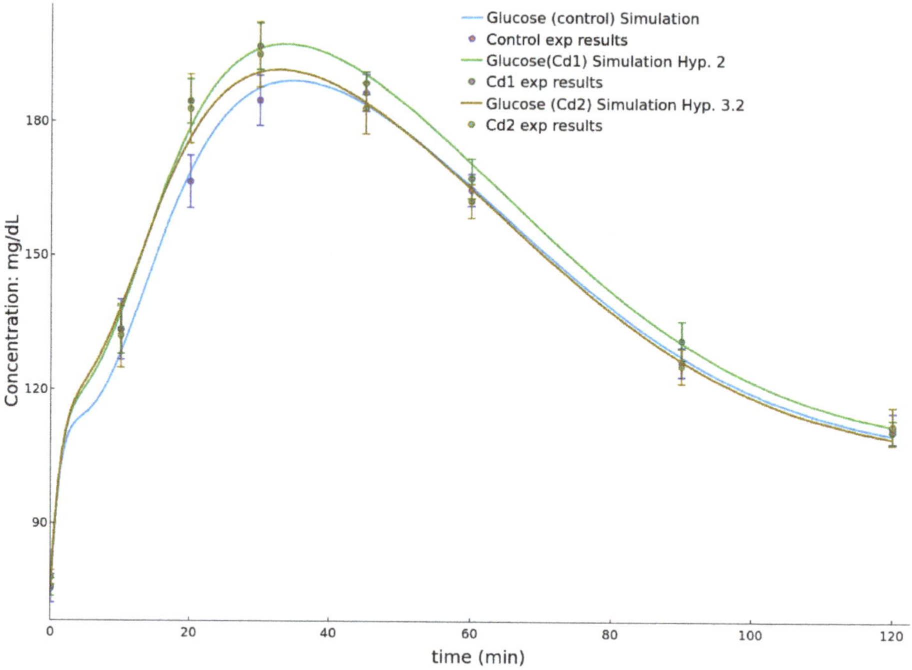

Figure 5. Simulations of the OGTT at PND26 for the control group, Cd1 and Cd2 groups.

Table 7. Initial condition determined for the control group and groups Cd1 and Cd2 at PND26.

Variable	Value	Unit
G(0)	76.0	mg/dL
X(0)	0.0	min^{-1}
I(0)	34.0	nU/dL
$I_s(0)$	5950.0	nU/dL

Table 8. Goodness of fit from Equation (5) of each hypothesis applied to the datasets of groups Cd1 and Cd2 at PND26.

Hypothesis	Cd1	Cd2
No Hyp.	0.00972	0.00600
Hyp 1.1	0.00411	0.00444
Hyp 1.2	0.00410	0.00435
Hyp 1.3	0.00398	0.00434
Hyp 2	0.00395	0.00442
Hyp 3.1	0.00762	0.00584
Hyp 3.2	0.00638	0.00388
Hyp 3.3	0.00819	0.00465

For group Cd2, we first observe that the higher variance on the experimental results leads to a lower error associated to the control parameter set (denoted no Hyp. in Table 8). In addition, even though Hypothesis 3.2 (reduction in the RRP release rate) yields the best goodness of fit, there is no clear distinction with the other hypotheses because of the increased variance. It follows that the previous interpretation given for group Cd1, namely that of a cadmium effect on the sensitivity of tissues to insulin or the hormone turnover, may still be valid.

Table 9. Parameters values fitted for the control group as well as groups Cd1 and Cd2 at PND26 (considering Hypothesis 3.2 for Cd2 and Hypothesis 2 for Cd1).

Parameters	Ctrl	Cd1	Cd2	Unit
p_1	0.01	–	–	min^{-1}
G_b	100.0	–	–	mg/dL
p_2	0.61	–	–	min^{-1}
p_3	0.0245	–	–	$(dL/nU)min^{-2}$
I_b	05.0	–	–	nU/dL
n	09.44	9.93	–	min^{-1}
γ	0.0110	–	–	$(nU/dL)min^{-2}$
h	79.0	–	–	mg/dL
p_4	0.0215	–	0.201	min^{-1}
r_{Cd}	1.0	–	–	N.U.

3.2.3. Results at PND60

Finally, considering the initial conditions from Table 10, the parameter set fitted to the datasets at PND60 are given in Table 11. The goodness of fit of the control group dataset is 0.00251 (see Table 6). It can be observed in Figure 6 that group Cd1 from mothers with medium cadmium burden and group Cd2 from the most intoxicated mothers show opposite behaviors with respect to the control curve. Whereas group Cd1 behaved in a similar fashion to the previous results at PND26 with a higher glucose peak than the control glucose response, the results of group Cd2 are characterized by a lower glucose peak.

In Table 12, we notice for group Cd1 that except Hypotheses 3.1 and 3.3, none of the other hypotheses have improved significantly the goodness of fit. However, Hypotheses 3.1 and 3.3 are not among the ones providing an important improvement of the fit for the results associated to group Cd1 at PND26. This raises the possibility of a delayed effect of cadmium on the function of β–cells after exposure during the perinatal period, in agreement with the variations of the C-peptide observed with the same animals [18].

For the results associated with group Cd2, the first three data points are below their control equivalent (see Figure 6). That means that, at PND60, group Cd2 (the one born of mothers with the highest cadmium burden) has a faster removal of glucose from the circulation in the first 40 min. In the simulation, it corresponds to an increase of the parameter $p4$ (Hypothesis 3.2) which best fits this evolution. All the other hypotheses demonstrate only marginal, or no, improvements.

Table 10. Initial condition determined for the control group and groups Cd1 and Cd2 at PND60.

Variable	Value	Unit
G(0)	95.0	mg/dL
X(0)	0.0	min^{-1}
I(0)	34.0	nU/dL
$I_s(0)$	5950.0	nU/dL

Table 11. Parameter values fitted for the control group as well as groups Cd1 and Cd2 at PND60 (considering Hypothesis 3.3 for Cd2 and Hypothesis 3.2 for Cd1).

Parameters	Ctrl	Cd1	Cd2	Unit
p_1	0.01	–	–	min^{-1}
G_b	100.0	–	–	mg/dL
p_2	0.79	–	–	min^{-1}
p_3	0.0335	–	–	$(\text{dL/nU})\text{min}^{-2}$
I_b	06.0	–	–	nU/dL
n	8.35	–	–	min^{-1}
γ	0.0078	–	–	$(\text{nU/dL})\text{min}^{-2}$
h	65.0	73.0	–	mg/dL
p_4	0.0170	–	0.0180	min^{-1}
r_{Cd}	1.0	–	–	N.U.

Table 12. Goodness of fit from Equation (5) of each hypothesis applied to the datasets of groups Cd1 and Cd2 at PND60.

Hypothesis	Cd1	Cd2
No Hyp.	0.00440	0.00403
Hyp 1.1	0.00395	0.00304
Hyp 1.2	0.00395	0.00304
Hyp 1.3	0.00396	0.00312
Hyp 2	0.00374	0.00325
Hyp 3.1	0.00267	–
Hyp 3.2	0.00439	0.00194
Hyp 3.3	0.00204	0.00402

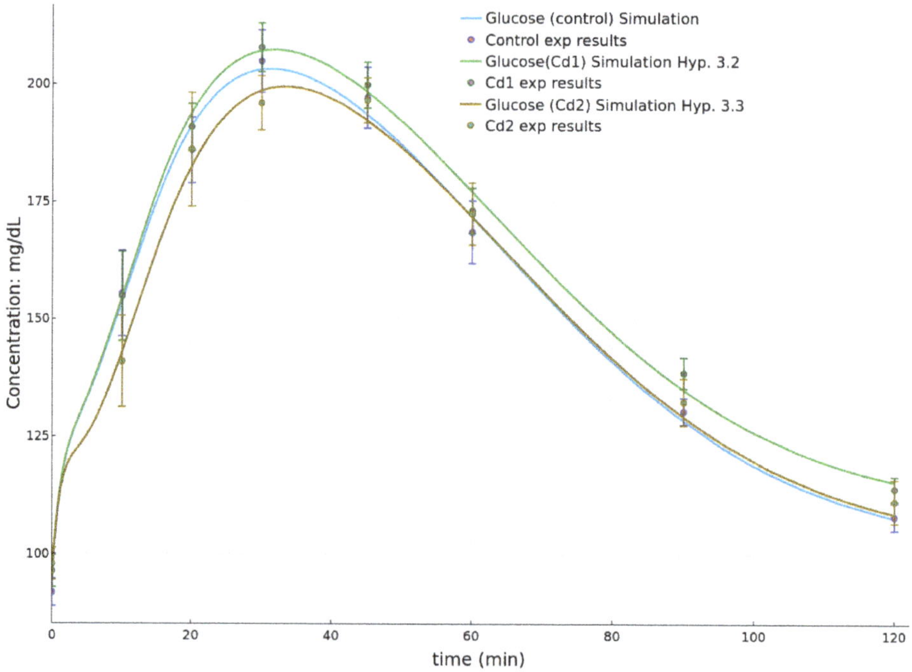

Figure 6. Simulations of the OGTT at PND60 for the control group and groups Cd1 and Cd2.

4. Discussion

As shown in the previous section, we tested through simulations various hypotheses that may explain the cadmium influence on the glucose regulation mechanism by insulin. To this aim, we started from a model reproducing correctly the control experiment with pups from mothers that were not intentionally exposed to cadmium. Then, we tested each hypothesis by varying a single parameter until it best fitted the dataset associated with the studied group of cadmium exposed pups. For this reason, we can only provide insight on the effect of one mechanism at a time.

An apparent weakness of our approach might be the risk of overfitting a single curve with at least 10 parameters for four variables. However, once the initial conditions have been set, the procedure aims at testing a series of hypotheses by varying a single parameter at a time to optimize fitting of a complex curve. This way a clear trend may appear, as for the probed data at weaning (PND21), or not. Thus, it is possible to safely avoid over-interpreting the simulations. The main practical interest of the modeling effort is to readily help sorting out the most relevant effects of a perturbation of glucose homeostasis.

For the experiments at PND21, we observed that, for both groups Cd1 and Cd2, it is the hypothesis of a decreased response to glucose during the slow phase of production that best represents the changes between the control group and the more exposed groups. On the experimental datasets, this is noticeable by an increased plasma glucose concentration over the $[30, 90]$ min interval, which previously led to increased AUC [18]. The fitted simulations under Hypothesis 3.1 show a good fitting especially on this interval.

However, a few noticeable points of the experimental datasets are not correctly represented by the simulation with Hypothesis 3.1. In particular for group Cd2, the points at 10 and 120 min are not correctly fitted by this single assumption on γ. The experimental point at 10 min, being higher than the simulation, suggests an additional effect in the first phase of insulin secretion. This is represented in our model by the parameter p_4. However, this parameter should be affected together with γ, as Table 3 shows that Hypothesis 3.2 (p_4 varies alone) does not correctly fit the data. Insights on the differences for the point at 120 min are more difficult to explain as they can be due to multiple reasons such as: a too coarse approximation of the glucose rate of appearance at 120 min, an effect on a mechanism not represented in the model such as gluconeogenesis, the role of other hormones than insulin, or a competition between multiple opposing effects that are not represented by our single hypothesis. In any case, the present results can be compared with the observations made in [18]. Few biochemical parameters were found to vary and consequently it was not possible to provide a robust explanation to the changes of the OGTT results and associated AUC. Here, simulations of these curves point to the decreased sensitivity of β-cells to glucose as the underlying factor. This decreased sensitivity is proportional to the dams' cadmium burden (Table 4), and it influences lipid metabolism [18]. The result applies to pups at weaning, i.e., at an age when the endocrine pancreas has yet to fully mature.

The experimental results at PND26 and PND60 represent the evolution of the three groups without additional exposure to cadmium through feeding beyond weaning: they show the lasting effect on the metabolism of a previous cadmium exposure, even though the AUC derived from OGTT were no longer significantly different between animal groups [18].

At PND26, we can already observe a slight behavioral difference with the previous datasets at PND21: whereas at PND21 the glucose concentration of Cd2 is always significantly above Cd1 and control ([18], Figure 5), at PND26, all groups share similar results. Looking to the mean values, one observes that the dataset of group Cd2 is closer to control than Cd1, which is confirmed in the simulation by the lower fitting error for Cd2 compared to Cd1 in absence of hypothesis (see Table 8). Even with this bias in favor of mean points, it is hard to reach any strong conclusion. The experimental results of group Cd1 are best fitted under the hypotheses of a reduced sensitivity to insulin of the glucose withdrawing tissues, or a faster degradation rate of insulin (Hypotheses 1.1–2). The experimental results of group Cd2 are so close to the control experimental results that no hypothesis seems much better than another.

Finally, at PND60, the differences among the three groups are not statistically significant ([18], Figure 9). This is witnessed by the small error associated with the entry without hypothesis in Table 12. When looking to the mean values, it is surprising to note that they are lower for group Cd2, and larger than control for Cd1. The best fit for group Cd1 are Hypotheses 3.1 and 3.3 that are modeling a negative effect on the slow phase of insulin production. The best fit for group Cd2 is the Hypothesis 3.2 modeling a positive effect on the first phase of insulin production.

5. Conclusions

In this work, we propose an extension of the MINMOD model [21] to simulate the circulating glucose evolution during OGTT. We fitted OGTT experimental results performed on rats at different ages after cadmium exposure through their mothers. Using these fitted models, we checked various different hypotheses on the effect of cadmium on the glucose response, by comparing the implementation of these hypotheses in the model to the experimental OGTT results for rats exposed to cadmium.

These simulations indicate that dams' exposure to cadmium negatively affects the slow phase of insulin release in response to glucose in pups at weaning. For the other experimental results at PND26 and PND60, there are no significant differences, yet the modeling approach agrees with the proposed long-lasting effects of cadmium in young animals, long after the indirect exposure via their mothers has ceased.

The results of this study may be extended by the development of a more complex model to better approximate the glucose appearance rate in the context of an OGTT, as well as the mechanism affected by Hypothesis 3.1. For this purpose, the comprehensive modeling of metabolism leading to insulin secretion [33] should be included when relevant experimental data become available. In this paper, we only propose a single fitting parameter set, but probing more complete datasets with more exhaustive and costly methods should be performed in order to further assert our conclusions. Finally, this model has only fitted the experimental glucose response, but not the evolution of insulin plasma concentration over time during OGTT in young rats: combining such more extensive datasets would be important to develop the modeling approach to be used in a more quantitative manner.

Author Contributions: Methodology, A.R. and E.F.; Software, A.R.; Formal analysis, A.R. and E.F.; Resources, E.F. and J.-M.M.; Writing—original draft preparation, A.R.; Writing—review and editing, E.F. and J.-M.M.; Supervision, E.F.; Project administration, E.F. and J.-M.M.; and Funding acquisition, E.F. and J.-M.M. All authors have read and agreed to the published version of the manuscript.

Funding: This research was supported in part by a grant from Agence Nationale de la Recherche ANR-13-CESA-008-Cadmidia.

Conflicts of Interest: The authors declare no conflict of interest.

Abbreviations

The following abbreviations are used in this manuscript:

PND21	Post-Natal Day 21
PND26	Post-Natal Day 26
PND60	Post-Natal Day 60
RRP	Readily Releasable Pool
OGTT	Oral Glucose Tolerance Test
AUC	Area Under the Curve
MINMOD	Minimal Model

References

1. Hannon, T.S.; Kahn, S.E.; Utzschneider, K.M.; Buchanan, T.A.; Nadeau, K.J.; Zeitler, P.S.; Ehrmann, D.A.; Arslanian, S.A.; Caprio, S.; Edelstein, S.L.; et al. Review of methods for measuring β-cell function: Design considerations from the Restoring Insulin Secretion (RISE) Consortium. *Diabetes Obes. Metab.* **2018**, *20*, 14–24. [CrossRef] [PubMed]

2. Schwartz, G.G.; Il'yasova, D.; Ivanova, A. Urinary cadmium, impaired fasting glucose, and diabetes in the NHANES III. *Diabetes Care* **2003**, *26*, 468–470. [CrossRef] [PubMed]
3. Barregard, L.; Bergström, G.; Fagerberg, B. Cadmium exposure in relation to insulin production, insulin sensitivity and type 2 diabetes: A cross-sectional and prospective study in women. *Environ. Res.* **2013**, *121*, 104–109. [CrossRef]
4. Guo, F.F.; Hu, Z.Y.; Li, B.Y.; Qin, L.Q.; Fu, C.; Yu, H.; Zhang, Z.L. Evaluation of the association between urinary cadmium levels below threshold limits and the risk of diabetes mellitus: A dose-response meta-analysis. *Environ. Sci. Pollut. Res. Int.* **2019**, 1–10. [CrossRef] [PubMed]
5. Kuo, C.C.; Moon, K.; Thayer, K.A.; Navas-Acien, A. Environmental chemicals and type 2 diabetes: An updated systematic review of the epidemiologic evidence. *Curr. Diab. Rep.* **2013**, *13*, 831–849. [CrossRef]
6. Li, Y.; Zhang, Y.; Wang, W.; Wu, Y. Association of urinary cadmium with risk of diabetes: A meta-analysis. *Environ. Sci. Pollut. Res. Int.* **2017**, *24*, 10083–10090. [CrossRef]
7. Moon, S.S. Association of lead, mercury and cadmium with diabetes in the Korean population: The Korea National Health and Nutrition Examination Survey (KNHANES) 2009–2010. *Diabet Med.* **2013**, *30*, e143–e148. [CrossRef]
8. Noor, N.; Zong, G.; Seely, E.W.; Weisskopf, M.; James-Todd, T. Urinary cadmium concentrations and metabolic syndrome in US adults: The National Health and Nutrition Examination Survey 2001–2014. *Environ. Int.* **2018**, *121*, 349–356. [CrossRef]
9. Tinkov, A.A.; Filippini, T.; Ajsuvakova, O.P.; Aaseth, J.; Gluhcheva, Y.G.; Ivanova, J.M.; Bjørklund, G.; Skalnaya, M.G.; Gatiatulina, E.R.; Popova, E.V.; et al. The role of cadmium in obesity and diabetes. *Sci. Total Environ.* **2017**, *601*, 741–755. [CrossRef]
10. Wallia, A.; Allen, N.B.; Badon, S.; El Muayed, M. Association between urinary cadmium levels and prediabetes in the NHANES 2005–2010 population. *Int. J. Hyg. Environ. Health* **2014**, *217*, 854–860. [CrossRef]
11. Rahman, A.; Kumarathasan, P.; Gomes, J. Infant and mother related outcomes from exposure to metals with endocrine disrupting properties during pregnancy. *Sci. Total Environ.* **2016**, *569*, 1022–1031. [CrossRef] [PubMed]
12. Shapiro, G.; Dodds, L.; Arbuckle, T.; Ashley-Martin, J.; Fraser, W.; Fisher, M.; Taback, S.; Keely, E.; Bouchard, M.; Monnier, P.; et al. Exposure to phthalates, bisphenol A and metals in pregnancy and the association with impaired glucose tolerance and gestational diabetes mellitus: The MIREC study. *Environ. Int.* **2015**, *83*, 63–71. [CrossRef] [PubMed]
13. Huang, C.C.; Kuo, C.Y.; Yang, C.Y.; Liu, J.M.; Hsu, R.J.; Lee, K.I.; Su, C.C.; Wu, C.C.; Lin, C.T.; Liu, S.H.; et al. Cadmium exposure induces pancreatic β-cell death via a Ca2+-triggered JNK/CHOP-related apoptotic signaling pathway. *Toxicology* **2019**, *425*, 152252. [CrossRef] [PubMed]
14. Li, X.; Li, M.; Xu, J.; Xiao, W.; Zhang, Z. Decreased insulin secretion but unchanged glucose homeostasis in cadmium-exposed male C57BL/6 mice. *J. Toxicol.* **2019**, *2019*. [CrossRef]
15. Jacquet, A.; Ounnas, F.; Lenon, M.; Arnaud, J.; Demeilliers, C.; Moulis, J.M. Chronic exposure to low-level cadmium in diabetes: Role of oxidative stress and comparison with polychlorinated biphenyls. *Curr. Drug Targets* **2016**, *17*, 1385–1413. [CrossRef] [PubMed]
16. Barry, E.; Roberts, S.; Oke, J.; Vijayaraghavan, S.; Normansell, R.; Greenhalgh, T. Efficacy and effectiveness of screen and treat policies in prevention of type 2 diabetes: Systematic review and meta-analysis of screening tests and interventions. *BMJ* **2017**, *356*, i6538. [CrossRef]
17. Jacquet, A. Conséquences d'une Exposition Chronique à des Doses Modérées de Cadmium sur le Métabolisme du Glucose de Rats à Différents Stades de la vie. Ph.D. Thesis, Université Grenoble Alpes, Saint-Martin-d'Hères, France, 2017.
18. Jacquet, A.; Barbeau, D.; Arnaud, J.; Hijazi, S.; Hazane-Puch, F.; Lamarche, F.; Quiclet, C.; Couturier, K.; Fontaine, E.; Moulis, J.M.; et al. Impact of maternal low-level cadmium exposure on glucose and lipid metabolism of the litter at different ages after weaning. *Chemosphere* **2019**, *219*, 109–121. [CrossRef]
19. Jacquet, A.; Arnaud, J.; Hininger-Favier, I.; Hazane-Puch, F.; Couturier, K.; Lénon, M.; Lamarche, F.; Ounnas, F.; Fontaine, E.; Moulis, J.M.; et al. Impact of chronic and low cadmium exposure of rats: Sex specific disruption of glucose metabolism. *Chemosphere* **2018**, *207*, 764–773. [CrossRef]

20. Pacini, G.; Bergman, R.N. MINMOD: A computer program to calculate insulin sensitivity and pancreatic responsivity from the frequently sampled intravenous glucose tolerance test. *Comput. Methods Prog. Biomed.* **1986**, *23*, 113–122. [CrossRef]
21. Nittala, A.; Ghosh, S.; Stefanovski, D.; Bergman, R.; Wang, X. Dimensional analysis of MINMOD leads to definition of the disposition index of glucose regulation and improved simulation algorithm. *Biomed. Eng. Online* **2006**, *5*, 44. [CrossRef]
22. Rackauckas, C.; Nie, Q. DifferentialEquations.jl—A performant and feature-rich ecosystem for solving differential equations in Julia. *J. Open Res. Softw.* **2017**, *5*. [CrossRef]
23. Kang, H.; Han, K.; Choi, M. Mathematical model for glucose regulation in the whole-body system. *Islets* **2012**, *4*, 84–93. [CrossRef] [PubMed]
24. Breda, E.; Cavaghan, M.K.; Toffolo, G.; Polonsky, K.S.; Cobelli, C. Oral glucose tolerance test minimal model indexes of β-cell function and insulin sensitivity. *Diabetes* **2001**, *50*, 150–158. [CrossRef] [PubMed]
25. Breda, E.; Toffolo, G.; Polonsky, K.S.; Cobelli, C. Insulin release in impaired glucose tolerance: Oral minimal model predicts normal sensitivity to glucose but defective response times. *Diabetes* **2002**, *51*, S227–S233. [CrossRef] [PubMed]
26. Dalla Man, C.; Campioni, M.; Polonsky, K.S.; Basu, R.; Rizza, R.A.; Toffolo, G.; Cobelli, C. Two-hour seven-sample oral glucose tolerance test and meal protocol. *Diabetes* **2005**, *54*, 3265–3273. [CrossRef]
27. Dalla Man, C.; Caumo, A.; Basu, R.; Rizza, R.; Toffolo, G.; Cobelli, C. Measurement of selective effect of insulin on glucose disposal from labeled glucose oral test minimal model. *Am. J. Physiol. Endocrinol. Metab.* **2005**, *289*, E909–E914. [CrossRef]
28. Dalla Man, C.; Rizza, R.A.; Cobelli, C. Meal simulation model of the glucose-insulin system. *IEEE Trans. Biomed. Eng.* **2007**, *54*, 1740–1749. [CrossRef]
29. Cobelli, C.; Dalla Man, C.; Toffolo, G.; Basu, R.; Vella, A.; Rizza, R. The oral minimal model method. *Diabetes* **2014**, *63*, 1203–1213. [CrossRef]
30. Wielinga, P.Y.; Wachters-Hagedoorn, R.E.; Bouter, B.; van Dijk, T.H.; Stellaard, F.; Nieuwenhuizen, A.G.; Verkade, H.J.; Scheurink, A.J. Hydroxycitric acid delays intestinal glucose absorption in rats. *Am. J. Physiol. Gastrointest. Liver Physiol.* **2005**, *288*, G1144–G1149. [CrossRef]
31. Constable, B. Changes in blood volume and blood picture during the life of the rat and guinea-pig from birth to maturity. *J. Physiol.* **1963**, *167*, 229–238. [CrossRef]
32. Henquin, J.C.; Nenquin, M.; Stiernet, P.; Ahren, B. In vivo and in vitro glucose-induced biphasic insulin secretion in the mouse: Pattern and role of cytoplasmic Ca2+ and amplification signals in β-cells. *Diabetes* **2006**, *55*, 441–451. [CrossRef] [PubMed]
33. Salvucci, M.; Neufeld, Z.; Newsholme, P. Mathematical model of metabolism and electrophysiology of amino acid and glucose stimulated insulin secretion: In vitro validation using a β-cell line. *PLoS ONE* **2013**, *8*. [CrossRef] [PubMed]

toxics

MDPI

Article

Associations between Maternal Cadmium Exposure with Risk of Preterm Birth and Low Birth Weight: Effect of Mediterranean Diet Adherence on Affected Prenatal Outcomes

Sarah Gonzalez-Nahm [1,*], Kiran Nihlani [2], John S. House [3], Rachel L. Maguire [4], Harlyn G. Skinner [4] and Cathrine Hoyo [4]

1 Department of Nutrition, University of Massachusetts Amherst, Amherst, MA 01003, USA
2 Department of Statistics, University of Pittsburgh, Pittsburgh, PA 15260, USA; kiran.nihlani@pitt.edu
3 National Institute of Environmental Health Sciences, Durham, NC 27709, USA; john.house@nih.gov
4 Department of Biological Sciences, North Carolina State University, Raleigh, NC 27606, USA; rlmaguir@ncsu.edu (R.L.M.); harlyn.skinner@ncsu.edu (H.G.S.); choyo@ncsu.edu (C.H.)
* Correspondence: snahm@umass.edu

Received: 15 September 2020; Accepted: 16 October 2020; Published: 20 October 2020

Abstract: Prenatal cadmium exposure at non-occupational levels has been associated with poor birth outcomes. The intake of essential metals, such as iron and selenium, may mitigate cadmium exposure effects. However, at high levels, these metals can be toxic. The role of dietary patterns rich in these metals is less studied. We used a linear and logistic regression in a cohort of 185 mother–infant pairs to assess if a Mediterranean diet pattern during pregnancy modified the associations between prenatal cadmium exposure and (1) birth weight and (2) preterm birth. We found that increased cadmium exposure during pregnancy was associated with lower birth weight ($\beta = -210.4$; 95% CI: −332.0, −88.8; $p = 0.008$) and preterm birth (OR = 0.11; 95% CI: 0.01, 0.72; $p = 0.04$); however, these associations were comparable in offspring born to women reporting high adherence to a Mediterranean diet ($\beta = -274.95$; 95% CI: −701.17, 151.26; $p = 0.20$) and those with low adherence ($\beta = -64.76$; 95% CI: −359.90, 230.37; $p = 0.66$). While the small sample size limits inference, our findings suggest that adherence to a Mediterranean dietary pattern may not mitigate cadmium exposure effects. Given the multiple organs targeted by cadmium and its slow excretion rate, larger studies are required to clarify these findings.

Keywords: cadmium; heavy metals; birth weight; preterm birth; diet pattern; Mediterranean diet; pregnancy

1. Introduction

Although cadmium is a naturally occurring heavy metal, its increased use in numerous industrial applications has made it one of the most abundant environmental pollutants present in atmospheric, terrestrial, and aquatic systems [1,2]. Cadmium is classified as a probable carcinogen [3] and its lack of degradation in the environment facilitates its persistence and enables sustained human exposure [2,4]. While contaminated air from industrial processes is the most cited source of occupational exposure [2], non-occupational cadmium exposure can occur through the inhalation of tobacco smoke and dust. Cadmium is also present in some commercial fertilizers [5–8] and contamination of agricultural soils results in the ingestion of cadmium through dietary staples [2,4]. In the US and other regulated societies, dietary cadmium intake is estimated at ~1 µg/day [1,9]. The slow excretion of cadmium leads to accumulation in the body over time [4].

Early-life cadmium exposure in children and pregnant women has been associated with low birth weight (either due to growth restriction or shorter gestation) [10–13], childhood disorders including neurodevelopmental disorders, and indicators of metabolic dysfunction such as obesity—which have been recapitulated in zebrafish [14]. Low birth weight and preterm birth are public health concerns, as they are risk factors for early mortality and the onset of later disease and co-morbidities [15]. Approximately 8% of infants in the US are born with a low birth weight (≤2500 g) [16] and approximately 10% of infants are born preterm (prior to 37 weeks gestation) [17] with increased frequencies for African-American infants [17] The management of low birth weight and preterm birth and associated co-morbidities poses a large financial burden on families and the healthcare system [18].

Dietary supplementation with essential metals including iron, calcium and selenium, has been recommended by multiple environmental health agencies to mitigate the effects of cadmium exposure, in part because cadmium influx occurs with metal transporters for these essential metals [19–21]. However, appropriate doses are unclear, as these essential metals can be toxic at high doses [20,21]. Polyphenols and other antioxidants in the diet have also shown the potential to reduce the negative consequences of cadmium exposure [20,21]. As humans typically consume combinations of nutrients as a part of meals or whole foods, the study of dietary patterns is an important tool to understand how public health recommendations can help reduce the risk from prenatal cadmium exposure. The Mediterranean diet pattern which is characterized by a high intake of iron, selenium, and antioxidants can be easily studied and translated to public health guidelines. Maternal adherence to a Mediterranean diet during pregnancy has been found to be associated with a reduced risk of gestational diabetes [22], normal birth weight [23–26] and longer gestational age [26,27], as well as favorable behavioral patterns [28], and other positive child outcomes [26]. Although there is an abundance of evidence suggesting multiple health benefits from adhering to a Mediterranean diet pattern [29–33], the potential role of this diet in mitigating the effects of prenatal cadmium exposure and birth outcomes has not yet been described. These analyses aim to explore the effect measure modification of Mediterranean diet pattern adherence during pregnancy in the association between elevated prenatal cadmium exposure and birth outcomes, including birth weight and preterm birth, and exploratory analyses of the association between prenatal cadmium exposure and Apgar scores and infant ponderal index at birth.

2. Materials and Methods

We used data from participants of the Newborn Epigenetics Study (NEST), a cohort of women–infant dyads from central North Carolina. Enrollment details have been described elsewhere [34]. In brief, 1700 women enrolled during pregnancy between 2009 and 2011 at qualifying prenatal clinics. Women met the following inclusion criteria: 18 years of age or older, plan to deliver in one of two birthing facilities in Durham county, and English or Spanish speaking. We excluded women who planned to give up custody of their child and those who did not carry offspring to term. Of the 1700 enrolled, 1304 remained after additional exclusions ($n = 115$ experienced a fetal death, $n = 281$ refused further participation or an inability to follow-up with the participant). We collected blood and obtained cadmium measures for the first $n = 310$ women. Of the 310, $n = 298$ had non-missing values for birth weight, and $n = 185$ women completed a food frequency questionnaire (FFQ). The median gestational age at enrollment was 11–12 weeks. We have previously shown that the 310 mother–infant pairs in whom cadmium was measured did not vary significantly from the remainder of the cohort [14]. The $n = 185$ on whom FFQ data were available also did not differ from the 310 with respect to sex, race/ethnicity and maternal obesity distribution ($p > 0.05$). Those included were, however, more likely to have a higher educational level and older maternal age at delivery ($p < 0.05$). These factors were adjusted for in the analysis. The women in our cohort were not significantly different with respect to covariates from the women in the overall NEST cohort ($p > 0.05$). This study was approved by the Duke University Institutional Review Board (#Pro00014548) on 19 February 2020.

2.1. Cadmium Exposure

We measured cadmium in whole blood for the first 310 enrolled women at a median gestation age of 12 weeks, using ICP-MS and methods previously described in detail [11,13]. Because cadmium co-occurs with other environmental pollutants [35], we also measured lead and arsenic. Briefly, we measured prenatal cadmium concentrations in whole blood donated at enrollment as nanograms per gram (ng/g; 1000 ng/g = 1035 ng/μL) of blood weight using well-accepted solution-based ICP-MS methods. We homogenized temperature equilibrated whole blood samples (0.2 mL) and pipetted them into a trace metal-clean test tube. We used a calibrated mass balance to confirm the samples gravimetrically to ±0.001mg, and we spiked samples with internal standards consisting of known quantities (10 and 1 ng/g, respectively) of indium (In) and bismuth (Bi) (SCP Science, USA), used to correct for instrument drift. We then diluted the solutions with water purified to 18.2 MΩ/cm resistance, which we will refer to as Milli-Q water (Millipore, Bedford, MA, USA) and acidified the solutions using ultra-pure 12.4 mol/L hydrochloric acid to result in a final concentration of 2% hydrochloric acid (by volume). We prepared all standards, including aliquots of the certified NIST 955c, and procedural blanks using the same process. We measured Cd concentrations using a Perkin Elmer DRC II (Dynamic Reaction Cell) axial field ICP-MS at Duke School of the environment, Durham, NC, USA. Calibration standards used to assess metals in blood included aliquots of Milli-Q water, and NIST 955c SRM spiked with known quantities of each metal in a linear range from 0.025 to 10 ng/g. We prepared standards from 1000 mg/L single element standards (SCP Science, USA). We calculated method detection limits (MDLs) consistent with the two-step approach using the t99SLLMV method (USEPA, 1993) at 99% CI (t = 3.71). The MDLs generated values of 0.006, 0.005, and 0.071 μg/dL, for cadmium, lead and arsenic, respectively. The thresholds of detection (LODs) were 0.002, 0.002, and 0.022 μg/dL, for Cd, Pb and As, respectively, and limits of quantification (LOQs) (according to Long and Winefordner, 1983) were 0.0007, 0.0006, and 0.0073 μg/dL for Cd, Pb, and As, respectively. The number of samples below the LOD for Cd, Pb, and As were two, two, and one, respectively.

2.2. Mediterranean Diet

We measured overall diet using a modified food frequency questionnaire (FFQ) [36] at enrollment. Women were asked to report their usual intake over the past 3 months, allowing us to capture the periconceptional period. We scored women's diets using the data-driven Mediterranean Diet Score (MDS) [37]. The MDS assesses adherence to a Mediterranean diet pattern based on the reported intake of foods that are deemed to be beneficial: fruit, vegetables, fish, dairy, whole grains, legumes, nuts, and monounsaturated fatty acids, and foods that are deemed detrimental: meat. We excluded alcohol from the diet score, as alcohol is not generally recommended during pregnancy and the reported alcohol intake in our cohort was low. Women who reported an intake of a beneficial foods at or above the median for the study population received a score of 1 and 0 otherwise. Those who reported an intake of detrimental foods below the median received a score of 1 or 0 otherwise. The MDS ranges from 0 to 9, with 0 representing the lowest possible adherence to a Mediterranean diet pattern and 9 representing the highest adherence to a Mediterranean diet pattern. We assessed maternal Mediterranean diet adherence as low (MDS at or below 4) and high (MDS above 4).

2.3. Birth Outcomes

At delivery, we abstracted parturition data, including infant birth weight and gestational age, from medical records. We used standard definitions for low birth weight (≤2500 g) and preterm birth (<37 weeks). We assessed birth weight continuously and preterm birth categorically (>37 weeks gestation/≤37 weeks gestation). We assessed infant Apgar scores continuously (1–10), with a higher score reflecting a greater level of health at birth. We also assessed birth length (cm), and derived the infant ponderal index (PI) at birth. PI is a measure of the proportionality of body growth and is calculated using the formula: weight (g) × (100/length (cm^3)).

2.4. Statistical Analysis

We used a linear regression to assess the association between elevated cadmium exposure during pregnancy and birth weight, and a logistic regression to assess the association between elevated cadmium exposure and preterm birth. In our study, cadmium was severely right-skewed. Despite log transformation, the skewness did not improve (results using the continuous log Cd variables are available in Supplemental Tables S1 and S2). As cadmium exposure is ubiquitous, we assessed cadmium in quartiles and defined high cadmium exposure as having a cadmium blood level in the highest quartile (mean Cd (ng/g) per quartile: 25th percentile: 0.12, 50th percentile: 0.24, 75th percentile: 0.46). We identified potential confounders a priori based on the literature and substantive knowledge and selected a final set of confounders using Bayesian Information Criteria (BIC). We included prepregnancy BMI, smoking during pregnancy, and sex of the infant as confounders in our final models. In our analysis of birth weight, we also included gestational age as a confounder and in our analysis of preterm birth we included birth weight as a confounder in the model. We assessed effect measure modification by Mediterranean diet adherence by including an interaction term in our models and by stratification of high and low maternal Mediterranean diet adherence. Effect measure modification analyses are limited to the 185 women who completed first trimester FFQs and had cadmium measures available. We conducted supplemental analysis to explore possible changes in the association between prenatal cadmium exposure and birth outcomes using different cut points for high and low Mediterranean diet adherence. Additionally, we explored the association between prenatal cadmium exposure and (1) infant Apgar score, (2) infant ponderal index at birth.

3. Results

We present study participant demographic factors overall, and by birth weight (Table 1) and Mediterranean diet adherence (Table 2). Of the 298 women included in our sample, 36% were Black, 28% were white, 32% were Latina or Hispanic, and 4% were of other race/ethnicities. Approximately one-quarter of women had a BMI of 30 or greater, and about 75% of obese women were either African American or Hispanic. Over half of our sample (55%) had a high school diploma. Among infants in our study, 6% were born prior to 37 weeks gestation and 5.7% weighed 2500 g or less at birth. Approximately 20% of mothers in our study reported smoking during pregnancy. The median (IQR) of cadmium concentration in blood was 0.24 (0.34) ug/g of blood weight, and MDS scores were normally distributed and ranged from 0 to 9 and approximately half of the women in our study had a score at or below 4. Women who did not deliver a low birth weight infant were more likely to be white, non-smokers, and have a college degree.

3.1. Cadmium Exposure and Birth Weight

Results of the associations between cadmium and birth weight are summarized in Table 3. After adjustment for prepregnancy BMI, smoking during pregnancy, gestational age, and sex of the infant, we observed that the women in the highest quartile of cadmium exposure during the prenatal period had infants whose birth weights were 210 g lower ($\beta = -210.4$; 95% CI: −332.0, −88.8; $p = 0.008$) than those in the lower three quartiles. Further including other co-occurring metals, lead and arsenic, that also have been linked to lower birth weights did not alter these associations. We explored removing gestational age from these models, as it may be on the causal pathway. This somewhat attenuated the association, however, it remained statistically significant ($\beta = -161.6$; 95% CI: −311.3, −11.9; $p = 0.04$). Further adjusting the co-occurrence of other metals, including lead or arsenic, did not materially alter these findings (data not shown).

Table 1. Sociodemographic characteristics of study participants by birth weight.

Characteristics	Overall	Low Birth Weight (<2500 g)	Non-Low Birth Weight (≥2500 g)
Ethnicity	N (%)	N (%)	N (%)
White	84 (28.2)	3 (17.6)	81 (28.8)
Black	108 (36.2)	11 (64.7)	97 (34.5)
Hispanic	94 (31.5)	2 (11.8)	92 (32.7)
Other	12 (4)	1 (5.9)	11 (3.9)
Maternal obesity before pregnancy			
<30	219 (73.5)	13 (76.4)	206 (73.3)
30+	76 (25.5)	4 (23.5)	72 (25.6)
Missing	3 (1.0)	–	3 (1.1)
Sex			
Male	149 (50.0)	8 (47.0)	141 (50.2)
Female	149 (50.0)	9 (52.9)	140 (49.8)
Gestational age at delivery			
<37 weeks	18 (6.0)	12 (70.6)	6 (2.1)
37+ weeks	280 (94.0)	5 (29.4)	275 (97.8)
Cigarette smoking during pregnancy			
No	242 (81.2)	9 (52.9)	233 (82.9)
Yes	46 (15.4)	8 (47.1)	38 (13.5)
Missing	10 (3.4)	–	10 (3.6)
Maternal educational attainment			
College Graduate and some college	134 (45.0)	6 (3.5)	128 (45.6)
High school or less	164 (55.0)	11 (64.7)	153 (54.4)
Cadmium categories			
Low	224 (75.2)	8 (47.1)	216 (76.9)
High	74 (24.8)	9 (52.9)	65 (23.1)
Cadmium concentrations (Median and interquartile range)			
Cd	0.24 (0.34)	0.67 (0.61)	0.23 (0.29)
Mediterranean diet adherence			
Low (≤4)	92 (30.9)	8 (47.1)	84 (29.9)
High (>4)	92 (30.9)	3 (17.6)	89 (31.7)
Missing	114 (38.2)	6 (35.3)	108 (38.4)

– No missing data in this category.

Table 2. Sociodemographic characteristics of study participants by Mediterranean diet adherence.

Characteristics	Overall	Low Mediterranean Adherence (≤4)	High Mediterranean Adherence (>4)
Ethnicity	N (%)	N (%)	N (%)
White	70 (37.8)	24 (26.1)	46 (49.5)
Black	54 (29.2)	38 (41.3)	16 (17.2)
Hispanic	51 (27.6)	26 (28.2)	25 (26.9)
Other	10 (5.4)	4 (4.3)	6 (6.4)
Maternal obesity before pregnancy			
<30	143 (77.3)	69 (75.0)	74 (79.6)
30+	41 (22.2)	22 (23.9)	19 (20.4)
Missing	1 (0.5)	1 (1.1)	–
Sex			
Male	101 (54.6)	52 (56.5)	49 (52.7)
Female	84 (45.4)	40 (43.5)	44 (47.3)
Gestational age at delivery			
<37 weeks	13 (7.0)	9 (9.8)	4 (4.3)
37+ weeks	172 (93.0)	83 (90.2)	89 (95.7)
Cigarette smoking during pregnancy			
No	158 (85.4)	73 (79.3)	85 (91.4)
Yes	22 (11.9)	16 (17.4)	6 (6.5)
Missing	5 (2.7)	3 (3.3)	2 (2.1)
Maternal educational attainment			
College Graduate and some college	86 (46.5)	53 (57.6)	33 (35.5)
High school or less	99 (53.5)	39 (41.9)	60 (64.5)
Birth Weight			
<2500 g	11 (6.0)	8 (8.7)	3 (3.2)
2500+ grams	173 (93.5)	84 (91.3)	89 (95.7)
Missing	1 (0.5)	–	1 (1.1)
Cadmium categories			
Low	147 (79.5)	69 (75.0)	78 (83.9)
High	38 (20.5)	23 (25.0)	15 (16.1)
Metal concentrations (Median and interquartile range)			
Cd	0.1892 (0.34)	0.2319 (0.36)	0.1723 (0.21)

– No missing data in this category.

We also regressed gestational age at birth on cadmium exposure, controlling for the same covariates (Table 4). We found that preterm birth is marginally associated with prenatal cadmium exposure ($\beta = -0.11$; 95% CI: 0.01, 0.72; $p = 0.04$) (Table 2). We included birth weight as a confounder in our main analysis and explored the effect of removing it in a supplemental analysis. When birth weight was removed from the model, the association between elevated prenatal cadmium exposure and preterm birth was no longer statistically significant ($\beta = 1.2$; 95% CI: 0.37, 3.31; $p = 0.74$). Again, further adjustment for the co-occurring metals, lead and arsenic, did not alter these findings, suggesting that growth restriction, rather than preterm birth, may be the major contributor to these birth outcomes.

Table 3. Regression coefficients and 95% confidence intervals for the association/relationship between, cadmium exposure and weight.

Factor	β	95% CI	p
Birth weight [a]	−210.38	(−332.00, −88.78)	0.0008
Birth weight, no gestational age [d]	−161.596	(−311.33, −11.86)	0.04
Birth weight, low Med adherence (≤4) [b]	−64.76	(−359.89, 230.37)	0.66
Birth Weight, high Med adherence (>4) [c]	−126.46	(−453.14, 200.22)	0.44

[a] Adjusted for smoking during pregnancy, prepregnancy BMI, gestational age and sex of the infant. [b] Adjusted for smoking during pregnancy, prepregnancy BMI, gestational age and sex of the infant, among mothers with a Mediterranean diet score at or below 4. [c] Adjusted for smoking during pregnancy, prepregnancy BMI, gestational age and sex of the infant, among mothers with a Mediterranean diet score above 4. [d] Adjusted for smoking during pregnancy, prepregnancy BMI, and sex of the infant.

Table 4. Odds ratio and 95% confidence intervals of the association between elevated prenatal cadmium exposure and preterm birth.

Factor	Odds Ratio	95% CI	p
Preterm birth [a]	0.11	(0.01, 0.72)	0.04
Preterm birth, no birth weight [d]	1.20	(0.37, 3.31)	0.74
Preterm birth, low Med adherence (≤4) [b]	0.07	(0.0008, 1.31)	0.14
Preterm birth, high Med adherence (>4) [c]	0.01	(0, 1.59)	0.20

[a] Adjusted for smoking during pregnancy, prepregnancy BMI, birth weight and sex of the infant. [b] Adjusted for smoking during pregnancy, prepregnancy BMI, birth weight and sex of the infant, among mothers with a Mediterranean diet score at or below 4. [c] Adjusted for smoking during pregnancy, prepregnancy BMI, birth weight and sex of the infant, among mothers with a Mediterranean diet score above 4. [d] Adjusted for smoking during pregnancy, prepregnancy BMI, and sex of the infant.

3.2. *Stratification by Mediterranean Diet Adherence*

To determine whether these associations were modified by adherence to a Mediterranean diet pattern, we first dichotomized the MDS below the median (a score of 4 of 9) among the n = 185 of 310 pregnant women who also completed the food frequency questionnaire. We examined cadmium-birth outcome associations among low and high adherers to the Mediterranean diet. We found no evidence for effect measure modification by Mediterranean diet adherence in the association between prenatal cadmium exposure and either gestational age or birth weight. Among women who reported high adherence to a Mediterranean diet pattern during pregnancy, the magnitude of the association between prenatal cadmium exposure and birth weight ($\beta = -126.46$; 95%CI: −453.14, 200.22; $p = 0.44$) was indistinguishable from the $\beta = -210.38$ observed among all participants. Similarly, the association between prenatal cadmium exposure and birth weight among women with low Mediterranean adherence was not statistically significant ($\beta = -64.76$; 95% CI: −359.90, 230.37; $p = 0.66$) (Table 3). However, these risk estimates lacked precision as confidence intervals were wide. We also observed no evidence for effect measure modification by maternal Mediterranean diet adherence on the association between prenatal cadmium exposure and preterm birth (high adherence: β: 0.01; 95% CI: 0, 1.59; $p = 0.20$; low adherence: β: 0.07; 95% CI: 0.0008, 1.31; $p = 0.14$) (Table 4). As expected from stratified analyses, including the interaction term of the Mediterranean diet adherence score and cadmium exposure did not alter these findings. The p-values for the interaction terms of cadmium and MDS in the overall birthweight or preterm birth models were not significant ($p > 0.15$). Defining "high Mediterranean adherence" with a more stringent cut-off of MDS of 5, 6 or 7 did alter these findings (data not shown).

3.3. Exploratory Analyses: Apgar Scores and PI

In our exploratory analyses we found no association between elevated prenatal cadmium exposure and Apgar scores ($\beta = -0.009$; 95% CI: −0.13, 0.12; $p = 0.89$) or PI ($\beta = -0.03$; 95% CI: −0.11, 0.06; $p = 0.51$). Results available in Supplemental Table S3.

4. Discussion

Understanding the effects of cadmium in early life is important, as this toxic metal is ubiquitous in the environment. With no set upper threshold for children, the accepted tolerable limits based on body weight are likely detrimental to children whose body weight is also smaller. In these analyses, we evaluated the extent to which adherence to a Mediterranean diet modified the association of cadmium and poor birth outcomes. We found that elevated prenatal cadmium exposure was associated with a lower birth weight compared to infants born to mothers with average or low cadmium exposure during pregnancy. These associations persisted after further adjusting for other co-occurring toxic metals that have been previously associated with these poor birth outcomes. Furthermore, after removing gestational age as a confounder, the association between prenatal cadmium exposure and birth weight remained significant. However, the association between prenatal cadmium exposure and preterm birth lost significance after removing birth weight. We found no association between prenatal cadmium exposure and Apgar score or infant PI at birth.

Our findings are consistent with previous data from our group and others that have demonstrated that prenatal exposure to cadmium, at non-occupational levels, is associated with lower birth weight [10–12] and is not associated with preterm birth [10,38]. These findings are, however, not consistent with the hypothesis that dietary patterns rich in iron, selenium, and folate may mitigate exposure. We did not find evidence to support our hypothesis that adherence to a Mediterranean diet prenatally modifies the associations between cadmium exposure and poor birth outcomes, regardless of the cut-off used to define "high Mediterranean adherence". While sample size limits inference, these data suggest that, in this population, at these cadmium levels, adherence to a Mediterranean dietary pattern may not modify the effects of prenatal cadmium exposure on birth outcomes. We were also interested in understanding whether the association between prenatal cadmium exposure and adverse birth outcomes was related to growth restriction or shortened gestation. In our exploratory analysis, the association between cadmium exposure and birth weight remained significant after excluding gestational age from the model; however, the association between cadmium exposure and preterm birth was no longer significant after excluding birth weight. This suggests that cadmium exposure may influence birth weight through growth restriction rather than shortened gestation.

To our knowledge, this is the first attempt to determine the effects of the Mediterranean diet on the association between prenatal cadmium concentrations and documented poor birth outcomes in humans. Previous animal- and cell-based studies have shown that a dietary intake of iron, calcium, selenium, and folate can reduce toxicity from cadmium exposure [20,21]. The Mediterranean diet pattern has been found to be a rich source of iron, folate, and selenium [39]. Thus, our analysis showing that adherence to a Mediterranean diet pattern during pregnancy did not change the association between prenatal cadmium exposure and birth weight or preterm birth was surprising. The average intake of selenium in the US is high at 108.5 mcg/day [40], the intake of iron and calcium from food is lower than recommended at 11.5–13.7 mg/day [40] and 748 to 968 mg/day (females) [41], respectively, and the intake of folate is insufficient for pregnancy at 455 mcg DFE/day (females) [40]. It is possible that usual eating patterns in the US may not provide sufficient amounts of these nutrients to mitigate elevated cadmium exposure; therefore, diet interventions that encourage following a diet pattern with higher levels of iron, calcium, and folate may be warranted. Interventions focused on dietary modifications may hold better prospects for implementation and adherence in exposed populations when compared to interventions focused on costly landscape remediation. Additionally, dietary intervention does not carry the health risks associated with cadmium chelation using agents such as EDTA.

The inability to find associations could be due to one of several possibilities, some related to how cadmium is estimated, and others related to the measurement of diet. For example, maternal circulating levels of cadmium may not reflect cadmium levels that the offspring may be exposed to, as there is evidence in support of cadmium being sequestered by the placenta [42]. Secondly, because in the United States the main source of cadmium in the diet is lettuce, milk and cookies [43], it is possible that the additional exposure to cadmium may overwhelm the nutritive benefits of this diet. It is also possible that women's intake in our sample may not represent a true Mediterranean diet pattern, even at high MDS values, as food choices and availability may differ by country [44]. Additionally, it may be that adherence to a Mediterranean diet pattern does reduce the effects of cadmium exposure on lower birth weight, yet we were underpowered to detect the associations. Although we were unable to establish a modifying effect of Mediterranean diet on the association between prenatal cadmium exposure and birth outcomes, the Mediterranean diet has been shown to protect against a number of diseases and inflammatory processes in the body [45], thus providing a rationale for its continued study. Given the ubiquity of this toxic metal in the environment, the effects of cadmium on birth outcomes, and the plausibility that a Mediterranean diet may mitigate the adverse effects, repeating these analyses in larger data sets is warranted.

Our study findings should be interpreted in the context of the study limitations. In addition to being underpowered to detect a significant effect measure modification that may have existed, both the measurement of Mediterranean diet adherence and our inability to "remove" the effects of dietary items such as lettuce and milk, which are major sources of cadmium in the US, is a limitation. An analysis of these relationships in different populations may clarify these findings. Furthermore, although implausible values were excluded from analyses, the Mediterranean diet was computed from self-reported diet data, which may have led to misclassified food intake that may be further biased by social desirability. This may have led to the under-reporting of unhealthy foods and the over-reporting of healthy foods. An additional limitation is the use of the MDS to assess diet. Although widely used and associated with a number of health outcomes, the MDS does not assess many foods that are thought to be "detrimental", such as sugar or highly processed convenience foods.

Despite this, our study also exhibits strengths. We used prospectively collected data, therefore we can establish the timing of exposure, modifiers, and outcomes. Another important strength of this study is that it assessed maternal dietary patterns rather than the intake of single nutrients. Humans consume most of their nutrients through foods and combinations of nutrients, therefore it is important to assess the role of dietary patterns in the potential mitigation of negative consequences from toxic exposures.

5. Conclusions

These limitations notwithstanding, this study contributes to the growing literature on the effects of toxic exposures during pregnancy and adds information on the potential role of diet in preventing adverse birth outcomes. Although our study did not support that maternal adherence to a Mediterranean diet pattern may mitigate exposure, it is possible that other dietary patterns may in fact help mitigate the association between elevated prenatal cadmium exposure and lower birth weights. Future research should focus on finding dietary patterns that can mitigate prenatal cadmium risk and that can be easily translatable into public health recommendations.

Supplementary Materials: The following are available online at http://www.mdpi.com/2305-6304/8/4/90/s1, Table S1: Regression coefficients and 95% confidence intervals for the association/relationship between, cadmium exposure (log cd) and birth weight; Table S2: Odds ratio and 95% confidence intervals for the association/relationship between cadmium exposure (log cd) and preterm birth; Table S3: Regression coefficients and 95% confidence intervals for the association/relationship between, cadmium exposure (high/low) and (1) Apgar score, (2) Ponderal index.

Author Contributions: Conceptualization, C.H. and S.G.-N.; methodology and analysis, C.H., K.N, S.G.-N.; writing—original draft preparation, S.G.-N. and C.H.; writing—review and editing, S.G.-N., K.N., J.S.H., R.L.M., H.G.S., C.H.; funding acquisition, C.H. All authors have read and agreed to the published version of the manuscript.

Funding: This research was funded by grant R24ES028531, R01MD011746 andP30ES025128, and supported in part by the division of intramural research at NIH, National Institute of Environmental Health Sciences.

Acknowledgments: The authors thank participants of the NEST study and Cheyenne Bradford for her help with the literature review.

Conflicts of Interest: The authors declare no conflict of interest.

References

1. World Health Organization. *Cadmium*; World Health Organization: Geneva, Switzerland, 1992.
2. United States Department of Health and Human Services; Agency for Toxic Substances and Disease Registry. *Toxicological Profile for Cadmium*; Centers for Disease Control and Prevention: Atlanta, GA, USA, 2012.
3. Straif, K.; Benbrahim-Tallaa, L.; Baan, R.; Grosse, Y.; Secretan, B.; El Ghissassi, F.; Bouvard, V.; Guha, N.; Freeman, C.; Galichet, L.; et al. A review of human carcinogens-Part C: Metals, arsenic, dusts, and fibres. *Lancet Oncol.* **2009**, *10*, 453–454. [CrossRef]
4. Satarug, S. Dietary Cadmium Intake and Its Effects on Kidneys. *Toxics* **2018**, *6*, 15. [CrossRef] [PubMed]
5. Webb, S.F. Simultaneous Determination of Arsenic, Cadmium, Calcium, Chromium, Cobalt, Copper, Iron, Lead, Magnesium, Manganese, Molybdenum, Nickel, Selenium, and Zinc in Fertilizers by Microwave Acid Digestion and Argon Inductively Coupled Plasma-Optical Emission Spectrometry Detection: Single-Laboratory Validation, First Action 2017.02. *J. AOAC Int.* **2018**, *101*, 383–384. [CrossRef] [PubMed]
6. Xu, Y.; Tang, H.; Liu, T.; Li, Y.; Huang, X.; Pi, J. Effects of long-term fertilization practices on heavy metal cadmium accumulation in the surface soil and rice plants of double-cropping rice system in Southern China. *Environ. Sci. Pollut. Res. Int.* **2018**, *25*, 19836–19844. [CrossRef]
7. Dharma-Wardana, M.W.C. Fertilizer usage and cadmium in soils, crops and food. *Environ. Geochem. Health* **2018**, *40*, 2739–2759. [CrossRef]
8. Rao, Z.X.; Huang, D.Y.; Wu, J.S.; Zhu, Q.H.; Zhu, H.H.; Xu, C.; Xiong, J.; Wang, H.; Duan, M.M. Distribution and availability of cadmium in profile and aggregates of a paddy soil with 30-year fertilization and its impact on Cd accumulation in rice plant. *Environ. Pollut.* **2018**, *239*, 198–204. [CrossRef]
9. World Health Organization. *Cadmium Chapter 6.3. Air Quality Guidelines*; World Health Organization: Geneva, Switzerland, 2000.
10. Johnston, J.E.; Valentiner, E.; Maxson, P.; Miranda, M.L.; Fry, R.C. Maternal cadmium levels during pregnancy associated with lower birth weight in infants in a North Carolina cohort. *PLoS ONE* **2014**, *9*, e109661. [CrossRef]
11. Vidal, A.C.; Semenova, V.; Darrah, T.; Vengosh, A.; Huang, Z.; King, K.; Nye, M.D.; Fry, R.; Skaar, D.; Maguire, R.; et al. Maternal cadmium, iron and zinc levels, DNA methylation and birth weight. *BMC Pharmacol. Toxicol.* **2015**, *16*, 20. [CrossRef]
12. Lin, C.M.; Doyle, P.; Wang, D.; Hwang, Y.H.; Chen, P.C. Does prenatal cadmium exposure affect fetal and child growth? *Occup. Environ. Med.* **2011**, *68*, 641–646. [CrossRef]
13. Wang, H.; Liu, L.; Hu, Y.F.; Hao, J.H.; Chen, Y.H.; Su, P.Y.; Yu, Z.; Fu, L.; Tao, F.B.; Xu, D.X. Association of maternal serum cadmium level during pregnancy with risk of preterm birth in a Chinese population. *Environ. Pollut.* **2016**, *216*, 851–857. [CrossRef]
14. Green, A.J.; Hoyo, C.; Mattingly, C.J.; Luo, Y.; Tzeng, J.Y.; Murphy, S.K.; Buchwalter, D.B.; Planchart, A. Cadmium exposure increases the risk of juvenile obesity: A human and zebrafish comparative study. *Int. J. Obes.* **2018**, *42*, 1285–1295. [CrossRef] [PubMed]
15. Gluckman, P.D.; Hanson, M.A.; Cooper, C.; Thornburg, K.L. Effect of in utero and early-life conditions on adult health and disease. *N. Engl. J. Med.* **2008**, *359*, 61–73. [CrossRef]
16. Martin, J.A.; Hamilton, B.E.; Osterman, M.J.K. Births in the United States, 2018. *NCHS Data Brief* **2019**, *346*, 1–8.
17. Martin, J.A.; Osterman, M.J.K. Describing the Increase in Preterm Births in the United States, 2014–2016. *NCHS Data Brief* **2018**, *312*, 1–8.
18. Beam, A.L.; Fried, I.; Palmer, N.; Agniel, D.; Brat, G.; Fox, K.; Kohane, I.; Sinaiko, A.; Zupancic, J.A.F.; Armstrong, J. Estimates of healthcare spending for preterm and low-birthweight infants in a commercially insured population: 2008–2016. *J. Perinatol.* **2020**, *40*, 1091–1099. [CrossRef] [PubMed]
19. Genchi, G.; Sinicropi, M.S.; Lauria, G.; Carocci, A.; Catalano, A. The Effects of Cadmium Toxicity. *Int. J. Environ. Res. Public Health* **2020**, *17*, 3782. [CrossRef] [PubMed]

20. Zwolak, I. The Role of Selenium in Arsenic and Cadmium Toxicity: an Updated Review of Scientific Literature. *Biol. Trace Elem. Res.* **2020**, *193*, 44–63. [CrossRef]
21. Zhai, Q.; Narbad, A.; Chen, W. Dietary strategies for the treatment of cadmium and lead toxicity. *Nutrients* **2015**, *7*, 552–571. [CrossRef]
22. Mijatovic-Vukas, J.; Capling, L.; Cheng, S.; Stamatakis, E.; Louie, J.; Cheung, N.W.; Markovic, T.; Ross, G.; Senior, A.; Brand-Miller, J.C.; et al. Associations of Diet and Physical Activity with Risk for Gestational Diabetes Mellitus: A Systematic Review and Meta-Analysis. *Nutrients* **2018**, *10*, 698. [CrossRef] [PubMed]
23. Timmermans, S.; Steegers-Theunissen, R.P.; Vujkovic, M.; den Breeijen, H.; Russcher, H.; Lindemans, J.; Mackenbach, J.; Hofman, A.; Lesaffre, E.E.; Jaddoe, V.V.; et al. The Mediterranean diet and fetal size parameters: the Generation R Study. *Br. J. Nutr.* **2012**, *108*, 1399–1409. [CrossRef]
24. Parlapani, E.; Agakidis, C.; Karagiozoglou-Lampoudi, T.; Sarafidis, K.; Agakidou, E.; Athanasiadis, A.; Diamanti, E. The Mediterranean diet adherence by pregnant women delivering prematurely: Association with size at birth and complications of prematurity. *J. Matern-Fetal Neonatal Med.* **2019**, *32*, 1084–1091. [CrossRef]
25. Chatzi, L.; Mendez, M.; Garcia, R.; Roumeliotaki, T.; Ibarluzea, J.; Tardón, A.; Amiano, P.; Lertxundi, A.; Iñiguez, C.; Vioque, J.; et al. Mediterranean diet adherence during pregnancy and fetal growth: INMA (Spain) and RHEA (Greece) mother-child cohort studies. *Br. J. Nutr.* **2012**, *107*, 135–145. [CrossRef] [PubMed]
26. Biagi, C.; Nunzio, M.D.; Bordoni, A.; Gori, D.; Lanari, M. Effect of Adherence to Mediterranean Diet during Pregnancy on Children's Health: A Systematic Review. *Nutrients* **2019**, *11*, 997. [CrossRef] [PubMed]
27. Peraita-Costa, I.; Llopis-Gonzalez, A.; Perales-Marin, A.; Diago, V.; Soriano, J.M.; Llopis-Morales, A.; Morales-Suarez-Varela, M. Maternal profile according to Mediterranean diet adherence and small for gestational age and preterm newborn outcomes. *Public Health Nutr.* **2020**, *29*, 1–13. [CrossRef] [PubMed]
28. House, J.S.; Mendez, M.; Maguire, R.L.; Gonzalez-Nahm, S.; Huang, Z.; Daniels, J.; Murphy, S.K.; Fuemmeler, B.F.; Wright, F.A.; Hoyo, C. Periconceptional Maternal Mediterranean Diet Is Associated With Favorable Offspring Behaviors and Altered CpG Methylation of Imprinted Genes. *Front. Cell Dev. Biol.* **2018**, *6*, 107. [CrossRef] [PubMed]
29. Martinez-Gonzalez, M.A.; Salas-Salvado, J.; Estruch, R.; Corella, D.; Fito, M.; Ros, E.; Predimed, I. Benefits of the Mediterranean Diet: Insights From the PREDIMED Study. *Prog. Cardiovasc. Dis.* **2015**, *58*, 50–60. [CrossRef] [PubMed]
30. Sofi, F.; Abbate, R.; Gensini, G.F.; Casini, A. Accruing evidence on benefits of adherence to the Mediterranean diet on health: An updated systematic review and meta-analysis. *Am. J. Clin. Nutr.* **2010**, *92*, 1189–1196. [CrossRef]
31. Chatzi, L.; Rifas-Shiman, S.L.; Georgiou, V.; Joung, K.E.; Koinaki, S.; Chalkiadaki, G.; Margioris, A.; Sarri, K.; Vassilaki, M.; Vafeiadi, M.; et al. Adherence to the Mediterranean diet during pregnancy and offspring adiposity and cardiometabolic traits in childhood. *Pediatric Obes.* **2017**, *12* (Suppl. 1), 47–56. [CrossRef] [PubMed]
32. Chatzi, L.; Garcia, R.; Roumeliotaki, T.; Basterrechea, M.; Begiristain, H.; Iniguez, C.; Vioque, J.; Kogevinas, M.; Sunyer, J. Mediterranean diet adherence during pregnancy and risk of wheeze and eczema in the first year of life: INMA (Spain) and RHEA (Greece) mother-child cohort studies. *Br. J. Nutr.* **2013**, *110*, 2058–2068. [CrossRef]
33. Sofi, F.; Macchi, C.; Abbate, R.; Gensini, G.F.; Casini, A. Mediterranean diet and health status: An updated meta-analysis and a proposal for a literature-based adherence score. *Public Health Nutr.* **2014**, *17*, 2769–2782. [CrossRef]
34. Liu, Y.; Murphy, S.K.; Murtha, A.P.; Fuemmeler, B.F.; Schildkraut, J.; Huang, Z.; Overcash, F.; Kurtzberg, J.; Jirtle, R.; Iversen, E.S.; et al. Depression in pregnancy, infant birth weight and DNA methylation of imprint regulatory elements. *Epigenetics* **2012**, *7*, 735–746. [CrossRef] [PubMed]
35. Iwai-Shimada, M.; Kameo, S.; Nakai, K.; Yaginuma-Sakurai, K.; Tatsuta, N.; Kurokawa, N.; Nakayama, S.F.; Satoh, H. Exposure profile of mercury, lead, cadmium, arsenic, antimony, copper, selenium and zinc in maternal blood, cord blood and placenta: the Tohoku Study of Child Development in Japan. *Environ. Health Prev. Med.* **2019**, *24*, 35. [CrossRef] [PubMed]
36. Gonzalez-Nahm, S.; Mendez, M.A.; Robinson, W.R.; Murphy, S.K.; Hoyo, C.; Hogan, V.K.; Rowley, D.L. Low maternal adherence to a Mediterranean diet is associated with increase in methylation at the MEG3-IG differentially methylated region in female infants. *Environ. Epigenet.* **2017**, *3*, 1–10. [CrossRef] [PubMed]
37. Trichopoulou, A.; Costacou, T.; Bamia, C.; Trichopoulos, D. Adherence to a Mediterranean diet and survival in a Greek population. *N. Engl. J. Med.* **2003**, *348*, 2599–2608. [CrossRef] [PubMed]

38. Yildirim, E.; Derici, M.K.; Demir, E.; Apaydin, H.; Kocak, O.; Kan, O.; Gorkem, U. Is the Concentration of Cadmium, Lead, Mercury, and Selenium Related to Preterm Birth? *Biol. Trace Elem. Res.* **2019**, *191*, 306–312. [CrossRef] [PubMed]
39. Serra-Majem, L.; Bes-Rastrollo, M.; Roman-Vinas, B.; Pfrimer, K.; Sanchez-Villegas, A.; Martinez-Gonzalez, M.A. Dietary patterns and nutritional adequacy in a Mediterranean country. *Br. J. Nutr.* **2009**, *101* (Suppl. 2), S21–S28. [CrossRef] [PubMed]
40. U.S. Department of Agriculture, Agricultural Research Service. *What We Eat in America: NHANES 2013-2014*; U.S. Department of Agriculture: Beltsville, MD, USA, 2016.
41. Bailey, R.L.; Dodd, K.W.; Goldman, J.A.; Gahche, J.J.; Dwyer, J.T.; Moshfegh, A.J.; Sempos, C.T.; Picciano, M.F. Estimation of total usual calcium and vitamin D intakes in the United States. *J. Nutr.* **2010**, *140*, 817–822. [CrossRef]
42. Needham, L.L.; Grandjean, P.; Heinzow, B.; Jørgensen, P.J.; Nielsen, F.; Patterson, D.G., Jr.; Sjödin, A.; Turner, W.E.; Weihe, P. Partition of environmental chemicals between maternal and fetal blood and tissues. *Environ. Sci. Technol.* **2011**, *45*, 1121–1126. [CrossRef]
43. Kim, K.; Melough, M.M.; Vance, T.M.; Noh, H.; Koo, S.I.; Chun, O.K. Dietary Cadmium Intake and Sources in the US. *Nutrients* **2018**, *11*, 2. [CrossRef]
44. Hoffman, R.; Gerber, M. Evaluating and adapting the Mediterranean diet for non-Mediterranean populations: A critical appraisal. *Nutr. Rev.* **2013**, *71*, 573–584. [CrossRef]
45. Mentella, M.C.; Scaldaferri, F.; Ricci, C.; Gasbarrini, A.; Miggiano, G.A.D. Cancer and Mediterranean Diet: A Review. *Nutrients* **2019**, *11*, 2059. [CrossRef] [PubMed]

toxics

MDPI

Article

Early-Life Dietary Cadmium Exposure and Kidney Function in 9-Year-Old Children from the PROGRESS Cohort

Edna Rodríguez-López [1], Marcela Tamayo-Ortiz [1,2,*], Ana Carolina Ariza [1], Eduardo Ortiz-Panozo [3], Andrea L. Deierlein [4], Ivan Pantic [5], Mari Cruz Tolentino [6], Guadalupe Estrada-Gutiérrez [7], Sandra Parra-Hernández [7], Aurora Espejel-Núñez [7], Martha María Téllez-Rojo [1], Robert O. Wright [8,9] and Alison P. Sanders [8,9,*]

1. Center for Nutrition and Health Research, National Institute of Public Health (INSP), Cuernavaca 62100, Morelos, Mexico; edds.rdz@gmail.com (E.R.-L.); carolina.ariza@insp.mx (A.C.A.); mmtellez@insp.mx (M.M.T.-R.)
2. National Council of Science and Technology (CONACyT), Mexico City 03940, Mexico
3. Center for Population Health Research, National Institute of Public Health (INSP), Cuernavaca 62100, Morelos, Mexico; eduardo.ortiz@insp.mx
4. Public Health Nutrition, School of Global Public Health, New York University, New York, NY 10012, USA; ald8@nyu.edu
5. Department of Developmental Neurobiology, National Institute of Perinatology, Mexico City 11000, Mexico; ivandpantic@gmail.com
6. Department of Nutrition and Bio programming, National Institute of Perinatology, Mexico City 11000, Mexico; cruz_tolentino@yahoo.com.mx
7. Department of Immunobiochemistry, National Institute of Perinatology, Mexico City 11000, Mexico; gpestrad@gmail.com (G.E.-G.); rebe1602@hotmail.com (S.P.-H.); aurora_espnu@yahoo.com.mx (A.E.-N.)
8. Department of Environmental Medicine and Public Health, Icahn School of Medicine at Mount Sinai, New York, NY 10029, USA; robert.wright@mssm.edu
9. Department of Pediatrics, Icahn School of Medicine at Mount Sinai, New York, NY 10029, USA

* Correspondence: marcela.tamayo@insp.mx (M.T.-O.); alison.sanders@mssm.edu (A.P.S.)

Received: 21 August 2020; Accepted: 23 September 2020; Published: 7 October 2020

Abstract: Cadmium (Cd) is a toxic metal associated with adverse health effects, including kidney injury or disease. The aims of this study were to estimate dietary Cd exposure during childhood, and to evaluate the association of early-life dietary Cd with biomarkers of glomerular kidney function in 9-year-old Mexican children. Our study included 601 children from the Programming Research in Obesity, Growth, Environment and Social Stressors (PROGRESS) cohort with up to five follow-up food frequency questionnaires from 1 to 9 years of age; and 480 children with measures of serum creatinine, cystatin C, and blood nitrogen urea (BUN), as well as 9-year-old estimated glomerular filtration rate. Dietary Cd was estimated through food composition tables. Multiple linear regression models were used to analyze the association between 1 and 9 years, cumulative dietary Cd, and each kidney parameter. Dietary Cd exposure increased with age and exceeded the tolerable weekly intake (TWI = 2.5 μg/kg body weight) by 16–64% at all ages. Early-life dietary Cd exposure was above the TWI and we observed inverse associations between dietary Cd exposure and kidney function parameters. Additional studies are needed to assess kidney function trajectories through adolescence. Identifying preventable risk factors including environmental exposures in early life can contribute to decreasing the incidence of adult kidney disease.

Keywords: cadmium; children; diet; kidney function

1. Introduction

Cadmium (Cd) is a heavy metal found naturally in the environment that has been associated with adverse health effects, such as kidney failure, bone damage, cardiovascular disease, and cancer [1]. Children's exposure to Cd is of special concern as they may be more susceptible than adults to its toxic effects. Compared to adults, children's food and water intake per body weight is greater, and they have increased intestinal absorption and limited renal excretion [2]. Ingestion and inhalation are the primary routes of exposure to Cd—primarily through food, tobacco smoke, and dust. Cd accumulation occurs in different tissues and organs [3]. Among the possible target organs of Cd, the kidney is one of the most sensitive organs, wherein Cd exposure is associated with tubular dysfunction, hypercalciuria, polyuria, tubulointerstitial nephritis, and low-molecular-weight proteinuria, which could lead to kidney failure in later stages [4–6].

There is evidence to suggest that Cd exposure plays a role in the development of chronic kidney disease (CKD) and that Cd can be nephrotoxic at environmental levels [5,7]. A recent exposure-wide association study of over 250 chemicals found that Cd was associated with CKD [8]. Therefore, identifying preventable risk factors, including environmental exposures in childhood, could contribute to our knowledgebase of early-life intervenable factors for decreasing the incidence of CKD [9]. Estimates suggest that 8–16% of the global population is affected by some form of CKD [7]. Few epidemiological studies have evaluated the association between dietary Cd and kidney function in children; however, it has been suggested that the mechanism is similar to that of adults for whom there is evidence of dietary Cd exposure and prevalence of CKD [10,11].

Regarding dietary Cd exposure, previous studies have shown elevated tolerable weekly intakes (TWI = 2.5 μg/kg body weight) in children, wherein regularly consumed food items were an important source of Cd [12,13]. A study in Uruguayan children found that Cd levels increased with age [14], and notably, a recent study in Mexican children reported an association between dietary Cd intake and urinary Cd [15]. Despite the existing evidence that children's dietary Cd exposure is elevated, and the importance of early detection of risk factors that may affect children's kidney health, no studies in Mexico have evaluated longitudinal dietary Cd exposure and its association with kidney function in childhood. Therefore, the aims of this study were: (1) To estimate the dietary exposure of Cd during childhood and identify the primary foods contributing to children's Cd exposure; and (2) to evaluate the association of early-life dietary Cd exposure with biomarkers of kidney function in 9-year-old Mexican children.

2. Materials and Methods

2.1. Study Population

This analysis included children from the Programming Research in Obesity, Growth, Environment and Social Stressors (PROGRESS) cohort from Mexico City, which has been previously described in more detail [16]. Briefly, pregnant women receiving care at clinics of the Mexican Institute of Social Security were invited to participate between July 2007 and February 2011. Women were eligible if they were 18 years or older, at <20 weeks of gestation, free of heart or kidney disease, did not use steroids or anti-epilepsy drugs, did not consume alcohol on a daily basis, had access to a telephone, and planned to reside in Mexico City for the following three years.

Children were seen at our research facilities at the National Institute of Perinatology, Mexico City (INPer) at 5 follow-up visits when they were 1 year (min 0.98 years, max 1.16 years), 2 years (min 1.95 years, max 2.58 years), 4 years (min 4.00 years, max 6.75 years), 6 years (min 5.96 years, max 9.65 years), and 9 years (min 8.08 years, max 12.06 years). To estimate dietary Cd exposure, we included 601 children who had at least 1 food frequency questionnaire (FFQ) from follow-up visits. For the analysis of kidney function, 480 children with measures of creatinine, cystatin C, blood nitrogen urea (BUN), and estimated glomerular filtration rate (eGFR) at 9 years were included. We excluded children with very low birth weight (<1500 g) and/or born preterm (<37 weeks gestation) (n = 27).

All participants provided written informed consent at the start of the study visit. The study was approved by the internal review boards of the Icahn School of Medicine at Mount Sinai (#12-00751) and the National Institute of Public Health Mexico (project #560), 31 October 2017.

2.2. Diet Data Collection

Children's diet was assessed using a semiquantitative FFQ that collected food and beverage intake during the previous 7 days [17]. The questionnaire included 101 foods grouped into 14 categories (dairy products, fruits, vegetables, fast food, meat, fish, legumes, cereals, corn products, beverages, snacks, soups, miscellaneous, and tortillas). Frequency values ranged from never consumed, to consumed 7 days per week, as well as times per day that they were consumed with values ranging from consumed 1 to 6 times per day. Serving size (small, medium, large, and very large) and the number of servings consumed were reported. The questionnaire was administered by an interviewer at each of the study visits and answered by the child's mother or caregiver.

Dietary Cadmium

To estimate dietary Cd, we carried out a search of composition tables reporting Cd levels in food, based on the Total Diet Study (TDS) methodology, which consists of reporting concentrations of contaminants in food [18]. As Mexico lacks such tables, we used tables from the United States, The European Food Safety Authority, Australia, Hong Kong, and Canada. We also used available Cd concentrations measured in selected meat products (ham, sausage, and chorizo) by a study in Mexico City [19]. Each food and beverage item in our FFQ was matched with each of the items found in the Cd composition tables of the different countries. We used the composition tables to obtain an average Cd concentration for each food item, i.e., when the food item was included in all five tables, the average Cd concentration from the tables was used, and so on, if the food item was included in only one table that value was used. In some cases, more than one food item was inquired as the same item on our FFQ (e.g., "broccoli and cauliflower"); for those cases, we used the average Cd for each of the food items from the composition tables. Cd from dishes and prepared foods was estimated (per 100 g of preparation) using a standardized method that accounts for grams of each ingredient in the recipe. Cd levels were estimated in μg/day and were reported for each study visit, as well as the "top ten" foods that contribute the most to the Cd intake according to their frequency of consumption.

We also created a dichotomous variable for children's Cd exposure at each study visit according to the European Food Safety Authority TWI for Cd of 2.5 μg/kg body weight. If the child's Cd intake was above the TWI: High = 1, or below the TWI: Low = 0 [20]. Finally, to account for approximate cumulative Cd exposure, we generated an ordinal Cd score by adding the Cd TWI high or low from all study visits (scores ranged from 0 = low exposure in all study visits, to 5 = high exposure in all study visits). This was done only for children who had dietary information for all five study visits (n = 182).

2.3. Kidney Function Parameters

Kidney function parameters were determined at 9 years by standardized and trained staff in the Nutrition and Bio-programming Research, and the Immunochemistry department's laboratories at INPer. Fasting blood samples were collected in BD Vacutainer tubes, and serum was separated according to the standard protocol and stored at −70 °C until the analysis. The laboratory analyses were carried out using the following methods:

Serum creatinine (SCr) was measured through the kinetic test without deproteinization according to the Jaffé method [21]. *Cystatin C (Cys C)* was measured by Quantikine Human Cystatin C enzyme-linked immunosorbent assay. *Blood urea nitrogen (BUN)* was calculated with the following formula: Serum urea (mg/dL)/2.14; serum urea was determined through the Urease—GLDH test: Enzymatic UV test [22]. *Estimated glomerular filtration rate (eGFR)* was calculated using two formulae: (1) Schwartz formula: $eGFR_{Schwartz} = (k \times \text{height})/SCr$, where k is 0.55 for children under 13 years, height is measured in cm, and SCr is in mg/dL [23]; and (2) the 2012 Cystatin C-based equation: $eGFR_{Cystatin\ C} = 70.69 \times (CysC)^{-0.931}$, where cystatin C is in mg/L [24].

2.4. Covariates

Information on secondhand tobacco exposure was obtained by questionnaire; mothers reported the minutes per day that children spent with smokers at 4, 6, and 9 years. Children were weighed with the least amount of clothing possible and without footwear using an InBody230, and height was measured with a SECA stadiometer without footwear. The z-score for body mass index (BMI) was estimated according to WHO guidelines [25]: Underweight, normal weight, overweight, and obesity were defined as <-2SD, >-2SD to $\leq+1$SD, $>+1$SD to $+2$SD, and $>+2$SD, respectively. As there were few underweight children, these observations were collapsed to the normal weight category. Physical activity was measured with the International Physical Activity Questionnaire (IPAQ) that was answered by the child's mother at 4, 6, and 9 years. We considered moderate to vigorous activities such as play in the park, run, walk, ride a bike, and dance to estimate minutes of aerobic activities per day. Maternal socioeconomic status was collected at the time of enrollment using a questionnaire according to the Mexican Association of Market Intelligence and Public Opinion Agencies (AMAI, 2007 version). The AMAI classifies Mexican households into seven levels (very low, low, middle-low, middle, middle-high, and high) according to their ability to satisfy the needs of their members. In this study, we collapsed the AMAI levels into three categories: lower, middle, and higher.

2.5. Statistical Analysis

We performed descriptive analyses to identify the food items at each study visit that most contributed to the estimated total dietary Cd intake and reported them as percentages.

We analyzed the distributions and descriptive statistics for each kidney parameter and log-transformed variables for cystatin C, BUN, and eGFR. We used multivariable linear regression models to analyze associations between dietary Cd at 1 and 9 years with kidney parameters at 9 years. In a subset of children with dietary information across all five study visits, we derived an ordinal cumulative Cd score. The ordinal score was derived as follows: A score of 0 indicated no exposure throughout the study visits, a score of 1 indicated a high dietary Cd in one study visit and so forth, and 5 indicated high dietary Cd in all ages (i.e., 1, 2, 4, 6, and 9 years). We incorporated the ordinal score as a discrete and categorical variable in models and examined associations with each kidney function parameter. Final models were adjusted for sex, age in months (to account for the wider age range at the study visit), BMI z-score, physical activity, secondhand tobacco exposure, and socioeconomic status. All statistical analyses were performed in Stata Statistical Software: Release 14. College Station, TX: StataCorp LP.

3. Results

Table 1 shows the participant characteristics at each study visit. Just over half of the children were male, and the age ranged from 12.2 ± 0.28 months at the 1-year visit to 116 ± 8.2 months at the 9 year visit. Most of the children were of normal weight between 1 and 6 years; however, at 9 years, almost half of the children were overweight (24.8%) or obese (22.0%). Physical activity at 4 and 6 years was 65.8 ± 30.0 and 69.73 ± 29.3 min/day on average, respectively, and decreased to 21.0 ± 7.10 min/day at 9 years. The majority of children (more than 80% at 4, 6, and 9 years) were not exposed to secondhand tobacco smoke and were of middle or lower socioeconomic status.

Table 1. Participant characteristics at follow-up study visits.

Study Visit	1-Year Visit n = 566	2-Year Visit n = 530	4-Year Visit n = 582	6-Year Visit n = 573	9-Year Visit n = 544
Characteristic	Mean ± SD or n (%)	Mean ± SD or n (%)	Mean ± SD or n (%)	Mean ± SD or n (%)	Mean ± SD or n (%)
Sex Male	285 (50.3%)	278 (52.4%)	293 (50.3%)	293 (51.2%)	280 (51.4%)
Age (months)	12.2 ± 0.28	24.4 ± 0.54	58.5 ± 6.7	82.1 ± 7.2	116 ± 8.2
BMI Z-score [a]					
Underweight	15 (2.6%)	2 (0.38%)	2 (0.34%)	7 (1.2%)	3(0.53%)
Normal weight	455 (80.3%)	352 (66.4%)	474 (81.4%)	407 (71.0%)	286 (52.5%)
Overweight	73 (12.9%)	130 (24.5%)	68 (11.6%)	92 (16.0%)	135 (24.8%)
Obesity	23 (4.0%)	46 (8.6%)	38 (6.5%)	67 (11.6%)	120 (22.0%)
Physical activity (min/day) [b]	N/A	N/A	65.8 ± 30.0	69.73 ± 29.3	21.02 ± 7.10
Aerobic activities					
Second-hand smoking (daily) [c]	N/A	N/A			
Yes			58 (10%)	75 (13%)	98 (18.1%)
No			517 (90%)	486 (86.6%)	442 (81.8%)
Socioeconomic Status [d]					
Lower	292 (51.5%)				
Middle	218 (38.5%)				
Higher	56 (9.8%)				

[a]: Classification according to BMI/age z-score (Underweight <−2SD, normal >−2SD to ≤+1SD, overweight >+1SD to +2SD, obesity >+2SD); [b]: Aerobic activities: Play in the park, run, walk, ride a bike, dance, stage 48–n = 7 missing observations; [c]: Classification according to the minutes that children expend with smokers, stage 48–n = 7 missing observations, stage 72–n = 12 missing observations, stage 96–n = 4 missing observations; [d]: Classification according to the AMAI index; data from the enrollment.

Table 2 shows kidney function parameters measured at 9 years; the mean cystatin C was 0.730 ± 0.17 mg/dL, while the mean BUN was 12.20 ± 3.09 mg/dL. Using the $eGFR_{CystatinC}$ formula, there were two children below 60 mL/min/1.73 m^2 and 75 children in the 60–90 mL/min/1.73 m^2 range, while for the $eGFR_{Schwartz}$, a single child was between 60 and 90 and the rest had and eGFR ≥ 90 mL/min/1.73 m^2. We note that while fewer children had SCr measures, this observation is in line with evidence that SCr-based equations may overestimate eGFR [26].

Table 2. Kidney function parameters from 9-year-old children.

Kidney Function Parameter	n	Mean ± SD	(5–95%)
Serum Creatinine (mg/dL)	380	0.434 ± 0.09	(0.28–0.59)
Cystatin C (mg/L)	455	0.730 ± 0.17	(0.48–1.03)
BUN (mg/dL)	379	12.20 ± 3.09	(7.71–17.9)
$eGFR_{Schwartz}$ (mL/min/1.73 m^2)	379	180.91 ± 41.65	(125.43–261.8)
$eGFR_{Cystatin\ C}$ (mL/min/1.73 m^2)	455	116.55 ± 28.41	(77.93–166.79)

Figure 1 shows the primary foods contributing to the estimated dietary intake of Cd from 1 to 9 years of age. At 1 and 2 years, the top contributors were leafy greens (1 year: 16.0%, 2 years: 9.0%), milk (1 year: 10.1%, 2 years: 9.8%), and carrots (1 year: 8.8%, 2 years: 7.9%); at 4 years, the top contributors were sweets (6.8%), milk (6.1%), and carrots (4.8%); at 6 years, the top contributors were lettuce (6.8%), sandwich (6.6%), and sweets (6.4%); and at 9 years, the top contributors were lettuce (6.0%), pasta soup (5.7%), and sweets (5.5%). Total dietary Cd intake was 4.43 ± 2.53 µg/d at 1 year; 4.65 ± 2.45 μg/d at 2 years; 6.00 ± 3.45 μg/d at 4 years; 6.83 ± 3.15 μg/d at 6 years; and 8.09 ± 4.33 μg/d at 9 years. According to the TWI, Cd intakes were exceeded by children at all study visits (study visit, % children): 1 year, 64%; 2 years, 49%; 4 years, 35%; 6 years, 28%; and 9 years, 16%. For the cumulative Cd score (n = 175 children with information on dietary Cd in all study visits), we saw that 23 children had low Cd across all study visits; 38 children had high Cd in one study visit; 57 children had high Cd in two study visits; 31 children had high Cd in three study visits; 16 children had high Cd in four study visits; and 10 children had high Cd intake in all five study visits.

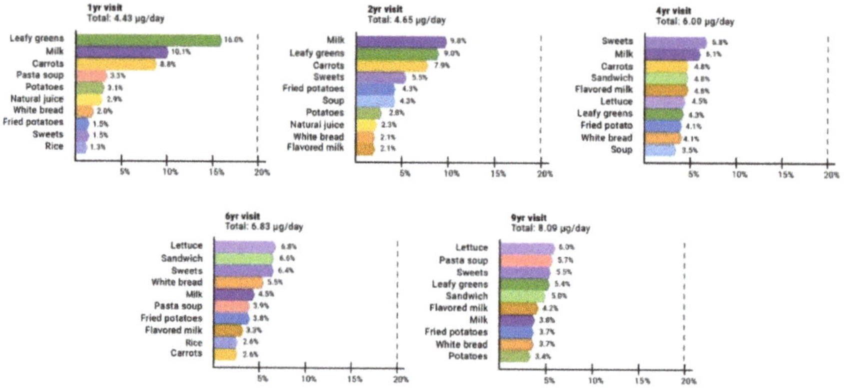

Figure 1. Primary foods contributing to estimated dietary Cd intake in 1–9-year-old children.

For the cross-sectional associations between higher 9-year dietary Cd and kidney parameters (Table 3), we observed an inverse association between dietary Cd and BUN (β = −0.077 (95% CI: [−0.151, −0.003])) and, marginally, with $eGFR_{CystatinC}$ (β = −0.046 (95% CI: [−0.107, 0.014])).

Table 3. Association between tolerable weekly intake (TWI) [a] dietary cadmium exposure at 9 years and concurrent kidney function parameters in children.

		Unadjusted			**Adjusted** [b]
	n	Low CdD	High CdD β (95% CI)	n	High CdD β (95% CI)
SCr [c] (mg/dL)	375	Ref	−0.021 (−0.047, 0.005)	342	−0.013 (−0.041, 0.015)
Cystatin C (mg/L)	447	Ref	0.057 (0.001, 0.113)	409	0.049 (−0.010, 0.109)
BUN (mg/dL)	375	Ref	−0.038 (−0.111, 0.033)	342	−0.077 (−0.151, −0.003)
$eGFR_{Schwartz}$ (mL/min/1.73 m^2)	376	Ref	0.020 (−0.043, 0.084)	343	0.022 (−0.046, 0.091)
$eGFR_{Cystatin\ C}$ (mL/min/1.73 m^2)	449	Ref	−0.053 (−0.110, 0.004)	411	−0.046 (−0.107, 0.014)

[a] Tolerable Weekly Intake: High ≥2.5 μg/kg body weight, low: <2.5 μg/kg body weight. [b] adjusted for sex, age, z-score BMI, physical activity, secondhand smoke, and socioeconomic status. [c] Serum creatinine.

We observed no significant associations between 1-year dietary Cd and subsequent children's kidney function (Table 4).

Table 4. Association between TWI dietary cadmium exposure (high vs. low) [a] at 1-year and kidney function parameters in 9-year-old children.

	Unadjusted			Adjusted [b]	
		Low CdD	High CdD		High CdD
	n		β (95% CI)	n	β (95% CI)
SCr [c] (mg/dL)	229	Ref	−0.012 (−0.039, 0.013)	208	−0.003 (−0.031, 0.025)
Cystatin C (mg/L)	274	Ref	−0.051 (−0.110, 0.007)	248	−0.026 (−0.089, 0.036)
BUN (mg/dL)	229	Ref	−0.055 (−0.125, 0.014)	208	−0.011 (−0.081, 0.059)
$eGFR_{Schwartz}$ (mL/min/1.73 m^2)	230	Ref	0.027 (−0.035, 0.090)	209	−0.003 (−0.072, 0.065)
$eGFR_{Cystatin\ C}$ (mL/min/1.73 m^2)	276	Ref	0.065 (0.004, 0.125)	250	0.034 (−0.029, 0.098)

[a] Tolerable Weekly Intake: High ≥2.5 μg/kg body weight, low: <2.5 μg/kg body weight. [b] adjusted for sex, age, z-score BMI, physical activity, secondhand smoke, and socioeconomic status. [c] Serum creatinine.

Finally, we assessed associations with cumulative Cd intake using an ordinal score, analyzed as discrete and categorical (Table 5). We again identified an inverse association with BUN when using the score as a discrete variable; however, no associations with the other parameters were observed. Using the score as categorical, we observed an inverted "U-shaped" relationship with cystatin C where estimates decreased with an increasing cumulative Cd score to 3 and then increased with the cumulative Cd score from 4 and 5; and a negative dose-response for BUN where, as the score increased, the model estimates decreased progressively from −0.006 to −0.187 (Table 5).

Table 5. Association between estimated cumulative dietary Cd score (as a discrete and categorical variable) and 9-year kidney function parameters [a].

Kidney Function Parameter	SCr [b] (n = 124)	Cystatin C (n = 140)	BUN (n = 124)	$eGFR_{Schwartz}$ (n = 124)	$eGFR_{CystatinC}$ (n = 142)
Score	β (95% CI)	β (95% CI)	β (95% CI)	β (95% CI)	β (95% CI)
Discrete	−0.011 (−0.025, 0.002)	−0.019 (−0.050, 0.010)	−0.037 (−0.072, −0.003)	0.025 (−0.007, 0.058)	0.020 (−0.011, 0.051)
0 (n = 23)	Ref	Ref	Ref	Ref	Ref
1 (n = 38)	0.017 (−0.047, 0.081)	0.063 (−0.083, 0.211)	−0.006 (−0.168, 0.154)	−0.028 (−0.182, 0.126)	−0.064 (−0.216, 0.088)
2 (n = 57)	−0.015 (−0.075, 0.044)	0.053 (−0.087, 0.193)	−0.041 (−0.191, 0.107)	0.048 (−0.094, 0.190)	−0.072 (−0.216, 0.071)
3 (n = 31)	−0.039 (−0.0105, 0.026)	−0.082 (−0.241, 0.075)	−0.092 (−0.257, 0.073)	0.104 (−0.053, 0.262)	0.081 (−0.082, 0.244)
4 (n = 16)	0.000 (−0.081, 0.081)	−0.028 (−0.209, 0.151)	−0.129 (−0.332, 0.073)	0.011 (−0.182, 0.204)	0.027 (−0.159, 0.213)
5 (n = 10)	−0.051 (−0.147, 0.044)	−0.007 (−0.202, 0.187)	−0.187 (−0.428, 0.052)	0.100 (−0.128, 0.328)	0.009 (−0.192, 0.210)

[a] adjusted for sex, age, z-score BMI, physical activity, secondhand smoke, and socioeconomic status. [b] Serum creatinine.

4. Discussion

In this longitudinal study of 601 Mexican children, we found that the estimated dietary Cd exposure increased with age, from ~4.4 μg/d at 1 year to 8.1 μg/d at 9 years. The main food sources of Cd changed across all study visits; at 1 and 2 years, leafy greens, milk, and carrots were the primary dietary contributors, and beginning at 4 years, we observed a dietary transition to sweets, lettuce, and sandwiches as the primary contributors. This transition most likely reflects maternal control of the child's dietary intake during the first two years of life and then the child's food preferences influencing intake at older ages. TWI was exceeded at all study visits, with 64% at 1 year decreasing to 16% in 9-year children consuming more Cd than is recommended. Finally, we found inverse associations between dietary 9-year high Cd intake, as well as the cumulative score and BUN β = −0.077 (95% CI: (−0.151, −0.003)) and β = −0.037 (−0.072, −0.003), respectively.

Our results are similar to the Cd intake observed among 4–12-year-old Australian children where the Cd intake was 4.0 ± 2.2 (0.98–9.5) μg/d [27] but higher than a study from the United States where the mean Cd intake in 2 to 10-year-old children was 2.96 (2.83, 3.10) μg/d [28]. Regarding the main food contributors, these results are similar to a previous study in the United States where the top Cd contributors to children's diet at 10–11 years old were milk, lettuce, and cookies [28]. The TWIs are in line with a study in France that observed that diets of 5–6-year-old children exceeded the Cd TWI by 12–15% [12], while diets of 1 to 3-year-old and 6-year-old Finnish children exceeded the TWI by 88% and 64%, respectively [13].

Cd intake was comparable to other populations, suggesting that at these daily intakes, the kidney parameters we studied are not altered in 9-year-old children. There are several possible interpretations of our findings. It is possible that at this early stage of childhood (age 8–12), potential changes in kidney function are not yet apparent. This is likely given that glomerular function, as assessed via eGFR and less specifically with BUN, may not show a marked decrease until substantial dysfunction has occurred [29]. Thus, we note with interest the marginally significant inverse associations with eGFR as early as age 8–12 observed in this study. The earliest indication of kidney damage in humans is typically an increased excretion of low-molecular-weight proteins, such as β2-microglobulin, α1-microglobulin, retinol binding protein, and N-acetyl-β-glucosaminidase, among others; and increased excretion of calcium and metallothionein [30]. We also note that BUN is a nonspecific biomarker that can vary independently of the GFR. BUN can be associated with other factors such as liver dysfunction [31], and low or high BUN may be related to undesirable states like malnutrition, starvation, dehydration, high protein intake, among others [32]. Future studies should assess biomarkers of subclinical injury, including urinary proteins like β2-microglobulin and additional assessment of liver function.

Another interpretation is that there is no kidney damage at these Cd intake concentrations. We would not anticipate 'normal' dietary levels of Cd to cause clinically apparent kidney dysfunction. However, there is evidence that when Cd reaches between 50 and 300 μg/g wet weight in the kidney cortex, the amount of Cd not bound to metallothionein becomes sufficiently high to cause tubular damage [30]. Studies have estimated that to reach these Cd levels, a Cd intake of >200 μg/day or lifetime intake of 1300 mg is necessary [33]. Lastly, it is possible that a compensatory mechanism exists, where kidney function in healthy children can cope with this level of Cd insult, while high levels of Cd are nephrotoxic [34].

An important limitation of our study is the estimation of dietary Cd using FFQs, as these can introduce measurement error from maternal recall. It is unlikely though that this could have led to bias as mothers were unaware of the research question (i.e., did not answer the questionnaire in terms of Cd exposure or kidney function). Nonetheless, FFQs are also subject to measurement error as, beyond maternal recall, children spend time in school or in other contexts where they consume food items most likely not reported in the FFQ. Furthermore, we did not measure the concentrations directly in food items. Except for Cd concentrations for a few food items (processed meat) reported in a study of adults in Mexico City [19], we used data from nutrient composition tables from different countries, where the Cd concentrations reported for food items may be different from Mexico. Ideally, our study would have measured the Cd concentrations in food items reported in the FFQ and purchased samples in local markets; however, this was beyond the scope of this study. By using food content tables from the United States, The European Food Safety Authority, Australia, Hong Kong, and Canada, we aimed at having a higher diversity of food items, as well as a higher variability for the Cd concentrations, also considering the reality of globalized food supply chains and the availability of international food products in Mexican markets.

We therefore cannot rule out that we either under- or over-estimated Cd intake; however, the results are in line with levels reported in previous studies. For example, a study conducted by the United States Food and Drug Administration showed that the top contributors to dietary Cd were grains, prepared foods (e.g., hamburgers, pizza, lasagna, soups), and vegetables [2]; a study of French children showed that the main contributors to dietary Cd were bread and potatoes [35]; and a study of Chinese children found that the three greatest contributors to dietary Cd were rice, leafy vegetables, and wheat flour [36]. Further, Cd intake estimated by FFQ does not reflect its absorption, metabolism, or excretion. Cd absorption differs between individuals based on their nutritional status, particularly levels of zinc and iron. For this study, we lacked data on indicators of children's nutritional status of these micronutrients. We also lacked urinary Cd measurement, which is an indicator of body burden [37]. PROGRESS has archived urine samples in which Cd concentrations will be analyzed in future studies.

Among the strengths of this study are the repeated measurements of diet at five stages ranging from 1 to 9 years of age. An important observation of this study was the marked increase in children with overweight or obesity; at 4 years, only 18% of the children presented with overweight or obesity, but by age 9 years, this increased to 46.8%. We also observed an important decrease in physical activity between 6 and 9 years. Both obesity and physical activity are important metabolic risk factors that could modify the association between Cd exposure and kidney parameters [33,38]. Future studies will directly assess the role of obesity and physical activity as risk factors for longitudinal childhood kidney function trajectories.

Although we did not observe significant associations between children's Cd intake and kidney parameters, the TWI for Cd was exceeded at all study visits, from 1 to 9 years of age. The TWI for Cd is based on preventing downstream effects on kidney, bone, and cardiovascular health in adulthood because it can accumulate throughout life. Follow-ups of this study population at later life stages will elucidate possible Cd nephrotoxicity.

Author Contributions: Conceptualization, E.R.-L., M.T.-O., A.C.A. and A.P.S.; data curation, A.P.S.; formal analysis, E.R.-L., M.T.-O., A.C.A., E.O.-P., G.E.-G. and A.P.S.; funding acquisition, M.M.T.-R., R.O.W. and A.P.S.; investigation, E.R.-L. and M.T.-O.; methodology, E.R.-L., M.T.-O., A.C.A., E.O.-P., M.C.T., G.E.-G., S.P.-H., A.E.-N. and A.P.S.; project administration, M.T.-O., I.P., M.M.T.-R., R.O.W. and A.P.S.; resources, I.P. and R.O.W.; supervision, M.T.-O., A.C.A., E.O.-P., M.M.T.-R. and A.P.S.; writing—original draft, E.R.-L., M.T.-O., A.C.A., E.O.-P. and A.P.S.; writing—review and editing, E.R.-L., M.T.-O., A.C.A., E.O.-P., A.L.D., I.P., M.C.T., G.E.-G., S.P.-H., A.E.-N., M.M.T.-R., R.O.W. and A.P.S. All authors have read and agreed to the published version of the manuscript.

Funding: This work was supported in part by funding from the NIH/NIEHS: K99ES027508, R00ES027508, R01ES013744, R01ES020268, and R01ES021357.

Acknowledgments: Authors thank the National Institute of Perinatology, Mexico for the support provided by its facilities.

Conflicts of Interest: The authors declare no conflict of interest.

References

1. Wang, Z.; Pan, L.; Liu, G.; Zhang, H.; Zhang, J.; Jiang, J. Dietary exposure to cadmium of Shenzhen adult residents from a total diet study. *Food Addit. Contam. Part A* **2018**, *35*, 706–714. [CrossRef]
2. Spungen, J.H. Children's exposures to lead and cadmium: FDA total diet study 2014–2016. *Food Addit. Contam. Part A Chem. Anal. Control. Expo. Risk Assess* **2019**, *36*, 893–903. [CrossRef] [PubMed]
3. Nikic, D.; Stankovic, A. Estimated daily intake of cadmium by children living in the city of Nis, Serbia. *Turk J. Pediatr* **2009**, *51*, 257–263. [PubMed]
4. Goyer, R.A. Mechanisms of lead and cadmium nephrotoxicity. *Toxicol. Lett.* **1989**, *46*, 153–162. [CrossRef]
5. Prozialeck, W.C.; Edwards, J.R. Mechanisms of cadmium-induced proximal tubule injury: New insights with implications for biomonitoring and therapeutic interventions. *J. Pharmacol. Exp. Ther.* **2012**, *343*, 2–12. [CrossRef]
6. de Burbure, C.; Buchet, J.P.; Leroyer, A.; Nisse, C.; Haguenoer, J.M.; Mutti, A.; Smerhovský, Z.; Cikrt, M.; Trzcinka-Ochocka, M.; Razniewska, G.; et al. Renal and neurologic effects of cadmium, lead, mercury, and arsenic in children: Evidence of early effects and multiple interactions at environmental exposure levels. *Environ. Health Perspect.* **2006**, *114*, 584–590. [CrossRef]
7. Orr, S.E.; Bridges, C.C. Chronic Kidney Disease and Exposure to Nephrotoxic Metals. *Int. J. Mol. Sci.* **2017**, *18*, 1039.
8. Lee, J.; Oh, S.; Kang, H.; Kim, S.; Lee, G.; Li, L.; Kim, C.T.; An, J.N.; Oh, Y.K.; Lim, C.S.; et al. Environment-wide association study of CKD. *Clin. J. Am. Soc. Nephrol.* **2020**, *15*, 766–775. [CrossRef]
9. Zheng, L.Y.; Sanders, A.P.; Saland, J.M.; Wright, R.O.; Arora, M. Environmental exposures and pediatric kidney function and disease: A systematic review. *Environ. Res.* **2017**, *158*, 625–648. [CrossRef]
10. Shi, Z.; Taylor, A.W.; Riley, M.; Byles, J.; Liu, J.; Noakes, M. Association between dietary patterns, cadmium intake and chronic kidney disease among adults. *Clin. Nutr.* **2017**, *37*, 276–284. [CrossRef]

11. Ferraro, P.M.; Costanzi, S.; Naticchia, A.; Sturniolo, A.; Gambaro, G. Low level exposure to cadmium increases the risk of chronic kidney disease: Analysis of the NHANES. *BMC Public Health* **2010**, *10*, 304. [CrossRef] [PubMed]
12. Jean, J.; Sirot, V.; Hulin, M.; Le Calvez, E.; Zinck, J.; Noël, L.; Vasseur, P.; Nesslany, F.; Gorecki, S.; Guérin, T.; et al. Dietary exposure to cadmium and health risk assessment in children—Results of the French infant total diet study. *Food Chem. Toxicol.* **2018**, *115*, 358–364. [CrossRef] [PubMed]
13. Mykkänen, H.; Räsänen, L.; Ahola, M.; Kimppa, S. Dietary intakes of mercury, lead, cadmium and arsenic by Finnish children. *Hum. Nutr. Appl. Nutr.* **1986**, *40*, 32–39.
14. Burganowski, R.; Vahter, M.; Queirolo, E.I.; Peregalli, F.; Baccino, V.; Barcia, E.; Mangieri, S.; Ocampo, V.; Mañay, N.; Martínez, G.; et al. A cross-sectional study of urinary cadmium concentrations in relation to dietary intakes in Uruguayan school children. *Sci. Total Environ.* **2019**, *658*, 1239–1248. [CrossRef] [PubMed]
15. Moynihan, M.; Peterson, K.E.; Cantoral, A.; Song, P.X.K.; Jones, A.; Solano-González, M.; Meeker, J.D.; Basu, N.; Téllez-Rojo, M.M. Dietary predictors of urinary cadmium among pregnant women and children. *Sci. Total Environ.* **2017**, *575*, 1255–1262. [CrossRef] [PubMed]
16. Braun, J.M.; Wright, R.J.; Just, A.C.; Power, M.C.; Tamayo-Ortiz, M.; Schnaas, L.; Hu, H.; Wright, R.O.; Tellez-Rojo, M.M. Relationships between lead biomarkers and diurnal salivary cortisol indices in pregnant women from Mexico City: A cross-sectional study. *Environ. Health* **2014**, *13*, 50. [CrossRef] [PubMed]
17. Rodríguez-Ramírez, S.; Mundo-Rosas, V. Methodology for the analysis of dietary data from the Mexican National Health and Nutrition Survey 2006. *Salud Publica Mex.* **2009**, *51*, 523–529. [CrossRef]
18. Kim, C.I.; Lee, J.; Kwon, S.; Yoon, H.J. Total diet study: For a closer-to-real estimate of dietary exposure to chemical substances. *Toxicol. Res.* **2015**, *31*, 227–240. [CrossRef]
19. Torres-Sánchez, L.; Vázquez-Salas, R.A.; Vite, A.; Galván-Portillo, M.; Cebrián, M.E.; Macias-Jiménez, A.P.; Ríos, C.; Montes, S. Blood cadmium determinants among males over forty living in Mexico City. *Sci. Total Environ.* **2018**, *637–638*, 686–694. [CrossRef]
20. Panel, E.; Chain, F. Statement on tolerable weekly intake for cadmium. *EFSA J.* **2011**, *9*, 1975.
21. Jaffe, M. Ueber den Niederschlag, welchen Pikrinsäure in normalem Harn erzeugt und über eine neue Reaction des Kreatinins. *Z. Für Physiol. Chem.* **1886**, *10*, 391–400.
22. Sarkar, R. Establishment of Biological Reference Intervals and Reference Curve for Urea by Exploratory Parametric and Non-Parametric Quantile Regression Models. *EJIFCC* **2013**, *24*, 61–67. [PubMed]
23. Schwartz, G.J.; Muñoz, A.; Schneider, M.F.; Mak, R.H.; Kaskel, F.; Warady, B.A.; Furth, S.L. New equations to estimate GFR in children with CKD. *J. Am. Soc. Nephrol.* **2009**, *20*, 629–637. [CrossRef] [PubMed]
24. Schwartz, G.J.; Schneider, M.F.; Maier, P.S.; Moxey-Mims, M.; Dharnidharka, V.R.; Warady, B.A.; Furth, S.L.; Mũoz, A. Improved equations estimating GFR in children with chronic kidney disease using an immunonephelometric determination of cystatin C. *Kidney Int.* **2012**, *82*, 445–453. [CrossRef]
25. WHO Multicentre Growth Reference Study Group. *WHO Child Growth Standards: Methods and Development*; WHO: Geneva, Switzerland, 2014; p. 312.
26. Pottel, H.; Hoste, L.; Dubourg, L.; Ebert, N.; Schaeffner, E.; Eriksen, B.O.; Melsom, T.; Lamb, E.J.; Rule, A.D.; Turner, S.T.; et al. An estimated glomerular filtration rate equation for the full age spectrum. *Nephrol. Dial. Transpl.* **2016**, *31*, 798–806. [CrossRef] [PubMed]
27. Tinggi, U.; Schoendorfer, N. Analysis of lead and cadmium in cereal products and duplicate diets of a small group of selected Brisbane children for estimation of daily metal exposure. *J. Trace Elem. Med. Biol.* **2018**, *50*, 671–675. [CrossRef]
28. Kim, K.; Melough, M.M.; Vance, T.M.; Noh, H.; Koo, S.I.; Chun, O.K. Dietary cadmium intake and sources in the US. *Nutrients* **2019**, *11*, 2. [CrossRef]
29. Greenberg, J.H.; Kakajiwala, A.; Parikh, C.R.; Furth, S. Emerging biomarkers of chronic kidney disease in children. *Pediatr. Nephrol.* **2018**, *33*, 925–933. [CrossRef]
30. ATSDR. *Toxicological Profile for Cadmium*; US Department of Health and Humans Services, Public Health Service: Atlanta, GA, USA, 2012.
31. Lopez-Giacoman, S. Biomarkers in chronic kidney disease, from kidney function to kidney damage. *World J. Nephrol.* **2015**, *4*, 57. [CrossRef]
32. Hosten, A.O. *BUN and Creatinine. Clinical Methods: The History, Physical, and Laboratory Examinations*, 3rd ed.; Butterworths: Boston, MA, USA, 1990; ISBN 040990077X.
33. Satarug, S. Dietary cadmium intake and its effects on kidneys. *Toxics* **2018**, *6*, 15. [CrossRef]

34. Saif, M.; Rahman, U.R.; Ali, M.U.; Shoaib, M.; Amin, M.A. Cadmium Induced Nephrotoxicity: Advances and Perspectives. *Trends Biosci.* **2015**, *8*, 5167–5175.
35. Marín, S.; Pardo, O.; Báguena, R.; Font, G.; Yusà, V. Dietary exposure to trace elements and health risk assessment in the region of Valencia, Spain: A total diet study. *Food Addit. Contam.* **2017**, *34*, 228–240. [CrossRef] [PubMed]
36. Song, Y.; Wang, Y.; Mao, W.; Sui, H.; Yong, L.; Yang, D.; Jiang, D.; Zhang, L.; Gong, Y. Dietary cadmium exposure assessment among the Chinese population. *PLoS ONE* **2017**, *12*, e0177978. [CrossRef] [PubMed]
37. International Program on Chemical Safety; Friberg, L.; Elinder, C.-G.; Kjellström, T.; United Nations Environment Programme; International Labour Organisation; World Health Organization; International Program on Chemical Safety. *Cadmium–Environmental Health Criteria 134*; World Health Organization: Geneva, Switzerland, 1992; ISBN 9241571349.
38. Sowers, J.R. Metabolic risk factors and renal disease. *Kidney Int.* **2007**, *71*, 719–720. [CrossRef]

toxics

MDPI

Article

A Comparison of the Nephrotoxicity of Low Doses of Cadmium and Lead

Soisungwan Satarug [1,2], Glenda C. Gobe [2,3,4], Pailin Ujjin [1,5] and David A. Vesey [2,6,*]

1 National Research Centre for Environmental Toxicology, The University of Queensland, Coopers Plains, Brisbane 4108, Australia; sj.satarug@yahoo.com.au (S.S.); upailin@gmail.com (P.U.)
2 Kidney Disease Research Collaborative, The University of Queensland Faculty of Medicine and Translational Research Institute, Woolloongabba, Brisbane 4102, Australia; g.gobe@uq.edu.au
3 School of Biomedical Sciences, The University of Queensland, Brisbane 4072, Australia
4 NHMRC Centre of Research Excellence for CKD.QLD, UQ Health Sciences, Royal Brisbane and Women's Hospital, Brisbane 4029, Australia
5 Department of Laboratory Medicine, Chulalongkorn University Faculty of Medicine, Bangkok 10330, Thailand
6 Department of Nephrology, Princess Alexandra Hospital, Brisbane 4075, Australia
* Correspondence: david.vesey@health.qld.gov.au

Received: 13 January 2020; Accepted: 25 February 2020; Published: 2 March 2020

Abstract: Environmental exposure to moderate-to-high levels of cadmium (Cd) and lead (Pb) is associated with nephrotoxicity. In comparison, the health impacts of chronic low-level exposure to Cd and Pb remain controversial. The aim of this study was to therefore evaluate kidney dysfunction associated with chronic low-level exposure to Cd and Pb in a population of residents in Bangkok, Thailand. The mean age and the estimated glomerular filtration rate (eGFR) for 392 participants (195 men and 197 women) were 34.9 years and 104 mL/min/1.73 m^2, respectively, while the geometric mean concentrations of urinary Cd and Pb were 0.25 µg/L (0.45 µg/g of creatinine) and 0.89 µg/L (1.52 µg/g of creatinine), respectively. In a multivariable regression analysis, the eGFR varied inversely with blood urea nitrogen in both men ($\beta = -0.125$, $p = 0.044$) and women ($\beta = -0.170$, $p = 0.008$), while inverse associations of the eGFR with urinary Cd ($\beta = -0.132$, $p = 0.043$) and urinary Pb ($\beta = -0.130$, $p = 0.044$) were seen only in women. An increased urinary level of Cd to the median level of 0.38 µg/L (0.44 µg/g of creatinine) was associated with a decrease in the eGFR by 4.94 mL/min/1.73 m^2 ($p = 0.011$). The prevalence odds of a reduced eGFR rose 2.5-, 2.9- and 2.3-fold in the urinary Cd quartile 3 ($p = 0.013$), the urinary Cd quartile 4 ($p = 0.008$), and the urinary Pb quartile 4 ($p = 0.039$), respectively. This study suggests that chronic exposure to low-level Cd is associated with a decline in kidney function and that women may be more susceptible than men to nephrotoxicity due to an elevated intake of Cd and Pb.

Keywords: cadmium; creatinine clearance; creatinine excretion; glomerular filtration rate; lead; nephrotoxicity

1. Introduction

Cadmium (Cd) and lead (Pb) are environmental toxicants of significant public health concern due to their widespread environmental pollution and persistence, as well as their known adverse impacts on human health, including an enhanced risk of chronic kidney disease (CKD) and various types of cancer [1–5]. The International Agency for Research on Cancer has established Cd as a human carcinogen [6], while the carcinogenicity of chronic Pb exposure in workplace settings has been observed in two large prospective cohort studies [7,8]. Co-exposure to low levels of environmental Cd and Pb has been reported in large population-based studies in the U.S. [9–12], Canada [13], Taiwan [14], and Korea [15]. About half of the participants in the U.S. National Health and Nutrition Examination Surveys (NHANES) 2007–2012, aged ≥6 years, had blood or urinary levels of Cd and Pb above reported median levels [11].

CKD is the cause of significant human morbidity and mortality. Its high worldwide prevalence and escalating treatment costs make developing strategies to prevent CKD of global importance [16–18]. CKD is characterized by albuminuria and/or a decrease of the glomerular filtration rate (GFR) to 60 mL/min/1.73 m^2 that persists for at least three months [19–21]. In theory, the GFR reflects the number of surviving nephrons × the average GFR per nephron [21]. Accordingly, GFR is considered to best indicate nephron function. In practice, the GFR is estimated from equations, including the Chronic Kidney Disease Epidemiology Collaboration (CKD-EPI) equations [19–22], and is reported as an estimated GFR (eGFR). Prospective cohort studies in Sweden have linked low-level Pb exposure to decreases in the GFR, CKD onset, and end-stage kidney disease [4,23]. In addition, cross-sectional studies have implicated low-level environmental exposure to Cd as a risk factor for CKD in Spain [24], Korea [25], and the U.S. [26–29].

Elevated dietary Cd intake has been associated with an increased risk of CKD in China [30]. A marked decrease in the GFR has also been observed in residents of an area with Cd pollution in Thailand [2,31–35], as well as in Cd-exposed workers [36,37]. Likewise, marked GFR decreases have been noted in workers and residents of Pb-smelter communities [38]. However, the variable effect of low-level environmental exposure to Cd and Pb on GFR has caused some controversy. Consequently, governments worldwide have not established the necessary regulations to protect their populations. An inverse association has been seen between the GFR and urinary Cd and/or blood Cd [9,28,39,40]. In the opposite direction, other studies have observed a positive association between GFR and urinary Cd [9,12,41,42]. Inverse associations of blood urea nitrogen (BUN) with blood Cd and Pb were noted in a prospective cohort study of premenopausal U.S. women [43]. However, a cross-sectional analysis of data from adolescents (n = 2709, aged 12–19 years) who were enrolled in NHANES 2009–2014 reported positive associations of urinary Cd and Pb with an increased eGFR and BUN in models that incorporated urinary creatinine as a covariate [42]. A common practice of normalizing urinary concentrations of Cd to urinary concentrations of creatinine may have caused these disparate findings [33,35,44,45].

The most frequently reported adverse effects of chronic Cd exposure in the general population have included tubular injury and reduced tubular re-absorption, as reflected by elevated urinary N-acetyl-β-D-glucosaminidase (NAG) and β_2-microglobulin (β_2MG) levels, respectively [5]. However, despite numerous reports, the observed Cd-linked tubular dysfunction has not been considered to be clinically relevant [5]. Thus, the present study aimed to clarify the impact on kidney function of long-term environmental exposure to low levels of Cd and Pb with a focus on the GFR, a reliable clinical measure of kidney function and diagnosis of CKD. We used the CKD-EPI equations to derive the eGFR and excretion of Cd (E_{Cd}) as indicators of body burden. The associations of the eGFR with E_{Cd} and the excretion of Pb (E_{Pb}), age, gender, smoking, body iron stores, and BUN (another indicator of kidney effect) were evaluated. For a comparative analysis, E_{Cd} and E_{Pb} were normalized to both the creatinine clearance (C_{cr}) and the excretion of creatinine (E_{cr}).

2. Materials and Methods

2.1. Study Population

We assembled archived data from participants who were drawn from residential areas in the Bangkapi suburb of Bangkok, Thailand, between 2001 and 2003. Our Thai urban population project was undertaken based on the global food monitoring system database, which indicated dietary Cd and Pb may exceed the tolerable intake levels 7 μg Cd/kg body weight/week and 25 μg Pb/kg body weight/week in some countries, Thailand included [46]. The Institutional Ethical Committee, Chulalongkorn Medical Faculty Hospital, Chulalongkorn University, Bangkok, Thailand, approved the study protocol (Approval No. 142/2544, 5 October 2001). All participants were apparently healthy and had no history of exposure to Cd or Pb in the workplace. Participants took part in the study after giving informed consent. The health status of participants was assessed by a physical examination and was confirmed by routine urinary and blood chemistry analysis. Smoking, diabetes, hypertension, the regular use of medications, educational level, occupation and family health history were obtained by questionnaires. After the exclusion of participants with incomplete datasets, 392 persons (195 men and 197 women) formed the study cohort.

2.2. Specimen Collection and Analysis

Blood samples were collected within 1 h after drinking 300 mL of water following an overnight fast. Urine samples were collected within 3 h of blood sampling. Urine and blood samples were transported on ice to the Department of Laboratory Medicine, Chulalongkorn University Hospital, where plasma samples were prepared for routine chemistry by using an automated system. The assay for plasma and urinary creatinine concentrations was based on the Jaffe reaction, while the plasma ferritin assay was based on an electrochemiluminescence immunoassay (Boehringer Mannheim Elecsys 1010, Roche Diagnostics GmbH, Mannheim, Germany). Aliquots of urine, with 5 mL per aliquot, were shipped on dry ice and kept frozen throughout shipment period. They were delivered to the National Research Centre for Environmental Toxicology, Australia, where they were stored at −80 °C for later analysis. Urinary concentrations of Cd and Pb were determined with inductively-coupled plasma/mass spectrometry (ICP/MS, Agilent 7500, Agilent Technologies, Santa Clara, CA, USA), which had been calibrated with multi-element standards (EM Science, EM Industries, Inc., NJ, USA). Quality assurance and control were conducted with simultaneous analyses of samples of the reference urine Lyphochek® (Bio-Rad, Gladesville, New South Wales, Australia), which contained low- and high-range Cd and Pb levels. A coefficient of variation value of 2.5% was obtained for Cd and Pb in the reference urine. The low limit of detection (LOD) was 0.05 μg/L for urinary Cd and 0.03 μg/L for urinary Pb. The urine samples containing Cd and Pb levels below the LOD were assigned as the LOD divided by the square root of 2. Fifty-eight subjects (14.8%) had urinary Cd levels below the LOD, while 26 subjects (6.6%) had urinary Pb levels below the LOD.

2.3. Estimation of Excretion Rates

The procedures for the simultaneous collection of blood and urine samples enabled the normalization of the excretion rates of metals to creatinine clearance (C_{cr}) by using the following equation: $E_x/C_{cr} = [x]_u[cr]_p/[cr]_u$, where E_x/C_{cr} = excretion of x per volume of filtrate; $[x]_u$ = urine concentration of x (mass/volume); $[cr]_p$ = plasma creatinine concentration (mg/dL); and $[cr]_u$ = urine creatinine concentration (mg/dL) [33,35,47]. The normalization of E_x to C_{cr} circumvents the effect of muscle mass on E_x/E_{cr} and $[x]_u/[cr]_u$ while nullifying urine volume (V_u) as a confounder on concentration ($[x]_u$).

As is typical, the excretion of Cd (E_{Cd}) was normalized to the excretion of creatinine (E_{cr}) as $[Cd]_u/[cr]_u$, where $[Cd]_u$ = urine concentration of Cd (μg/L), and $[cr]_u$ = urine creatinine concentration (mg/dL). The ratio $[Cd]_u/[cr]_u$ was expressed as μg/g of creatinine. This allows for the correction of the urine flow rate (V_u) on concentration ($[x]_u$). However, it introduces another confounder or bias given that E_{cr} is affected by muscle mass and many other factors unrelated to nephron function [48].

2.4. Estimated Glomerular Filtration Rates

The eGFR was calculated by using the CKD-EPI equations [19,21]. The male eGFR = 141 × [serum creatinine / 0.9]^{Y} × 0.993^{age}, where Y = −0.411 if serum creatinine ≤ 0.9 mg/dL, Y = −1.209 if serum creatinine > 0.9 mg/dL. The female eGFR = 144 × [serum creatinine / 0.7]^{Y} × 0.993^{age}, where Y = −0.329 if serum creatinine ≤ 0.7 mg/dL, Y = −1.209 if serum creatinine > 0.7 mg/dL. CKD is defined as an eGFR <60 mL/min/1.73 m^2 for three months or more [19,22]. CKD stages 1, 2, 3, 4, and 5 corresponded to an eGFR of 90–119, 60–89, 30–59, 15–29, and <15 mL/min/1.73 m^2, respectively [19,21].

2.5. Statistical Analysis

Data were analyzed with SPSS 17.0 (SPSS Inc., Chicago, IL, USA, 2008). The Mann–Whitney U test was used to compare the mean differences between men and women, while the Pearson chi-squared test was used to compare the percentage differences between men and women. The one-sample Kolmogorov–Smirnov test was used to examine departures from a normal distribution of continuous variables, and a base-10 logarithmic transformation was applied to the variables that showed rightward skewing. A multivariable regression model analysis was used to evaluate the association of the eGFR with independent variables including the excretion of Cd and Pb. For each regression model, the coefficient of determination (R^2) value was obtained together with standardized β. A generalized linear model analysis was used to estimate the mean eGFR with adjustment for age, covariates and interactions. Logistic regression analysis was used to estimate the prevalence odds ratio (POR) for the reduced eGFR across the quartiles of excretion of Cd and Pb. The p-values ≤0.05 for two-sided tests were assumed to indicate statistical significance.

3. Results

3.1. Descriptive Characteristics of Study Population

The demographic data, including the blood and urinary biochemistry and other clinical features for the study population of 392 Thai subjects, are shown in Table 1. The overall mean age was 34.9 years. Men were on average 4.1 years younger than women ($p < 0.001$). The mean urinary concentrations of Cd and Pb were 0.25 μg/L (0.45 μg/g of creatinine) and 0.89 μg/L (1.52 μg/g of creatinine), respectively. The mean eGFR (range) was 105 (70–139) mL/min/1.73 m^2. The percentage of the eGFR <90mL/min/1.73 m^2 was similar in men and women (12.3% vs. 13.7%, respectively). The percentage of woman with low iron stores (ferritin levels ≤30 μg/L) were six times that of men (22.3% vs 3.6%, $p < 0.001$). Half of the men (49.7%) smoked (8.9 cigarettes per day), with an average duration of 10 years. There was no record of smoking in any of the women.

Table 1. Descriptive characteristics of study population.

Parameters/Factors	All Subjects $n = 392$	Men $n = 195$	Women $n = 197$	p-Values
Age, years	34.9 ± 9.6 (16–60)	32.8 ± 8.8 (16–57)	36.9 ± 10 (19–60)	<0.001 *
Smoking (%)	24.7	49.7	0	<0.001 *
Serum ferritin, μg/L	89.0 ± 134 (3–378)	159 ± 153 (14–978)	50.0 ± 61.3 (3–353)	<0.001 *
Low body iron stores (%) [a]	13.0	3.6	22.3	<0.001 *
eGFR, mL/min/1.73 m^2 [b]	105 ± 14 (70–139)	104 ± 14 (70–138)	106 ± 13 (72–139)	0.170
eGFR <90 mL/min/1.73 m^2	13.0	12.3	13.7	0.681
BUN, mg/dL	11.1 ± 2.8 (5–24)	11.8 ± 2.8 (5–24)	10.4 ± 2.8 (5–19)	<0.001 *
Total plasma protein, g/dL	7.85 ± 0.46 (6–9.1)	7.86 ± 0.46 (6–9.1)	7.84 ± 0.47 (6.9–9.1)	0.385
Plasma creatinine, mg/dL	0.82 ± 0.16 (0.5–1.3)	0.95 ± 0.11 (0.5–1.3)	0.71 ± 0.10 (0.5–1.0)	<0.001 *
Urine creatinine, mg/dL	59.5 ± 68.4 (7.2–377)	74.2 ± 79.1 (11–377)	47.8 ± 49.1 (7.2–294)	<0.001 *
Total urine protein, mg/dL	1.60 ± 8.41 (0.02–70)	1.80 ± 9.14 (0.02–65)	1.43 ± 7.57 (0.02–75)	0.162
Urinary concentrations				
Cd, μg/L	0.25 ± 0.68 (0.04–9.4)	0.28 ± 0.84 (0.04–9.4)	0.23 ± 0.49 (0.04–4.2)	0.117
Pb, μg/L	0.89 ± 1.73 (0.02–19)	0.80 ± 1.66 (0.02–13)	1.00 ± 1.80 (0.1–19)	0.239
Urinary metals normalized to excretion of creatinine				
E_{Cd}/E_{cr}, μg/g of creatinine	0.45 ± 0.46 (0.03–3.8)	0.39 ± 0.46 (0.03–3.8)	0.51 ± 0.46 (0.04–2.4)	<0.001 *
E_{Pb}/E_{cr}, μg/g of creatinine	1.52 ± 2.16 (0.05–33)	1.10 ± 1.42 (0.05–13)	2.10 ± 2.62 (0.05–33)	<0.001 *
Urinary metals normalized to creatinine clearance				
$E_{Cd}/C_{cr} \times 100$, μg/L	0.35 ± 0.38 (0.03–3.1)	0.36 ± 0.42 (0.03–3.1)	0.34 ± 0.34 (0.03–1.9)	0.842
$E_{Pb}/C_{cr} \times 100$, μg/L	1.23 ± 1.70 (0.04–27)	1.02 ± 1.20 (0.04–19)	1.48 ± 2.08 (0.04–27)	0.062

[a] Low body iron stores were defined as plasma ferritin ≤30 μg/L. [b] eGFR = estimated glomerular filtration rate, determined with Chronic Kidney Disease Epidemiology Collaboration (CKD–EPI) equations [19,21]. Data for age and the eGFR are arithmetic mean values ± standard deviation (SD). Data for all other continuous variables are geometric mean ± SD values. Numbers in parentheses are range. * $p \leq 0.05$ indicate mean or % differences between men and women based on the Mann–Whitney U-test or the Pearson chi-squared test, respectively.

The mean BUN, serum creatinine, and urinary creatinine were higher in men than women with p values of less than 0.001. The mean plasma protein concentration in men and women was similar ($p = 0.385$), as was the mean urinary protein concentration ($p = 0.162$). E_{Cd}/E_{cr} and E_{Pb}/E_{cr} showed marked differences between men and women. The mean E_{Cd}/E_{cr} was 1.3-fold lower in men than women (0.39 vs. 0.51 μg/g of creatinine, $p < 0.001$), while the mean E_{Pb}/E_{cr} was 1.9-fold lower in men than women (1.10 vs. 2.10 μg/g of creatinine, $p < 0.001$). Notably, E_{Cd}/C_{cr} and E_{Pb}/C_{cr} showed little gender differences. The mean for $E_{Cd}/C_{cr} \times 100$ in men (0.36 μg/L) was nearly identical to that of women (0.34 μg/L), while the mean $E_{Pb}/C_{cr} \times 100$ in men of showed a tendency to be lower than in women (1.02 vs. 1.48 μg/L, $p = 0.062$).

3.2. Predictors of eGFR

In the multivariable regression analysis for the eGFR with metal excretion rates normalized to C_{cr} (Table 2), the independent variables (urinary Cd, urinary Pb, age, BUN, serum ferritin, gender and smoking) accounted for 27.2%, 33.4%, 25.9%, 25.4% and 40.2% of the eGFR variability in the entire group, men, women, non-smokers, and smokers, respectively, with the p value being <0.001 for the entire group and all subgroups. In the entire group, the eGFR was not associated with urinary Pb ($p = 0.115$), but it showed an inverse association with age (β = −0.436, $p < 0.001$), BUN (β = −0.157, $p = 0.001$) and urinary Cd (β = −0.126, $p = 0.006$).

Table 2. Predictors of the estimated glomerular filtration rate (eGFR).

Independent Variables	eGFR, mL/min/1.73 m^2									
	All, $n = 392$		Men, $n = 195$		Women, $n = 197$		Non-Smokers, $n = 295$		Smokers, $n = 97$	
	β	p	β	p	β	p	β	p	β	p
Age	−0.436	<0.001 *	−0.501	<0.001 *	−0.378	<0.001 *	−0.405	<0.001 *	−0.510	<0.001
BUN	−0.157	0.001 *	−0.125	0.044 *	−0.170	0.008 *	−0.135	0.012 *	−0.207	0.016 *
Urine Cd	−0.126	0.006 *	−0.082	0.219	−0.132	0.043 *	−0.119	0.026 *	−0.122	0.182
Urine Pb	−0.072	0.115	−0.060	0.333	−0.130	0.044	−0.092	0.092	−0.056	0.513
Ferritin	0.076	0.156	0.147	0.017 *	0.002	0.969	0.059	0.330	0.101	0.227
Gender	0.222	0.001 *	−	−	−	−	0.208	0.001 *	−	−
Smoking	0.075	0.166	0.062	0.317	−	−	−	−	−	−
Adjusted R^2	0.272	<0.001 †	0.334	<0.001 †	0.259	<0.001 †	0.254	<0.001 †	0.402	<0.001 †

The eGFR is a continuous dependent variable. Independent variables are listed in the first column, including urine Cd as log [$(E_{Cd}/C_{cr}) \times 10^5$], μg/L and urine Pb as log [$(E_{Pb}/C_{cr}) \times 10^5$]. A standardized regression coefficient β indicates the strength of an association between the eGFR and an independent variable. * $p \leq 0.05$ identifies statistically significant associations. An adjusted R^2 value indicates the fraction of eGFR variation explained by independent variables. † $p \leq 0.05$ indicates that the model explained a significant variability of eGFR levels.

In a subgroup analysis, the eGFR was inversely associated with urinary Cd (β = −0.132, $p = 0.043$) and urinary Pb (β = −0.130, $p = 0.044$), only in women. In contrast, the eGFR was not associated with urinary Cd ($p = 0.219$) or with urinary Pb ($p = 0.333$) in men, but it showed a positive association with plasma ferritin (β = 0.147, $p = 0.017$). Inverse associations of the eGFR with age and BUN were evident in all subgroups. The strength of an association between the eGFR and BUN was relatively stronger in male smokers (β −0.207, $p = 0.016$), compared with other subgroups, with β values being −0.125 in men ($p = 0.044$), −0.170 in women ($p = 0.008$), and −0.135 in non-smokers ($p = 0.012$).

In an equivalent multivariable regression analysis of the eGFR with metal excretion rates that were normalized to the excretion of creatinine (Table S1), an association between the eGFR and urinary Cd was not evident in the entire group or in any subgroups, as was the association of the eGFR and urinary Pb.

3.3. Quantitation of Effects of Cadmium and Lead on the Decline of eGFR

Figure 1 provides the results of a quantitative analysis of changes in the eGFR that was done by using metal excretion rates that were normalized to creatinine clearance. In the scatterplot of the eGFR against E_{Cd}/C_{cr}, a moderate inverse association was evident (β −0.249, $p < 0.001$) (Figure 1A).

Six point two % of the eGFR reduction ($R^2 = 0.062$) could be attributed to Cd. An inverse association was evident also from the scatterplot of the eGFR against E_{Pb}/C_{cr} (Figure 1B). However, the strength of eGFR-E_{Pb}/C_{cr} association was insignificant ($p = 0.314$), and as little as 0.3% of eGFR variation could be attributed to Pb.

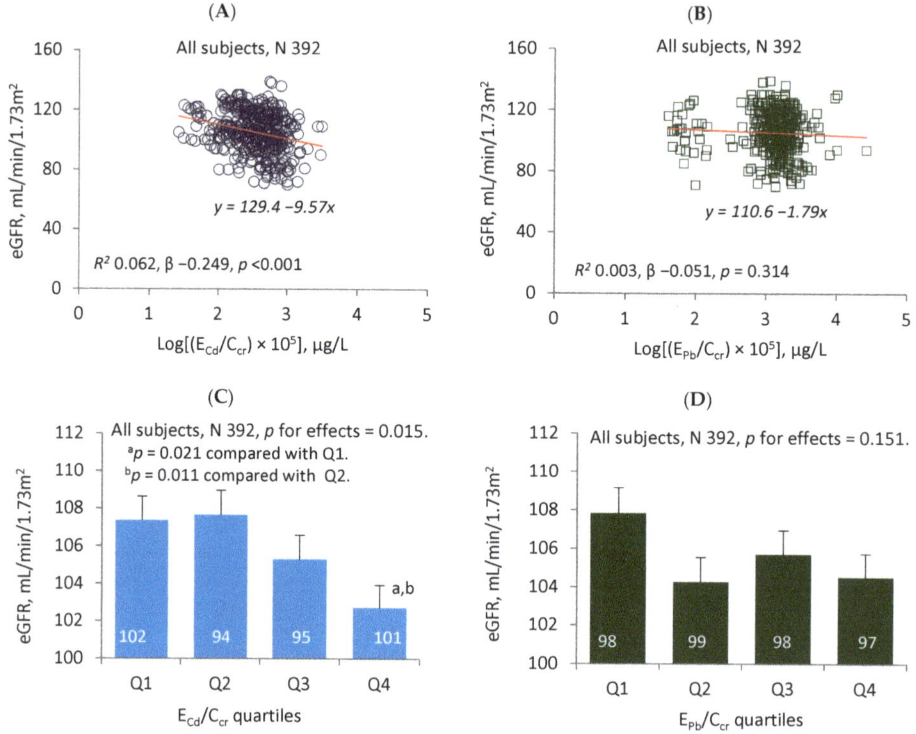

Figure 1. Comparing effects of cadmium and lead on eGFR change. The scatterplots show the relationship between the eGFR and log [excretion of Cd (E_{Cd})/creatinine clearance (C_{cr})) $\times 10^5$] and between the eGFR and log [excretion of Pb (E_{Pb})/C_{cr}) $\times 10^5$] in all subjects (**A**,**B**). The linear equations and coefficients of determination (R^2) are provided together with standardized β and *p*-values. The bars represent the mean values for the eGFR across urinary Cd and urinary Pb quartiles (**C**,**D**) with adjustments for various covariates and potential interactions. The numbers of subjects are provided for all subgroups. The geometric mean (GM) values (standard deviation) for $E_{Cd}/C_{cr} \times 100$ in urinary Cd quartiles 1, 2, 3 and 4 were 0.12 (0.05), 0.30 (0.05), 0.48 (0.07) and 0.88 (0.44) μg/L, respectively. The GM (SD) for $E_{Pb}/C_{cr} \times 100$ in urinary Pb quartiles 1, 2, 3 and 4 are 0.41 (0.36), 1.26 (0.10), 1.63 (0.14) and 2.73 (2.86) μg/L, respectively.

A generalized linear model (GLM) was then used to estimate the mean eGFR values for subgroups stratified by the quartiles of E_{Cd}/C_{cr} (Figure 1C) and the quartiles of E_{Pb}/C_{cr} (Figure 1D). After adjustments for age, covariates and the interactions, a negative effect of Cd on the eGFR was evident ($p = 0.015$). The estimated mean eGFR (standard error of mean, SEM) for males and females with urinary Cd in the fourth quartile was, respectively, 4.65 (1.72) and 4.94 (1.70) mL/min/1.73 m^2 lower than those with urine Cd in the first quartile ($p = 0.021$) and with urine Cd in the second quartile ($p = 0.011$), respectively. Distinct from Cd, the relationship between Pb and the eGFR was negligible and insignificant ($p = 0.151$) (Figure 1D).

Figure S1 provides the results of an equivalent quantitative analysis of changes in the eGFR that was done by using metal excretion rates that were normalized to the excretion of creatinine.

In the scatterplot of the eGFR against E_{Cd}/E_{cr} (Figure S1A), an inverse association between the eGFR and E_{Cd}/E_{cr} was evident (β = −0.104, p = 0.040), but this relationship was weakened and became insignificant (p = 0.763) after adjustments for age, covariates and interactions (Figure S1C). In contrast, the scatterplot of the eGFR against E_{Pb}/E_{cr} indicated a marginal but non-significant positive association between the eGFR and E_{Pb}/E_{cr} (β = 0.080, p = 0.115) (Figure S1B). After adjustments for age, covariates and interactions, there were significant increases in eGFR levels across E_{Pb}/E_{cr} quartiles (p = 0.010) (Figure S1D). The estimated mean eGFR (SEM) for subjects with E_{Pb}/E_{cr} in the fourth quartile was 5.89 (1.77) mL/min/1.73 m^2 higher than those with E_{Pb}/E_{cr} in the second quartile (p = 0.003).

3.4. The Prevalence Odds of Reduced eGFR across the Quartiles of Urinary Cd and Urinary Pb

Table 3 provides the results of a logistic regression analysis of the POR for the reduced eGFR, defined as the eGFR at the 25th percentile or below (≤96 mL/min/1.73 m^2). The POR for the reduced eGFR showed an inverse association with age (β= −0.071, p < 0.001) and gender (β = −1.020, p = 0.003). In addition, the POR for the reduced eGFR appeared to rise with urinary Cd in a dose-dependent manner. The POR for the reduced eGFR was 2.87 (95% CI: 1.32, 6.24), 2.51 (95% CI: 1.22, 5.18) and 1.70 (95% CI: 0.875, 3.29) in the urinary Cd quartile 4 (p = 0.008), quartile 3 (p =0.013) and quartile 1 (p = 0.117), respectively. The POR for the reduced eGFR was not associated with the urinary Pb quartile 2 (p = 0.198) or quartile 3 (p = 0.744), but it rose to 2.23 (95% CI: 1.04, 4.78) in the urinary Pb quartile 4 (p = 0.039).

Table 3. Prevalence odds ratios for the reduced eGFR across the E_{Cd}/C_{cr} and E_{Pb}/C_{cr} quartiles.

Independent Variables/Factors	eGFR Levels <96 mL/min/1.73 m^2				
	β Coefficients (SE)	POR [a]	95% CI for POR Lower	Upper	p Value
Age (years)	−0.071 (0.015)	0.931	0.904	0.959	<0.001
Gender	−1.020 (0.345)	0.361	0.184	0.709	0.003
Smoking	−0.475 (0.367)	0.622	0.303	1.277	0.195
Low body iron store status [b]	−0.015 (0.437)	0.985	0.418	2.320	0.972
E_{Cd}/C_{cr} × 100, μg/L					
Q1 (0.03−0.21)	Referent	1.000	1.000	1.000	
Q2 (0.22−0.38)	0.529 (0.338)	1.697	0.875	3.291	0.117
Q3 (0.39−0.61)	0.920 (0.370)	2.510	1.216	5.181	0.013
Q4 (0.62−3.10)	1.053 (0.396)	2.867	1.319	6.236	0.008
E_{Pb}/C_{cr} × 100, μg/L					
Q1 (0.04−1.07)	Referent	1.000	1.000	1.000	
Q2 (1.08−1.42)	0.469 (0.365)	1.598	0.782	3.265	0.198
Q3 (1.43−1.93)	0.115 (0.535)	1.122	0.562	2.241	0.744
Q4 (1.94−26.5)	0.803 (0.388)	2.233	1.043	4.780	0.039

[a] POR = prevalence odds ratios for eGFR levels ≤96 mL/min/1.73 m^2. The eGFR 96 mL/min/1.73 m^2 corresponds to the 25th percentile eGFR. [b] Low iron store status was defined as serum ferritin levels ≤ 30μg/L. * p ≤ 0.05 indicates a statistically significant increment of POR, compared with the reference. The GM (SD) for E_{Cd}/C_{cr} and E_{Pb}/C_{cr} together with number of subjects in all urinary Cd and urinary Pb quartiles are as in Figure 1.

Table S2 provides the results of an equivalent logistic regression analysis for the reduced eGFR that was done by using urinary Cd and urinary Pb that were normalized to the excretion of creatinine. In this analysis, the POR for the reduced eGFR only showed an inverse association with age (β = −0.080, p < 0.001). No associations were seen between the reduced eGFR and urinary Cd or Pb in any quartiles of urinary Cd or Pb.

4. Discussion

None of the participants in the present study had been exposed to metals in the workplace, and their urinary concentrations of Cd and Pb were thus presumed to reflect environmental sources, notably diet [5,49]. The urinary Cd and Pb concentrations were similar to the data obtained from population-based studies in the U.S. [9–12], Canada [13], Taiwan [14] and Korea [15]. The eGFR was calculated by using CKD-EPI equations, which are considered to be the most accurate equations for the eGFR [20,22]. The CKD-EPI equations have been validated by using inulin clearance [22]. The overall mean eGFR for participants was 105 mL/min/1.73 m^2, ranging between 70 and 139 mL/min/1.73 m^2. The wide range of variation in the eGFR was congruent with the notion that a normal level of the GFR could vary widely [20]. Both physiological and pathological conditions are known to affect the GFR, and the mean GFR in young adult Caucasians is approximately 125 mL/min/1.73 m^2 [20].

In a regression model in which all subjects were included, the eGFR levels varied inversely with age, BUN and E_{Cd}/C_{cr}, but they did not vary with E_{Pb}/C_{cr} (Table 2). The inverse association between the eGFR and BUN was expected, as urea is one of the metabolic waste products that is eliminated through kidneys. Of note, however, while the inverse associations of the eGFR with age and BUN were present in all subgroups, the association between the eGFR and E_{Cd}/C_{cr} reached statistical significance levels in non-smokers (men and women). In addition, the eGFR levels in women varied inversely with both E_{Cd}/C_{cr} ($\beta = -0.170$, $p = 0.008$) and E_{Pb}/C_{cr} ($\beta = -0.132$, $p = 0.043$). These data could be interpreted to suggest that levels of Cd and Pb intake from the diet were sufficient to produce adverse effects on nephrons and subsequently reduce the elimination rate of urea. They also suggested that women may be more susceptible than men to renal effects of elevated Cd and Pb intake levels. Supporting this argument is the fact that blood Cd and Pb both were associated with BUN in a prospective study in the U.S. that included 259 premenopausal women, where one-third of them had eGFR levels <90 mL/min/1.73 m^2 and stage 1 CKD [43]. In addition, urinary Cd and Pb were associated with increased BUN in adolescents enrolled in NHANES 2009–2014 [42].

In a multivariable regression analysis that was done by using urinary Cd and Pb that were normalized to the excretion of creatinine (Table S1), the eGFR did not show significant relationships with E_{Cd}/E_{cr} or E_{Pb}/E_{cr} in any subgroups. Normalizing to the excretion of creatinine was done to correct for urine dilution. This practice, however, inevitably introduces confounders and often creates gender bias. In general, men have a higher muscle mass than women, and, consequently, the mean E_{Cd}/E_{cr} was lower in men than women (Table 1). In effect, the health risks associated with Cd exposure in men could have been underestimated. The mean E_{Cd}/C_{cr} in men was almost identical to that of women (Table 1). It is increasingly recognized that creatinine adjustment is problematic, and urine specific gravity has been used to correct for dilution effects [9,44,45,50–52]. Herein, we have demonstrated the utility of normalizing excretion rate of metals to creatinine clearance that only required simultaneous urine and blood sampling together with the equations, given in Section 2.3 [33,35].

In a quantitative analysis for an effect of Pb, a non-significant association between the eGFR and E_{Pb}/C_{cr} was evident (Figure 1D). Furthermore, the POR for the reduced eGFR did not increase with E_{Pb}/C_{cr} in a dose-dependent manner (Table 3). Though urinary Pb is not a good indicator of Pb body burden, it does not rule out the possibility for a glomerular effect of Pb. Blood Pb levels ≥2.4 µg/dL were associated with a 1.56-fold increase in risk of eGFR levels of <60 mL/min/1.73 m^2 in adults who enrolled in NHANES 1999–2006 [26]. However, the absence of a dose–response relationship between the E_{Pb}/C_{cr} quartiles and POR for the reduced eGFR may suggest that the levels of environmental exposure to Pb that were experienced by participants in this study were below a nephrotoxicity threshold limit for Pb.

In a quantitative analysis for an effect of Cd (Figure 1C), an increment of E_{Cd}/C_{cr} to the median level (0.38 µg/L) was associated with a significant decrease in the eGFR (an approximate of 5 mL/min/1.73 m^2). An increment of E_{Cd}/C_{cr} to the 75th percentile level (0.62 µg/L) was not associated with a further decrease in the eGFR level. In the logistic regression analysis (Table 3), the POR for the reduced eGFR rose by 2.51 and 2.87 fold as the E_{Cd}/C_{cr} rose to the median level and the 75th percentile, respectively. The median E_{Cd}/C_{cr} level could thus be considered to represent the lowest urinary Cd level that was associated with observed adverse effect among the participants in the present study. The median and 75th percentile levels of E_{Cd}/Ecr corresponded to 0.44 and 0.76 µg/g of creatinine, respectively.

Of relevance, urinary Cd level of 0.8 µg/g of creatinine has been found to be associated with a significant eGFR decrease in Swedish women, aged 53–64 years [39]. In addition, U.S. population studies (NHANES) have provided a rich data source that links Cd and Pb exposure indicators to increased risk of CKD. In NHANES 1999–2006, urinary Cd levels ≥1 µg/L and blood Cd levels ≥0.6 µg/L were associated, respectively, with 1.48- and 1.32-fold increases in the risk of a low eGFR, defined as an eGFR <60 mL/min/1.73 m^2 [26,27]. In NHANES 2011–2012, blood Cd levels >0.53 µg/L were associated with 2.21-fold increases in risk of low eGFR [53].

In NHANES 2007–2012, blood Cd levels >0.61 µg/L were associated with a 1.80-fold increase in the risk of a low GFR [28]. In addition, the mean eGFR in women with hypertension and blood Cd in the highest quartile was 5.77 mL/min/1.73 m^2 lower than that of normotensive women who had blood Cd in the lowest quartile [28]. Of interest, an additional effect of hypertension on Cd-related GFR reduction has been seen in residents of an area of Thailand with Cd pollution: Those with hypertension, on average, had a 4.6 mL/min/1.73 m^2 lower eGFR compared with the mean eGFR of normotensive subjects who had similarly high urinary Cd levels [33].

In a Swedish women study, urinary Cd levels associated with a glomerular effect (eGFR decline) of 0.8 µg/g of creatinine were close to urinary Cd levels of 0.67 µg/g of creatinine that were associated with tubular injury based on urinary NAG levels [39]. These data challenge a long-held view that tubular effects occur long before the glomerular effect becomes apparent. A recent quantitative analysis of excreted Cd in relation to levels of the eGFR, urinary NAG, and β_2MG suggested a decrease in the GFR to be an early effect, given that excreted Cd emanates from injured tubular cells and that the injury leads to nephron atrophy, a decreased eGFR, and impaired reabsorption of filtered β_2MG [35]. Accordingly, it can be hypothesized that sufficient tubular injury induced by Cd disables glomerular filtration, destroys nephrons, and causes glomerulosclerosis, interstitial inflammation, fibrosis and CKD [35,54].

A lack of association between the eGFR and urinary Cd was reported in a cross-sectional study in Japan [55] in which eGFR values were derived for 1200 women by using a serum creatinine-based eGFR estimating equation for Japanese women. In this Japanese study, 222 women who were aged 42–79 years (mean 61.9) were drawn from a control area without Cd pollution, based on the Cd content in rice, which is a dietary staple, while 636 and 355 women of the similar age range were drawn from two areas with Cd pollution. Though the Cd intake levels from rice in the two Cd pollution areas were higher than those of the control group, the mean eGFR values in these three areas were similar. In addition, the eGFR levels were unrelated to urinary Cd, but they were related to age. These data suggested that the eGFR was not associated with Cd body burden in the Japanese population with relatively high levels of Cd intake [55]. A longitudinal study is required to dispute or confirm the observation made in this Japanese study. It is noteworthy, however, that a prospective study in a Cd pollution area in Thailand reported a progressive decrease in the eGFR over a five-year observation period [31].

Distinct from the Japanese study, an inverse association between the eGFR and urinary Cd was observed in the present study. The study Thai women were younger (the mean age of 36.9) and had lower urinary Cd levels (mean urinary of 0.51 µg/g of creatinine) compared to the Japanese women in the control area (mean age of 61.9) and mean urinary Cd of 3.03 µg/g of creatinine. The mean eGFR (range) was 106 (72−139) and 79.8 (30.6−130) mL/min/1.73 m^2 in the Thai and Japanese studies, respectively. The eGFR-urinary Cd association in the Thai study could have been due to younger age and lower Cd intake levels compared with the Japanese study. In addition, it is conceivable that the functional expressions of Cd-induced nephrotoxicity in low-dose and high-dose exposure conditions are different. For instance, a low-level environmental exposure to Cd has been implicated in the pathogenesis of hypertension, a known cause and consequence of CKD, in a longitudinal study in the U.S. [56], while blood Cd as low as 0.4 µg/L was associated, respectively, with 1.54- and 2.38-fold increases in risk of hypertension in Caucasian women and Mexican-American women who were aged ≥20 years and enrolled in NHANES 1999–2006 [57]. In stark contrast, a chronic high-dose Cd exposure has not been found to be associated with hypertension in Japanese population studies [58,59].

In the present study, chronic low-level exposure to Cd, indicated by a urinary Cd level as low as 0.44 μg/g of creatinine was associated with a decrease in the eGFR by 5 mL/min/1.73m^2. This low urinary Cd level was also associated with a 2.5 fold increase in the prevalence odds of eGFR levels <96 mL/min/1.73 m^2.These findings support the large number of population-based studies that have suggested that low-environmental exposure to Cd may increase the risk of CKD, thereby raising the possibility for a role of Cd exposure in current epidemics of CKD. It is noteworthy that the reported toxic urinary Cd levels did not exceed the toxicity threshold limit of 5.24 μg/g of creatinine that was established by the Food and Agriculture Organization of the United Nations (FAO) World Health Organization (WHO) [49,60]. We suggest that the current urinary Cd threshold limit does not afford health protection and should be lowered.

A small observable decrease in the eGFR that is attributable to long-term environmental exposure to Cd was expected, as the participants in our study were relatively young, with an overall mean age of 34.9 years. However, because dietary exposure to Cd and Pb is inevitable for most people, exposure to these toxic metals is likely to continue, leading to a further reduction in the GFR. In addition, the GFR may continue to decrease presumably due to mobilization of liver Cd and bone Pb to kidneys [5]. Even a small increase in the risk of CKD can result in many affected people, given that environmental exposure to Cd and Pb is widespread.

In conclusion, our analysis of archived data provides evidence that links environmental exposure to Cd to GFR decline, even when dietary intake levels of Cd are low. This glomerular effect of low-level environmental exposure to Cd was demonstrable only when urinary Cd concentrations that were normalized to creatinine clearance. Women appeared to be more susceptible than men to toxicity due to an elevated dietary intake of Cd and Pb.

5. Strengths and Limitations

The strengths of this study include the community-based recruitment of apparently healthy women and men who were relatively young, as well as the fact that simultaneous blood and urine sampling was undertaken at the same time of the day, thereby reducing diurnal variation of the GFR. The normalization of excretion rates of Cd and Pb to creatinine clearance was an additional strength because confounding effects of muscle mass and urine flow rate were both eliminated. Furthermore, environmental sources of Cd and Pb were relatively homogenous, as none of the participants had occupational exposure to metals. The limitations of this study were archived data with no availability to access the same people for long term comparisons, a modest sample size, and a cross-sectional design, which limited a causal inference of Cd and Pb exposure on the observed GFR reduction.

Supplementary Materials: The following are available online at http://www.mdpi.com/2305-6304/8/1/18/s1, Figure S1: Comparing effects of E_{Cd}/E_{cr} and E_{Pb}/E_{cr} on eGFR change; Table S1: Multivariable regression analysis for association of eGFR with E_{Cd}/E_{cr} and E_{Pb}/E_{cr}; Table S2: Prevalence odds ratios for reduced eGFR across E_{Cd}/E_{cr} quartiles and E_{Pb}/E_{cr} quartiles.

Author Contributions: S.S., D.A.V., P.U. and G.C.G. formulated study protocols. P.U. obtained ethical institutional clearance, recruited participants and organized the collection of biologic specimens and their shipment for metal analysis by the ICP/MS in Australia. S.S. prepared an initial draft of a manuscript. D.A.V. and G.G. provided intellectual input and revised the manuscript. All authors have read and agreed to the published version of the manuscript.

Funding: This research project received no external funding.

Acknowledgments: This work was partially supported by the Chulalongkorn University Medical Faculty, Bangkok, Thailand and the Commission for Higher Education, Thailand Ministry of Education. Additionally, it was supported with resources of the Department of Nephrology, Princess Alexandra Hospital, and the Kidney Disease Research Centre, the University of Queensland Faculty of Medicine and Translational Research Institute.

Conflicts of Interest: The authors have declared no potential conflicts of interest.

References

1. Satarug:, S.; Garrett, S.H.; Sens, M.A.; Sens, D.A. Cadmium, environmental exposure, and health outcomes. *Environ. Health Perspect.* **2010**, *118*, 182–190. [CrossRef] [PubMed]
2. Satarug, S.; Ruangyuttikarn, W.; Nishijo, M.; Ruiz, P. Urinary cadmium threshold to prevent kidney disease development. *Toxics* **2018**, *6*, 26. [CrossRef] [PubMed]
3. Shefa, S.T.; Héroux, P. Both physiology and epidemiology support zero tolerable blood lead levels. *Toxicol. Lett.* **2017**, *280*, 232–237. [CrossRef] [PubMed]
4. Harari, F.; Sallsten, G.; Christensson, A.; Petkovic, M.; Hedblad, B.; Forsgard, N.; Melander, O.; Nilsson, P.M.; Borné, Y.; Engström, G.; et al. Blood lead levels and decreased kidney function in a population-based cohort. *Am. J. Kidney Dis.* **2018**, *72*, 381–389. [CrossRef] [PubMed]
5. Satarug, S. Dietary cadmium intake and its effects on kidneys. *Toxics* **2018**, *6*, 15. [CrossRef] [PubMed]
6. IARC (International Agency for Research on Cancer). Cadmium and cadmium compounds. In *Beryllium, Cadmium, Mercury and Exposures in the Glass Manufacturing Industry*; IARC: Lyon, France, 1993; Volume 58, pp. 120–238.
7. Liao, L.M.; Friesen, M.C.; Xiang, Y.B.; Cai, H.; Koh, D.H.; Ji, B.T.; Yang, G.; Li, H.L.; Locke, S.J.; Rothman, N.; et al. Occupational lead exposure and associations with selected cancers: The Shanghai men's and women's health study cohorts. *Environ. Health Perspect.* **2016**, *124*, 97–103. [CrossRef] [PubMed]
8. Steenland, K.; Barry, V.; Anttila, A.; Sallmén, M.; McElvenny, D.; Todd, A.C.; Straif, K. A cohort mortality study of lead-exposed workers in the USA, Finland and the UK. *Occup. Environ. Med.* **2017**, *74*, 785–791. [CrossRef]
9. Buser, M.C.; Ingber, S.Z.; Raines, N.; Fowler, D.A.; Scinicariello, F. Urinary and blood cadmium and lead and kidney function: NHANES 2007–2012. *Int. J. Hyg. Environ. Health* **2016**, *219*, 261–267. [CrossRef]
10. Wang, W.; Schaumberg, D.A.; Park, S.K. Cadmium and lead exposure and risk of cataract surgery in U.S. adults. *Int. J. Hyg. Environ. Health* **2016**, *219*, 850–856. [CrossRef]
11. Shim, Y.K.; Lewin, M.D.; Ruiz, P.; Eichner, J.E.; Mumtaz, M.M. Prevalence and associated demographic characteristics of exposure to multiple metals and their species in human populations: The United States NHANES, 2007–2012. *J. Toxicol. Environ. Health A* **2017**, *80*, 502–512. [CrossRef]
12. Jin, R.; Zhu, X.; Shrubsole, M.J.; Yu, C.; Xia, Z.; Dai, Q. Associations of renal function with urinary excretion of metals: Evidence from NHANES 2003–2012. *Environ. Int.* **2018**, *121*, 1355–1362. [CrossRef] [PubMed]
13. Saravanabhavan, G.; Werry, K.; Walker, M.; Haines, D.; Malowany, M.; Khoury, C. Human biomonitoring reference values for metals and trace elements in blood and urine derived from the Canadian Health Measures Survey 2007–2013. *Int. J. Hyg. Environ. Health* **2017**, *220*, 189–200. [CrossRef] [PubMed]
14. Liao, K.W.; Pan, W.H.; Liou, S.H.; Sun, C.W.; Huang, P.C.; Wang, S.L. Levels and temporal variations of urinary lead, cadmium, cobalt, and copper exposure in the general population of Taiwan. *Environ. Sci. Pollut. Res. Int.* **2019**, *26*, 6048–6064. [CrossRef] [PubMed]
15. Kim, N.S.; Ahn, J.; Lee, B.K.; Park, J.; Kim, Y. Environmental exposures to lead, mercury, and cadmium among South Korean teenagers (KNHANES 2010–2013): Body burden and risk factors. *Environ. Res.* **2017**, *156*, 468–476. [CrossRef] [PubMed]
16. De Nicola, L.; Zoccali, C. Chronic kidney disease prevalence in the general population: Heterogeneity and concerns. *Nephrol. Dial. Transplant.* **2016**, *31*, 331–335. [CrossRef]
17. Glassock, R.J.; David, G.; Warnock, D.G.; Delanaye, P. The global burden of chronic kidney disease: Estimates, variability and pitfalls. *Nat. Rev. Nephrol.* **2017**, *13*, 104–114. [CrossRef]
18. George, C.; Mogueo, A.; Okpechi, I.; Echouffo-Tcheugui, J.B.; Kengne, A.P. Chronic kidney disease in low-income to middle-income countries: The case for increased screening. *BMJ Glob. Health* **2017**, *2*, e000256. [CrossRef]
19. Levey, A.S.; Stevens, L.A.; Schmid, C.H.; Zhang, Y.; Castro, A.F., III; Feldman, H.I.; Kusek, J.W.; Eggers, P.; Van Lente, F.; Greene, T.; et al. A new equation to estimate glomerular filtration rate. *Ann. Intern. Med.* **2009**, *150*, 604–612. [CrossRef]
20. Levey, A.S.; Inker, L.A.; Coresh, J. GFR estimation: From physiology to public health. *Am. J. Kidney Dis.* **2014**, *63*, 820–834. [CrossRef]
21. Levey, A.S.; Becker, C.; Inker, L.A. Glomerular filtration rate and albuminuria for detection and staging of acute and chronic kidney disease in adults: A systematic review. *JAMA* **2015**, *313*, 837–846. [CrossRef]

22. White, C.A.; Allen, C.M.; Akbari, A.; Collier, C.P.; Holland, D.C.; Day, A.G.; Knoll, G.A. Comparison of the new and traditional CKD-EPI GFR estimation equations with urinary inulin clearance: A study of equation performance. *Clin. Chim. Acta* **2019**, *488*, 189–195. [CrossRef]
23. Sommar, J.N.; Svensson, M.K.; Björ, B.M.; Elmståhl, S.I.; Hallmans, G.; Lundh, T.; Schön, S.M.; Skerfving, S.; Bergdahl, I.A. End-stage renal disease and low level exposure to lead, cadmium and mercury; a population-based, prospective nested case-referent study in Sweden. *Environ. Health* **2013**, *12*, 9. [CrossRef]
24. Grau-Perez, M.; Pichler, G.; Galan-Chilet, I.; Briongos-Figuero, L.S.; Rentero-Garrido, P.; Lopez-Izquierdo, R.; Navas-Acien, A.; Weaver, V.; García-Barrera, T.; Gomez-Ariza, J.L.; et al. Urine cadmium levels and albuminuria in a general population from Spain: A gene-environment interaction analysis. *Environ. Int.* **2017**, *106*, 27–36. [CrossRef]
25. Myong, J.P.; Kim, H.R.; Baker, D.; Choi, B. Blood cadmium and moderate-to-severe glomerular dysfunction in Korean adults: Analysis of KNHANES 2005–2008 data. *Int. Arch. Occup. Environ. Health* **2012**, *85*, 885–893. [CrossRef]
26. Navas-Acien, A.; Tellez-Plaza, M.; Guallar, E.; Muntner, P.; Silbergeld, E.; Jaar, B.; Weaver, V. Blood cadmium and lead and chronic kidney disease in US adults: A joint analysis. *Am. J. Epidemiol.* **2009**, *170*, 1156–1164. [CrossRef]
27. Ferraro, P.M.; Costanzi, S.; Naticchia, A.; Sturniolo, A.; Gambaro, G. Low level exposure to cadmium increases the risk of chronic kidney disease: Analysis of the NHANES 1999–2006. *BMC Public Health* **2010**, *10*, 304. [CrossRef]
28. Madrigal, J.M.; Ricardo, A.C.; Persky, V.; Turyk, M. Associations between blood cadmium concentration and kidney function in the U.S. population: Impact of sex, diabetes and hypertension. *Environ. Res.* **2018**, *169*, 180–188. [CrossRef]
29. Zhu, X.J.; Wang, J.J.; Mao, J.H.; Shu, Q.; Du, L.Z. Relationships between cadmium, lead and mercury levels and albuminuria: Results from the National Health and Nutrition Examination Survey Database 2009–2012. *Am. J. Epidemiol.* **2019**, *188*, 1281–1287. [CrossRef]
30. Shi, Z.; Taylor, A.W.; Riley, M.; Byles, J.; Liu, J.; Noakes, M. Association between dietary patterns, cadmium intake and chronic kidney disease among adults. *Clin. Nutr.* **2017**, *5614*, 31366–31368.
31. Swaddiwudhipong, W.; Limpatanachote, P.; Mahasakpan, P.; Krintratun, S.; Punta, B.; Funkhiew, T. Progress in cadmium-related health effects in persons with high environmental exposure in northwestern Thailand: A five-year follow-up. *Environ. Res.* **2012**, *112*, 194–198. [CrossRef]
32. Swaddiwudhipong, W.; Nguntra, P.; Kaewnate, Y.; Mahasakpan, P.; Limpatanachote, P.; Aunjai, T.; Jeekeeree, W.; Punta, B.; Funkhiew, T.; Phopueng, I. Human health effects from cadmium exposure: Comparison between persons living in cadmium-contaminated and non-contaminated areas in northwestern Thailand. *Southeast Asian J. Trop. Med. Public Health* **2015**, *46*, 133–142.
33. Satarug, S.; Boonprasert, K.; Gobe, G.C.; Ruenweerayut, R.; Johnson, D.W.; Na-Bangchang, K.; Vesey, D.A. Chronic exposure to cadmium is associated with a marked reduction in glomerular filtration rate. *Clin. Kidney J.* **2018**, *12*, 468–475. [CrossRef]
34. Satarug, S.; Vesey, D.A.; Nishijo, M.; Ruangyuttikarn, W.; Gobe, G.C. The inverse association of glomerular function and urinary β2-MG excretion and its implications for cadmium health risk assessment. *Environ. Res.* **2019**, *173*, 40–47. [CrossRef]
35. Satarug, S.; Vesey, D.A.; Ruangyuttikarn, W.; Nishijo, M.; Gobe, G.C.; Phelps, K.R. The source and pathophysiologic significance of excreted cadmium. *Toxics* **2019**, *7*, 4. [CrossRef]
36. Roels, H.A.; Lauwerys, R.R.; Buchet, J.P.; Bernard, A.M.; Vos, A.; Oversteyns, M. Health significance of cadmium induced renal dysfunction: A five year follow up. *Occup. Environ. Med.* **1989**, *46*, 755–764. [CrossRef]
37. Jarup, L.; Persson, B.; Elinder, C.G. Decreased glomerular filtration rate in solderers exposed to cadmium. *Occup. Environ. Med.* **1995**, *52*, 818–822. [CrossRef]
38. Reilly, R.; Spalding, S.; Walsh, B.; Wainer, J.; Pickens, S.; Royster, M.; Villanacci, J.; Little, B.B. Chronic environmental and occupational lead exposure and kidney function among African Americans: Dallas Lead Project II. *Int. J. Environ. Res. Public Health* **2018**, *15*, 12. [CrossRef]
39. Akesson, A.; Lundh, T.; Vahter, M.; Bjellerup, P.; Lidfeldt, J.; Nerbrand, C.; Samsioe, G.; Strömberg, U.; Skerfving, S. Tubular and glomerular kidney effects in Swedish women with low environmental cadmium exposure. *Environ. Health Perspect.* **2005**, *113*, 1627–1631. [CrossRef]

40. Hwangbo, Y.; Weaver, V.M.; Tellez-Plaza, M.; Guallar, E.; Lee, B.K.; Navas-Acien, A. Blood cadmium and estimated glomerular filtration rate in Korean adults. *Environ. Health Perspect.* **2011**, *119*, 1800–1805. [CrossRef]
41. Weaver, V.M.; Kim, N.S.; Jaar, B.G.; Schwartz, B.S.; Parsons, P.J.; Steuerwald, A.J.; Todd, A.C.; Simon, D.; Lee, B.K. Associations of low-level urine cadmium with kidney function in lead workers. *Occup. Environ. Med.* **2011**, *68*, 250–256. [CrossRef]
42. Sanders, A.P.; Mazzella, M.J.; Malin, A.J.; Hair, G.M.; Busgang, S.A.; Saland, J.M.; Curtin, P. Combined exposure to lead, cadmium, mercury, and arsenic and kidney health in adolescents age 12–19 in NHANES 2009–2014. *Environ. Int.* **2019**, *131*, 104993. [CrossRef] [PubMed]
43. Pollack, A.Z.; Mumford, S.L.; Mendola, P.; Perkins, N.J.; Rotman, Y.; Wactawski-Wende, J.; Schisterman, E.F. Kidney biomarkers associated with blood lead, mercury, and cadmium in premenopausal women: A prospective cohort study. *J. Toxicol. Environ Health A* **2015**, *78*, 119–131. [CrossRef] [PubMed]
44. Weaver, V.M.; Vargas, G.G.; Silbergeld, E.K.; Rothenberg, S.J.; Fadrowski, J.J.; Rubio-Andrade, M.; Parsons, P.J.; Steuerwald, A.J.; Navas-Acien, A.; Guallar, E. Impact of urine concentration adjustment method on associations between urine metals and estimated glomerular filtration rates (eGFR) in adolescents. *Environ. Res.* **2014**, *132*, 226–232. [CrossRef] [PubMed]
45. Weaver, V.M.; Kotchmar, D.J.; Fadrowski, J.J.; Silbergeld, E.K. Challenges for environmental epidemiology research: Are biomarker concentrations altered by kidney function or urine concentration adjustment? *J. Expo. Sci. Environ. Epidemiol.* **2016**, *26*, 1–8. [CrossRef]
46. Galal-Gorchev, H. Dietary intake, levels in food and estimated intake of lead, cadmium, and mercury. *Food Addit. Contam.* **1993**, *10*, 115–128. [CrossRef]
47. Phelps, K.R.; Stote, K.S.; Mason, D. Tubular calcium reabsorption and other aspects of calcium homeostasis in primary and secondary hyperparathyroidism. *Clin. Nephrol.* **2014**, *82*, 83–91. [CrossRef]
48. Heymsfield, S.B.; Arteaga, C.; McManus, C.; Smith, J.; Moffitt, S. Measurement of muscle mass in humans: Validity of the 24-h urinary creatinine method. *Am. J. Clin. Nutr.* **1983**, *37*, 478–494. [CrossRef]
49. Satarug, S.; Vesey, D.A.; Gobe, G.C. Health risk assessment of dietary cadmium intake: Do current guidelines indicate how much is safe? *Environ. Health Perspect.* **2017**, *125*, 284–288. [CrossRef]
50. Jenny-Burri, J.; Haldiman, M.; Bruschweiler, B.J.; Bochud, M.; Burnier, M.; Paccaud, F.; Dudler, V. Cadmium body burden of the Swiss population. *Food Addit. Contam. Part Anal. Chem. Control Expo. Risk Assess.* **2015**, *32*, 1265–1272. [CrossRef]
51. De Craemer, S.; Croes, K.; van Larebeke, N.; De Henauw, S.; Schoeters, G.; Govarts, E.; Loots, I.; Nawrot, T.; Nelen, V.; Den Hond, E.; et al. Metals, hormones and sexual maturation in Flemish adolescents in three cross-sectional studies (2002–2015). *Environ. Int.* **2017**, *102*, 190–199. [CrossRef]
52. Barr, D.B.; Wilder, L.C.; Caudill, S.P.; Gonzalez, A.J.; Needham, L.L.; Pirkle, J.L. Urinary creatinine concentrations in the U.S. population: Implications for urinary biologic monitoring measurements. *Environ. Health Perspect.* **2005**, *113*, 192–200. [CrossRef] [PubMed]
53. Lin, Y.S.; Ho, W.C.; Caffrey, J.L.; Sonawane, B. Low serum zinc is associated with elevated risk of cadmium nephrotoxicity. *Environ. Res.* **2014**, *134*, 33–38. [CrossRef]
54. Schnaper, H.W. The tubulointerstitial pathophysiology of progressive kidney disease. *Adv. Chronic Kidney Dis.* **2017**, *24*, 107–116. [CrossRef] [PubMed]
55. Horiguchi, H.; Oguma, E.; Sasaki, S.; Okubo, H.; Murakami, K.; Miyamoto, K.; Hosoi, Y.; Murata, K.; Kayama, F. Age-relevant renal effects of cadmium exposure through consumption of home-harvested rice in female Japanese farmers. *Environ. Int.* **2013**, *56*, 1–9. [CrossRef] [PubMed]
56. Oliver-Williams, C.; Howard, A.G.; Navas-Acien, A.; Howard, B.V.; Tellez-Plaza, M.; Franceschini, N. Cadmium body burden, hypertension, and changes in blood pressure over time: Results from a prospective cohort study in American Indians. *J. Am. Soc. Hypertens.* **2018**, *12*, 426–437. [CrossRef] [PubMed]
57. Scinicariello, F.; Abadin, H.G.; Murray, H.E. Association of low-level blood lead and blood pressure in NHANES 1999–2006. *Environ. Res.* **2011**, *111*, 1249–1257. [CrossRef]
58. Nakagawa, H.; Nishijo, M. Environmental cadmium exposure, hypertension and cardiovascular risk. *J. Cardiovasc. Risk* **1996**, *3*, 11–17. [CrossRef]

59. Kurihara, I.; Kobayashi, E.; Suwazono, Y.; Uetani, M.; Inaba, T.; Oishiz, M.; Kido, T.; Nakagawa, H.; Nogawa, K. Association between exposure to cadmium and blood pressure in Japanese peoples. *Arch. Environ. Health* **2004**, *59*, 711–776. [CrossRef]
60. Food and Agriculture Organization of the United Nations (FAO) World Health Organization (WHO) Summary and Conclusions. In Proceedings of the Joint FAO/WHO Expert Committee on Food Additives Seventy-Third Meeting, Geneva, Switzerland, 8–17 June 2010. Available online: http://www.who.int/foodsafety/publications/chem/summary73.pdf (accessed on 13 January 2020).

toxics

MDPI

Article

The Source and Pathophysiologic Significance of Excreted Cadmium

Soisungwan Satarug [1,*], David A. Vesey [1,2], Werawan Ruangyuttikarn [3], Muneko Nishijo [4], Glenda C. Gobe [1,2,5,6] and Kenneth R. Phelps [7]

1 Kidney Disease Research Collaborative, The University of Queensland Faculty of Medicine and Translational Research Institute, Woolloongabba, Brisbane 4102, Australia; David.Vesey@health.qld.gov.au (D.A.V.); g.gobe@uq.edu.au (G.C.G.)

2 Department of Nephrology, Princess Alexandra Hospital, Brisbane 4075, Australia

3 Division of Toxicology, Department of Forensic Medicine, Chiang Mai University, Chiang Mai 50200, Thailand; ruangyuttikarn@gmail.com

4 Department of Public Health, Kanazawa Medical University, Uchinada, Ishikawa 920-0293, Japan; ni-koei@kanazawa-med.ac.jp

5 School of Biomedical Sciences, The University of Queensland, Brisbane 4072, Australia

6 NHMRC Centre of Research Excellence for CKD.QLD, UQ Health Sciences, Royal Brisbane and Women's Hospital, Brisbane 4029, Australia

7 Stratton Veterans' Affairs Medical Center and Albany Medical College, Albany, NY 12208, USA; Kenneth.Phelps@va.gov

* Correspondence: sj.satarug@yahoo.com.au

Received: 10 August 2019; Accepted: 16 October 2019; Published: 18 October 2019

Abstract: In theory, the identification of the source of excreted cadmium (Cd) might elucidate the pathogenesis of Cd-induced chronic kidney disease (CKD). With that possibility in mind, we studied Thai subjects with low, moderate, and high Cd exposure. We measured urine concentrations of Cd, ($[Cd]_u$); N-acetyl-β-D-glucosaminidase, a marker of cellular damage ($[NAG]_u$); and β_2-microglobulin, an indicator of reabsorptive dysfunction ($[\beta_2MG]_u$). To relate excretion rates of these substances to existing nephron mass, we normalized the rates to creatinine clearance, an approximation of the glomerular filtration rate (GFR) (E_{Cd}/C_{cr}, E_{NAG}/C_{cr}, and $E_{\beta 2MG}/C_{cr}$). To link the loss of intact nephrons to Cd-induced tubular injury, we examined linear and quadratic regressions of estimated GFR (eGFR) on E_{Cd}/C_{cr}, eGFR on E_{NAG}/C_{cr}, and E_{NAG}/C_{cr} on E_{Cd}/C_{cr}. Estimated GFR varied inversely with both ratios, and E_{NAG}/C_{cr} varied directly with E_{Cd}/C_{cr}. Linear and quadratic regressions of $E_{\beta 2MG}/C_{cr}$ on E_{Cd}/C_{cr} and E_{NAG}/C_{cr} were significant in moderate and high Cd-exposure groups. The association of E_{NAG}/C_{cr} with E_{Cd}/C_{cr} implies that both ratios depicted cellular damage per surviving nephron. Consequently, we infer that excreted Cd emanated from injured tubular cells, and we attribute the reduction of eGFR to the injury. We suggest that E_{Cd}/C_{cr}, E_{NAG}/C_{cr}, and eGFR were associated with one another because each parameter was determined by the tubular burden of Cd.

Keywords: β_2-microglobulin; cadmium; creatinine clearance; glomerular filtration; N-acetyl-β-D-glucosaminidase; nephron mass; nephrotoxicity

1. Introduction

Cadmium (Cd), a divalent metal used for industrial purposes, is an important environmental pollutant in some regions of the world [1–5]. The metal is conveyed to humans in food, air, and tobacco smoke, and subsequently gains access to the circulation through the gut and lungs [5]. Salts of ionized Cd are absorbed in the duodenum; in addition, complexes of Cd with plant metallothioneins (MT) and phytochelatins (PC) may be absorbed in the colon after liberation by bacteria [6]. In the bloodstream, Cd is bound to red blood cells, albumin, glutathione (GSH), sulfur-containing amino acids, MT, and

PC [6–10]. In the liver, hepatocytes take up Cd not bound to MT [10], synthesize MT in response to the metal, and store complexes of CdMT. These complexes are subsequently released from hepatocytes and transported to the kidneys [8,11,12]. Cd in plasma is filterable by glomeruli if it is bound to GSH, amino acids, MT, or PC [8,9], but the fraction of circulating Cd that enters the filtrate is unknown. The proximal tubule reabsorbs and retains most or all of the filtered Cd with an array of channels, solute carriers, and mediators of endocytosis [7,10,13–16]. Basolateral uptake may also add to the cellular content of Cd in the proximal tubule [16–18].

It is currently assumed that the magnitude of a gradually acquired burden determines the toxicity of Cd in tubular cells [19]. The emergence of Cd from lysosomes induces robust intracellular synthesis of MT, which greatly mitigates the injury inflicted by free Cd through complexation of the metal [20]. Nevertheless, a fraction of Cd remains unbound to MT and is presumed to promote autophagy, apoptosis, and necrosis as accumulation of Cd progresses [19,21]. Manifestations of renal toxicity include increased excretion of cellular proteins, impaired reabsorption of filtered substances, histologically demonstrable tissue injury, loss of intact nephrons, and reduction of the glomerular filtration rate (GFR) [5,8,21–27]. GFR may continue to fall for many years after exogenous exposure ceases [22,24], presumably because traffic of CdMT from the liver to kidneys persists.

In human studies of Cd-induced nephropathy, the most commonly assayed marker of tubular cell damage is the lysosomal enzyme N-acetyl-β-D-glucosaminidase (NAG). Because NAG is too large to be filtered by glomeruli, excessive excretion (E_{NAG}) signifies tubular injury [28]. The most commonly measured indicator of impaired reabsorption is β_2-microglobulin (β_2MG). This small circulating protein is extremely filterable by glomeruli [29]; ordinarily, more than 99% of filtered β_2MG is reabsorbed [30], but that percentage falls early in the course of tubular injury [31].

Although the urinary excretion rate of Cd (E_{Cd}) is believed to reflect the body burden of the metal [5], the precise source and pathophysiologic significance of excreted Cd have not been clarified. One possibility is that Cd is excreted because it is filtered and not reabsorbed; an alternate possibility is that excretion reflects liberation of Cd into filtrate from injured or dying tubular cells [32]. This distinction is important because the source of urinary Cd is central to the relationship between Cd accumulation and progression of chronic kidney disease (CKD). Herein, we present evidence that excreted Cd emanates from cells that it has injured. The injury leads to the loss of intact nephrons, reduction of GFR, and impaired reabsorption of filtered β_2MG.

2. Materials and Methods

2.1. Study Subjects

The Institutional Ethical Committees of Chulalongkorn University, Chiang Mai University and the Mae Sot Hospital approved the study protocol (Approval No. 142/2544, 5 October 2001) [33]. All participants gave informed consent before participation. Subjects were recruited from urban communities in Bangkok in 2001/2002 and from subsistence farming areas in Mae Sot District, Tak Province, Thailand in 2004/2005 [33]. They had lived at their current addresses for at least 30 years. Exclusion criteria were pregnancy, breast-feeding, a history of metal work, and a hospital record or physician's diagnosis of an advanced chronic disease. Because occupational exposure was an exclusion criterion, we presumed that all participants had acquired Cd from the environment.

Cd exposure was low in Bangkok and moderate or high in Mae Sot [33,34]. Determination of exposure was based on reported levels of Cd in rice grains grown in the Cd-affected areas of the Mae Sot District [35,36]. After exclusion of subjects with incomplete datasets, we studied 172, 310, and 222 persons from the low, moderate, and high exposure areas, respectively.

2.2. Collection of Biological Specimens and Laboratory Analyses

Second morning-void urine samples were collected after an overnight fast. Within three hours after urine sampling, specimens of whole blood were obtained and serum samples were prepared. Aliquots of urine, whole blood, and serum were transported on ice from a mobile clinic to a laboratory and stored at −20 °C or −80 °C for later analysis. The assay for urine and serum creatinine concentrations ($[cr]_u$, $[cr]_p$) was based on the Jaffe reaction. The urine NAG assay was based on colorimetry (NAG test kit, Shionogi Pharmaceuticals, Sapporo, Japan). The urine β_2MG assay was based on the latex immunoagglutination method (LX test, Eiken 2MGII; Eiken and Shionogi Co., Tokyo, Japan). When the urine concentration of β_2MG ($[\beta_2MG]_u$) was below the limit of detection (LOD), 0.5 μg/L, the value assigned to $[\beta_2MG]_u$ was LOD/(square root of 2).

For the Bangkok group, $[Cd]_u$ was determined by inductively-coupled plasma mass spectrometry (ICP/MS, Agilent 7500, Agilent Technologies), because it had the high sensitivity required to measure Cd concentrations below the detectable limit of atomic absorption spectrophotometry. Multi-element standards (EM Science, EM Industries, Inc., Newark, NJ, USA) were used to calibrate Cd analyses. The accuracy and precision of those analyses were evaluated with reference urine (Lyphochek®, Bio-Rad, Sydney, Australia). When $[Cd]_u$ was less than the detection limit of 0.05 μg/L, the concentration assigned was the detection limit divided by the square root of 2.

For the Mae Sot groups, $[Cd]_u$ was determined by atomic absorption spectrophotometry (Shimadzu Model AA-6300, Kyoto, Japan). Urine standard reference material No. 2670 (National Institute of Standards, Washington, DC, USA) was used for quality assurance and control purposes. None of the urine samples from the Mae Sot groups were found to have $[Cd]_u$ below the detection limit.

2.3. *Estimated Glomerular Filtration Rate (eGFR)*

The glomerular filtration rate was estimated with equations from the Chronic Kidney Disease Epidemiology Collaboration (CKD-EPI) [37,38]. CKD stages 1, 2, 3, 4, and 5 corresponded to eGFR of 90–119, 60–89, 30–59, 15–29, and <15 mL/min/1.73 m^2, respectively. For dichotomous comparisons, CKD was defined as eGFR < 60 mL/min/1.73 m^2.

2.4. *Normalization of Excretion Rates to Creatinine Clearance (C_{cr})*

Excretion rates of Cd, NAG, and β_2MG were normalized to C_{cr} to yield the ratios E_{Cd}/C_{cr}, E_{NAG}/C_{cr}, and $E_{\beta 2MG}/C_{cr}$ in units of mass (amount excreted) per volume of filtrate. For x = Cd, NAG, or β_2MG, E_x/C_{cr} was calculated as $[x]_u[cr]_p/[cr]_u$ ([39]; Supplementary Materials).

2.5. *Statistical Analysis*

Data were analyzed with SPSS 17.0 (SPSS Inc., Chicago, IL, USA). Distributions of excretion rates for Cd, NAG, and β_2MG were examined for skewness, and those showing rightward skewing were subjected to base-10 logarithmic transformation before analysis. Departure of a given variable from normal distribution was assessed with the one-sample Kolmogorov–Smirnov test. For continuous variables not conforming to a normal distribution, the Kruskal–Wallis test was used to determine differences among the three localities in E_{Cd}/C_{cr}, E_{NAG}/C_{cr}, $E_{\beta 2MG}/C_{cr}$, and other parameters. The Mann–Whitney *U*-test was used to compare mean differences between two groups. The Chi-Square test was used to determine differences in percentage and prevalence data. p-values ≤ 0.05 for two-tailed tests were assumed to indicate statistical significance.

Polynomial regression was used to fit lines and curves to the scatterplots of five pairs of variables, including eGFR versus E_{Cd}/C_{cr}, eGFR versus E_{NAG}/C_{cr}, E_{NAG}/C_{cr} versus E_{Cd}/C_{cr}, $E_{\beta 2MG}/C_{cr}$ versus E_{Cd}/C_{cr}, and E_{NAG}/C_{cr} versus $E_{\beta 2MG}/C_{cr}$. A linear model, $y = a + bx$, was adopted if the relationship was monotonic. A quadratic model (second-order polynomial), $y = a + b_1x + b_2x^2$, was used if there was a significant change in the direction of the slope (b_1 to b_2) for prediction of the dependent variable y. In both types of equations, a represented the y-intercept.

The relationships between x and y were assessed with R^2 (the coefficient of determination) and with unstandardized and standardized β coefficients. In linear and quadratic models, R^2 is the fraction of variation in y that is explained by the variation in x. In linear models, the unstandardized β coefficient is the slope of the linear regression, and the standardized β coefficient indicates the strength of the association between y and x on a uniform scale. To examine quadratic curves relating eGFR to E_{Cd}/C_{cr} and E_{NAG}/C_{cr}, we performed slope change analyses with a linear regression method.

3. Results

Table 1 presents data concerning age, gender, blood pressure, smoking status, and renal function of subjects with low, moderate, and high environmental exposure to Cd. There were significant differences in age and percentages of women and smokers across the three exposure subsets. Female gender was overrepresented in the moderate exposure group. More than half of subjects in the high exposure group were smokers. Blood pressures were recorded in the low and moderate exposure groups; systolic and mean pressures were significantly higher in the latter.

Table 1. Study subjects drawn from three localities.

Descriptors	All Subjects	Locality		
		Low Cd	Moderate Cd	High Cd
Number of subjects	704	172	310	222
Women (%)	60.7	47.7	72.9	53.6 *
Smoking (%)	43.6	23.8	40.6	63.1 *
Age (years)	48.34 ± 11.11	38.72 ± 10.29	47.24 ± 4.72	57.34 ± 11.13 †
SBP (mmHg)	122.7 ± 13.5	120.1 ± 10.4	124.2 ± 14.7 ¶	–
DBP (mmHg)	78.9 ± 9.5	78.1 ± 7.6	79.4 ± 10.4	–
MBP (mmHg)	93.5 ± 9.9	92.1 ± 7.9	94.3 ± 3.3 ¶¶	–
eGFR (mL/min/1.73 m^2)	90.32 ± 21.84	105.46 ± 15.05	95.72 ± 16.13	71.05 ± 19.65 †
CKD prevalence (%)	9.5	0	3.5	25.2
Kidney disease stage (%)				
Stage 1	54.8	84.1	66.5	16.2 *
Stage 2	36.6	15.9	31.0	59.9 *
Stage 3	7.7	0	2.6	20.7 **
Stage 4	1.0	0	0	3.2
Serum creatinine (mg/dL)	0.80 (0.70, 1.0)	0.8 (0.7, 0.9)	0.8 (0.7, 0.9)	1.0 (0.9, 1.2) †
Urine creatinine (mg/dL)	97 (53, 156)	52 (32, 106)	110 (62, 171)	115 (69, 158) †
Urine Cd (μg/L)	3.7 (1.1, 8.3)	0.2 (0.1, 0.6)	3.9 (2.4, 7.2)	8.3 (4.7, 13.9) †
Urine NAG (units/L)	6.4 (2.4, 16.6)	1.8 (1.3, 2.9)	11.9 (7.1, 19)	5.3 (2.7, 9.2) †
Urine β_2MG (μg/L)	154 (33, 778)	9.5 (0.3, 42)	400 (134, 1118)	171 (64, 1368) †
E_{Cd}/C_{cr} × 100, μg/L	3.1 (1.1, 7.0)	0.3 (0.3, 0.6)	3.0 (1.7, 5.0)	8.2 (4.8, 15) †
E_{NAG}/C_{cr} × 100, units/L	5.6 (3.4, 9.4)	3.2 (2.0, 4.1)	8.0 (5.8, 12)	4.9 (3.1. 8.3) †
$E_{\beta 2MG}/C_{cr}$ × 100, μg/L	137 (29, 604)	17 (0.4, 36)	368 (92, 808)	162 (64, 176) †

SBP = systolic blood pressure; DBP = diastolic blood pressure; MBP = Mean arterial pressure; CKD = chronic kidney disease; eGFR = estimated glomerular filtration rate; NAG = N-acetyl-β-D-glucosaminidase. MBP = DBP + (pulse pressure)/3, where pulse pressure = SBP − DBP. Data for age and eGFR are arithmetic mean values ± standard deviation (SD). Data for blood pressure are geometric mean values ± SD. Data for all other continuous variables are the median (25th, 75th percentile) values. * Significant % differences among three groups ($p < 0.05$, Pearson Chi-Square test). ** Significant % differences between two groups ($p < 0.001$, Pearson Chi-Square test). † Significant mean differences among three groups ($p < 0.001$, Kruskal–Wallis test). ¶ Significant difference from the low exposure group ($p = 0.003$, Mann–Whitney U-test). ¶¶ Significant difference from the low exposure group ($p = 0.014$, Mann–Whitney U-test).

Mean eGFR fell and the percentages of stages 2 and 3 CKD rose with intensity of exposure. The mean serum creatinine concentration was higher in the high-Cd locality. In general, urine concentrations of Cd, NAG, and β_2MG rose with Cd exposure, but $[NAG]_u$ and $[\beta_2MG]_u$ were higher in the moderate Cd group than in the other two. E_{Cd}/C_{cr}, E_{NAG}/C_{cr}, and $E_{\beta 2MG}/C_{cr}$ followed the same pattern.

Figure 1A–D present scatterplots of eGFR against log(E_{Cd}/C_{cr}) in each exposure subset and the entire sample. In each subset, significant linear and quadratic relationships were documented, and quadratic R^2 values were slightly higher. Quadratic R^2 was 0.228 in the low-Cd group, 0.083 in the moderate-Cd group, 0.154 in the high-Cd group, and 0.378 in the entire sample. In the linear model, standardized β was −0.467 in the low-Cd group, −0.259 in the moderate-Cd group, −0.361 in the high-Cd group, and −0.598 in the entire sample.

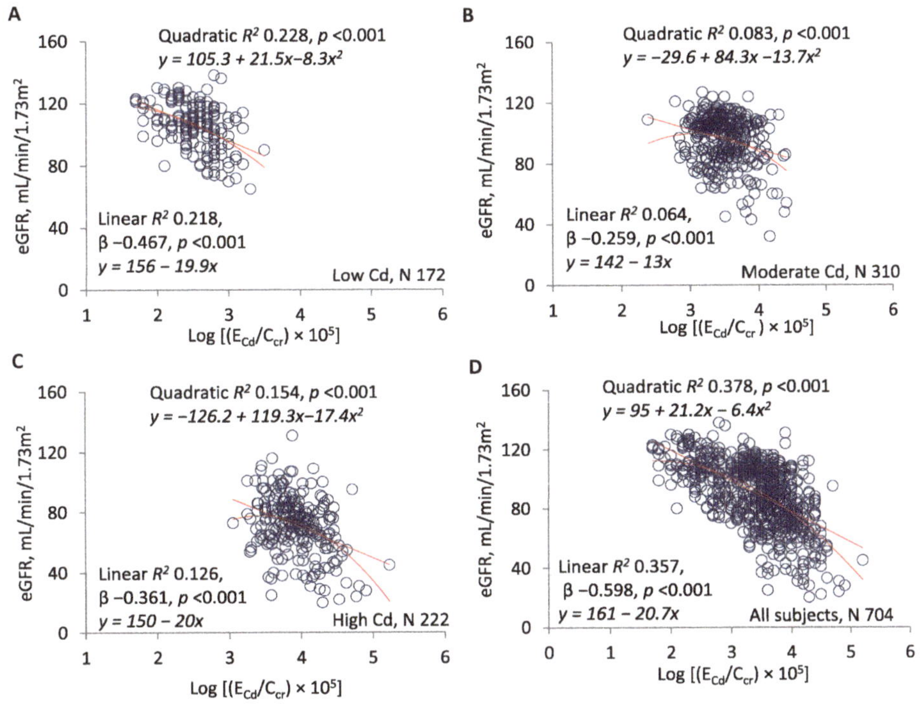

Figure 1. E_{Cd}/C_{cr} as a predictor of the estimated glomerular filtration rate (eGFR). Scatterplots compare eGFR to $\log[(E_{Cd}/C_{cr}) \times 10^5]$ in subjects grouped by locality (**A–C**) and in all subjects (**D**). Quadratic and linear coefficients of determination (R^2) are provided together with corresponding equations, standardized β coefficients, and *p*-values.

Figure 2A–D present scatterplots of eGFR against $\log(E_{NAG}/C_{cr})$. As in Figure 1, significant, inverse linear and quadratic relationships were documented in subsets and the entire sample, and quadratic R^2 values were slightly higher. Quadratic R^2 was 0.055 in the low-Cd group, 0.216 in the moderate-Cd group, 0.381 in the high-Cd group, and 0.139 in the entire sample. In the linear model, standardized β was −0.206 in the low-Cd group, −0.447 in the moderate-Cd group, −0.605 in the high-Cd group, and −0.361 in the entire sample.

The quadratic curves in Figures 1D and 2D indicated that slopes describing rates of GFR reduction varied over the ranges of $\log[(E_{Cd}/C_{cr}) \times 10^5]$ and $\log[(E_{NAG}/C_{cr}) \times 10^3]$. We assumed that $\log[(E_{Cd}/C_{cr}) \times 10^5]$ of 3.0 and $\log[(E_{NAG}/C_{cr}) \times 10^3]$ of 1.5 represented the excretion rates of Cd and NAG at which the rates of GFR reduction increased. Table 2 confirms that the slopes changed significantly at these points on the *x*-axes.

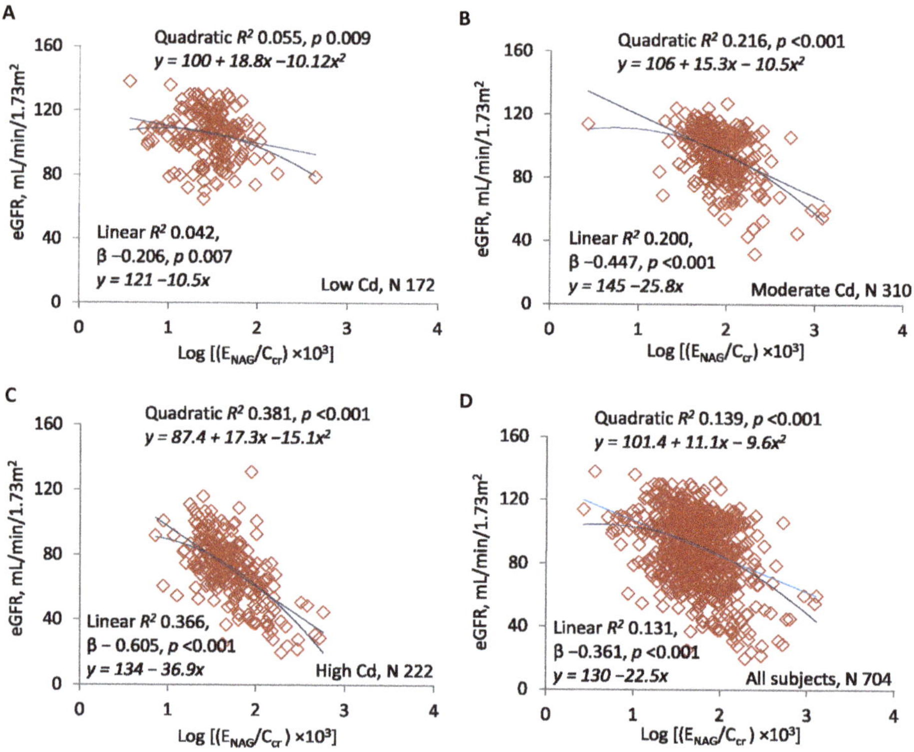

Figure 2. E_{NAG}/C_{cr} as a predictor of eGFR. Scatterplots compare eGFR to $\log[(E_{NAG}/C_{cr}) \times 10^3]$ in subjects grouped by locality (**A–C**) and in all subjects (**D**). Quadratic and linear coefficients of determination (R^2) are provided together with corresponding equations, standardized β coefficients, and *p*-values.

Table 2. Slope analysis for comparing rates of eGFR reduction.

Excretion Rates of Cd or NAG	Number of Subjects	eGFR vs. $\log[(E_{Cd}/C_{cr}) \times 10^5]$ or $\log[(E_{NAG}/C_{cr}) \times 10^3]$ β Coefficients: Slope (Unstandardized β) ± SE	Standardized β	R^2	*p* Value
$\log[(E_{Cd}/C_{cr}) \times 10^5]$					
<3	168	−17.62 ± 3.20	−0.392	0.154	<0.001
≥3	536	−27.71 ± 2.06	−0.503	0.253	<0.001
All subjects	704	−20.86 ± 1.06	−0.598	0.357	<0.001
$\log[(E_{NAG}/C_{cr}) \times 10^3]$					
<1.5	153	−15.91 ± 7.62	−0.168	0.028	0.038
≥1.5	551	−28.35 ± 3.35	−0.339	0.115	<0.001
All subjects	704	−22.49 ± 2.19	−0.361	0.131	<0.001

The standardized β coefficient indicates the strength of the association of eGFR with $\log[(E_{Cd}/C_{cr}) \times 10^5]$ or $\log[(E_{NAG}/C_{cr}) \times 10^3]$. R^2 values are coefficients of determination that indicate the fraction of eGFR variation explained by E_{Cd}/C_{cr} or E_{NAG}/C_{cr}. $p \le 0.05$ identifies statistically significant eGFR reduction rates or associations of eGFR with urinary Cd or NAG excretion.

Figure 3A–D present scatterplots of log(E_{NAG}/C_{cr}) against log(E_{Cd}/C_{cr}) in the exposure subsets and the entire sample. In all subsets, the two ratios varied directly, significant linear and quadratic relationships were documented, and quadratic R^2 values were slightly higher. Quadratic R^2 was 0.108 in the low-Cd group, 0.114 in the moderate-Cd group, 0.269 in the high-Cd group, and 0.229 in the entire sample. In the linear model, standardized β was 0.325 in the low-Cd group, 0.327 in the moderate-Cd group, 0.507 in the high-Cd group, and 0.471 in the entire sample.

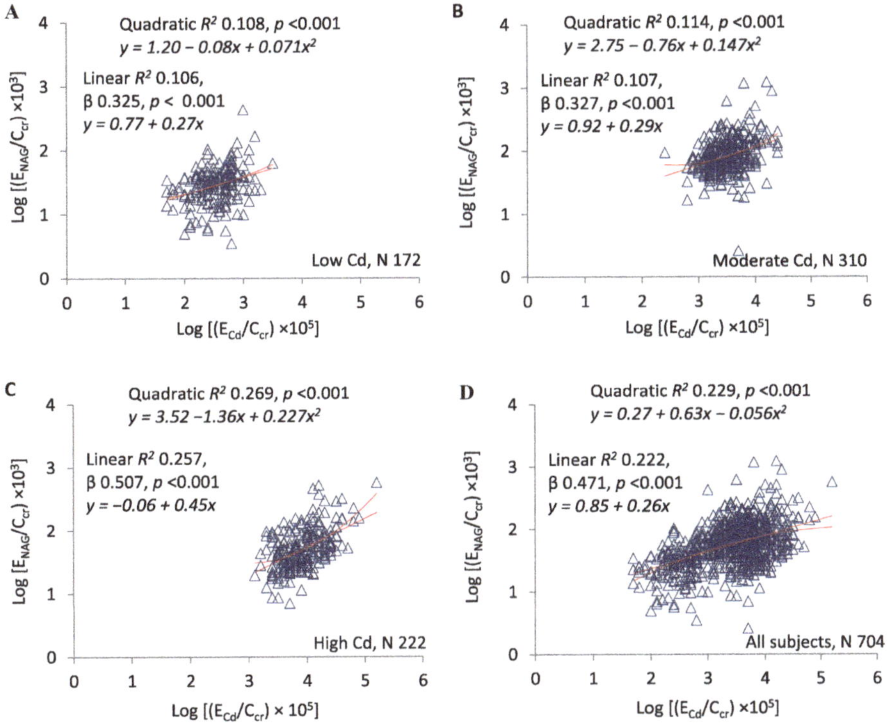

Figure 3. E_{Cd}/C_{cr} as a predictor of E_{NAG}/C_{cr}. Scatterplots compare log[(E_{NAG}/C_{cr}) × 10^3] to log[(E_{Cd}/C_{cr}) × 10^5] in subjects grouped by locality (**A–C**) and in all subjects (**D**). Quadratic and linear coefficients of determination (R^2) are provided together with corresponding equations, standardized β coefficients, and *p*-values.

Figure 4A–D present scatterplots of log($E_{\beta 2MG}/C_{cr}$) against log(E_{Cd}/C_{cr}) in the exposure subsets and the entire sample. Figure 4A demonstrates the absence of a relationship at the lowest Cd exposure (quadratic $R^2 = 0.028$, $p = 0.088$). At moderate and high exposure, the two ratios were directly related, significant linear and quadratic relationships were documented, and quadratic R^2 values were slightly higher (Figure 4B,C). Quadratic R^2 was 0.126 in the moderate exposure group, 0.204 in the high exposure group, and 0.370 in the entire sample. Quadratic and linear relationships in the entire sample were virtually identical (Figure 4D). In the linear model, standardized β was 0.067 in the low-Cd group, 0.334 in the moderate-Cd group, 0.450 in the high-Cd group, and 0.608 in the entire sample.

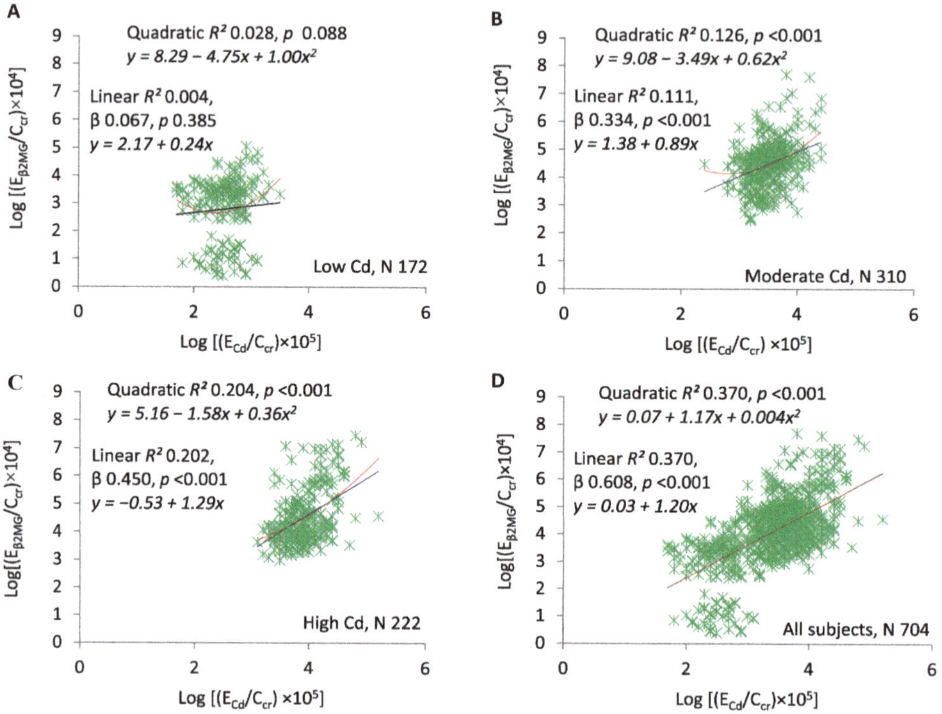

Figure 4. ECd/C_{cr} as a predictor of $E_{\beta 2MG}/C_{cr}$. Scatterplots compare $\log[(E_{\beta 2MG}/C_{cr}) \times 10^4]$ to $\log[(E_{Cd}/C_{cr}) \times 10^5]$ in subjects grouped by locality (**A–C**) and in all subjects (**D**). Quadratic and linear coefficients of determination (R^2) are provided together with corresponding equations, standardized β coefficients, and *p*-values.

Figure 5A–D present scatterplots of $\log(E_{\beta 2MG}/C_{cr})$ against $\log(E_{NAG}/C_{cr})$. Figure 5A demonstrates the absence of a relationship at the lowest Cd exposure (linear $R^2 = 0.009$, $p = 0.225$). At moderate and high exposure, the two ratios were directly related, significant linear and quadratic regressions were documented, and quadratic R^2 values were slightly higher (Figure 5B,C). Quadratic R^2 was 0.152 in the moderate exposure group, 0.426 in the high exposure group, and 0.288 in the entire sample. In the linear model, standardized β was 0.093 in the low-Cd group, 0.360 in the moderate-Cd group, 0.647 in the high-Cd group, and 0.536 in the entire sample.

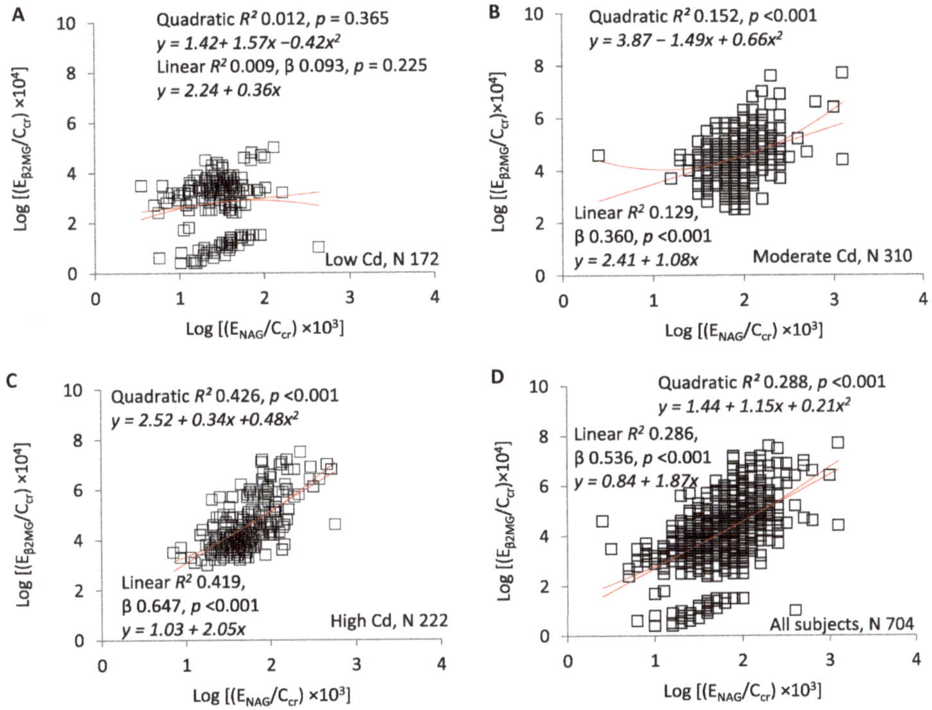

Figure 5. E_{NAG}/C_{cr} as a predictor of $E_{\beta 2MG}/C_{cr}$. Scatterplots compare log[(E_{NAG}/C_{cr}) × 10^3] to log[($E_{\beta 2MG}/C_{cr}$) × 10^4] in subjects grouped by locality (**A–C**) and in all subjects (**D**). Quadratic and linear coefficients of determination (R^2) are provided together with corresponding equations, standardized β coefficients, and p-values.

4. Discussion

Our goals in the present study were to elucidate the source of urinary Cd and to relate that source to the pathogenesis of Cd nephropathy. Data were obtained from clinically healthy Thai subjects residing in areas with low, moderate, or high exposure to Cd. In Mae Sot District, Tak Province, intensity of exposure was determined from the Cd content of rice grains [35,36]. Exposure in Bangkok was assumed to be low on the basis of food analyses and dietary histories [33].

Subjects in the three subsets were demographically dissimilar (Table 1). Both age and percentage of smokers rose with intensity of exposure. The percentage of women was particularly high in the moderate exposure group, and some women were of childbearing age. Because iron and Cd share a transporter in intestinal epithelium, menstruating women in this group may have absorbed Cd with exceptional avidity and incurred exceptional tubular toxicity secondarily (Table 1). In the high exposure subset, increased age may have conferred additional reasons for deterioration of GFR, and smoking may have provided a second environmental source of Cd. Whether smoking itself could have accelerated the progression of CKD is unresolved [40–42]. Neither age, nor smoking per se, nor the source of exogenous Cd obscured the significant relationship between eGFR and E_{Cd}/C_{cr}.

Table 1 shows that with the increasing intensity of exposure, E_{Cd}/C_{cr} rose and eGFR fell in stepwise fashion. In contrast, both E_{NAG}/C_{cr} and $E_{\beta 2MG}/C_{cr}$ were higher in the moderate than in the high exposure group. Although one might expect a direct relationship between NAG excretion and the number of intact nephrons, the higher E_{NAG}/C_{cr} in the moderate group implies that the median excretion of NAG *per intact nephron* was also higher in these subjects. At the same time, the overlap of E_{NAG}/C_{cr} between the moderate and high exposure groups was substantial (Figures 2 and 5), and consistent relationships among E_{Cd}/C_{cr}, E_{NAG}/C_{cr}, and eGFR were demonstrable at all intensities of exposure (Figures 1–3). We speculate that the number of menstruating women in the moderate exposure subset was sufficient to increase Cd absorption and tubular toxicity in the entire group, but insufficient to disrupt the statistical relationships seen in all groups among E_{Cd}/C_{cr}, E_{NAG}/C_{cr}, and eGFR.

Analogous statements can be made about β_2MG. As impaired reabsorption of this protein is an early sign of proximal tubular injury, it is not surprising that median $E_{\beta 2MG}/C_{cr}$ tracked with median E_{NAG}/C_{cr} (Table 1). As would be expected, $E_{\beta 2MG}/C_{cr}$ varied directly with E_{NAG}/C_{cr} in the moderate and high exposure groups, but also varied directly with E_{Cd}/C_{cr}, which increased progressively with the intensity of exposure (Figures 4 and 5).

Although CKD-EPI equations estimate GFR imprecisely [37,38], each exposure group differed significantly from the others with respect to eGFR (Table 1). Estimated GFR was inversely related to E_{Cd}/C_{cr} and E_{NAG}/C_{cr} in the entire sample and each subset (Figures 1 and 2), and E_{NAG}/C_{cr} varied directly with E_{Cd}/C_{cr} (Figure 3). For all comparisons in Figures 1–3, both linear and quadratic relationships were significant, and with one exception (Figure 1B), R^2 rose with the exposure intensity. Standardized β followed the same pattern. Despite the statistical significance of all comparisons, some R^2 values indicated that the fractional contribution of E_{Cd}/C_{cr} or E_{NAG}/C_{cr} to eGFR was <10% (Figures 1B and 2A); simultaneously, however, standardized β indicated robust effects of changes in x on changes in y. Factors other than E_{Cd}/C_{cr} and E_{NAG}/C_{cr} affected eGFR, but variation in each ratio was associated with substantial variation in eGFR.

Taken together, the graphs in Figures 1–3 imply that in each subset, GFR was inversely related to the severity of cellular injury per nephron (E_{NAG}/C_{cr}), which in turn was associated with the amount of Cd excreted per nephron (E_{Cd}/C_{cr}). In addition, the quadratic relationships in Figures 1 and 2 suggest that small increments in the most advanced injury were accompanied by disproportionate reductions in GFR. Slope analyses of curves in Figures 1D and 2D confirm this inference (Table 2).

Other investigators have described direct relationships of $[NAG]_u/[cr]_u$ and eGFR to $[Cd]_u/[cr]_u$, but we have not found a synthesis of those relationships into a satisfactory pathophysiologic narrative [35,43–48]. A cogent interpretation of Figures 1–3 must explain how eGFR and E_{NAG}/C_{cr}—results of *cumulative* Cd sequestration—were related physiologically to E_{Cd}/C_{cr}, an indicator of Cd excretion *at the time of sampling*. Cd was excreted for two possible reasons; it was filtered and not reabsorbed, or it was released from tubular cells [32]. Although both processes may have occurred, we do not see how the first, excretion after filtration, could have produced a physiologic connection between E_{Cd}/C_{cr} and E_{NAG}/C_{cr} (Figure 3). In contrast, if Cd was released from damaged tubules, then Cd and NAG emanated from the same source, and both E_{Cd}/C_{cr} and E_{NAG}/C_{cr} measured cellular injury. This shared attribute of Cd and NAG explains the statistical association of the ratios.

Additional evidence for the tubular origin of excreted Cd is provided by demonstrated extrusions of MT into tubular lumens [49], documented correlations of E_{Cd} with renal tissue content of Cd [50–52], and direct relationships between E_{Cd} and GFR (number of intact nephrons) [53–55]. Experiments in rabbits demonstrated a high tubular maximum for reabsorption of CdMT that would preclude excretion of filtered Cd in the typically intoxicated human [56].

In addition to addressing the likely source of excreted Cd, we must also ask why declining eGFR, the result of continuous loss of intact nephrons over time, was associated in the present study with parameters of *current* cellular injury, E_{Cd}/C_{cr} and E_{NAG}/C_{cr}. To address this paradox, we propose that eGFR, E_{Cd}/C_{cr}, and E_{NAG}/C_{cr} were simultaneous consequences of the tubular content of Cd. As the content rose, cellular injury per nephron and the rate of nephron loss increased proportionately; at any moment in a subject's exposure history, the three variables were quantitatively associated because they were traceable to the same burden of sequestered Cd.

β_2MG, a small protein made by nucleated cells, is almost completely filtered by glomeruli [29]. Ordinarily, the proximal tubule reabsorbs and degrades over 99% of filtered β_2MG [30]. Because tubulopathies increase $E_{\beta 2MG}$ [31], excessive $E_{\beta 2MG}$ is conventionally interpreted as evidence of reabsorptive dysfunction [35,57,58]. This interpretation is understandable, but we suspect that it is an oversimplification. One reason is that endogenous production of β_2MG may be increased by chronic inflammatory conditions, solid tumors, lymphatic malignancies, and multiple myeloma [59]. If tubular degradation ($TD_{\beta 2MG}$) remains constant as production rises, $E_{\beta 2MG}$ also rises even though $TD_{\beta 2MG}$ has not fallen (SM). Moreover, if both β_2MG production and $TD_{\beta 2MG}$ per volume of filtrate ($TD_{\beta 2MG}/C_{cr}$) remain constant as GFR falls, $TD_{\beta 2MG}$ also falls, and $E_{\beta 2MG}$ rises (SM). Although these inferences are unproven, it seems likely that a combination of reabsorptive dysfunction and reduced GFR caused associations of $E_{\beta 2MG}/C_{cr}$ with E_{Cd}/C_{cr} and E_{NAG}/C_{cr} (Figures 4 and 5).

An additional observation requires explanation. In the low exposure group, a cluster of subjects exhibited exceptionally low $E_{\beta 2MG}/C_{cr}$. At a fixed rate of β_2MG filtration (equal to endogenous production) and a fixed value of $TD_{\beta 2MG/Ccr}$, the rate of β_2MG reabsorption increases with the number of intact nephrons, and $E_{\beta 2MG}$ decreases simultaneously. In the isolated cluster, mean eGFR was 105.3 mL/min/1.73 m^2; in the remainder of subjects in the study, it was 89.3 mL/min/1.73 m^2. We suspect that extremely low $E_{\beta 2MG}/C_{cr}$ in the cluster was the result of high C_{cr}, high $TD_{\beta 2MG}$, and secondarily reduced $E_{\beta 2MG}$.

In the present study, we have continued the recently introduced practice of normalizing excretion of Cd, NAG, and β_2MG to creatinine clearance instead of creatinine excretion [26]. Because the resulting ratios express E_{Cd}, E_{NAG}, and $E_{\beta 2MG}$ as functions of intact nephron mass, they nullify sources of imprecision that accompany normalization to E_{cr} or $[cr]_u$. At any GFR, E_{cr} is primarily a function of muscle mass [60]; consequently, at a given E_{Cd} (for example), $[Cd]_u/[cr]_u$ may vary by a multiple over the range of human body size. Moreover, multiple groups have reported *direct* rather than inverse relationships between GFR and $[Cd]_u/[cr]_u$ after Cd exposure [5,53–55]. If the nephron number determines E_{Cd} at a given cellular burden of the metal, then $[Cd]_u/[cr]_u$ may exaggerate the burden at normal GFR and underestimate it at reduced GFR. Normalization of E_{Cd} to C_{cr}—that is, calculation of $[Cd]_u[cr]_p/[cr]_u$—eliminates the confounding effects of both muscle mass and nephron number on $[Cd]_u/[cr]_u$. In addition, because the required measurements are made in aliquots of urine and serum, the calculation quantifies amounts of Cd (or other substances) excreted per volume of filtrate while eliminating the need for timed urine collections and direct determinations of GFR. We plan to address optimal expression of excretion rates relevant to Cd nephropathy in a separate publication.

In summary, we draw the following conclusions from the significant regressions described herein. E_{NAG}/C_{cr} varied directly with E_{Cd}/C_{cr} because sequestered Cd induced the release of NAG and Cd from tubular cells into filtrate. Estimated GFR varied inversely with both ratios because all three parameters reflected the extent of tubular Cd accumulation. E_{NAG}/C_{cr} and E_{Cd}/C_{cr} quantified ongoing cellular injury, and eGFR quantified the loss of intact nephrons. We suspect that the significant regressions of $E_{\beta 2MG}/C_{cr}$ on E_{Cd}/C_{cr} and E_{NAG}/C_{cr} resulted from effects of Cd on both tubular reabsorption and nephron number.

Supplementary Materials: The following are available online at http://www.mdpi.com/2305-6304/7/4/55/s1, The equation for normalization to creatinine clearance.

Author Contributions: S.S., D.A.V., W.R., M.N., and G.C.G. formulated the study designs and protocols. S.S. and W.R. obtained ethical institutional clearances for research on human subjects and supervised the collection of biologic specimens in Thailand. S.S. organized and analyzed the data, created the tables and figures, and revised the manuscript for important intellectual content. K.R.P. proposed normalization of excretion rates to creatinine clearance, provided logical data interpretation, and was the primary author of the manuscript.

Funding: This research received no external funding.

Acknowledgments: This work was partially supported by the Commission for High Education, Thailand Ministry of Education, and the National Science and Technology Development Agency (NSTDA). Additionally, it was supported with resources of the Stratton Veterans' Affairs Medical Center, Albany, NY, USA, and was made possible by facilities at that institution. Opinions expressed in this paper are those of the authors and do not represent the official position of the United States Department of Veterans' Affairs.

Conflicts of Interest: The authors have no potential conflicts of interest to declare.

Abbreviations

Abbreviation	Meaning
Cd	Cadmium
GFR	Glomerular filtration rate, units of volume/time
eGFR	Estimated glomerular filtration rate, units of mL/min/1.73 m^2
CKD-EPI	Chronic kidney disease epidemiology collaboration
MT	Metallothionein
CdMT	Cadmium–metallothionein complex
PC	Phytochelatin
CdPC	Cadmium–phytochelatin complex
GSH	Glutathione
NAG	N-acetyl-β-D-glucosaminidase
β_2MG	Beta$_2$-microglobulin
C_{cr}	Creatinine clearance, units of volume/time
V_u	Urine flow rate, units of volume/time
E_x/C_{cr}	Excretion rate of x per volume of filtrate, units of mass/volume, where x = Cd, NAG, or β_2MG
$TD_{\beta 2MG}$	Rate of tubular degradation of β_2MG, units of mass/time
$TD_{\beta 2MG}/C_{cr}$	Amount of β_2MG degraded per volume of filtrate, units of mass/volume

References

1. ATSDR (Agency for Toxic Substances and Disease Registry). *Toxicological Profile for Cadmium;* Department of Health and Humans Services, Public Health Service, Centers for Disease Control and Prevention: Atlanta, GA, USA, 2012.
2. WHO. *IPCS (International Programme on Chemical Safety) Environmental Health Criteria 134: Cadmium;* WHO: Geneva, Switzerland, 1992.
3. Satarug, S.; Vesey, D.A.; Gobe, G.C. Current health risk assessment practice for dietary cadmium: Data from different countries. *Food Chem. Toxicol.* **2017**, *106*, 430–445. [CrossRef] [PubMed]
4. Satarug, S.; Vesey, D.A.; Gobe, G.C. Health risk assessment of dietary cadmium intake: Do current guidelines indicate how much is safe? *Environ. Health Perspect.* **2017**, *125*, 284–288. [CrossRef] [PubMed]
5. Satarug, S. Dietary cadmium intake and its effects on kidneys. *Toxics* **2018**, *6*, 15. [CrossRef] [PubMed]
6. Langelueddecke, C.; Lee, W.-K.; Thevenod, F. Differential transcytosis and toxicity of the hNGAL receptor ligands cadmium-metallothionein and cadmium-phytochelatin in colon-like Caco-2 cells: Implications for cadmium toxicity. *Toxicol. Lett.* **2014**, *226*, 228–235. [CrossRef] [PubMed]
7. Dorian, C.; Gattone, V.H., II; Klaassen, C.D. Discrepancy between the nephrotoxic potencies of cadmium-metallothionein and cadmium chloride and the renal concentration of cadmium in the proximal convoluted tubules. *Toxicol. Appl. Pharmacol.* **1995**, *130*, 161–168. [CrossRef]
8. Sabolic, I.; Breljak, D.; Skarica, M.; Herak-Kramberger, C.M. Role of metallothionein in cadmium traffic and toxicity in kidneys and other mammalian organs. *Biometals* **2010**, *23*, 897–926. [CrossRef]
9. Fujita, Y.; ElBelbasi, H.I.; Min, K.-S.; Onosaka, S.; Okada, Y.; Matsumoto, Y.; Mutoh, N.; Tanaka, K. Fate of cadmium bound to phytochelatin in rats. *Res. Commun. Chem. Pathol. Pharmacol.* **1993**, *82*, 357–365.
10. Sudo, J.-I.; Hayashi, T.; Soyama, M.; Fukata, M.; Kakuino, K. Kinetics of Cd2+ in plasma, liver and kidneys after single intravenous injection of Cd-metallothionein-II. *Eur. J. Pharmacol.* **1994**, *270*, 229–235. [CrossRef]
11. Chan, H.M.; Zhu, L.F.; Zhong, R.; Grant, D.; Goyer, R.A.; Cherian, M.G. Nephrotoxicity in rats following liver transplantation from cadmium-exposed rats. *Toxicol. Appl. Pharmacol.* **1993**, *123*, 89–96. [CrossRef]
12. Dudley, R.E.; Gammal, L.M.; Klaassen, C.D. Cadmium-induced hepatic and renal injury in chronically exposed rats: Likely role of hepatic cadmium-metallothionein in nephrotoxicity. *Toxicol. Appl. Pharmacol.* **1985**, *77*, 414–426. [CrossRef]
13. Dorian, C.; Gattone, V.H., II; Klaassen, C.D. Renal cadmium deposition and injury as a result of accumulation of cadmium-metallothionein (CdMT) by the proximal convoluted tubules—A light microscopic autoradiography study with ^{109}CdMT. *Toxicol. Appl. Pharmacol.* **1992**, *114*, 173–181. [CrossRef]

14. Barbier, O.; Jacquillet, G.; Tauc, M.; Poujeol, P.; Cougnon, M. Acute study of interaction among cadmium, calcium, and zinc transport along rat nephron in vivo. *Am. J. Physiol.* **2004**, *287*, F1067–F1075. [CrossRef] [PubMed]
15. Felley-Bosco, E.; Diezi, J. Fate of cadmium in rat renal tubules: A micropuncture study. *Toxicol. Appl. Pharmacol.* **1989**, *98*, 243–251. [CrossRef]
16. Thevenod, F.; Fels, J.; Lee, W.-K.; Zarbock, R. Channels, transporters and receptors for cadmium and cadmium complexes in eukaryotic cells: Myths and facts. *Biometals* **2019**, *32*, 469–489. [CrossRef] [PubMed]
17. Soodvilai, S.; Nantavishit, J.; Muanprasat, C.; Chatsudthipong, V. Renal organic cation transporters mediated cadmium-induced nephrotoxicity. *Toxicol. Lett.* **2011**, *204*, 38–42. [CrossRef] [PubMed]
18. Zalups, R.K. Evidence for basolateral uptake of cadmium in kidneys of rats. *Toxicol. Appl. Pharmacol.* **2000**, *164*, 15–23. [CrossRef]
19. Prozialeck, W.C.; Edwards, J.R. Mechanisms of cadmium-induced proximal tubule injury: New insights with implications for biomonitoring and therapeutic interventions. *J. Pharmacol. Exp. Ther.* **2012**, *343*, 2–12. [CrossRef]
20. Liu, Y.; Liu, J.; Habeebu, S.S.; Klaassen, C.D. Metallothionein protects against the nephrotoxicity produced by chronic CdMT exposure. *Toxicol. Sci.* **1999**, *50*, 221–227. [CrossRef]
21. Goyer, R.A.; Miller, C.R.; Zhu, S.-Y.; Victery, W. Non-metallothionein-bound cadmium in the pathogenesis of cadmium nephrotoxicity in the rat. *Toxicol. Appl. Pharmacol.* **1989**, *101*, 232–244. [CrossRef]
22. Jarup, L.; Persson, B.; Elinder, C.G. Decreased glomerular filtration rate in solderers exposed to cadmium. *Occup. Environ. Med.* **1995**, *52*, 818–822. [CrossRef]
23. Jarup, L.; Hellstrom, L.; Alfven, T.; Carlsson, M.D.; Grubb, A.; Persson, B.; Pettersson, C.; Spang, G.; Schutz, A.; Elinder, C.-G. Low level exposure to cadmium and early kidney damage: The OSCAR study. *Occup. Environ. Med.* **2000**, *57*, 668–672. [CrossRef] [PubMed]
24. Roels, H.A.; Lauwerys, R.R.; Buchet, J.P.; Bernard, A.M.; Vos, A.; Oversteyns, M. Health significance of cadmium induced renal dysfunction: A five year follow up. *Occup. Environ. Med.* **1989**, *46*, 755–764. [CrossRef] [PubMed]
25. Akesson, A.; Lundh, T.; Vahter, M.; Bjellerup, P.; Lidfeldt, J.; Nerbrand, C.; Samsioe, G.; Strömberg, U.; Skerfving, S. Tubular and glomerular kidney effects in Swedish women with low environmental cadmium exposure. *Environ. Health Perspect.* **2005**, *113*, 1627–1631. [CrossRef] [PubMed]
26. Satarug, S.; Boonprasert, K.; Gobe, G.C.; Ruenweerayut, R.; Johnson, D.W.; Na-Bangchang, K.; Vesey, D.A. Chronic exposure to cadmium is associated with a marked reduction in glomerular filtration rate. *Clin. Kidney J.* **2018**, *12*, 468–475. [CrossRef]
27. Swaddiwudhipong, W.; Limpatanachote, P.; Mahassakpan, P.; Krintratun, S.; Punta, B.; Funkhiew, T. Progress in cadmium-related health effects in persons with high environmental exposure in northwestern Thailand: A five-year follow-up. *Environ. Res.* **2012**, *112*, 194–198. [CrossRef]
28. Price, R.G. Measurement of N-acetyl-beta-glucosaminidase and its isoenzymes in urine: Methods and clinical applications. *Eur. J. Clin. Chem. Clin. Biochem.* **1992**, *30*, 693–705.
29. Portman, R.J.; Kissane, J.M.; Robson, A.M. Use of β2 microglobulin to diagnose tubulo-interstitial renal lesions in children. *Kidney Int.* **1986**, *30*, 91–98. [CrossRef]
30. Argyropoulos, C.P.; Chen, S.S.; Ng, Y.-H.; Roumelioti, M.-E.; Shaffi, K.; Singh, P.P.; Tzamaloukas, A.H. Rediscovering beta-2 microglobulin as a biomarker across the spectrum of kidney diseases. *Front. Med.* **2017**, *4*, 73. [CrossRef]
31. Peterson, P.A.; Evrin, P.-E.; Berggard, I. Differentiation of glomerular, tubular, and normal proteinuria: Determination of urinary excretion of β2-microglobulin, albumin, and total protein. *J. Clin. Investig.* **1969**, *48*, 1189–1198. [CrossRef]
32. Chaumont, A.; Voisin, C.; Deumer, G.; Haufroid, V.; Annesi-Maesano, I.; Roels, H.; Thijs, L.; Staessen, J.; Bernard, A. Associations of urinary cadmium with age and urinary proteins: Further evidence of physiological variations unrelated to metal accumulation and toxicity. *Environ. Health Perspect.* **2013**, *121*, 1047–1053. [CrossRef]
33. Satarug, S.; Swaddiwudhipong, W.; Ruangyuttikarn, W.; Nishijo, M.; Ruiz, P. Modeling cadmium exposures in low- and high-exposure areas in Thailand. *Environ. Health Perspect.* **2013**, *121*, 531–536. [CrossRef] [PubMed]

34. Swaddiwudhipong, W.; Nguntra, P.; Kaewnate, Y.; Mahasakpan, P.; Limpatanachote, P.; Aunjai, T.; Jeekeeree, W.; Punta, B.; Funkhiew, T.; Phopueng, I. Human health effects from cadmium exposure: Comparison between persons living in cadmium-contaminated and non-contaminated areas in northwestern Thailand. *Southeast Asian J. Trop. Med. Public Health* **2015**, *46*, 133–142.
35. Honda, R.; Swaddiwudhipong, W.; Nishijo, M.; Mahasakpan, P.; Teeyakasem, W.; Ruangyuttikarn, W.; Satarug, S.; Padungtod, C.; Nakagawa, H. Cadmium induced renal dysfunction among residents of rice farming area downstream from a zinc-mineralized belt in Thailand. *Toxicol. Lett.* **2010**, *198*, 26–32. [CrossRef] [PubMed]
36. Simmons, R.W.; Pongsakul, P.; Saiyasitpanich, D.; Klinphoklap, S. Elevated levels of cadmium and zinc in paddy soils and elevated levels of cadmium in rice grain downstream of a zinc mineralized area in Thailand: Implications for public health. *Environ. Geochem. Health* **2005**, *27*, 501–511. [CrossRef] [PubMed]
37. Levey, A.S.; Stevens, L.A.; Schmid, C.H.; Zhang, Y.; Castro, A.F., III; Feldman, H.I.; Kusek, J.W.; Eggers, P.; Van Lente, F.; Greene, T.; et al. A new equation to estimate glomerular filtration rate. *Ann. Intern. Med.* **2009**, *150*, 604–612. [CrossRef] [PubMed]
38. Levey, A.S.; Becker, C.; Inker, L.A. Glomerular filtration rate and albuminuria for detection and staging of acute and chronic kidney disease in adults: A systematic review. *JAMA* **2015**, *313*, 837–846. [CrossRef]
39. Phelps, K.R.; Stote, K.S.; Mason, D. Tubular calcium reabsorption and other aspects of calcium homeostasis in primary and secondary hyperparathyroidism. *Clin. Nephrol.* **2014**, *82*, 83–91. [CrossRef]
40. Ricardo, A.C.; Anderson, C.A.; Yang, W.; Zhang, X.; Fischer, M.J.U.; Dember, L.M.; Fink, J.C.; Frydrych, A.; Jensvold, N.; Lustigova, E.; et al. Healthy lifestyle and risk of kidney disease progression, atherosclerotic events, and death in CKD: Findings from the chronic renal insufficiency cohort (CRIC) study. *Am. J. Kidney Dis.* **2015**, *65*, 412–424. [CrossRef]
41. Staplin, N.; Haynes, R.; Herrington, W.G.; Reith, C.; Cass, A.; Fellstrom, B.; Jiang, L.; Kasiske, B.L.; Krane, V.; Levin, A.; et al. Smoking and adverse outcomes in patients with CKD: The study of heart and renal protection (SHARP). *Am. J. Kidney Dis.* **2016**, *68*, 371–380. [CrossRef]
42. Wang, J.; Wang, B.; Liang, M.; Wang, G.; Li, J.; Zhang, Y.; Huo, Y.; Cui, Y.; Xu, X.; Qin, X. Independent and combined effect of bilirubin and smoking on the progression of chronic kidney disease. *Clin. Epidemiol.* **2018**, *10*, 121–132. [CrossRef]
43. Zhang, Y.R.; Wang, P.; Liang, X.X.; Tan, C.S.; Tan, J.B.; Wang, J.; Huang, Q.; Huang, R.; Li, Z.X.; Chen, W.C.; et al. Associations between urinary excretion of cadmium and renal biomarkers in non-smoking females: A cross-sectional study in rural areas of South China. *Int. J. Environ. Res. Public Health* **2015**, *12*, 11988–12001. [CrossRef]
44. Bernard, A.; Thielemans, N.; Roels, H.; Lauwerys, R. Association between NAG-B and cadmium in urine with no evidence of a threshold. *Occup. Environ. Med.* **1995**, *52*, 177–180. [CrossRef] [PubMed]
45. Liu, C.X.; Li, Y.B.; Zhju, C.S.; Dong, Z.M.; Zhang, K.; Zhao, Y.B.; Xu, Y.L. Benchmark dose for cadmium exposure and elevated N-acetyl-β-D-glucosaminidase: A meta-analysis. *Environ. Sci. Pollut. Res.* **2016**, *23*, 20528–20538. [CrossRef]
46. Kawada, T.; Koyama, H.; Suzuki, S. Cadmium, NAG activity, and β2-microglobulin in the urine of cadmium pigment workers. *Occup. Environ. Med.* **1989**, *46*, 52–55. [CrossRef] [PubMed]
47. Kawada, T.; Shinmyo, R.R.; Suzuki, S. Urinary cadmium and N-acetyl-β-D-gluosaminidase excretion of inhabitants living in a cadmium-polluted area. *Int. Arch. Occup. Environ. Health* **1992**, *63*, 541–546. [CrossRef]
48. Koyama, H.; Satoh, H.; Suzuki, S.; Tohyama, C. Increased urinary cadmium excretion and its relationship to urinary N-acetyl-β-D-gluosaminidase activity in smokers. *Arch. Toxicol.* **1992**, *66*, 598–601. [CrossRef]
49. Sabolic, I.; Skarica, M.; Ljubojevic, M.; Breljak, D.; Herak-Kramberger, C.M.; Crljen, V.; Ljubesic, N. Expression and immunolocalization of metallothioneins MT1, MT2 and MT3 in rat nephron. *J. Trace Elem. Med. Biol.* **2018**, *46*, 62–75. [CrossRef] [PubMed]
50. Satarug, S.; Baker, J.R.; Reilly, P.E.B.; Moore, M.R.; Williams, D.J. Cadmium levels in the lung, liver, kidney cortex, and urine samples from Australians without occupational exposure to metals. *Arch. Environ. Health* **2002**, *57*, 69–77. [CrossRef]
51. Akerstrom, M.; Barregard, L.; Lundh, T.; Sallsten, G. The relationship between cadmium in kidney and cadmium in urine and blood in an environmentally exposed population. *Toxicol. Appl. Pharmacol.* **2013**, *268*, 286–293. [CrossRef]

52. Roels, H.A.; Lauwerys, R.; Dardenne, A.N. The critical level of cadmium in human renal cortex: A reevaluation. *Toxicol. Lett.* **1983**, *15*, 357–360. [CrossRef]
53. Buser, M.C.; Ingber, S.Z.; Raines, N.; Fowler, D.A.; Scinicariello, F. Urinary and blood cadmium and lead and kidney function: NHANES 2007-2012. *Int. J. Hyg. Environ. Health* **2016**, *219*, 261–267. [CrossRef] [PubMed]
54. Weaver, V.M.; Kim, N.-S.; Jaar, B.G.; Schwartz, B.S.; Parsons, P.J.; Steuerwald, A.J.; Todd, A.C.; Simon, D.; Lee, B.-K. Associations of low-level urine cadmium with kidney function in lead workers. *Occup. Environ. Med.* **2011**, *68*, 250–256. [CrossRef] [PubMed]
55. Jin, R.; Zhu, X.; Shrubsole, J.M.; Yu, C.; Xia, Z.; Dai, Q. Associations of renal function with urinary excretion of metals: Evidence from NHANES 2003-2012. *Environ. Int.* **2018**, *121*, 1355–1362. [CrossRef] [PubMed]
56. Nomiyama, K.; Foulkes, E.C. Reabsorption of filtered cadmium-metallothionein in the rabbit kidney. *Proc. Soc. Exp. Biol. Med.* **1977**, *156*, 97–99. [CrossRef]
57. Roels, H.A.; Bernard, A.M.; Buchet, J.P.; Lauwerys, R.R.; Hotter, G.; Ramis, I.U.; Mutti, A.; Franchini, I.; Bundschuh, I.; Stolte, H.; et al. Markers of early renal changes induced by industrial pollutants. III Application to workers exposed to cadmium. *Occup. Environ. Med.* **1993**, *50*, 37–48. [CrossRef]
58. Kim, Y.-D.; Yim, D.-H.; Eom, S.-Y.; Moon, S.-I.; Park, C.-H.; Kim, G.-B.; Uy, S.-D.; Choi, B.-S.; Park, J.-D.; Kim, H. Temporal changes in urinary levels of cadmium, N-acetyl-β-D-gluosaminidase and β2-miocroglobuilin in individuals in a cadmium-contaminated area. *Environ. Toxicol. Pharmacol.* **2015**, *39*, 35–41. [CrossRef]
59. Forman, D.T. Beta-2 microglobulin—An immunogenetic marker of inflammatory and malignant origin. *Ann. Clin. Lab. Sci.* **1982**, *12*, 447–451.
60. Heymsfield, S.B.; Arteaga, C.; McManus, C.; Smith, J.; Moffitt, S. Measurement of muscle mass in humans: Validity of the 24-hour urinary creatinine method. *Am. J. Clin. Nutr.* **1983**, *37*, 478–494. [CrossRef]

toxics

MDPI

Article

Association between Heavy Metals and Rare Earth Elements with Acute Ischemic Stroke: A Case-Control Study Conducted in the Canary Islands (Spain)

Florián Medina-Estévez [1], Manuel Zumbado [2], Octavio P. Luzardo [2], Ángel Rodríguez-Hernández [2], Luis D. Boada [2], Fernando Fernández-Fuertes [1], María Elvira Santandreu-Jimenez [1] and Luis Alberto Henríquez-Hernández [2,*]

1 Rehabilitation Service, Complejo Hospitalario Insular-Materno Infantil (CHUIMI), Avenida Marítima del Sur, 35016 Las Palmas de Gran Canaria, Spain; florianmed@gmail.com (F.M.-E.); fferfue@gobiernodecanarias.org (F.F.-F.); maviras@yahoo.es (M.E.S.-J.)

2 Toxicology Unit, Research Institute of Biomedical and Health Sciences (IUIBS), Department of Clinical Sciences, Universidad de Las Palmas de Gran Canaria (ULPGC), Paseo Blas Cabrera Felipe s/n, 35016 Las Palmas de Gran Canaria, Spain; manuel.zumbado@ulpgc.es (M.Z.); octavio.perez@ulpgc.es (O.P.L.); anrodrivet@gmail.com (Á.R.-H.); luis.boada@ulpgc.es (L.D.B.)

* Correspondence: luis.henriquez@ulpgc.es

Received: 7 August 2020; Accepted: 31 August 2020; Published: 2 September 2020

Abstract: The role of inorganic elements as risk factors for stroke has been suggested. We designed a case-control study to explore the role of 45 inorganic elements as factors associated with stroke in 92 patients and 83 controls. Nineteen elements were detected in >80% of patients and 21 were detected in >80% of controls. Blood level of lead was significantly higher among patients (11.2 vs. 9.03 ng/mL) while gold and cerium were significantly higher among controls (0.013 vs. 0.007 ng/mL; and 18.0 vs. 15.0 ng/mL). Lead was associated with stroke in univariate and multivariate analysis (OR = 1.65 (95% CI, 1.09–2.50) and OR = 1.91 (95% CI, 1.20–3.04), respectively). Gold and cerium showed an inverse association with stroke in multivariate analysis (OR = 0.81 (95% CI, 0.69–0.95) and OR = 0.50 (95% CI, 0.31–0.78)). Future studies are needed to elucidate the potential sources of exposure and disclose the mechanisms of action.

Keywords: stroke; cerebrovascular accident; heavy metal; rare earth element; case-control study

1. Introduction

Ischemic stroke is a sudden disorder of cerebral blood flow that temporarily or permanently alters the function of a certain region of the brain. According to the World Stroke Organization (WSO), age-adjusted rate for ischemic stroke per 100,000 populations was 142.34 in 2016. Over 9.5 million new cases were diagnosed during that year [1]. Prevalence of stroke in US population younger than 60 years old is around 2%, but this proportion rises to 6% and 15% in people older than 60 and 80 years old, respectively [2]. In Spain, it has been estimated a prevalence of stroke of 6.4% in subjects older than 70 years [3].

Age-adjusted incidence ranges from 50 to 250 per 100,000 populations in France and Portugal, respectively [4]. In our country, for a similar period, incidence ranged from 99 to 206 per 100,000 populations, depending on the region in which the study was conducted [4]. The Canary Islands are the second region of Spain with the lowest adjusted rate of stroke (25.33 per 100,000 men and 19.66 per 100,000 women) [3].

Stroke is the second leading cause of death worldwide, and the third leading cause of disability [5]. In Spain, mortality has decreased considerably during the past decades, standing at around 50 per

100,000 inhabits for both sexes [6]. The Canary Islands are the second autonomous community in Spain with the lowest adjusted rate of cerebrovascular deaths (25.3 per 100,000 males and 19.7 per 100,000 women) [3].

The main risk factors for stroke are mostly modifiable factors such as hypertension, dyslipidemia, diabetes, smoking, low physical activity levels, unhealthy diet and abdominal obesity [2]. Age, gender, race/ethnicity or genetics also have an important role for the disease [7]. New risk factors for stroke have been proposed during the last decades. Some of them have emerged as protective factors (i.e., antiplatelet therapy) while others seem to increase the risk of stroke (i.e., sleep apnea or lipoprotein levels) [2]. However, their contribution to stroke risk is less well defined and understood. This is the case of environmental pollutants. In addition to gaseous and particulate air pollutants [8], persistent organic pollutants (POPs) seem to play an important role in development of stroke [9]. Although the association had been seen for years, it has recently been observed that elevated serum POPs levels were associated with an increased risk of stroke, specifically for organochlorine pesticides (p,p′-DDE) and polychlorinated biphenyls (PCB-118, -156 and -138) [10], possibly due to an association with hypertension [11,12] and obesity [13].

Among environmental pollutants, toxic heavy metals and metalloids are among the most dangerous because they are also not biodegradable and tend to accumulate in environmental compartments [14]. According to their high degree of toxicity, arsenic, cadmium, lead and mercury are usually highlighted among others [14]. However, the Agency for Toxic Substances and Disease Registry (ATSDR) publishes a list of priority chemicals that are determined to represent the most significant potential threat to human health because of their known or suspected toxicity, together with the potential human exposure. Additionally, there are a number of elements, the rare earth elements (REE) and other minor elements (ME), which are increasingly coveted due to the large number of technological applications for which they are already indispensable [15]. This set of elements is of growing concern because its enormous range of applications makes them mobilized from the few sites where they are abundant to be distributed all over the planet [16], especially once the useful life of the devices containing them ends. Although some of these elements are relatively abundant in the Earth's crust (i.e., cerium is as abundant as copper), REEs have been included among the new and emerging occupational and environmental health risks by several international organizations [17]. Different studies have shown that some of these elements have an adverse effect on people's health [18–20], although the mechanisms of action are not clear [17,21].

Of all these inorganic elements, arsenic and lead have shown a relationship with stroke [22–25]. A significant dose-response relationship was observed between arsenic concentration in well water and prevalence of cerebrovascular disease [25] and a positive trend was reported between blood lead and stroke in a series of 88,000 workers from USA, Finland and UK [24]. However, the mechanisms of action are not clear and, for example, a potential role for arsenic methylation in the pathogenesis of stroke has been suggested [22].

It has to be highlighted that some inorganic elements are neurological disruptors with the capacity to cross the blood brain barrier [18]. While small concentrations of some elements are needed for life, most are considered non-essential and some are very toxic even at very low concentrations. Some elements follow a hormetic dose–response curve and may cause, at a very low dose, the opposite effect to a high dose [26]. Thus, the presence of these elements into neurons, even at low concentrations, seems to be able to modify brain homeostasis. This is the case of gadolinium and tantalum whose tissue concentrations were higher among patients with brain cancer compared to a control group [18]. The aim of the present study was to evaluate the contribution of 45 inorganic elements—including trace elements, elements included in the priority list of substances of the Agency for Toxic Substances and Disease Registry (ATSDR), and REE and other elements used in electronic devices—as factors associated with stroke.

2. Patients and Methods

2.1. Study Design and Participants

We designed a case-control study aimed to disclose the role of inorganic elements in the stroke. The study was approved by the Research Ethics Committee of the CHUIMI on 23 February 2017 (ID number: CEIm-CHUIMI-2017/907). For that, a total of 92 patients diagnosed with ischemic stroke and admitted into the Complejo Hospitalario Insular-Materno Infantil CHUIMI for rehabilitation were included in the study. The control group consisted of patients admitted to the rehabilitation service for other causes. The final number of control subjects was 83. The recruitment was made between April 2017 and April 2018. The inclusion criteria for cases were: (i) having been diagnosed of stroke in the 12 months prior to being referred to the Rehabilitation Service, (ii) ability to agree to participate in the study (signed informed consent) and (iii) being over 18 years old. The inclusion criteria for controls were: (i) admission diagnosis unrelated with stroke (i.e., traumatic diseases), (ii) never having been diagnosed with stroke, (iii) ability to agree to participate in the study (signed informed consent) and (iv) being over 18 years. Cases and controls were matched in terms of age and gender making a selection of cases in relation to the demographic characteristics of the cases.

Patients—cases and controls—were contacted and asked to participate in the study. All patients signed the informed consent before entering the study. The study was approved by the Research Ethics Committee of the CHUIMI (study number CEIm-CHUIMI-2017/907).

Barthel index, an instrument widely used to evaluate independency and measures the capacity of the person for the execution of ten basic activities in daily life [27], was recorded three months after the admission in the rehabilitation service. The demographic and clinical data of the patients included in the study were collected from the corresponding medical records and are shown in Table 1.

Table 1. Demographic characteristics of study participants.

	Cases *N* (%)	Controls *N* (%)	*p*-Value
All participants	92 (52.6)	83 (47.4)	
Gender			
Male	47 (51.1)	43 (51.8)	0.924 [a]
Female	45 (48.9)	40 (48.2)	
Age (years)			
Mean ± SD	64.1 ± 12.7	61.7 ± 14.8	0.472 [b]
Median	64	65	
Range	34–87	33–86	
Smoker (yes)	31 (33.7)	14 (16.9)	0.015 [a]
Diabetes (yes)	25 (27.2)	29 (34.9)	0.326 [a]
Arterial hypertension (yes)	61 (66.3)	28 (33.7)	<0.0001 [a]
Dyslipidemia (yes)	61 (66.3)	30 (36.1)	<0.0001 [a]
Coronary cardiopathy (yes)	30 (32.6)	13 (15.7)	0.013 [a]
Barthel index			
Mean ± SD	67.2 ± 32.7	93.2 ± 16.9 [c]	<0.0001 [b]
Median	75	100	
0–60 (severe dependence)	38 (41.3)	9 (11.0)	<0.0001 [a]
61–90 (moderate dependence)	20 (21.7)	6 (7.3)	
>90 (poor dependence/Independence)	34 (37.0)	67 (81.7)	

Abbreviations: SD, standard deviation. [a] Chi-squared test (two tail). [b] Mann–Whitney's U test (two tail). [c] 1 missed data.

Blood samples were obtained from all of the participants. Samples of blood were collected in 4 mL heparinized tubes (BD Vacutainer, LH 68 I.U. Lithium Heparin, BD-Plymouth, PL6 7BP, UK) and maintained at 4 °C. An aliquot of blood was stored at −80 °C until the chemical analysis, performed in the Toxicology Unit of the ULPGC.

2.2. Selection of Elements and Sample Preparation

Blood concentration levels of 45 inorganic elements were analyzed. We determined trace elements, heavy metals, rare earth elements (REEs) and other elements used in electronic devices, as we have previously reported [15,28].

Then, 100 mg of whole blood was weighed into quartz digestion tubes and then digested into 1 mL of acid solution (65% HNO_3) using a Milestone Ethos Up equipment (Milestone, Bologna, Italy). The digestion conditions were programmed as follows (power (W)–temperature (°C)–time (min): step 1: 1800–100–5; step 2: 1800–150–5; step 3: 1800–200–8; and step 4: 1800–200–7. After cooling, the digested samples were transferred and diluted. An aliquot of each sample was taken and the internal standard (ISTD) was added for the analysis.

The ISTD solution included scandium, germanium, rhodium and iridium (20 mg/mL each). Elements of standard purity (5% HNO_3, 100 mg/L) were purchased from CPA Chem (Stara Zagora, Bulgaria). Two standard curves (range = 0.005–20 ng/mL) were made: (a) one used a commercial multi-element mixture (CPA Chem Catalog number E5B8·K1.5N.L1, 21 elements) containing all the trace elements and the main heavy metals and (b) the other multi-element mixture included individual elements (CPA Chem) that contained the REEs and other elements used in electronic devices [18,19].

2.3. Analytical Procedure

An Agilent 7900 ICP-MS (Agilent Technologies, Tokyo, Japan) was used for quantification. Instrument configuration and optimization were previously reported [18]. The elements were quantified in the MassHunter v.4.2. ICP-MS Data Analysis software (Agilent Technologies).

The analytical method was previously validated [29]. The recoveries rates were 89–128% for REEs and other elements used in electronic devices, and 87—118% for ATSDR's toxic heavy elements and trace elements (regression coefficients > 0.998 for all elements). The limit of quantification (LOQ) was calculated by quantifying 6 replicates of blanks, consisting in 0.130 μL of alkaline solution, as the concentration of the element that produced a signal three times higher than that of the averaged blanks (Supplementary Materials 1). The accuracy and precision were assessed by substituting the sample with a fortified alkaline solution (0.05, 0.5 and 5 ng/mL). The calculated relative standard deviations (RSD) were lower than 8%, except for copper, nickel, selenium, iron, barium, zinc and samarium. However, at the lowest level of fortification, the RSD was higher than 15–16%.

2.4. Statistical Analysis

Descriptive analyses were conducted for all of the variables. Medians, ranges and the 5th–95th percentiles of the distribution were calculated for continuous variables. Proportions were calculated for categorical variables. Values below the LOQ were assigned a random value between 0 and the LOQ [18,30]. For this, a specific computational function was used (Microsoft Excel (2010), RANDBETWEEN function).

The normality of the data was assessed using the Kolmogorov–Smirnov test. Since most of the data (concentrations of elements) did not follow a normal distribution, comparisons between groups were performed using non-parametric tests (Kruskal–Wallis and Mann–Whitney U-test). Differences in the categorical variables were tested with the Chi-square test. The correlation of inorganic elements with continuous variables (age and Barthel index) was analyzed with Pearson's correlation test. Bivariate correlations among elements were done with Spearman's rho test. Univariate and multivariate analyses were done with logistic regression test. For multivariate logistic regression analysis, smoking, arterial hypertension, dyslipidemia and coronary cardiopathy were included as covariates. These variables were specifically included because they showed to be a significant risk factor for stroke in the present series (Figure 1). Values of elements were log transformed before the inclusion in logistic regression analyses. We used PASW Statistics v 19.0 (SPSS Inc., Chicago, IL, USA) to manage the database and to perform the statistical analyses. Probability levels of <0.05 (two-tailed) were considered statistically significant.

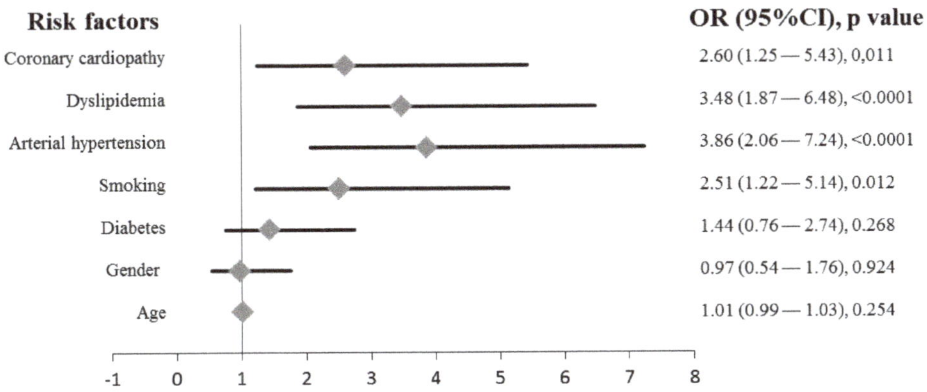

Figure 1. Forrest plot of odds ratios (ORs) with 95% confidence interval (CI) for factors associated with stroke. Each diamond represents the OR and the horizontal line indicates the 95% CI. For the binary logistic regression, patients were dichotomized into two groups as follows: patients who suffered stroke vs. patients who did not suffer the disease.

3. Results and Discussion

A total of 45 inorganic elements were measured. To better understand the main results, elements were separated into two different categories: (i) trace elements and inorganic elements included in the ATSDR's priority pollutant list, which includes heavy metal and other well-known toxic elements [28]; and (ii) RREs and other elements employed in the manufacture of electronic devices [15].

3.1. Clinical Characteristics of Cases and Controls

A total of 92 patients, admitted into the Rehabilitation Service after suffering a stroke, and 83 control patients were included in the study. No significant differences were detected in age and gender distribution (Table 1). Although it has been published that three quarters of strokes occur in patients over 65 [6], we observed that this proportion was 50.0% in our series (Data not shown).

The distribution of the main clinical factors associated to the stroke [7] were significantly different among cases and controls, with the exception of diabetes. Smoking, arterial hypertension, dyslipidemia and coronary cardiopathy appeared associated with stroke (Figure 1). We observed that hypertension was the factor that showed the highest significance (odds ratio (OR) = 3.86 (confidence interval (CI) 95%, 2.06–7.24), *p*-value < 0.0001; univariate analysis), as previously established [7]. Regarding diabetes, it has been published a 2-fold increased risk in stroke for diabetic patients, and stroke accounts for approximately 20% of deaths in diabetics [7]. However, we did not observe this trend in our series. Canary Islands have one of the highest ratios of diabetes in Spain [31]. In that sense, while 27.2% of cases were diabetics, this proportion was higher (34.9%) among controls (Table 1). This pattern of distribution makes difficult to observe the role of diabetes in our study population. Cigarette smoking remains a major factor for stroke [32]. We absolutely agree with that observation and an OR = 2.51 (Figure 1) was observed in the present series.

Mean value of Barthel index was 67.8 and 93.2 among cases and controls, respectively ($p < 0.0001$, Mann–Whitney U-test), and 41.3% of patients who suffered a stroke showed a severe dependence (Table 1). This profile is similar to other studies focused in the evaluation of disability after a stroke [33].

3.2. *ATSDR's Priority Elements in Stroke*

A total of 19 inorganic elements including in the ATSDR's priority pollutant list [28] were analyzed in the whole blood of cases and controls. Serum is the matrix of choice for the determination of inorganic elements, mainly for trace elements whose reference values are those of the serum. However, in an effort to prioritize the toxic elements whose presence is mostly found in blood cells (i.e., lead or mercury), whole blood was the matrix of study [18]. We observed a high frequency of detection in both groups, where most of the elements were present in more than 75% of the series (Table 2). The less frequently detected elements were beryllium in the control group (8.4%), and palladium among stroke patients (9.8%).

In general, we do not observe any influence of age on the distribution of these elements, with the exception of antimony and thorium that showed a significant positive correlation in cases and controls (Pearson's r = 0.26, *p*-value = 0.012 and Pearson's r = 0.24, *p*-value = 0.026, respectively; Supplementary Materials 2). Among patients in the control group, women presented slightly higher levels of silver, cadmium, cobalt, copper, manganese, strontium and uranium; however, among cases, this list was reduced to beryllium, cobalt and copper (Supplementary Materials 3). Since age did not seem to be a determining factor for the accumulation of these substances, these differences could be attributable to other environmental factors such as diet or unhealthy habits [34–37]. However, although it is known that the smoking habit is a source of exposure of inorganic elements, we do not observe this trend in our series (Supplementary Materials 3), possibly due to the low proportion of smokers (25.7% of the series was smoker) and the lack of determining covariates such as the intensity of the habit or its duration [38].

Among the 19 inorganic elements included in the ATSDR's priority pollutant list, 2 of them had a higher blood concentration among cases (beryllium and lead); and 2 showed higher blood concentration among the controls (barium and uranium). Of these 4 elements, 3 (barium, lead and uranium) were detected in 100% of the subjects. Given the low frequency of detection, the result referring to beryllium should be taken with caution (Table 2). In univariate analysis, barium and lead were significantly associated with stroke (OR = 0.34, 95% CI 0.19–0.60, *p*-value < 0.001; and OR = 1.65, 95% CI 1.09–2.50, *p*-value = 0.019, respectively; Table 3). No significant results were observed for uranium (Data not shown). In multivariate analysis, barium and lead kept their significant tendency (Table 3).

Neither of these two elements (barium or lead) were significantly influenced by any of the known risk factors for stroke. That is, neither in the case group nor in the group of controls, was barium or lead differentially affected by diabetes, dyslipidemia, smoking or the presence of arterial hypertension (Supplementary Materials 3). From this it follows that both elements can be considered independent factors associated with stroke, something plausible given the capacity of these substances to cross the blood–brain barrier and, therefore, exert an effect on brain tissue [18]. The role that inorganic elements have in relation to stroke has been studied, above all, in relation to heavy metals and major metalloids, with disparate and, sometimes, contradictory results [39]. It has to be taken into account that some toxic elements have been associated to well-known risk factors for stroke, establishing an indirect association with the disease. This is the case of arsenic, lead and specific RREs found in indoor air pollution affecting the risk of suffering hypertension [40]; or the case of arsenic, lead, cadmium and copper, whose exposure is associated with an increased risk of cardiovascular disease [23,41].

Arsenic has been previously associated with stroke [42]. In the present study, no significant differences were observed regarding to the blood concentration of arsenic among cases and controls (Table 2), possible due to the limit size of our series. Wen et al. (2019) reported median values of arsenic—among 1277 cases and 1277 controls—of 1.48 and 1.18 ng/mL, respectively [42], being significant that subtle difference of concentration. In our series, median values of arsenic were 1.61 and 1.69 ng/mL among 92 cases and 83 controls, respectively (*p*-value = 0.546; Table 2).

Table 2. Blood concentration (ng/mL) of inorganic elements including in the ATSDR's priority pollutant list (2017) [a], among cases and controls.

	Controls (n = 83)			Cases (n = 92)			
	Frequency of Detection (%)	Median	(p5th–p95th)	Frequency of Detection (%)	Median	(p5th–p95th)	p-Value [b]
Ag (silver)	79.5	0.006	(0–0.37)	80.4	0.064	(0–0.29)	0.429
As (arsenic)	100	1.69	(0.45–7.74)	100	1.61	(0.38–5.50)	0.546
Ba (barium)	100	207.0	(111.9–669.3)	100	173.5	(96.3–324.8)	<0.0001
Be (beryllium)	8.4	0.002	(0–0.20)	12.0	0.005	(0–0.57)	0.006
Cd (cadmium)	100	0.25	(0.09–1.32)	100	0.26	(0.12–1.06)	0.359
Co (cobalt)	97.6	0.19	(0.11–0.38)	100	0.19	(0.11–0.45)	0.742
Cu (copper) [c,d]	100	0.60	(0.42–0.89)	100	0.62	(0.49–0.80)	0.293
Hg (mercury)	98.8	3.74	(1.01–17.4)	100	3.65	(0.92–11.9)	0.793
Mn (manganese) [c]	96.4	8.48	(0.16–14.5)	97.8	7.85	(4.55–16.8)	0.591
Ni (nickel)	92.8	1.08	(0.048–52.6)	93.5	0.98	(0.052–76.5)	0.534
Pb (lead)	100	9.03	(4.21–20.0)	100	11.2	(4.01–25.3)	0.011
Pd (palladium)	19.3	0.002	(0–0.083)	9.8	0.004	(0–0.25)	0.352
Se (selenium) [c]	100	126.1	(73.0–205.3)	100	128.3	(79.6–169.2)	0.589
Sb (antimony)	33.7	0.027	(0.003–1.14)	26.1	0.022	(0.002–1.31)	0.151
Sr (strontium)	100	16.6	(11.2–25.0)	100	15.4	(9.93–28.7)	0.101
Th (thorium)	92.8	0.071	(0.001–0.22)	89.1	0.061	(0.001–0.12)	0.082
U (uranium)	100	0.082	(0.051–0.21)	100	0.072	(0.037–0.16)	0.024
V (vanadium)	59.0	0.011	(0.001–0.44)	35.9	0.008	(0–0.56)	0.221
Zn (zinc) [c,d]	100	5.13	(3.7–8.06)	100	5.29	(3.77–6.53)	0.652

[a] Complete list available at https://www.atsdr.cdc.gov/spl/. [b] Mann-Whitney U test (two tails). [c] Also considered as trace elements. [d] Data reported in µg/mL.

Table 3. Inorganic elements significantly associated with stroke.

Element	Odds Ratio	95% CI	*p*-Value [a]
Univariate analyses			
Ba (barium)	0.34	(0.19–0.60)	<0.001
Pb (lead)	1.65	(1.09–2.50)	0.019
Au (gold)	0.81	(0.70–0.95)	0.007
Ce (cerium)	0.61	(0.42–0.90)	0.012
Ga (gallium)	0.64	(0.46–0.88)	0.007
Multivariate analyses			
Ba (barium)	0.28	(0.15–0.55)	<0.001
Pb (lead)	1.91	(1.20–3.04)	0.006
Au (gold)	0.81	(0.69–0.95)	0.011
Ce (cerium)	0.50	(0.31–0.78)	0.003
Ga (gallium)	0.58	(0.40–0.86)	0.006

[a] *p*-values were calculated by binary logistic regression. Inorganic elements are log transformed and included in the models as continuous variables. For multivariate analyses, smoking, arterial hypertension, dyslipidemia and coronary cardiopathy are included as covariables.

Lead was associated with stroke in univariate and multivariate analysis (Table 3). In that sense, lead-exposed workers showed higher mortality rate by stroke—and other diseases, a result that supports those obtained in the present study [24]. The association of ischemic stroke and lead has been shown in other studies [41,43]. However, other studies did not report any association between lead—or arsenic—and stroke [39]. Reference values (RV95s) for arsenic and lead are 2.0 and 33 ng/mL, respectively, for adult population [44]. In the present series, 35.9% (n = 33) and 39.8% (n = 33) of cases and controls, respectively, showed values of arsenic higher than RV95s (Chi-square test, $p = 0.641$; data not shown). Nobody was above RV95s for lead. This profile of distribution of elements is similar to the general population of Spain [45].

Previous publications have observed that the levels of certain inorganic elements are higher in the control group than among stroke patients [39]. This is the case of barium in the present study (Table 2). Barium is a compound frequently used in medical tests as a contrast, which makes it necessary to know details of the clinical history that were not considered in the present study. To our knowledge, this is the first time that any type of association between barium and stroke has been observed. However, this is a modest result that would require further investigation in larger series to elucidate the mechanism of action behind this association.

3.3. REEs and Other Inorganic Elements in Stroke

A total of 26 rare earth elements (RREs) and other elements used in the manufacturing of high tech devices [15] were analyzed in the whole blood of cases and controls. Cerium, iron and gallium were detected in 100% of subjects (Table 4). Lutetium, tantalum, terbium and thulium were detected in less than 15% of cases and/or controls. We did not observe any influence of age in relation to the blood concentration of these elements among controls. However, we observed a positive correlation of some of these elements with age among cases (Supplementary Materials 2): dysprosium (Pearson's $r = 0.26$, *p*-value = 0.013), erbium (Pearson's $r = 0.30$, *p*-value = 0.003), europium (Pearson's $r = 0.25$, *p*-value = 0.014), holmium (Pearson's $r = 0.29$, *p*-value = 0.005), neodymium (Pearson's $r = 0.28$, *p*-value = 0.008), praseodymium (Pearson's $r = 0.24$, *p*-value = 0.020), thulium (Pearson's $r = 0.23$, *p*-value = 0.024), yttrium (Pearson's $r = 0.23$, *p*-value = 0.027) and ytterbium (Pearson's $r = 0.26$, *p*-value = 0.014). Blood concentration of iron was significantly lower among women, in cases and controls (270.4 vs. 292.4 ng/mL, *p*-value = 0.002; 264.3 vs. 301.1 ng/mL, *p*-value = 0.004; respectively). We did not detect significant differences between RREs and clinical variables (Supplementary Materials 3).

Table 4. Blood concentration (ng/mL) of rare earth elements (REE) and elements used in high tech devices [a], among cases and controls.

	Controls (n = 83)			Cases (n = 92)			
	Frequency of Detection (%)	Median	(p5th–p95th)	Frequency of Detection (%)	Median	(p5th–p95th)	p-Value [b]
Au (gold)	57.8	0.013	(0.001–0.80)	30.4	0.007	(0–0.28)	0.001
Bi (bismuth)	86.7	0.11	(0.001–0.33)	63.0	0.085	(0–0.16)	0.001
Ce (cerium)	100	18.0	(8.02–81.7)	100	15.0	(7.23–47.2)	0.010
Dy (dysprosium)	86.7	0.017	(0–0.062)	84.8	0.018	(0–0.037)	0.459
Er (erbium)	57.8	0.002	(0–0.027)	41.3	0	(0–0.015)	0.806
Eu (europium)	45.8	0	(0–0.022)	58.7	0.007	(0–0.017)	0.047
Fe (iron) [c,d]	100	275.5	(187.6–427.6)	100	277.8	(203.4–357.9)	0.860
Ga (gallium)	100	0.61	(0.27–4.47)	100	0.49	(0.20–1.58)	0.014
Gd (gadolinium)	69.9	0.036	(0–0.15)	63.0	0.032	(0–0.089)	0.207
Ho (holmium)	26.5	0	(0–0.010)	43.5	0	(0–0.007)	0.079
In (indium)	20.5	0	(0–0.035)	64.1	0.001	(0–0.040)	0.000
La (lanthanum)	47.0	0.010	(0.002–0.30)	22.8	0.007	(0–0.28)	0.002
Lu (lutetium)	12.0	0	(0–0.003)	7.6	0	(0–0.002)	0.425
Nb (niobium)	49.4	0.014	(0.001–0.58)	29.3	0.011	(0.001–0.57)	0.159
Nd (neodymium)	53.0	0.006	(0.001–0.28)	50.0	0.005	(0.001–0.22)	0.275
Os (osmium)	81.9	0.002	(0–0.023)	66.3	0.001	(0–0.053)	0.000
Pr (praseodymium)	48.2	0.001	(0–0.070)	50.0	0.002	(0–0.051)	0.727
Pt (platinum)	30.1	0	(0–0.014)	45.7	0	(0–0.010)	0.001
Ru (ruthenium)	60.2	0.001	(0–0.002)	22.8	0	(0–0.002)	0.000
Sm (samarium)	83.1	0.001	(0–0.067)	79.3	0.001	(0–0.045)	0.109
Sn (tin)	54.2	0.17	(0.017–4.16)	42.4	0.11	(0.018–8.58)	0.680
Ta (tantalum)	9.6	0.003	(0.001–0.28)	8.7	0.004	(0.001–0.35)	0.107
Tb (terbium)	22.9	0	(0–0.014)	8.7	0	(0–0.009)	0.410
Tm (thulium)	3.6	0	(0–0.003)	19.6	0	(0–0.003)	0.009
Y (yttrium)	54.2	0.004	(0–0.26)	56.5	0.004	(0–0.17)	0.756
Yb (ytterbium)	19.3	0	(0–0.015)	26.1	0	(0–0.012)	0.001

Abbreviations: p5th-p95th, percentiles 5 and 95 of the distribution. [a] Complete list available from B. Tansel et al. Environment International 98 (2017) 35-45. [b] Mann–Whitney U test (two tails). Significant differences are highlighted in bold. [c] Also considered as trace elements. [d] Data reported in μg/mL.

Of the 26 RREs, 12 showed a statistically different blood concentration between cases and controls. However, trying to guarantee a minimum statistical power, only elements with detection frequencies higher than 80% were considered. Thus, blood concentration of bismuth, cerium, gallium and osmium were higher among controls (Table 4). In univariate analysis, cerium and gallium showed an association with stroke (Table 3). No significant results were observed for bismuth and osmium (data not shown). In multivariate analysis, cerium and gallium kept their significant tendency (Table 3), which suggests that, apart from the ability to cross the blood–brain barrier [18], these elements could play a protective effect on stroke. The effect that gallium may have on stroke is difficult to assess since it is usually used as a contrast in various medical tests. It is necessary to know details of the clinical history to be able to discriminate the true effect of the association observed in the present study.

The role of these minority elements seems to be more important than initially thought. Thus, it has been recently published that gold nanoclusters penetrate the blood–brain barrier and have neuroprotective effects, suggesting the possibility of utilizing this nanoparticles to regulate microglial polarization and improve neuronal regeneration in central nervous system [46]. In the present study, blood concentration of gold was significantly higher among controls (Table 4) and the association with stroke was also found in multivariate analysis (Table 3). Although the frequency of detection of gold did not meet the quality standards imposed to guarantee a minimum statistical power, the present result agrees with others which suggest that gold is an interesting factor to consider for the treatment of stroke [46]. The neuroprotective role of cerium has been previously reported [47,48]. Cerium oxide nanoparticles, known as nanoceria, show a promising potential in diverse disorders such as stroke. The mechanism behind this effect is closely related to the antioxidant capacity of these particles [49]. Thus, the neuroprotective effects of nanoceria are due to a modest reduction in reactive oxygen species and to a reduction of the levels of ischemia-induced 3-nitrotyrosine, a modification to tyrosine residues in proteins induced by the peroxynitrite radical [47]. Optimal doses of nanoceria reduce infarct volumes and the rate of ischemic cell death [48,49] and may be useful as a therapeutic intervention to reduce oxidative and nitrosative damage after a stroke [47]. The findings observed in this regard in our series may contribute to improve the knowledge about the role of gold and cerium in relation to stroke.

3.4. Strengths and Limitations of the Study

The present study is a case control study aimed to evaluate the role of inorganic elements in stroke. One of the main limitations for this type of studies is the design of the groups. In that sense, we tried to minimize the impact of non-modifiable risk factors for stroke. Thus, gender and age were comparable among cases and controls. However, modifiable risk factors were different between groups, which suppose a bias that must be taken into account when interpreting the results. Ideally, the control group should exclude patients with hypertension, dyslipidemia, smokers and other obvious risk factors for stroke. Despite this, the fact that the main results were not influenced by these types of factors lends credibility to them. Sample size is a clear limitation in this type of studies. Our series included 92 cases and 83 controls, a modest number that can limit the statistical confidence. However, while it is true that similar studies have been done with a greater number of patients, other studies included smaller patient groups [39]. In any case, we tried to increase the statistical confidence by performing multivariate analysis—taken into account cofounding variables—, elements were included in the analyses after log transformation and we considered elements that showed high detection frequencies (>80%). However, we are aware that variables such as diet, details about smoking habit (intensity, duration type of tobacco and even label, which could be a significant source of inorganic elements [36]), other toxic habits like alcohol or illicit drugs intake, clinical endpoints associated with stroke (medical tests and other clinical variables like blood pressure), pharmacological treatments (antihypertensive drugs among controls) and other variables related with lifestyle (sedentary lifestyle) were avoided and could be of relevance. Similarly, we do not know the combined effect that these elements may have on human health, especially considering that exposure to many of these elements correlates with exposure to others [45]. We observed a significant amount of correlations between the elements, most of them positive (Supplementary Materials 4). Moreover, the patterns of correlation appeared to be different in cases and controls (Supplementary Materials 4, see correlation maps), suggesting the existence of different exposure profiles [37,50]. This finding is similar to previous published studies [45,50] and encourage exploring the combined action of contaminants. Finally, due to the characteristics of the study design, the mechanism of action behind our results can only be hypothesized. Therefore, the present study should be considered as a hypothesis generator.

According to the analyses carried out, the series seems robust both in its conformation and in its distribution, which gives value to the observed results. The methodology is equally robust and has been validated in previous studies [29]. Finally, to our knowledge, it is the first time that such a quantity of inorganic elements is measured in relation to this disease, which can contribute to broadening knowledge about a disease of such wide distribution and mortality.

4. Conclusions

Our study was the first to evaluate a large amount of inorganic elements in relation to stroke, including 19 inorganic elements belonging to the ATSDR's priority pollutant list and 26 rare earth elements and other elements used in the manufacturing of high tech devices. The findings of this study indicated that patients with stroke had higher levels of lead and lower levels of bismuth, cerium, gallium and osmium. These findings provided new evidence of the potential association of dysregulated heavy metals and other elements in patients with stroke, whose ability to cross the blood brain barrier has been previously suggested. While lead was as a risk factor for stroke, barium, gold, cerium and gallium appeared as protective factors for the disease. Given the high persistence of these elements in the environment and the significant technological dependence on them, future studies are needed to elucidate the potential sources of exposure and disclose the mechanisms of action of the identified elements in the prevalence and prognosis of stroke.

Supplementary Materials: The following are available online at http://www.mdpi.com/2305-6304/8/3/66/s1. Supplementary material 1: Limit of quantification (LOQ)a of elements of inorganic elements included in the study, Supplementary material 2: Bivariate correlations between inorganic elements and continuous demographic variables, Supplementary material 3: Bivariate correlations between inorganic elements and categorical variables. Significant associations are highlighted in bold. Data reported in ng/mL, except for copper, zinc and iron (ug/mL), Supplementary material 4a: Bivariate Spearman correlations between the inorganic elements among controls ($n = 83$), Supplementary material 4b: Bivariate Spearman correlations between the inorganic elements among cases ($n = 92$).

Author Contributions: Conceptualization, F.M.-E., L.D.B. and L.A.H.-H.; methodology, M.Z. and Á.R.-H. formal analysis, L.A.H.-H.; data curation, F.M.-E., F.F.-F. and M.E.S.-J.; writing—original draft preparation, L.A.H.-H.; writing—review and editing, O.P.L. and L.D.B.; supervision, O.P.L.; project administration, L.D.B. All authors have read and agreed to the published version of the manuscript.

Funding: This research received no external funding.

Acknowledgments: The authors would also like to thank all participants, without whom this study would not have been possible.

Conflicts of Interest: The authors declare that they have no competing interests.

References

1. WSO. Global Stroke Fact Sheet. 2016. Available online: https://www.world-stroke.org/assets/downloads/WSO_Global_Stroke_Fact_Sheet.pdf (accessed on 20 August 2020).
2. Guzik, A.; Bushnell, C. Stroke Epidemiology and Risk Factor Management. *Continuum. (Minneap. Minn.)* **2017**, *23*, 15–39. [CrossRef] [PubMed]
3. SCS. *Guía de Atención al Ictus*; Asistenciales, D.G.d.P., Ed.; Servicio Canario de la Salud (SCS): Canary Islands, Spain, 2013.
4. Thrift, A.G.; Thayabaranathan, T.; Howard, G.; Howard, V.J.; Rothwell, P.M.; Feigin, V.L.; Norrving, B.; Donnan, G.A.; Cadilhac, A.D. Global stroke statistics. *Int. J. Stroke* **2017**, *12*, 13–32. [CrossRef] [PubMed]

5. Johnson, W.; Onuma, O.; Owolabi, M.; Sachdev, S. Stroke: A global response is needed. *Bull. World Health Organ.* **2016**, *94*, 634. [CrossRef] [PubMed]
6. SNS. *Estrategia en Ictus del Sistema Nacional de Salud*; Ministerio de Sanidad y Política Social: Madrid, Spain, 2009.
7. Boehme, A.K.; Esenwa, C.; Elkind, M.S. Stroke Risk Factors, Genetics, and Prevention. *Circ. Res.* **2017**, *120*, 472–495. [CrossRef] [PubMed]
8. Shah, A.S.; Lee, K.K.; McAllister, D.A.; Hunter, A.; Nair, H.; Whiteley, W.; Langrish, J.P.; Newby, D.E.; Mills, N.L. Short term exposure to air pollution and stroke: Systematic review and meta-analysis. *BMJ* **2015**, *350*, h1295. [CrossRef]
9. Lee, D.H.; Lind, P.M.; Jacobs, D.R., Jr.; Salihovic, S.; van Bavel, B.; Lind, L. Background exposure to persistent organic pollutants predicts stroke in the elderly. *Environ. Int.* **2012**, *47*, 115–120. [CrossRef]
10. Lim, J.E.; Lee, S.; Jee, S.H. Serum persistent organic pollutants levels and stroke risk. *Environ. Pollut.* **2018**, *233*, 855–861. [CrossRef]
11. Henriquez-Hernandez, L.A.; Luzardo, O.P.; Zumbado, M.; Camacho, M.; Serra-Majem, L.; Alvarez-Leon, E.E.; Boada, L.D. Blood pressure in relation to contamination by polychlorobiphenyls and organochlorine pesticides: Results from a population-based study in the Canary Islands (Spain). *Environ. Res.* **2014**, *135*, 48–54. [CrossRef]
12. Henriquez-Hernandez, L.A.; Luzardo, O.P.; Zumbado, M.; Serra-Majem, L.; Valeron, P.F.; Camacho, M.; Alvarez-Perez, J.; Salas-Salvado, J.; Boada, L.D. Determinants of increasing serum POPs in a population at high risk for cardiovascular disease. Results from the PREDIMED-CANARIAS study. *Environ. Res.* **2017**, *156*, 477–484. [CrossRef]
13. Henriquez-Hernandez, L.A.; Luzardo, O.P.; Valeron, P.F.; Zumbado, M.; Serra-Majem, L.; Camacho, M.; Gonzalez-Antuna, A.; Boada, L.D. Persistent organic pollutants and risk of diabetes and obesity on healthy adults: Results from a cross-sectional study in Spain. *Sci. Total Environ.* **2017**, *607–608*, 1096–1102. [CrossRef]
14. Hussain, M.; Mumtaz, S. E-waste: Impacts, issues and management strategies. *Rev. Environ. Health* **2014**, *29*, 53–58. [CrossRef] [PubMed]
15. Tansel, B. From electronic consumer products to e-wastes: Global outlook, waste quantities, recycling challenges. *Environ. Int.* **2017**, *98*, 35–45. [CrossRef] [PubMed]
16. Bozlaker, A.; Prospero, J.M.; Fraser, M.P.; Chellam, S. Quantifying the contribution of long-range Saharan dust transport on particulate matter concentrations in Houston, Texas, using detailed elemental analysis. *Environ. Sci. Technol.* **2013**, *47*, 10179–10187. [CrossRef] [PubMed]
17. Pagano, G.; Aliberti, F.; Guida, M.; Oral, R.; Siciliano, A.; Trifuoggi, M.; Tommasi, F. Rare earth elements in human and animal health: State of art and research priorities. *Environ. Res.* **2015**, *142*, 215–220. [CrossRef] [PubMed]
18. Gaman, L.; Radoi, M.P.; Delia, C.E.; Luzardo, O.P.; Zumbado, M.; Rodriguez-Hernandez, A.; Stoian, I.; Gilca, M.; Boada, L.D.; Henriquez-Hernandez, L.A. Concentration of heavy metals and rare earth elements in patients with brain tumours: Analysis in tumour tissue, non-tumour tissue, and blood. *Int. J. Environ. Health Res.* **2019**, 1–14. [CrossRef] [PubMed]
19. Henriquez-Hernandez, L.A.; Boada, L.D.; Carranza, C.; Perez-Arellano, J.L.; Gonzalez-Antuna, A.; Camacho, M.; Almeida-Gonzalez, M.; Zumbado, M.; Luzardo, O.P. Blood levels of toxic metals and rare earth elements commonly found in e-waste may exert subtle effects on hemoglobin concentration in sub-Saharan immigrants. *Environ. Int.* **2017**, *109*, 20–28. [CrossRef] [PubMed]
20. Cabrera-Rodriguez, R.; Luzardo, O.P.; Gonzalez-Antuna, A.; Boada, L.D.; Almeida-Gonzalez, M.; Camacho, M.; Zumbado, M.; Acosta-Dacal, A.C.; Rial-Berriel, C.; Henriquez-Hernandez, L.A. Occurrence of 44 elements in human cord blood and their association with growth indicators in newborns. *Environ. Int.* **2018**, *116*, 43–51. [CrossRef]
21. Pagano, G.; Guida, M.; Tommasi, F.; Oral, R. Health effects and toxicity mechanisms of rare earth elements-Knowledge gaps and research prospects. *Ecotoxicol. Environ. Saf.* **2015**, *115*, 40–48. [CrossRef]
22. Tsinovoi, C.L.; Xun, P.; McClure, L.A.; Carioni, V.M.O.; Brockman, J.D.; Cai, J.; Guallar, E.; Cushman, M.; Unverzagt, F.W.; Howard, V.J.; et al. Arsenic Exposure in Relation to Ischemic Stroke: The Reasons for Geographic and Racial Differences in Stroke Study. *Stroke* **2018**, *49*, 19–26. [CrossRef]

23. Moon, K.A.; Oberoi, S.; Barchowsky, A.; Chen, Y.; Guallar, E.; Nachman, K.E.; Rahman, M.; Sohel, N.; D'Ippoliti, D.; Wade, T.J.; et al. A dose-response meta-analysis of chronic arsenic exposure and incident cardiovascular disease. *Int. J. Epidemiol.* **2017**, *46*, 1924–1939. [CrossRef]
24. Steenland, K.; Barry, V.; Anttila, A.; Sallmen, M.; McElvenny, D.; Todd, A.C.; Straif, K. A cohort mortality study of lead-exposed workers in the USA, Finland and the UK. *Occup. Environ. Med.* **2017**, *74*, 785–791. [CrossRef] [PubMed]
25. Chiou, H.Y.; Huang, W.I.; Su, C.L.; Chang, S.F.; Hsu, Y.H.; Chen, C.J. Dose-response relationship between prevalence of cerebrovascular disease and ingested inorganic arsenic. *Stroke* **1997**, *28*, 1717–1723. [CrossRef] [PubMed]
26. Tchounwou, P.B.; Yedjou, C.G.; Patlolla, A.K.; Sutton, D.J. Heavy metal toxicity and the environment. *Exp. Suppl.* **2012**, *101*, 133–164. [PubMed]
27. Cid-Ruzafa, J.; Damian-Moreno, J. Disability evaluation: Barthel's index. *Rev. Esp. Salud. Publica* **1997**, *71*, 127–137. [CrossRef] [PubMed]
28. ATSDR. Agency for Toxic Substances and Disease Registry. 2018. Available online: https://www.atsdr.cdc.gov/ (accessed on 27 January 2020).
29. Gonzalez-Antuna, A.; Camacho, M.; Henriquez-Hernandez, L.A.; Boada, L.D.; Almeida-Gonzalez, M.; Zumbado, M.; Luzardo, O.P. Simultaneous quantification of 49 elements associated to e-waste in human blood by ICP-MS for routine analysis. *MethodsX* **2017**, *4*, 328–334. [CrossRef]
30. Lubin, J.H.; Colt, J.S.; Camann, D.; Davis, S.; Cerhan, J.R.; Severson, R.K.; Bernstein, L.; Hartge, P. Epidemiologic evaluation of measurement data in the presence of detection limits. *Environ. Health Perspect.* **2004**, *112*, 1691–1696. [CrossRef]
31. Orozco-Beltran, D.; Sanchez, E.; Garrido, A.; Quesada, J.A.; Carratala-Munuera, M.C.; Gil-Guillen, V.F. Trends in Mortality From Diabetes Mellitus in Spain: 1998–2013. *Rev. Esp. Cardiol. (Engl. Ed.)* **2017**, *70*, 433–443. [CrossRef]
32. Wolf, P.A.; D'Agostino, R.B.; Belanger, A.J.; Kannel, W.B. Probability of stroke: A risk profile from the Framingham Study. *Stroke* **1991**, *22*, 312–318. [CrossRef]
33. Musa, K.I.; Keegan, T.J. The change of Barthel Index scores from the time of discharge until 3-month post-discharge among acute stroke patients in Malaysia: A random intercept model. *PLoS ONE* **2018**, *13*, e0208594. [CrossRef]
34. Furst, A. Can nutrition affect chemical toxicity? *Int. J. Toxicol.* **2002**, *21*, 419–424. [CrossRef]
35. Starling, P.; Charlton, K.; McMahon, A.T.; Lucas, C. Fish intake during pregnancy and foetal neurodevelopment—A systematic review of the evidence. *Nutrients* **2015**, *7*, 2001–2014. [CrossRef] [PubMed]
36. Zumbado, M.; Luzardo, O.P.; Rodriguez-Hernandez, A.; Boada, L.D.; Henriquez-Hernandez, L.A. Differential exposure to 33 toxic elements through cigarette smoking, based on the type of tobacco and rolling paper used. *Environ. Res.* **2019**, *169*, 368–376. [CrossRef] [PubMed]
37. Badea, M.; Luzardo, O.P.; Gonzalez-Antuna, A.; Zumbado, M.; Rogozea, L.; Floroian, L.; Alexandrescu, D.; Moga, M.; Gaman, L.; Radoi, M.; et al. Body burden of toxic metals and rare earth elements in non-smokers, cigarette smokers and electronic cigarette users. *Environ. Res.* **2018**, *166*, 269–275. [CrossRef] [PubMed]
38. Mezynska, M.; Brzoska, M.M. Environmental exposure to cadmium-a risk for health of the general population in industrialized countries and preventive strategies. *Environ. Sci. Pollut. Res. Int.* **2018**, *25*, 3211–3232. [CrossRef] [PubMed]
39. Lin, C.H.; Hsu, Y.T.; Yen, C.C.; Chen, H.H.; Tseng, C.J.; Lo, Y.K.; Chan, J.Y.H. Association between heavy metal levels and acute ischemic stroke. *J. Biomed. Sci.* **2018**, *25*, 49. [CrossRef] [PubMed]
40. Wang, B.; Zhu, Y.; Pang, Y.; Xie, J.; Hao, Y.; Yan, H.; Li, Z.; Ye, R. Indoor air pollution affects hypertension risk in rural women in Northern China by interfering with the uptake of metal elements: A preliminary cross-sectional study. *Environ. Pollut.* **2018**, *240*, 267–272. [CrossRef]
41. Chowdhury, R.; Ramond, A.; O'Keeffe, L.M.; Shahzad, S.; Kunutsor, S.K.; Muka, T.; Gregson, J.; Willeit, P.; Warnakula, S.; Khan, H.; et al. Environmental toxic metal contaminants and risk of cardiovascular disease: Systematic review and meta-analysis. *BMJ* **2018**, *362*, k3310. [CrossRef]
42. Wen, Y.; Huang, S.; Zhang, Y.; Zhang, H.; Zhou, L.; Li, D.; Xie, C.; Lv, Z.; Guo, Y.; Ke, Y.; et al. Associations of multiple plasma metals with the risk of ischemic stroke: A case-control study. *Environ. Int.* **2019**, *125*, 125–134. [CrossRef]

43. Wang, W.; Liu, C.; Ying, Z.; Lei, X.; Wang, C.; Huo, J.; Zhao, Q.; Zhang, Y.; Duan, Y.; Chen, R.; et al. Particulate air pollution and ischemic stroke hospitalization: How the associations vary by constituents in Shanghai, China. *Sci. Total Environ.* **2019**, *695*, 133780. [CrossRef]
44. Saravanabhavan, G.; Werry, K.; Walker, M.; Haines, D.; Malowany, M.; Khoury, C. Human biomonitoring reference values for metals and trace elements in blood and urine derived from the Canadian Health Measures Survey 2007–2013. *Int. J. Hyg. Environ. Health* **2017**, *220*, 189–200. [CrossRef]
45. Henriquez-Hernandez, L.A.; Romero, D.; Gonzalez-Antuna, A.; Gonzalez-Alzaga, B.; Zumbado, M.; Boada, L.D.; Hernandez, A.F.; Lopez-Flores, I.; Luzardo, O.P.; Lacasana, M. Biomonitoring of 45 inorganic elements measured in plasma from Spanish subjects: A cross-sectional study in Andalusian population. *Sci. Total Environ.* **2020**, *706*, 135750. [CrossRef] [PubMed]
46. Xiao, L.; Wei, F.; Zhou, Y.; Anderson, G.J.; Frazer, D.M.; Lim, Y.C.; Liu, T.; Xiao, Y. Dihydrolipoic Acid-Gold Nanoclusters Regulate Microglial Polarization and Have the Potential to Alter Neurogenesis. *Nano Lett.* **2020**, *20*, 478–495. [CrossRef] [PubMed]
47. Estevez, A.Y.; Pritchard, S.; Harper, K.; Aston, J.W.; Lynch, A.; Lucky, J.J.; Ludington, J.S.; Chatani, P.; Mosenthal, W.P.; Leiter, J.C.; et al. Neuroprotective mechanisms of cerium oxide nanoparticles in a mouse hippocampal brain slice model of ischemia. *Free Radic. Biol. Med.* **2011**, *51*, 1155–1163. [CrossRef] [PubMed]
48. Kim, C.K.; Kim, T.; Choi, I.Y.; Soh, M.; Kim, D.; Kim, Y.J.; Jang, H.; Yang, H.S.; Kim, J.Y.; Park, H.K.; et al. Ceria nanoparticles that can protect against ischemic stroke. *Angew. Chem. Int. Ed. Engl.* **2012**, *51*, 11039–11043. [CrossRef]
49. Zhou, D.; Fang, T.; Lu, L.Q.; Yi, L. Neuroprotective potential of cerium oxide nanoparticles for focal cerebral ischemic stroke. *J. Huazhong Univ. Sci. Technolog. Med. Sci.* **2016**, *36*, 480–486. [CrossRef]
50. Hou, Q.; Huang, L.; Ge, X.; Yang, A.; Luo, X.; Huang, S.; Xiao, Y.; Jiang, C.; Li, L.; Pan, Z.; et al. Associations between multiple serum metal exposures and low birth weight infants in Chinese pregnant women: A nested case-control study. *Chemosphere* **2019**, *231*, 225–232. [CrossRef]

toxics

MDPI

Article

Mercury Exposure and Associations with Hyperlipidemia and Elevated Liver Enzymes: A Nationwide Cross-Sectional Survey

Seungho Lee [1], Sung-Ran Cho [2], Inchul Jeong [1], Jae Bum Park [1], Mi-Yeon Shin [3], Sungkyoon Kim [3,*,†] and Jin Hee Kim [4,*,†]

1 Department of Occupational & Environmental Medicine, Ajou University School of Medicine, Suwon 16499, Korea; lgydr@aumc.ac.kr (S.L.); icjeong0101@aumc.ac.kr (I.J.); jbpark@ajou.ac.kr (J.B.P.)

2 Department of Laboratory Medicine, Ajou University School of Medicine, Suwon 16499, Korea; sungran@aumc.ac.kr

3 Department of Environmental Health Sciences, Graduate School of Public Health, Seoul National University, Seoul 08826, Korea; damage7@snu.ac.kr

4 Department of Integrative Bioscience & Biotechnology, Sejong University, Seoul 05006, Korea

* Correspondence: ddram2@snu.ac.kr (S.K.); jhkim777@sejong.ac.kr (J.H.K.)

† Sungkyoon Kim and Jin Hee Kim contributed equally to this study.

Received: 3 June 2020; Accepted: 29 June 2020; Published: 1 July 2020

Abstract: Mercury (Hg) has obesogenic properties. However, the associated health outcomes of population-level mercury exposure were unclear. This study investigated the relationships between blood mercury levels and obesity-related outcomes such as hyperlipidemia and elevated liver enzymes. Using the second cycle of the Korean National Environmental Health Survey (n = 6454), we performed logistic regression to examine the effects of Hg on hyperlipidemia and elevated liver enzymes. The blood mercury levels were significantly higher in the hyperlipidemia group (n = 3699, male: 4.03 μg/L, female: 2.83 μg/L) compared to the non-hyperlipidemia group (n = 2755, male: 3.48 μg/L, female: 2.69 μg/L), and high blood mercury levels were associated with an 11% higher risk of hyperlipidemia. The elevated liver enzymes group had higher mean blood mercury levels (n = 1189, male: 4.38 μg/L, female: 3.25 μg/L) than the normal group (n = 5265, male: 3.64 μg/L, female: 2.70 μg/L), and elevated blood mercury was associated with a 35% higher risk of elevated liver enzymes. Moreover, the effect was constant after adjusting for personal medications. These results indicate that mercury exposure is significantly associated with hyperlipidemia and elevated liver enzymes.

Keywords: mercury; obesogen; lipid profiles; hyperlipidemia; elevated liver enzymes

1. Introduction

Obesity is a major risk factor for several chronic diseases, including hypertension, diabetes, and hyperlipidemia, and is a growing concern worldwide. The prevalence of metabolic syndromes in Korea is approximately 30% due to increasing obesity [1]. A Westernized diet, lifestyle patterns, and exposure to environmental pollutants are involved in the development of obesity. Endocrine-disrupting chemicals such as phthalates, phenols, polychlorinated biphenyl (PCBs), and polybrominated diphenyl ether (PBDEs) are well-known obesogens [2], and several studies have reported that mercury (Hg) is also associated with metabolic syndromes [3,4].

According to the first cycle of the Korean National Environmental Health Survey [5], the geometric mean (GM) of blood Hg among Koreans was 3.08 μg/L, which is high compared to the US (mean: 0.68 μg/L) [6] and Canada (mean: 0.59 μg/L) [7]. Blood Hg levels in Korea have been decreasing for the last ten years, but approximately 25% of the Korean population still has high levels over 5.00 μg/L, which represents the control value for blood Hg (HBM-I) [8].

The main reason for high blood Hg levels in the Korean population is frequent seafood consumption, due to the country's geographical characteristics [9]. A previous study reported that methyl mercury (MeHg) exposure is approaching the reference dose within the Korean population, which is the allowable daily intake [10].

Exposure to Hg induces oxidative stress, lipid peroxidation, and mitochondrial dysfunction [11,12], and γ-glutamyltransferase (GGT), a well-known biological marker of oxidative stress, is significantly associated with blood Hg [13]. Interestingly, GGT levels may reflect insulin resistance [14] and cardiovascular risk because of the relationship with lipoprotein cholesterol oxidation [15]. In a cohort study from Japan, the risk of metabolic syndrome and diabetes increased with the levels of hepatic enzymes, such as alanine aminotransferase (ALT), aspartate aminotransferase (AST), and GGT, among the metabolic syndrome–free participants [16]. Thus, the hepatic enzymes may serve as surrogate markers of obesity.

Several studies have investigated the associations between Hg and health, but the population-level health effects of Hg exposure remain unclear. Therefore, we hypothesized that Hg exposure induces obesity-related outcomes and investigated the relationships between blood Hg and hyperlipidemia and elevated liver enzymes. We used national biomonitoring data to identify the variables that influence blood Hg and analyzed the relationships between blood Hg and the lipid profiles and hepatic enzymes. Finally, we assessed the effects of Hg on hyperlipidemia and elevated liver enzymes.

2. Material and Methods

2.1. Survey Data

The Korean National Environmental Health Survey (KoNEHS) is a nationwide cross-sectional biomonitoring survey that aims to monitor the trends of environmental chemicals, including blood Hg, and to identify major exposure sources. Approximately 2000 subjects (≥19 years) were annually recruited via stratified multistage sampling units to represent the residential distributions of geographical area, sex, and age. A total of 6454 participants provided blood and urine samples and questionnaire responses, including demographic information and lifestyle. The KoNEHS was approved by the Research Ethics Committee of the National Institute of Environmental Research (NIER #2014-01-01-074, date of approval: 20 March 2014), Korea. Written informed consents were obtained from all participants. Detailed study information is provided in a prior publication [17]. The present study used data from the second cycle of the KoNEHS, conducted between 2012 and 2014.

2.2. Measurement

The participant blood samples were collected in EDTA-containing tubes. After mixing, the blood samples were aliquoted into cryo-tubes and stored at −20 °C. The blood chemistry markers were measured by Seoul Clinical Laboratories (SCL, Yongin, South Korea), with a reference laboratory service [18]. Briefly, the serum concentrations of total cholesterol, high-density lipoprotein (HDL) cholesterol, and triglycerides (TG) were measured by an enzymatic method using auto analyzer ADVIA 1800 (Siemens Medical Solutions, USA). Serum low-density lipoprotein (LDL) cholesterol concentrations were calculated from Friedewald's equation [19]. Calculated LDL values less than zero were designated as 0 (n = 37). The hepatic enzymes (ALT, AST, and GGT) were measured on an auto-analyzer ADVIA 1800 (Siemens Medical Solutions, Malvern, PA, USA).

Total Hg was measured by flow injection cold-vapor atomic absorption spectrometry (DMA 80, Milestone, Bergamo, Italy) using whole blood samples. The limit of detection (LOD) for blood Hg was 0.10 μg/L. A value below the LOD (n = 1) was included as LOD divided by the square root of 2. External quality control was performed twice per year by the Korean Association of Quality Assurance for Clinical Laboratory (KSLM) and the German External Quality Assessment Scheme for analysis of heavy metals in biological materials (G-EQUAS) [17].

2.3. Criteria for Hyperlipidemia and Definition of the Elevated Liver Enzymes

The criteria for hyperlipidemia were taken from the National Cholesterol Education Program—Adult Treatment Panel III (NCEP-ATP III) [20]. Based on these guidelines, hyperlipidemia was defined as lipid profiles showing high LDL (above 130 mg/dL), high total cholesterol (above 200 mg/dL), or high triglycerides (above 150 mg/dL). Elevated liver enzymes were defined by the reference ranges provided by SCL; ALT concentrations above 49 U/L, AST concentrations above 34 U/L, or GGT concentrations above 73 U/L (for men, above 38 U/L for women) [21].

2.4. Statistical Analyses

Subjects with missing records of blood Hg, lipid profiles, and hepatic enzymes were excluded (n = 24). The final dataset contained 6454 personal records, and the distribution of blood Hg was calculated using sampling weights and survey strata information. The blood Hg distribution was right-skewed, so a log-transformation was performed to satisfy the assumptions of normality. Bivariate analyses were initially performed to evaluate the demographic variables, including sex (male, female), age group (19–29, 30–39, 40–49, 50–59, 60–69, and >70), BMI (underweight: <18.5, normal: 18.5–23, overweight: 23–25, and obese: >25), smoking status (non-smoker, past-smoker, or current smoker), alcohol consumption frequency (never, <1 time/month, 1–3 times/month, 1–2 times/week, >3 times/week, or daily), household monthly income (<USD 1500, USD 1500–USD 3000, USD 3000–USD 5000, USD 5000–USD 10000, and ≥USD 10000), and fish consumption (rarely, 1–3 times/month, 1–3 times/week, or 4–6 times/week). We divided the blood Hg levels into three groups based on the interquartile range, low (blood Hg < 25th), middle (25th ≤ blood Hg < 75th), high (blood Hg ≥ 75th), and compared the blood lipid levels and hepatic enzymes among groups. Each marker was regressed on blood Hg with sex, age, BMI, smoking status, alcohol frequency, and income using sampling weights and survey strata information. Analysis of variance (ANOVA) by sex and analysis of covariance (ANCOVA) with age were used to assess the associations between blood Hg and criteria status of each clinical chemistry marker.

Logistic regression analyses were performed to examine the effect of Hg on hyperlipidemia and elevated liver enzymes. Self-reported personal medications were considered to adjust for the effect of medicine and individual health status. The corresponding health question was open-ended, so we extracted information for hyperlipidemia-associated diseases by including the following terms: 'hyperlipidemia', 'dyslipidemia', 'high blood pressure', 'hypertension', and 'diabetes'. The terms 'fatty liver', 'hepatitis', 'liver cirrhosis', 'liver disease', and 'elevated liver enzymes' were included to represent personal medications for liver diseases. The final models were selected via model fit scores, such as the Akaike information criteria (AIC) and Bayesian information criteria (BIC). The main effects of sex, age, BMI, smoking status, alcohol frequency, and fish consumption, and the two-way interaction of sex and alcohol frequency were included in the final model with the Hg levels. Personal medication information was included in the logistic regression model as a covariate. Finally, the correlations between liver enzymes and lipid profiles were analyzed across the blood Hg groups as part of the sensitivity analysis. The significance level (alpha) was set to 0.05, and all of the statistical analyses were performed in SAS version 9.4 (SAS Institute Inc., Cary, NC, USA, 2013).

3. Results

3.1. The Distribution of Blood Hg

The geometric mean (GM) and 95th percentile of blood Hg among all participants were 3.11 μg/L and 9.01 μg/L, respectively. The blood Hg levels were significantly higher in males (GM = 3.70 μg/L) than in females (GM = 2.63 μg/L; Table 1). Blood Hg levels increased until the participants were in their 60s. The blood Hg levels also increased as the BMI, alcohol frequency, and household income increased.

Fish consumption > 4 times per week was associated with blood Hg levels that were approximately twice as high as those who rarely ate fish (GM = 4.04 μg/L vs. GM = 2.17 μg/L). Smoking, alcohol consumption frequency and amount, cooking types, education, marital status, parity, and menopause were also significantly related to blood HG, but herbal medicine had no influence (Supplementary Materials Table S1).

Table 1. Blood Hg distributions by demographic variables (μg/L).

Variables	N	GM	95 % Confidence Interval	P75	P95	p-Value [a]
All	**6454**	**3.11**	**(3.02, 3.20)**	**4.69**	**9.01**	-
Sex						<0.0001
Male	2767	3.70	(3.57, 3.84)	5.48	10.2	
Female	3687	2.63	(2.54, 2.72)	3.83	7.11	
Age						<0.0001
19–29	536	2.37	(2.23, 2.52)	3.22	6.93	
30–39	1053	3.18	(3.04, 3.33)	4.71	8.10	
40–49	1224	3.58	(3.43, 3.75)	5.25	9.56	
50–59	1434	3.64	(3.47, 3.82)	5.21	10.4	
60–69	1326	3.23	(3.05, 3.43)	4.85	9.17	
70+	881	2.54	(2.38, 2.71)	3.86	8.40	
BMI						<0.0001
<18.5	159	2.13	(1.85, 2.45)	2.76	5.61	
18.5 to < 23.0	2209	2.74	(2.64, 2.85)	4.08	7.61	
23.0 to < 25.0	1602	3.27	(3.13, 3.41)	4.90	9.05	
≥25.0	2484	3.54	(3.41, 3.68)	5.24	9.95	
Smoke						<0.0001
Non-smoker	4244	2.74	(2.65, 2.83)	4.03	7.62	
Past	1053	3.92	(3.71, 4.14)	5.82	11.0	
Current	1157	3.81	(3.64, 4.00)	5.71	10.03	
Alcohol frequency						<0.0001
Never	2219	2.68	(2.57, 2.79)	4.07	7.49	
<1 time/month	709	2.68	(2.53, 2.84)	3.78	6.90	
1–3 times/month	1033	2.94	(2.79, 3.09)	4.28	7.83	
1–2 times/week	1400	3.47	(3.30, 3.64)	5.25	9.67	
>3 times/week	612	4.03	(3.80, 4.27)	5.93	11.5	
Daily	481	4.08	(3.77, 4.43)	5.85	13.3	
Household income (USD/month)						<0.0001
<1500	1792	2.76	(2.62, 2.92)	4.29	8.98	
1500 to < 3000	1621	3.01	(2.84, 3.18)	4.52	8.79	
3000 to < 5000	1765	3.21	(3.08, 3.35)	4.70	7.91	
5000 to < 10,000	1103	3.37	(3.19, 3.56)	5.01	9.50	
≥10,000	173	3.47	(3.06, 3.92)	5.19	9.97	
Fish consumption frequency						<0.0001
Rarely	622	2.17	(2.03, 2.32)	3.07	6.95	
1–3 times/month	2030	2.88	(2.77, 2.99)	4.36	7.76	
1–3 times/week	3377	3.41	(3.30, 3.53)	5.03	9.37	
4–6 times/week	425	4.04	(3.68, 4.43)	6.20	11.2	

Note: GM, geometric mean; P75, 75th percentile; P95, 95th percentile. [a] p-Value obtained from bivariate analysis (SAS Proc SURVEYREG).

3.2. *The Distribution of Lipid Profiles and Hepatic Enzymes*

The blood Hg levels were categorized into three groups—low: ≤2.36 μg/L, medium: 2.36 < Hg ≤ 4.07 μg/L, and high: >4.07 μg/L. Approximately 45% of men and 24.6% of women were in the high blood Hg group. Table 2 shows the distribution of each marker across the blood Hg groups. The GMs of LDL, total cholesterol, and TG increased with blood Hg and was highest in the high blood Hg group for both sexes. HDL tended to decrease with increasing blood Hg in all populations, but the trend disappeared after stratifying by sex. The GMs of hepatic enzymes increased with blood Hg in both sexes, and blood Hg had a significant effect on all of the markers, except TG.

Table 2. Lipid profiles and hepatic enzymes among the blood Hg groups.

Biomarkers (units)	Blood Hg Group [a]	Male N	Male GM	Male (P5	Male P95)	Female N	Female GM	Female (P5	Female P95)	All N	All GM	All (P5	All P95)	*p*-Value [b]
LDL (mg/dL)	Low	613	82.7	(45.3	143)	1534	89.6	(52.1	144)	2156	87.3	(48.8	143)	0.0085
	Middle	895	84.5	(40.1	146)	1236	92.3	(53.8	150)	2142	88.4	(45.8	148)	
	High	1234	86.7	(40.1	146)	905	91.2	(50.0	152)	2156	88.2	(43.3	149)	
HDL (mg/dL)	Low	613	48.9	(33.2	73.6)	1534	56.0	(36.5	83.5)	2156	53.6	(35.0	80.6)	0.0012
	Middle	895	49.6	(33.6	72.8)	1236	56.4	(37.8	85.8)	2142	52.9	(34.7	80.5)	
	High	1234	49.2	(33.3	72.4)	905	55.7	(37.2	84.4)	2156	51.3	(34.1	77.1)	
Total cholesterol (mg/dL)	Low	613	171	(126	234)	1534	178	(129	240)	2156	176	(128	238)	<0.0001
	Middle	895	180	(129	244)	1236	183	(135	248)	2142	181	(132	246)	
	High	1234	184	(132	246)	905	186	(137	242)	2156	185	(134	245)	
TG (mg/dL)	Low	613	139	(49.6	370)	1534	119	(49.2	303)	2156	125	(49.4	331)	0.5822
	Middle	895	160	(63.2	496)	1236	127	(49.2	365)	2142	143	(56.5	415)	
	High	1234	176	(72.8	461)	905	134	(53.8	393)	2156	160	(62.6	437)	
ALT (U/L)	Low	613	22.2	(10.3	62.4)	1534	16.5	(8.54	33.8)	2156	18.2	(8.99	42.7)	0.0002
	Middle	895	25.5	(11.7	71.6)	1236	18.1	(9.39	38.2)	2142	21.5	(10.0	55.4)	
	High	1234	27.4	(12.6	69.7)	905	19.7	(9.93	45.0)	2156	24.5	(11.1	60.9)	
AST (U/L)	Low	613	24.0	(16.0	39.1)	1534	21.4	(14.1	32.9)	2156	22.2	(14.6	34.9)	0.0226
	Middle	895	25.8	(16.2	45.0)	1236	21.9	(15.0	34.2)	2142	23.8	(15.3	39.0)	
	High	1234	26.1	(16.7	46.0)	905	23.1	(15.0	36.5)	2156	25.0	(16.0	44.0)	
GGT (U/L)	Low	613	25.7	(11.1	106)	1534	15.9	(7.93	41.7)	2156	18.6	(8.36	56.5)	<0.0001
	Middle	895	32.6	(12.6	132)	1236	17.8	(8.60	51.5)	2142	24.0	(9.46	88.7)	
	High	1234	39.2	(13.9	152)	905	19.9	(9.04	58.2)	2156	31.1	(10.7	134)	

Note: GM, geometric mean; P5, 5th percentile; P95, 95th percentile. [a] Blood Hg was categorized into three groups - low: ≤ 2.36 μg/L, middle: 2.36 < Hg ≤ 4.07 μg/L, or high: > 4.07 μg/L. [b] *p*-Values are the significance of blood Hg levels for each clinical marker, and the regression model included sex, age, BMI, smoking frequency, alcohol frequency, and income.

3.3. Associations between the Blood Hg Levels and Lipid Profiles

Table 3 shows the GMs of the blood Hg levels and their associations with the lipid profiles. Blood Hg increased until LDL levels reached 'Borderline high'. Total cholesterol consistently increased with blood Hg in females, but the blood Hg levels decreased with a 'High' total cholesterol classification in males. The blood Hg levels significantly differed for each lipid profile after being adjusted for sex. However, the significant difference for HDL disappeared after considering age. According to the definitions for hyperlipidemia (LDL ≥ 130 mg/dL, total cholesterol ≥ 200 mg/dL, or TG ≥ 150 mg/dL), 61.8% of males (n = 1710) and 53.9% of females (n = 1989) were hyperlipidemia. The blood Hg levels were significantly higher in the hyperlipidemia group (male: 4.03 μg/L, female: 2.83 μg/L) compared to the non-hyperlipidemia group (male: 3.48 μg/L, female: 2.69 μg/L).

Table 3. The geometric means of blood Hg and the associations with hyperlipidemia (unit: μg/L).

Lipid Profiles		Criteria	Male		Female		p-Value [a]	p-Value [b]
			N	GM	N	GM		
LDL	<100	Optimal	1640	3.70	1982	2.70	0.0009	0.1054
	100–129	Above optimal	791	3.85	1161	2.84		
	130–159	Borderline high	285	4.31	434	2.80		
	160–189	High	40	4.19	95	3.13		
	≥190	Very high	11	4.05	15	2.79		
HDL	<40	Low	552	3.53	321	2.59	0.0004	0.1730
	40–60	Optimal	1658	3.87	2023	2.77		
	≥60	High	557	3.92	1343	2.82		
Total cholesterol	<200	Desirable	1955	3.64	2504	2.71	<0.0001	<0.0001
	200–239	Borderline high	654	4.28	909	2.86		
	≥240	High	158	4.13	274	2.95		
TG	<150	Normal	1286	3.59	2235	2.73	<0.0001	<0.0001
	150–199	Borderline high	519	4.01	599	2.71		
	200–499	High	854	4.00	794	2.94		
	≥500	Very high	107	4.02	58	2.63		
Hyperlipidemia [c]		No	1057	3.48	1698	2.69	<0.0001	<0.0001
		Yes	1710	4.03	1989	2.83		

Note: GM, geometric mean; LDL, low-density lipoprotein; HDL, high-density lipoprotein; TG, triglyceride. [a] p-Value obtained using two-way ANOVA of the lipid profiles and sex. [b] p-Value obtained by ANCOVA adjusted for age. [c] Hyperlipidemia was identified according to the following criteria - LDL ≥ 130, total cholesterol ≥ 200, or TG ≥ 150.

3.4. Association between Blood Hg and the Hepatic Enzymes

The blood Hg levels were higher in participants who fell outside of the reference range for the hepatic enzymes (Table 4). The levels differed significantly by sex, and the significance remained after adjustment for age. According to the criteria for elevated liver enzymes, 24.3% of males (n = 671; ALT > 49 U/L, AST ≥ 34 U/L, or GGT ≥ 73) and 14.0 % of females (n = 518; ALT > 49 U/L, AST ≥ 34 U/L, or GGT ≥ 38) had elevated liver enzymes. The blood Hg levels were significantly higher in the elevated liver enzymes group (male: 4.36 μg/L, female: 3.25 μg/L) compared to the normal liver enzymes group (male: 3.64 μg/L, female: 2.70 μg/L).

Table 4. The geometric means of blood Hg and the associations with elevated liver enzymes (unit: µg/L).

Hepatic Enzymes	Male			Female			*p*-Value [a]	*p*-Value [b]
	Criteria	N	GM	Criteria	N	GM		
ALT	≤49	2513	3.78	≤49	3583	2.75	<0.0001	<0.0001
	>49	254	4.14	>49	104	3.56		
AST	<34	2373	3.76	<34	3446	2.74	<0.0001	<0.0001
	≥34	394	4.14	≥34	241	3.22		
GGT	<73	2361	3.67	<38	3305	2.71	<0.0001	<0.0001
	≥73	406	4.73	≥38	382	3.30		
Elevated Liver enzymes [c]	No	2096	3.64	No	3169	2.70	<0.0001	<0.0001
	Yes	671	4.38	Yes	518	3.25		

Note: GM, geometric mean; [a] *p*-Value obtained by two-way ANOVA of the hepatic enzymes and sex. [b] *p*-Value obtained by ANCOVA adjusted for age. [c] Elevated liver enzymes were identified according to the following criteria - ALT > 49, AST ≥ 34, or GGT ≥ 73 for males, and ALT > 49, AST ≥ 34, or GGT ≥ 38 for females.

3.5. The Risks of Hyperlipidemia and Elevated Liver Enzymes

Figure 1 shows the number of participants reporting personal medications; 317 (4.91%) reported hyperlipidemia, 1175 (18.2%) reported hypertension, and 539 (8.35%) reported diabetes. One hundred and forty-four subjects took medication for hyperlipidemia and hypertension, both. And 49 subjects indicated that they took medication for hyperlipidemia, hypertension, and diabetes. Increased blood Hg was associated with a 1.105-fold increase in the odds of hyperlipidemia (95% CI: 1.013, 1.208) (Table 5). Thus, an increase of 1 µg/L blood Hg was associated with an 11 % risk of hyperlipidemia. The significance of the odds ratio (OR) estimates remained even after adjustment for personal medications related to hyperlipidemia. For those participants reporting hyperlipidemia and diabetes, the blood Hg GM was 3.60 µg/L, and blood Hg was associated with a 1.105-fold increase in the odds of hyperlipidemia (95% CI: 1.013, 1.207). This remained after adjusting for personal medications (hyperlipidemia and diabetes).

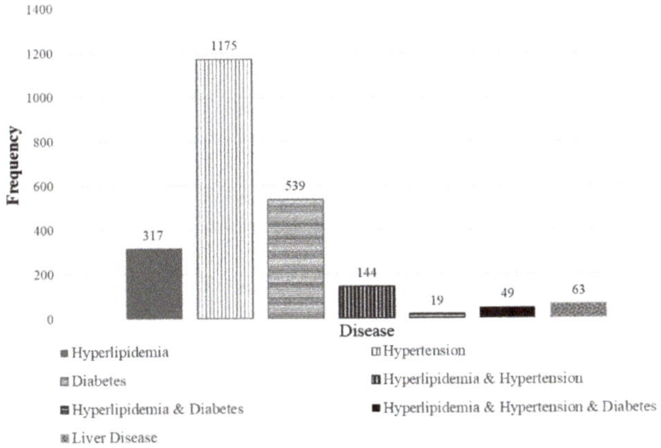

Figure 1. Frequency of the reported personal medications. Hyperlipidemia-associated diseases were extracted with the terms 'hyperlipidemia', 'dyslipidemia', 'high blood pressure', 'hypertension', and 'diabetes'. Liver diseases were categorized with the terms 'fatty liver', 'hepatitis', 'liver cirrhosis', 'liver disease', and 'elevated liver enzymes'.

Table 5. The relationships between blood Hg and hyperlipidemia and elevated liver enzymes.

Disease	Personal Medication [a]	GM	OR	95 % CI	*p*-Value [b]
Hyperlipidemia (n = 3699)					
	Unadjusted	3.33	1.105	(1.013, 1.206)	0.0252
	Hyperlipidemia	3.12	1.104	(1.012, 1.206)	0.0266
	Hyperlipidemia and Hypertension	2.95	1.104	(1.011, 1.205)	0.0275
	Hyperlipidemia and Diabetes	3.60	1.105	(1.013, 1.207)	0.0250
	Hyperlipidemia and Hypertension and Diabetes	3.16	1.104	(1.012, 1.206)	0.0263
	One of the Hyperlipidemia, Hypertension, Diabetes	3.19	1.100	(1.007, 1.201)	0.0335
Elevated liver enzymes (n = 1189)					
	Unadjusted	3.84	1.345	(1.206, 1.500)	<0.0001
	Liver disease	3.24	1.350	(1.210, 1.506)	<0.0001

Note: GM, geometric mean; OR, odds ratio; 95% CI, 95% confidence interval. [a] Personal medication information was included in the model from the self-reported response. [b] *p*-Value shows the significance of the odds ratio of blood Hg from logistic regression. The unadjusted model included the main effects of sex, age, BMI, smoke, alcohol frequency, fish consumption, and the two-way interaction of sex and alcohol frequency. Each personal medication information was included in the unadjusted model.

Sixty-three (0.98%) participants reported fatty liver, hepatitis, cirrhosis, liver disease, increased hepatic enzymes, or other liver-related diseases. Increased blood Hg induced a 1.345-fold increase in the odds of elevated liver enzymes (95% CI: 1.206, 1.500). Thus, high blood Hg induced a 35% greater odds of elevated liver enzymes. After adjustment for personal medications related to liver diseases, the OR showed a 1.350-fold risk of elevated liver enzymes.

3.6. Relationships between the Lipid Profiles and Hepatic Enzymes across Blood Hg Groups

The correlations between the lipid profiles and hepatic enzymes in each blood Hg group are presented in Figure 2. In general, the correlation coefficients showed no associations between the hepatic enzymes and lipid profiles, except for TG. The correlation coefficients between log TG and log hepatic enzymes were 0.28 for ALT, 0.14 for AST, and 0.35 for GGT, and did not differ across blood Hg levels.

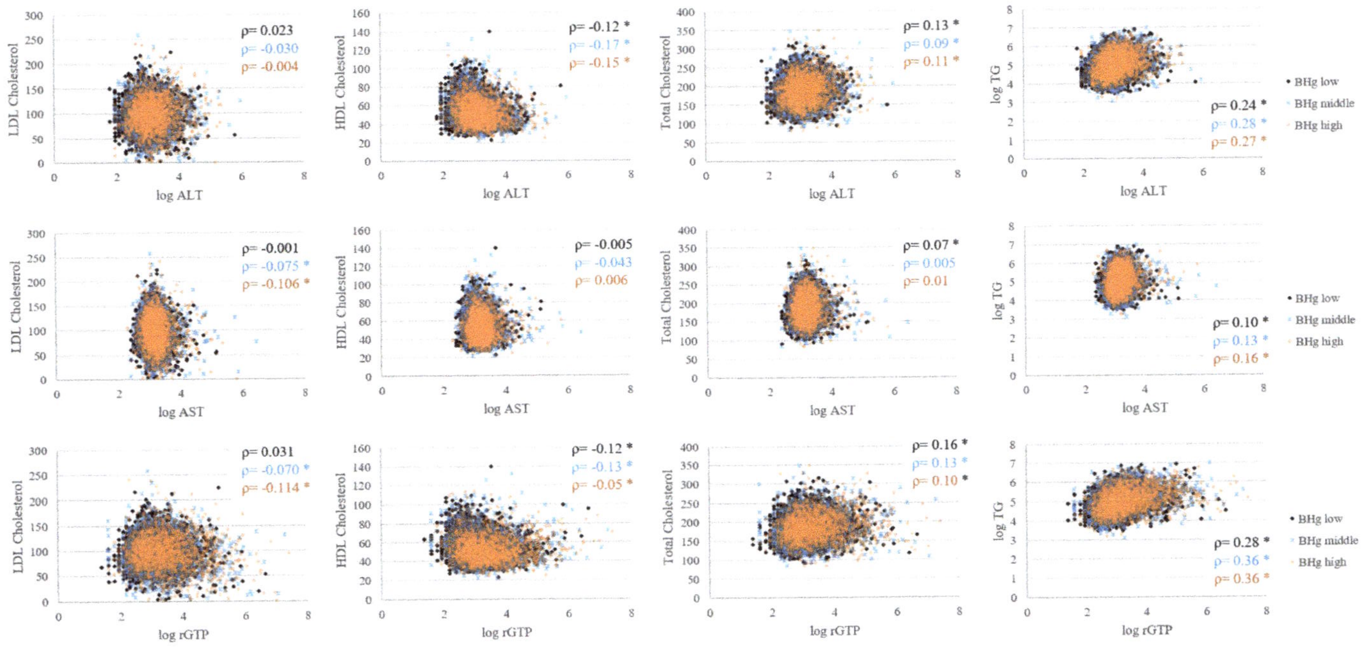

Figure 2. Correlations between the lipid profiles and hepatic enzymes in each blood Hg group. The x-axes represent the natural log scale of hepatic enzymes, and the y-axes represent the lipid profiles including natural log scale of TG. The black, blue, and orange colors indicate low, middle, and high blood Hg levels, respectively. 'ρ' represents the correlation coefficient, and * indicates the significance of the correlation coefficient ($p < 0.05$). BHg on the left side of the figure indicates blood Hg.

4. Discussion

This study used the second cycle of the KoNEHS (2012–2014) to examine the obesogenic properties of blood Hg as it relates to hyperlipidemia and elevated liver enzymes. The GM of blood Hg was high, up to 3.11 μg/L, and 57.3% of the survey population had hyperlipidemia. For participants aged 40 and above, 55–66% had hyperlipidemia, whereas 38% of the participants in their 20s and 50 % of the participants in their 30s had hyperlipidemia. The mean BMI of the hyperlipidemia group was 25.0 compared to 23.3 in the non-hyperlipidemia group. Moreover, the mean BMI was 24.0 in the normal group and 25.7 in the elevated liver enzymes group.

Approximately 32.1% of males (n = 889) and 15.4 % of females (n = 566) had blood Hg levels over 5.00 μg/L, which is the acceptable level for no adverse effects (HBM-I) [22]. These results are consistent with the first cycle of the KoNEHS (2009–2011), where 33.4% of males and 16.1% of females exceeded the HBM-I [10]. Many studies have investigated the high blood Hg levels in the Korean population. Some reported significant associations between Hg, high BMI, and metabolic syndromes [23,24], while others reported no associations or even negative associations [25–27]. Metabolic syndromes are associated with many factors, including dietary habits and living patterns, and some factors may have a stronger influence than Hg exposure. For example, alcohol consumption is a major risk factor for metabolic syndromes, and raw-fish and clam soup are popular menu items that are often consumed with alcohol in Korea. Thus, blood Hg is also significantly associated with drinking alcohol, and the frequency of alcohol intake should be accounted for when evaluating the relationship between Hg exposure and metabolic syndromes in Korea. In our study, 62.3% of males and 20.9% of females drank alcohol more than once a week. Therefore, we also included the interaction of alcohol consumption frequency and sex ($p < 0.0001$ for hyperlipidemia) when examining the obesogenic effects of Hg.

It is also possible that individual treatments for obesity attenuate the effects of Hg exposure. Those diagnosed with metabolic syndromes may actively control their lipid profiles and insulin resistance. Therefore, treatments including personal medications, could affect the associated markers and the diagnoses of metabolic syndromes. In the Table 5, we showed only the ORs of blood Hg after each medication. And the same analyses provided that taking personal medications for hyperlipidemia reduced the odds of hyperlipidemia by 29% (OR: 0.710, 95% CI: 0.559, 0.902), and taking personal medications for hyperlipidemia, hypertension, and diabetes was associated with 59% lower odds of hyperlipidemia (OR: 0.410, 95% CI: 0.029, 0.733). Nonetheless, Hg significantly affected to the odds of having hyperlipidemia.

Among the different forms of Hg, alkyl Hg is more lipid soluble and passes readily through biological membranes [28]. Especially, methylmercury (MeHg) among the alkyl Hg, is the dominant form in human blood [29] because the primary exposure source for the general population is fish consumption. MeHg exposure inhibits paraoxonase-1, which prevents the atherosclerotic process by metabolizing toxic oxidized lipids associated with LDL and HDL [30]. Therefore, Hg induces oxidative stress and disrupts gluconeogenesis, resulting in systemic inflammation that affects the accumulation of abnormal adipocytes [23,31]. Our results showed that the levels of blood Hg were significantly higher (p <.0001) in the hyperlipidemia group (male: 4.03 μg/L, female: 2.83 μg/L) than in the non-hyperlipidemia group (male: 3.48 μg/L, female: 2.69 μg/L), and that an increase of 1 μg/L blood Hg was associated with an 11% increase in the odds of hyperlipidemia, even after adjustment for personal medications.

Though bile is the major route of excretion, Hg can be reabsorbed into the blood via the enterohepatic system [12,32]. In particular, methylated Hg makes up most of the mercury in humans and can easily bind to cysteine residues [33], such as glutathione, and penetrate the cellular membranes [34]. The MeHg-cysteine complex can then enter the bile tract and be hydrolyzed by GGT and other dipeptides [13,33]. As a result, Hg induces hydrogen peroxide, depletes glutathione, and increases GGT levels. The association between Hg exposure and GGT, a marker of oxidative stress, is supported by several animal and human studies [35–37]. Our study also showed that the levels of blood Hg were significantly higher ($p < 0.0001$) in the elevated liver enzymes group (male: 4.36 μg/L, female:

3.25 μg/L) compared to the normal group (male: 3.64 μg/L, female: 2.70 μg/L). After adjustment for personal medications, blood Hg was associated with 35% higher odds of elevated liver enzymes.

This study has several limitations and strengths. The study design is a cross-sectional survey, and each measurement was analyzed from an individual spot sample. However, the dataset is representative of the entire Korean population. According to the previous studies, the intra-class correlation for blood Hg was 0.67~0.71 [38]. Moreover, diet is the major source of Hg, so we anticipate that the individual blood Hg levels would be constant. Secondly, individual health status or medical history data were unavailable. Instead, personal medication data were adjusted for the obesogenic effects of Hg. We also performed correlation analyses between the lipid profiles and hepatic enzymes to avoid overestimating the Hg effects. There were no associations between the lipid profiles and hepatic enzymes, nor were there any differences across blood Hg groups (Figure 2). This indicates that the effects of blood Hg on the lipid profiles were irrelevant to the hepatic enzymes and that the hepatic enzymes were not affected by the lipid profiles. Thus, correlation analyses demonstrate the significant effects of blood Hg on hyperlipidemia and elevated liver enzymes.

5. Conclusions

In this study, we investigated the obesogenic properties of blood Hg using lipid profiles and hepatic enzymes. Higher blood Hg levels were observed in the hyperlipidemia group than in the non-hyperlipidemia group, and the elevated liver enzymes group had higher mean blood Hg levels than the normal group. Blood Hg was associated with higher odds of hyperlipidemia and elevated liver enzymes, even after adjusting for personal medications. These results indicate that Hg exposure is associated with obesity-related outcomes and that other health effects due to low-level Hg exposure should be investigated.

Supplementary Materials: The following are available online at http://www.mdpi.com/2305-6304/8/3/47/s1, Table S1: Blood Hg distributions by influential variables.

Author Contributions: Conceptualization, S.L. and S.-R.C.; Methodology, I.J. and J.B.P.; Formal analysis, S.L.; Writing—Original Draft, S.L.; Writing—Review and Editing, M.-Y.S., S.-R.C., S.K., J.H.K.; Supervision, S.K. and J.H.K. All authors have read and agreed to the published version of the manuscript.

Funding: This research received no external funding.

Conflicts of Interest: The authors declare no conflict of interest.

References

1. Lee, S.E.; Han, K.; Kang, Y.M.; Kim, S.O.; Cho, Y.K.; Ko, K.S.; Park, J.Y.; Lee, K.U.; Koh, E.H. Taskforce Team of Diabetes Fact Sheet of the Korean Diabetes, A. Trends in the prevalence of metabolic syndrome and its components in South Korea: Findings from the Korean National Health Insurance Service Database (2009–2013). *PLoS ONE* **2018**, *13*, e0194490. [CrossRef]
2. Janesick, A.S.; Blumberg, B. Obesogens: An emerging threat to public health. *Am. J. Obstet. Gynecol.* **2016**, *214*, 559–565. [CrossRef] [PubMed]
3. Poursafa, P.; Ataee, E.; Motlagh, M.E.; Ardalan, G.; Tajadini, M.H.; Yazdi, M.; Kelishadi, R. Association of serum lead and mercury level with cardiometabolic risk factors and liver enzymes in a nationally representative sample of adolescents: The CASPIAN-III study. *Environ. Sci. Pollut. Res. Int.* **2014**, *21*, 13496–13502. [CrossRef] [PubMed]
4. Rothenberg, S.E.; Korrick, S.A.; Fayad, R. The influence of obesity on blood mercury levels for U.S. non-pregnant adults and children: NHANES 2007–2010. *Environ. Res.* **2015**, *138*, 173–180. [CrossRef] [PubMed]
5. National Institute of Environmental Research. *Integrated Report on Korean National Environmental Health Survey—The 1st Stage (2009–2011)*; National Institute of Environmental Research: Incheon, Korea, 2011.
6. Centers for Disease Control and Prevention. *Fourth National Report on Human Exposure to Environmental Chemicals, Updated Tables*; Centers for Disease Control and Prevention: Atlanta, GA, USA, 2017; Volume 1.

7. Health Canada. *Fourth Report on Human Biomonitoring of Environmental Chemicals in Canada*; Results of the Canadian Health Measures Survey Cycle 4 (2014–2015); Health Canada: Ottawa, ON, Canada, 2017.
8. Park, J.H.; Hwang, M.S.; Ko, A.; Jeong, D.H.; Kang, H.S.; Yoon, H.J.; Hong, J.H. Total mercury concentrations in the general Korean population, 2008–2011. *Regul. Toxicol. Pharm. RTP* **2014**, *70*, 681–686. [CrossRef] [PubMed]
9. Kim, N.Y.; Ahn, S.J.; Ryu, D.Y.; Choi, B.S.; Kim, H.; Yu, I.J.; Park, J.D. Effect of lifestyles on the blood mercury level in Korean adults. *Hum. Exp. Toxicol.* **2013**, *32*, 591–599. [CrossRef] [PubMed]
10. Lee, S.; Tan, Y.M.; Phillips, M.B.; Sobus, J.R.; Kim, S. Estimating Methylmercury Intake for the General Population of South Korea Using Physiologically Based Pharmacokinetic Modeling. *Toxicol. Sci.* **2017**, *159*, 6–15. [CrossRef]
11. Mergler, D.; Anderson, H.A.; Chan, L.H.; Mahaffey, K.R.; Murray, M.; Sakamoto, M.; Stern, A.H. Panel on Health, R.; Toxicological Effects of, M. Methylmercury exposure and health effects in humans: A worldwide concern. *Ambio* **2007**, *36*, 3–11. [CrossRef]
12. Hong, Y.S.; Kim, Y.M.; Lee, K.E. Methylmercury exposure and health effects. *J. Prev. Med. Public Health* **2012**, *45*, 353–363. [CrossRef]
13. Kim, S.-J.; Han, S.-W.; Lee, D.-J.; Kim, K.-M.; Joo, N.-S. Higher Serum Heavy Metal May Be Related with Higher Serum gamma-Glutamyltransferase Concentration in Koreans: Analysis of the Fifth Korea National Health and Nutrition Examination Survey (KNHANES V-1, 2, 2010, 2011). *Korean J. Fam. Med.* **2014**, *35*, 74–80. [CrossRef]
14. Oh, H.J.; Kim, T.H.; Sohn, Y.W.; Kim, Y.S.; Oh, Y.R.; Cho, E.Y.; Shim, S.Y.; Shin, S.R.; Han, A.L.; Yoon, S.J. Association of serum alanine aminotransferase and γ-glutamyltransferase levels within the reference range with metabolic syndrome and nonalcoholic fatty liver disease. *Korean J. Hepatol.* **2011**, *17*, 27–36. [CrossRef] [PubMed]
15. Mason, J.E.; Starke, R.D.; Van Kirk, J.E. Gamma-glutamyl transferase: A novel cardiovascular risk biomarker. *Prev. Cardiol.* **2010**, *13*, 36–41. [CrossRef] [PubMed]
16. Nakanishi, N.; Suzuki, K.; Tatara, K. Serum gamma-glutamyltransferase and risk of metabolic syndrome and type 2 diabetes in middle-aged Japanese men. *Diabetes Care* **2004**, *27*, 1427–1432. [CrossRef] [PubMed]
17. Choi, W.; Kim, S.; Baek, Y.W.; Choi, K.; Lee, K.; Kim, S.; Yu, S.D.; Choi, K. Exposure to environmental chemicals among Korean adults-updates from the second Korean National Environmental Health Survey (2012–2014). *Int. J. Hyg. Environ. Health* **2017**, *220*, 29–35. [CrossRef] [PubMed]
18. National Institute of Environmental Research. *Guideline for Biological Specimens Management on the Second Stage Korean National Environmental Health Survey*; National Institute of Environmental Research: Incheon, Korea, 2014.
19. Friedewald, W.T.; Levy, R.I.; Fredrickson, D.S. Estimation of the concentration of low-density lipoprotein cholesterol in plasma, without use of the preparative ultracentrifuge. *Clin. Chem.* **1972**, *18*, 499–502. [CrossRef] [PubMed]
20. National Institutes of Health. Third Report of the National Cholesterol Education Program (NCEP) Expert Panel on Detection, Evaluation, and Treatment of High Blood Cholesterol in Adults (Adult Treatment Panel III) Final Report. *Circulation* **2002**, *106*, 3143–3421.
21. National Institute of Environmental Research. *Manual for Laboratory Procedures on the Second Stage Korean National Environmental Health Survey (Heavy Metals)*; National Institute of Environmental Research: Incheon, Korea, 2015.
22. Schulz, C.; Angerer, J.; Ewers, U.; Kolossa-Gehring, M. The German Human Biomonitoring Commission. *Int. J. Hyg. Environ. Health* **2007**, *210*, 373–382. [CrossRef]
23. Eom, S.Y.; Choi, S.H.; Ahn, S.J.; Kim, D.K.; Kim, D.W.; Lim, J.A.; Choi, B.S.; Shin, H.J.; Yun, S.W.; Yoon, H.J.; et al. Reference levels of blood mercury and association with metabolic syndrome in Korean adults. *Int. Arch. Occup. Environ. Health* **2014**, *87*, 501–513. [CrossRef]
24. Bae, S.; Park, S.J.; Yeum, K.J.; Choi, B.; Kim, Y.S.; Joo, N.S. Cut-off values of blood mercury concentration in relation to increased body mass index and waist circumference in Koreans. *J. Investig. Med.* **2016**, *64*, 867–871. [CrossRef]
25. You, C.-H.; Kim, B.-G.; Kim, J.-M.; Yu, S.-D.; Kim, Y.-M.; Kim, R.-B.; Hong, Y.-S. Relationship between blood mercury concentration and waist-to-hip ratio in elderly Korean individuals living in coastal areas. *J. Prev. Med. Public Health* **2011**, *44*, 218. [CrossRef]

26. Park, S.; Lee, B.K. Body fat percentage and hemoglobin levels are related to blood lead, cadmium, and mercury concentrations in a Korean Adult Population (KNHANES 2008–2010). *Biol. Trace Elem. Res.* **2013**, *151*, 315–323. [CrossRef]
27. Moon, S.S. Additive effect of heavy metals on metabolic syndrome in the Korean population: The Korea National Health and Nutrition Examination Survey (KNHANES) 2009–2010. *Endocrine* **2014**, *46*, 263–271. [CrossRef] [PubMed]
28. IPCS. *International Programme on Chemical Safety-Methylmercury*; United Nations Environment Programme: Nairobi, Kenya; the International Labour Organisation and World Health Organization: Geneva, Switzerland, 1990; Available online: http://www.inchem.org/documents/ehc/ehc/ehc101.htm (accessed on 8 April 2019).
29. Jung, S.A.; Chung, D.; On, J.; Moon, M.H.; Lee, J.; Pyo, H. Correlation Between Total Mercury and Methyl Mercury-In Whole Blood of South Korean. *Bull. Korean Chem. Soc.* **2013**, *34*, 1101–1107. [CrossRef]
30. Ayotte, P.; Carrier, A.; Ouellet, N.; Boiteau, V.; Abdous, B.; Sidi, E.A.; Chateau-Degat, M.L.; Dewailly, E. Relation between methylmercury exposure and plasma paraoxonase activity in inuit adults from Nunavik. *Environ. Health Perspect* **2011**, *119*, 1077–1083. [CrossRef]
31. Maqbool, F.; Bahadar, H.; Niaz, K.; Baeeri, M.; Rahimifard, M.; Navaei-Nigjeh, M.; Ghasemi-Niri, S.F.; Abdollahi, M. Effects of methyl mercury on the activity and gene expression of mouse Langerhans islets and glucose metabolism. *Food Chem. Toxicol.* **2016**, *93*, 119–128. [CrossRef]
32. Agency for Toxic Substances and Disease Registry. *Toxicological Profile for Mercury*; Agency for Toxic Substances and Disease Registry: Atlanta, GA, USA, 1999.
33. Clarkson, T.W.; Vyas, J.B.; Ballatori, N. Mechanisms of mercury disposition in the body. *Am. J. Ind. Med.* **2007**, *50*, 757–764. [CrossRef] [PubMed]
34. Aschner, M.; Aschner, J.L. Mercury neurotoxicity: Mechanisms of blood-brain barrier transport. *Neurosci. Biobehav. Rev.* **1990**, *14*, 169–176. [CrossRef]
35. Singh, V.; Joshi, D.; Shrivastava, S.; Shukla, S. Effect of monothiol along with antioxidant against mercury-induced oxidative stress in rat. *Indian J. Exp. Biol.* **2007**, *45*, 1037–1044. [PubMed]
36. Wadaan, M.A. Effects of mercury exposure on blood chemistry and liver histopathology of male rats. *J. Pharmacol. Toxicol.* **2009**, *4*, 126–131. [CrossRef]
37. Schaefer, A.M.; Stavros, H.C.; Bossart, G.D.; Fair, P.A.; Goldstein, J.D.; Reif, J.S. Associations between mercury and hepatic, renal, endocrine, and hematological parameters in Atlantic bottlenose dolphins (Tursiops truncatus) along the eastern coast of Florida and South Carolina. *Arch. Environ. Con. Tox.* **2011**, *61*, 688–695. [CrossRef]
38. Lee, S.; Shin, M.; Hong, Y.C.; Kim, J.H. Temporal variability of blood lead, mercury, and cadmium levels in elderly panel study (2008–2014). *Int. J. Hyg. Environ. Health* **2017**, *220*, 407–414. [CrossRef]

toxics

MDPI

Article

Screening for Elevated Blood Lead Levels and Related Risk Factors among Thai Children Residing in a Fishing Community

Supabhorn Yimthiang [1,*], Donrawee Waeyang [1] and Saruda Kuraeiad [2]

1 School of Public Health, Walailak University, Thaiburi, Thasala, Nakhon Si Thammarat 80160, Thailand; donrawee.wae@gmail.com
2 School of Allied Health Sciences, Walailak University, Thaiburi, Thasala, Nakhon Si Thammarat 80160, Thailand; ksaruda@gmail.com
* Correspondence: ksupapor@mail.wu.ac.th; Tel.: +66-84852-5559

Received: 17 August 2019; Accepted: 8 October 2019; Published: 12 October 2019

Abstract: The present study explored environmental and behavioral factors associated with elevated blood lead (Pb) levels in 311 children (151 girls and 160 boys), aged 3–7 years, who lived in a coastal fishing community of the Pakpoon Municipality, Nakhon Si Thammarat, Thailand. The geometric mean for blood Pb was 2.81 μg/dL, ranging between 0.03 and 26.40 μg/dL. The percentage of high blood Pb levels, defined as blood Pb ≥ 5 μg/dL, was 10.0% in boys and 13.9% in girls. Parental occupation in producing fishing nets with lead weights was associated with a marked increase in the prevalence odds ratio (POR) for high blood Pb (POR 17.54, 95%; CI: 7.093, 43.390; $p < 0.001$), while milk consumption was associated with 61% reduction in the POR for high blood Pb (POR 0.393, 95%; CI: 0.166, 0.931; $p = 0.034$). High blood Pb was associated with an increased risk for abnormal growth (POR 2.042, 95%; CI: 0.999, 4.174; $p = 0.050$). In contrast, milk consumption was associated with a 43% reduction in POR for abnormal growth (POR 0.573, 95%; CI: 0.337, 0.976; $p = 0.040$). After adjustment for age, the mean (standard error of mean, SE) values for blood Pb were 6.22 (0.50) μg/dL in boys and 6.72 (0.49) μg/dL in girls of parents with an occupation in making fishing nets with lead weights. These mean blood Pb values were respectively 2.3 and 2.5 times higher than similarly aged boys and girls of parents with other occupations. These data are essential for setting surveillance and programmes to prevent toxic Pb exposure, especially in children of coastal fishing communities in southern Thailand.

Keywords: blood lead level; boatyard; childhood; lead poisoning; fishing community; lead weights

1. Introduction

Lead (Pb) is an environmental toxicant that causes serious harm to child health [1,2]. Children are highly susceptible to Pb toxicity due to hand-to-mouth behavior, high metal absorption rates, and the nervous system that is still in developing stage [3]. Pb enters the body through ingestion and breathing. It accumulates and causes toxicity in various tissues and organs that include the liver, kidneys, blood system, central nervous system (CNS), bone, and teeth [1]. Pb toxicity in the CNS cannot be restored to normal, and the World Health Organization considers mental retardation caused by excessive Pb exposure as one of the most serious environmental diseases [4]. There are no reports of blood Pb levels that are safe for children's health. Moreover, chronic Pb exposure in childhood may predispose individuals to various diseases later in life.

Chronic exposure to Pb among children has been observed in various nations, including China, Brazil, Ukraine, South Africa, United States of America, and Australia [5–12]. Previous studies have suggested that the main reason for Pb exposure in children is environmentally related [5–8].

Elevation of blood Pb levels have been seen in children living in areas with high Pb contaminations, and residential areas have often been found to be a determinant of high blood Pb in children [6–9]. Children living near an electronic waste disposal area in China were found to have blood Pb levels between 4.14 to 37.78 μg/dL [10], while children lived near zinc and lead mining areas in Zambia had blood Pb levels ranging from 5.4 to 427.8 μg/dL [11]. In other studies, children living in fishing villages near the coast of South Africa and Tasajera (Colombian Caribbean coast) were found to have blood Pb levels ranging from 2.2 to 22.4 μg/dL and 0.4 to 50.1 μg/dL, respectively [8,12].

Nakhon Si Thammarat Province situates in the southern part of the Gulf of Thailand, where fishing communities with mini-scale repair boatyards exist, especially in Pakpoon suburb. In the traditional boat repair method, plumboplumbic oxide (Pb_3O_4) has been used; the strands of cotton ropes coated with Pb_3O_4 are caulked between wooden planks as waterproofing and to prevent barnacles. In one study, boat-repair workers were found to have blood Pb levels ranging from 9 to 89 μg/dL, and 67% of the workers had blood Pb levels exceeding 40 μg/dL, the level of concern for Pb exposure [13]. Other studies detected substantial amounts of Pb in soil and house dust from areas in close proximity to repair boatyards [14–16]. Of concern, mothers who made fishing nets with lead weights at home can introduce an additional Pb source to family members, especially young children who are the most vulnerable. Data of blood Pb levels in children in these communities are lacking. Hence, the present study was undertaken to assess the levels of environmental exposure to Pb among young children, 3–7 years of age, as reflected by blood Pb levels. We used blood Pb levels $\geq$ 5 μg/dL as a warning level, established by the U.S. Center for Disease Control [17]. In addition, we aimed to explore a range of environmental and behavioral factors, known as determinants of children's blood Pb levels from the literature reports [5–12].

2. Materials and Methods

2.1. Study Design

The present study was in compliance with ethical standards. The Office of the Human Research Ethics Committee of Walailak University approved the study protocol (approval number 58/099, approval date 24 December 2015). The study was a community-based cross-sectional design that was undertaken from January 2016 to December 2018. Children, aged 3 to 7 years, were randomly chosen from the communities in Pakpoon suburb, where traditional wooden boat repairs were commonly practiced. The Taro Yamane equation was used to calculate the sample size, with a 5% level of significance and with a confidence coefficient of 95% [18]. The parents or guardians of all children provided written informed consent. We used structured interview questionnaires for information concerning a child's age, gender, birth weight, body weight, and height, together with children's behaviors including duration of outdoor play, home and school environment, diet, and health status.

2.2. Collection and Analysis of Blood Samples

The collection of children's blood samples was performed by trained nurses. Approximately 3 ml of venous blood was collected from each child with ethylene diamine tetra-acetic acid as an anticoagulant. In preventing contamination during storage and transport, blood samples were stored at −20 °C in a sealed compartment. Blood samples were transported to Bangkok RIA Laboratory, Thailand for an assay for blood Pb levels with graphite furnace atomic absorption spectrophotometry. The limit of detection is 0.03 μg/dL.

2.3. Assessment of Child Growth

To assess growth of individual children, we used the standard weight for height curves for Thai children, prescribed by Thailand Ministry of Public Health [19]. Abnormal growth is defined as underweight or overweight using weight for height standards in accordance the Thai criteria; $> +1.5$ SD to $> +3$ SD (overweight), -1.5 SD to $+1.5$ SD (normal), < -1.5 SD to < -2 SD (underweight).

2.4. Statistical Analysis

We analyzed data with the SPSS software (SPSS Inc., Chicago, IL, USA). We examined the distributions of all continuous variables (age, body weight, height, body mass index [BMI]) for skewness. Data of the variables showing rightward skewing were presented as geometric mean ± standard deviation (SD) values. We used age-adjusted logistic regression analysis to derive the prevalence odds ratio (POR) for high blood Pb levels (≥ 5 μg/dL) and for abnormal growth. We used the generalized linear model (GLM) analysis to derive the age-adjusted mean blood Pb and age-adjusted BMI. We also used GLM to evaluate an effect of parental occupation and the child's gender on blood Pb levels and BMI. p values ≤ 0.05 for two-tailed tests were assumed to identify statistical significance.

3. Results

3.1. Descriptive Characteristic of Study Children

A total of 311 children participated in the present study i.e., 160 were boys and 151 were girls. The average age was 4.67 years, ranging between 3 and 7 years (Table 1). The average body weight was 18.28 kg, the average height was 106 cm, and the average BMI was 16.6 kg/m^2. Of 311 study children, 14.8% had low birth weight and 36.7% showed abnormal growth, based on Thailand Ministry of Public Health weight for height standards [19]. The geometric mean blood Pb level was 2.81 μg/dL, and 11.9% of children had blood Pb levels ≥5 μg/dL. The highest blood Pb level was 26.40 μg/dL, and 0.03 μg/dL was the lowest.

Table 1. Descriptive characteristics of study children.

Parameters/Factors	Study Children			p Values
	All (n = 311)	Boys (n = 160)	Girls (n = 151)	
Age (years)	4.67 ± 1.14	4.67 ± 1.17	4.68 ± 1.11	0.776
Age range (years)	3–7	3–7	3–7	-
Body weight (kg)	18.28 ± 3.79	18.48 ±4.02	18.08 ±3.51	0.332
Height (cm)	106.0 ± 8.70	106.4 ± 9.50	105.6 ±7.80	0.466
Body mass index (kg/m^2)	16.6 ± 3.30	16.7 ± 3.50	16.5 ± 3.00	0.540
Blood Pb (μg/dL)	2.81 ± 3.39	2.81 ± 3.37	2.80 ± 3.42	0.947
Range (μg/dL)	0.03–26.40	0.80–26.40	0.03–20.40	-
Prevalence rate (%)				
Blood Pb levels ≥ 5 μg/dL	11.9	10.0	13.9	0.287
Birth weight < 2500 g	14.8	12.5	17.2	0.241
Abnormal growth [a]	36.7	36.9	36.4	0.934
Milk consumption	64.3	67.5	60.9	0.227
Seafood consumption	53.7	51.9	55.6	0.507
Living near repair boatyards	14.5	14.4	14.6	0.961
Parent occupation of producing fishing nets	23.5	22.5	24.5	0.677

Data for continuous variables are geometric means ± standard deviation (SD) values. [a] Abnormal growth is defined as underweight or overweight, based on the weight for height standard for Thai children; > +1.5 to > +3 SD (overweight), −1.5 SD to +1.5 SD (normal), < −1.5 SD to < −2 SD (underweight) (Nutrition Division Ministry of Public Health Thailand, 1999) [19]. p values ≤ 0.05 identify statistically significant differences between boys and girls. The Mann–Whitney U test was used to determine mean differences between boys and girls. The Chi-Square test was used to determine % differences between boy and girls.

The environmental and behavioral data showed that 14.5% of children lived near repair boatyards, whereas 23.5% had parents with an occupation in producing fishing nets at home. More than half of children consumed milk (64.3%) and seafoods (53.7%). There were no statistically significant differences between boys and girls with respect to all parameters/factors considered.

3.2. Predictors of Blood Lead Levels ≥ 5μg/dL

To screen for potential risk factors for high blood Pb levels in study children, we used age-adjusted logistic regression analysis. Table 2 presents the results of a final model that incorporated ten independent variables: gender, milk consumption, seafood consumption, signs of Pb toxicity, painted toys, use of painted ceramics, peeling of paint chips, living near a repair boatyard, and parent occupation. Of these ten incorporated variables, only two variables, namely parental occupation and milk consumption, were associated with the prevalence odds ratio (POR) for high blood Pb. Parental occupation in producing fishing cast nets with lead weights was associated with 17.54 (95%; CI: 7.093, 43.39) fold increase in POR for blood Pb levels ≥ 5µg/dL, compared with all other occupations ($p < 0.001$). In contrast, a child's milk consumption was associated with 61% reduction in the risk of having high blood Pb levels (POR = 0.393, 95%; CI: 0.166, 0.931; $p = 0.034$).

Table 2. Predictors of blood lead levels ≥ 5µg/dL.

Independent Variables/Factors	Blood Pb Levels ≥ 5µg/dL				
	β Coefficients (SE)	POR	95% CI		*p* Value
			Lower	Upper	
Age (years)	−0.154 (0.194)	0.857	0.586	1.255	0.429
Gender (boy = 1, girl = 2)	0.470 (0.426)	1.599	0.694	3.685	0.270
Milk consumption	−0.934 (0.440)	0.393	0.166	0.931	0.034 *
Seafood consumption	−0.101 (0.436)	0.904	0.385	2.124	0.817
Symptoms of Pb toxicity	0.490 (0.431)	1.632	0.701	3.799	0.256
Painted toys	0.351 (0.459)	1.420	0.578	3.489	0.444
Use of painted ceramics	0.081 (0.508)	1.085	0.400	2.938	0.873
Peeling of paint chips	0.279 (0.498)	1.322	0.498	3.504	0.575
Living near repair boatyard	0.093 (0.581)	1.098	0.352	3.428	0.872
Parent occupation of fishing net production	2.865 (0.462)	17.54	7.093	43.39	<0.001 *

POR = Prevalence odds ratio. High blood Pb is defined as blood Pb levels ≥ 5µg/dL. The POR for high blood Pb was derived from logistic regression in which high blood Pb was a categorical dependent variable. Independent variables were listed in the first column. * $p \leq 0.05$ identify the variable as a significant risk factor or predictor for high blood Pb levels.

3.3. *Predictors of Abnormal Growth*

We used also age-adjusted logistic regression to determine potential effects of high blood Pb levels on children's growth, defined as overweight or underweight in accordance with weight and height standards for Thai children. Table 3 presents the results of such analysis that incorporated seven independent categorical variables, including high blood Pb, milk and seafood consumptions, use of painted ceramics, living near a repair boatyard, and playing with painted toys. High blood Pb was associated with 2.042 (95%; CI: 0.999, 4.174) fold increase in POR for abnormal growth ($p = 0.050$). Seafood consumption was associated with 1.713 (95%; CI: 1.037, 2.831) fold increase in POR for abnormal growth ($p = 0.036$). In contrast, milk consumption was associated with 43% reduction in the risk of having abnormal growth (POR 0.573, 95%; CI: 0.337, 0.976; $p = 0.040$).

Table 3. Predictors of abnormal growth.

Independent Variables/Factors	Abnormal Growth [a]				
	β Coefficients (SE)	POR	95% CI		*p* Value
			Lower	Upper	
Age (years)	−0.084 (0.113)	0.920	0.737	1.148	0.459
Gender (boy = 1, girl = 2)	−0.116 (0.245)	0.891	0.551	1.440	0.637
Blood Pb levels ≥ 5 µg/dL	0.714 (0.365)	2.042	0.999	4.174	0.050 *
Milk consumption	−0.556 (0.271)	0.573	0.337	0.976	0.040 *
Seafood consumption	0.538 (0.256)	1.713	1.037	2.831	0.036 *

Table 3. *Cont.*

Independent Variables/Factors	Abnormal Growth [a]				
	β Coefficients (SE)	POR	95% CI		p Value
			Lower	Upper	
Use of painted ceramics	−0.552 (0.314)	0.576	0.311	1.066	0.079
Living near repair boatyards	0.561 (0.364)	1.753	0.860	3.574	0.123
Painted toys	0.277 (0.257)	1.319	0.798	2.181	0.281

POR = Prevalence odds ratio. [a] Abnormal growth is defined as underweight or overweight, based on weight for height standard for Thai children; > +1.5 SD to > +3 SD (overweight), −1.5 SD to +1.5 SD. (normal), < −1.5 SD to < −2 SD (underweight) (Nutrition Division Ministry of Public Health Thailand, 1999) [19]. * $p \leq 0.5$ identify significant associations between abnormal growth and variables/factors listed in the first column.

3.4. *Effect-Size Estimate*

We next used generalized linear model (GLM) analysis to quantify effects of parental occupation on blood Pb levels and body mass index (BMI) of children. Figure 1A shows blood Pb levels in boys and girls of parents with and without an occupation in producing fishing nets with lead weights. Age-adjusted mean ± SE values for blood Pb in boys and girls of parents with the occupation of making fishing nets of 6.22 ± 0.50 and 6.72 ± 0.49 μg/dL were respectively 2.3 and 2.5 times higher than the same age-adjusted mean ± SE in boys (2.67 ± 0.27) and girls (2.68 ± 0.28) of parents with other occupations ($p < 0.001$ for boys and girls, Bonferroni test).

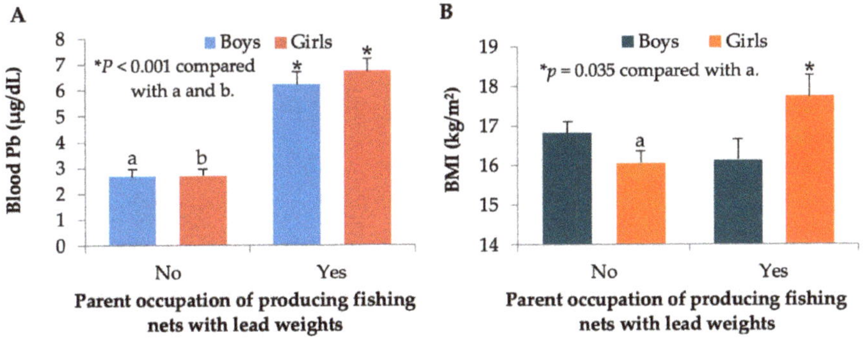

Figure 1. Blood Pb levels and BMI stratified by gender and parent occupation. Bars in (**A**) represent age-adjusted mean ± standard error of mean (SE) for blood Pb levels, while bars in (**B**) represent age-adjusted BMI ± SE in boys and girls from parents with and without an occupation of producing fishing nets with lead weights. * p values ≤ 0.05 identify statistical significance.

Of interest, Figure 1B indicated an effect of parental occupation on BMI in girls only. Age-adjusted mean ± SE values for BMI were 17.74 ± 0.53 kg/m^2 in girls of parents with the occupation of producing fishing nets and 16.12 ± 0.54 kg/m^2 in girls of parents with occupations other than making fishing nets ($p < 0.035$, Bonferroni test). On average, girls of parents with the occupation of producing fishing nets had a 9.1% higher BMI than the girls of parents of other occupations.

4. Discussion

In the present study, we examined environmental exposure to Pb among 3–7 years old children, living in Pakpoon suburb, Nakhon Si Thammarat Province. The study children were randomly selected from a fishing community, where repair boatyards were located (Figure 2). The results showed that blood Pb levels ranged from 0.03 to 26.40 μg/dL. Although the average blood Pb level of 2.81 μg/dL was below the level of concern of ≥ 5 μg/dL, set by the CDC [17], 11.9% of children had elevated blood

Pb levels ≥ 5 μg/dL. The blood Pb levels recorded for children in the present study appeared to be lower than the levels found in children living in fishing communities in the Tasajera and South Africa. Blood Pb levels in children in Tasajera, Colombian Caribbean coast, ranged from 0.4 to 50.1 μg/dL with 57.1% of study children having blood Pb levels ≥ 5 μg/dL [8]. Blood Pb levels in children of fishing communities in South Africa ranged from 2.2 to 22.4 μg/dL with 74% of study children having blood Pb levels > 5 μg/dL [12]. The 4.8 and 6.2 times higher percentages of high blood Pb in South Africa and Tasajera study might be due to different Pb exposure sources. The South Africa and Tasajera studies both found that living near a lead smelting area was strongly associated with children's high blood Pb levels [8,12]. In contrast, there was no melting of Pb weights in the process of making fishing nets in this Thai study.

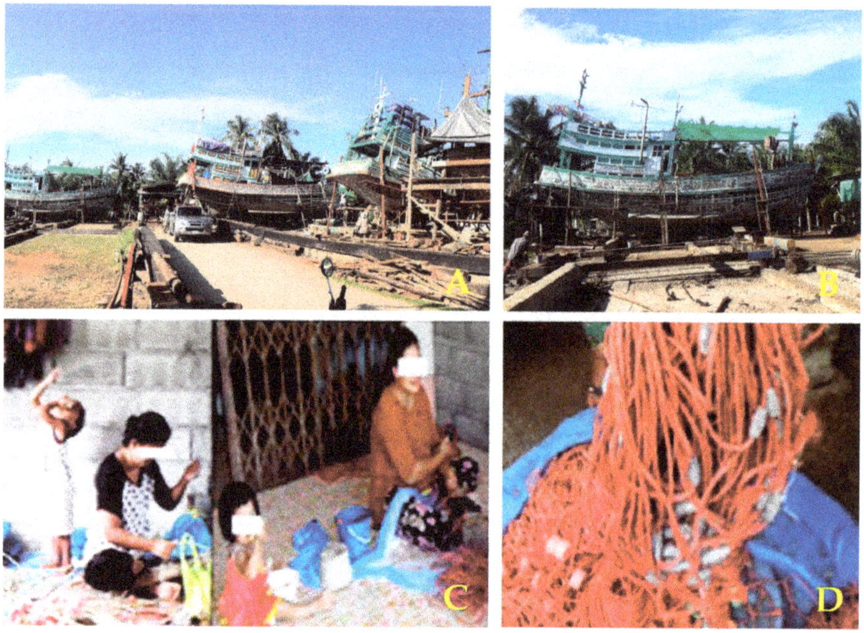

Figure 2. Boatyards, girls and working-at-home mothers, and a fishing net with lead weights. A total of 311 children were randomly selected from a fishing community in Pakpoon suburb, where repair boatyards existed (**A**,**B**). Girls were nearby while mothers were assembling lead weights to produce fishing nets (**C**). Approximately 180 lead weights are used to make a two-kg fishing net (**D**).

In the present study, we found that parent occupation involving lead weights was associated with 17.54 fold increase in risk of high blood Pb levels in children ($p < 0.001$). This might be attributable to environmental exposure via household Pb dust, water, and food contamination [20] from lead weights used in making fishing nets at home (Figure 2). However, living close to repair boatyards was not associated with high blood Pb levels ($p = 0.872$). Of note, blood Pb levels in both boys and girls of parents producing fishing nets were 2.3 and 2.5 times higher than similarly aged boys and girls of parents with other occupations ($p < 0.001$ for boys and girls). These data confirmed parents' occupation as a strong determinant of blood Pb levels. The levels of Pb in dust, water, and food contamination in the households that used lead weights require a further study. Blood Pb levels in mothers should also be investigated since Pb is readily transported through the placenta.

A child's milk consumption was associated with a 61% reduction in the risk for high blood Pb ($p = 0.034$) and a 43% reduction in the risk of having abnormal growth ($p = 0.040$). Milk has been reported to be a protective factor against Pb toxicity both in humans and experimental animals [21–24].

In an animal study, blood Pb levels decreased in lead-treated mice after nine weeks of daily milk intake. It is suggested that Pb absorption in gastrointestinal tract is reduced by the high calcium levels in milk, and that Pb absorption is enhanced by calcium deficiency [22,23]. In a longitudinal cohort study of children, aged 6–31 months [25], blood Pb levels were negatively correlated with calcium, magnesium, nickel, and zinc. It can be inferred that consumption of food rich in calcium and zinc can reduce Pb absorption. Another possible protective mechanism of milk might be due to organic substances that chelate Pb, thereby reducing Pb absorption and enhancing Pb excretion [21]. The synergism between Pb exposure levels and a lack of milk consumption is unknown. The present study indicated that milk is one of the factors that reduced the risk of high blood Pb levels in children. A quantitative study on milk intake is required.

Potential adverse effects of high blood Pb on children's growth was observed; high blood Pb was associated with 2.04 fold increase in the POR for abnormal growth ($p = 0.050$), while seafood consumption was associated with a 1.71 fold increase in the POR for abnormal growth ($p = 0.036$). Likewise, blood Pb and seafood consumption were associated with decreased growth rates in other studies [25,26]. A negative effect of Pb on children's growth may involve disruption of the endocrine system, causing circulating levels of insulin-like growth factor 1 to fall [27]. Pb may affect osteoblast and osteoclast development via 1, 25-dihydroxyvitamin D_3 [28,29]. Exposure to Pb during childhood could affect growth in adolescents and adults. This was observed in a longitudinal study in Russia, where children with blood Pb levels ≥5 μg/dL showed the most height decrease at 12–15 years of age [30]. An association between seafood consumption and abnormal growth may be attributable to methymercury in seafood [31]. Thus, children with abnormal growth rates should be monitored. Further information should be sought to identify specific types of seafood and frequencies of consumption.

Interestingly, an effect of Pb on BMI increase was seen in girls only. This is a new finding. Gender-specific neurological effects of Pb have been seen in prenatal and preschool age exposure conditions [32–34]. Such gender specific effects of Pb may be caused by gene-specific DNA methylation patterns in the brain [33]. The gender-specific difference in BMI needs confirmation. Nevertheless, the association seen between children BMI and parent occupation could be used in growth prediction and obesity prevention programs in children.

In conclusion, the present study provided baseline data on environmental Pb exposure levels experienced by boys and girls, aged 3–7 years together with factors associated with the high blood Pb levels. These data are useful in setting Pb surveillance and Pb toxicity mitigation programs for children of fishing communities. Aspects of environmental Pb contamination need a further investigation. A Pb primary prevention program should be implemented in conjunction with a nutritional promotion campaign.

Author Contributions: S.Y. designed the study protocol, obtained an approval from the Office of the Human Research Ethics Committee of Walailak University, and supervised the collection of demographic data and biologic specimens; S.Y., D.W. and S.K organized and analyzed the data, created the tables and figures, and revised the manuscript.

Funding: This research was funded by National Science and Technology Development Agency (NSTDA), Ministry of Science and Technology, Thailand, grant number FDA-CO-2559-1183-74. The APC was funded by Walailak University.

Acknowledgments: This work was cooperated with by the Pakpoon Health Promoting Hospital, Pakpoon Municipality, Nakhon Si Thammarat, Thailand. We thank Steve Nazar and George Kruzynski for editing the English. We also thanks Tanaporn Khamphaya for graphic design.

Conflicts of Interest: The authors have no potential conflicts of interest to declare.

References

1. Agency for Toxic Substances and Disease Registry (ATSDR). Toxicological Profile for Lead. ATSDR, Division of Toxicology and Environmental Medicine/Applied Toxicology Branch: Atlanta, GA, USA. 2007. Available online: http://www.atsdr.cdc.gov/ToxProfiles/tp13.pdf (accessed on 22 September 2019).
2. Cao, J.; Li, M.; Wang, Y.; Yu, G.; Yan, C. Environmental lead exposure among preschool children in Shanghai, China: Blood lead levels and risk factors. *PLoS ONE* **2014**, *9*, e113297. [CrossRef] [PubMed]
3. Jain, A.; Wolfe, L.; Jain, G. Impact of lead intoxication in children with iron deficiency anemia in low- and middle-income countries. *Blood* **2013**, *122*, 2288–2289. [CrossRef] [PubMed]
4. World Health Organization (WHO). Childhood Lead Poisoning. 2009. Available online: www.who.int/ceh/publications/leadguidance.pdf (accessed on 30 July 2019).
5. Zhang, X.Y.; Carpenter, D.O.; Song, Y.J.; Chen, P.; Qin, Y.; Wei, N.Y.; Lin, S.C. Application of the IEUBK model for linking children's blood lead with environmental exposure in a mining site, south China. *Environ. Pollut.* **2017**, *231*, 971–978. [CrossRef] [PubMed]
6. Dong, C.; Taylor, M.P.; Zahran, S. The effect of contemporary mine emissions on children's blood lead levels. *Environ. Int.* **2019**, *122*, 91–103. [CrossRef] [PubMed]
7. Taylor, M.P.; Isley, C.F.; Glover, J. Prevalence of childhood lead poisoning and respiratory disease associated with lead smelter emissions. *Environ. Int.* **2019**, *127*, 340–352. [CrossRef] [PubMed]
8. Alvarez-Ortega, N.; Caballero-Gallardo, K.; Olivero-Verbel, J. Toxicological effects in children exposed to lead: A cross-sectional study at the Colombian Caribbean coast. *Environ. Int.* **2019**, *130*, 104809. [CrossRef]
9. Lin, S.; Wang, X.; Yu, I.T.; Tang, W.; Miao, J.; Li, J.; Wu, S.; Lin, X. Environmental lead pollution and elevated blood lead levels among children in a rural area of China. *Am. J. Public Health* **2011**, *101*, 834–841. [CrossRef]
10. Zheng, L.; Wu, K.; Li, Y.; Qi, Z.; Han, D.; Zhang, B.; Gu, C.; Chen, G.; Liu, J.; Chen, S.; et al. Blood lead and cadmium levels and relevant factors among children from an e-waste recycling town in China. *Environ. Res.* **2008**, *108*, 15–20. [CrossRef]
11. Yabe, J.; Nakayama, S.M.M.; Ikenaka, Y.; Yohannes, Y.B.; Bortey-Sam, N.; Oroszlany, B.; Muzandu, K.; Choongo, K.; Kabalo, A.N.; Ntapisha, J.; et al. Lead poisoning in children from townships in the vicinity of a lead–zinc mine in Kabwe, Zambia. *Chemosphere* **2015**, *119*, 941–947. [CrossRef]
12. Mathee, A.; Khan, T.; Naicker, N.; Kootbodien, T.; Naidoo, S.; Becker, P. Lead exposure in young school children in South African subsistence fishing communities. *Environ. Res.* **2013**, *126*, 179–183. [CrossRef]
13. Thanapop, C.; Geater, A.F.; Robson, M.G.; Phakthongsuk, P.; Viroonudomphol, D. Exposure to lead among boatyard workers in southern Thailand. *J. Occup. Health* **2007**, *49*, 345–352. [CrossRef] [PubMed]
14. Thanapop, C.; Geater, A.F.; Robson, M.G.; Phakthongsuk, P. Elevated lead contamination in boat-caulkers' homes in southern Thailand. *Int. J. Occup. Environ. Health* **2009**, *15*, 282–290. [CrossRef] [PubMed]
15. Maharachpong, N.; Geater, A.; Chongsuvivatwong, V. Environmental and childhood lead contamination in the proximity of boat-repair yards in southern Thailand—I: Pattern and factors related to soil and household dust lead levels. *Environ. Res.* **2006**, *101*, 294–303. [CrossRef]
16. Untimanon, O.; Geater, A.; Chongsuvivatwong, V.; Saetia, W.; Utapan, S. Skin Lead Contamination of Family Members of Boat-caulkers in Southern Thailand. *Ind. Health* **2011**, *49*, 37–46. [CrossRef] [PubMed]
17. Centers for Disease Control and Prevention (CDC). Childhood Lead Poisoning Prevention Program. 2019. Available online: https://www.cdc.gov/nceh/lead/default.htm (accessed on 30 July 2019).
18. Yamane, Taro. *Statistics: An Introductory Analysis*, 2nd ed.; Harper and Row Publication: New York, NY, USA, 1973; Available online: https://www.gbv.de/dms/zbw/252560191.pdf (accessed on 25 January 2015).
19. Nutrition Division, Department of Health, Ministry of Public Health. *The Reference Guide for the Assessment of Weight and Height Growth of Thai Children Aged 1 Day–19 Years Old*; Ministry of Public Health: Nonthaburi, Thailand, 1999.
20. Chambial, S.; Shukla, K.K.; Dwivedi, S.; Bhardwaj, P.; Sharma, P. Blood Lead Level (BLL) in the Adult Population of Jodhpur: A Pilot Study. *Indian J. Clin. Biochem.* **2015**, *30*, 357–359. [CrossRef] [PubMed]
21. Zhang, Y.; Li, Q.; Liu, X.; Zhu, H.; Song, A.; Jiao, J. Antioxidant and micronutrient-rich milk formula reduces lead poisoning and related oxidative damage in lead-exposed mice. *Food Chem. Toxicol.* **2013**, *57*, 201–208. [CrossRef] [PubMed]
22. Kordas, K. The "Lead Diet": Can Dietary Approaches Prevent or Treat Lead Exposure? *J. Pediatr.* **2017**, *185*, 224–231. [CrossRef]

23. Kordas, K.; Casavantes, K.M.; Mendoza, C.; Lopez, P.; Ronquillo, D.; Rosado, J.L.; Vargas, G.G.; Stoltzfus, R.J. The association between lead and micronutrient status, and children's sleep, classroom behavior, and activity. *Arch. Environ. Occup. Health* **2007**, *62*, 105–112. [CrossRef]
24. Gulson, B.; Mizon, K.; Taylor, A.; Wu, M. Dietary zinc, calcium and nickel are associated with lower childhood blood lead levels. *Environ. Res.* **2019**, *168*, 439–444. [CrossRef]
25. Little, B.B.; Spalding, S.; Walsh, B.; Keyes, D.C.; Wainer, J.; Pickens, S.; Royster, M.; Villanacci, J.; Gratton, T. Blood lead levels and growth status among African–American and Hispanic children in Dallas, Texas – 1980 and 2002: Dallas Lead Project II. *Ann. Hum. Biol.* **2009**, *36*, 331–341. [CrossRef]
26. Yang, H.; Huo, X.; Yekeen, A.T.; Zheng, Q.; Zheng, M.; Xu, X. Effects of lead and cadmium exposure from electronic waste on child physical growth. *Environ. Sci. Pollut. Res. Int.* **2013**, *20*, 4441–4447. [CrossRef] [PubMed]
27. Ronis, M.J.; Badger, T.M.; Shema, S.J.; Roberson, P.K.; Templer, L.; Ringer, D.; Thomas, P.E. Endocrine mechanisms underlying the growth effects of developmental lead exposure in the rat. *J. Toxicol. Environ. Health A* **1998**, *54*, 101–120. [PubMed]
28. Berglund, M.; Akesson, A.; Bjellerup, P.; Vahter, M. Metal-bone interactions. *Toxicol. Lett.* **2000**, *113*, 219–225. [CrossRef]
29. Flora, G.; Gupta, D.; Tiwari, A. Toxicity of lead: A review with recent updates. *Interdiscip. Toxicol.* **2012**, *5*, 47–58. [CrossRef] [PubMed]
30. Burns, J.S.; Williams, P.L.; Lee, M.M.; Revich, B.; Sergeyev, O.; Hauser, R.; Korrick, S.A. Peripubertal blood lead levels and growth among Russian boys. *Environ. Int.* **2017**, *106*, 53–59. [CrossRef]
31. Chan, H.M. Advances in methylmercury toxicology and risk Assessment. *Toxics* **2019**, *7*, 20. [CrossRef] [PubMed]
32. Wang, J.; Gao, Z.Y.; Yan, J.; Ying, X.L.; Tong, S.L.; Yan, C.H. Sex differences in the effects of prenatal lead exposure on birth outcomes. *Environ. Pollut.* **2017**, *225*, 193–200. [CrossRef] [PubMed]
33. Singh, G.; Singh, V.; Wang, Z.; Voisin, G.; Lefebvre, F.; Navenot, J.-M.; Evans, B.; Verma, M.; Anderson, D.W.; Schneider, J.S. Effects of developmental lead exposure on the hippocampal methylome: Influences of sex and timing and level of exposure. *Toxicol. Lett.* **2018**, *290*, 63–72. [CrossRef]
34. Cecil, K.M.; Brubaker, C.J.; Adler, C.M.; Dietrich, K.N.; Altaye, M.; Egelhoff, J.C.; Wessel, S.; Elangovan, I.; Hornung, R.; Jarvis, K.; et al. Decreased brain volume in adults with childhood lead exposure. *PLoS Med.* **2008**, *5*, e112. [CrossRef]

toxics

MDPI

Article

The Immunotoxicity of Chronic Exposure to High Levels of Lead: An Ex Vivo Investigation

Kawinsaya Pukanha [1], Supabhorn Yimthiang [2] and Wiyada Kwanhian [1,*]

1 Department of Medical Technology, School of Allied Health Sciences, Walailak University, Nakhon Si Thammarat 80161, Thailand; p.kawinsaya@gmail.com
2 School of Public Health, Walailak University, Nakhon Si Thammarat 80160, Thailand; ksupapor@mail.wu.ac.th
* Correspondence: wiyadakwanhian@gmail.com

Received: 11 July 2020; Accepted: 12 August 2020; Published: 13 August 2020

Abstract: Lead (Pb) is a toxic metal known for its wide-ranging adverse health effects. However, a compound of Pb is still used in the caulking process to repair wooden fishing boats. The present study aimed to measure Pb exposure and its immunologic effects in boatyard workers in Nakhon Si Thammarat province, Thailand, in comparison with an age-matched control group of farmers. The age, body mass index, and smoking history in workers (n = 14) and controls (n = 16) did not differ. The median blood Pb concentration was 8.7-fold higher in workers than controls (37.1 versus 4.3 µg/dL, $p < 0.001$). Workers had 8.4% lower phagocytic active cells than controls (89.9% versus 98.1%, $p = 0.019$). In response to a mitogen stimulation, the peripheral blood mononuclear cells (PBMCs) from workers produced 2-fold higher ratios of interleukin-4 (IL-4) to interferon-γ than the PBMCs from controls ($p = 0.026$). Furthermore, Pb-exposed workers had 33.9% lower cytotoxic T (Tc) cells than controls (24.3% versus 36.8%, $p = 0.004$). In stark contrast, the percentage of regulatory T (Treg) cells in workers was 2.7-fold higher than controls (6.1% versus 2.3%, $p < 0.001$). In all subjects, blood Pb showed positive correlations with the percentages of Treg cells ($r = 0.843$, $p < 0.001$) and IL-4 ($r = 0.473$, $p = 0.041$) while showing an inverse correlation with the percentages of Tc cells ($r = -0.563$, $p = 0.015$). These findings indicate that chronic high Pb exposure may cause a shift towards humoral immune response, together with a suppression of cellular immunity, thereby suggesting an elevation in cancer risk in Pb-exposed workers.

Keywords: blood lead; cellular immunity; phagocytosis; humoral munity; immunosuppression

1. Introduction

Lead (Pb) is a heavy metal with versatile properties, including malleability, ductility, poor conductivity, softness, and corrosion resistance, and it has thus been used for several thousands of years, causing widespread distribution in the environment worldwide [1,2]. Due to its non-biodegradability, Pb accumulates in the environment and hazards increase over time, evident from numerous reports of Pb contamination in the environment by industrial, mining, and agricultural activities [1–3]. Pb has no known biological role, but it can accumulate in the body, causing toxicity in many tissues and organs, immune system included [1–12]. It is of concern that there is increasing evidence for the negative effects of chronic exposure to high-level Pb on cancer risk and mortality that has recently emerged from prospective cohort studies of Pb-exposed workers [13,14].

The immune system provides important defense mechanisms that reduce the potential adverse effects of exposure to harmful biological agents, mutant cells, and certain chemicals [15]. Studies in humans and experimental animals have demonstrated the adverse effects of Pb exposure on the body's immune system [16–21]. In one study, Pb-poisoned children were found to have lower numbers of CD4+CD8+ helper T cells (Th), while their CD3+CD8+ cytotoxic T cell (Tc) levels were higher than those of a control group [16]. Workers in a factory manufacturing lead stearate were found to have a decreased number of CD45RO+ memory T cells [17]. A decrease in lymphocyte proliferation was noted in another study of occupationally exposed workers [18]. A reduction in humoral immunity by 53.6% was observed in mice receiving Pb in drinking water [19]. In other studies, altered subpopulations of circulating CD4+ T cells (T cells) and CD8+ T cells (T cytotoxic cells) were noted, together with evidence for Th1 up-regulation occurring simultaneously with Th2 down-regulation [20,21].

Nakhon Si Thammarat Province, located in the southern region of Thailand, is not an industrial estate area. However, there are many shipyards in operation, especially in coastal areas such as the districts of Pak Phanang, Mueng, Thasala, and Si-Chon. Many occupations are associated with the shipyards, including boat caulkers and fishing net workers, using lead bars [22]. In a previous report published in 2007, 48% to 67% of caulkers, painters, and mechanics working in the shipyards of Pak Phanang and Thasala districts were found to have blood Pb concentrations >40 μg/dL [23]. The present study was undertaken to assess Pb exposure experienced by current boatyard workers by measuring their blood Pb concentrations. In addition, it examined the adverse effects of such exposure, with a focus on the function of immune cells, which included phagocytic activity, proliferation, and cytokine production, and T cell subpopulation profiles.

2. Materials and Methods

2.1. Study Subjects

The Committee on Human Rights Related to Research Involving Human Subjects at Walailak University approved all experimental protocols in the present study (approval no. 14/057, 1 August 2014). A total of fourteen Pb-exposed workers (boat caulkers and fishing net workers included) from Pak Phanang district, Nakhon Si Thammarat Province, Thailand, were enrolled in this study. Additional age-matched farmers (n = 16) were enrolled as controls. The main criterion for inclusion in the worker group was blood Pb concentration ≥25 μg/dL. For controls, blood Pb levels were <25 μg/dL. The blood Pb level of 25 μg/dL was an exposure limit for Pb-exposed workers, based on the Occupational Safety and Health Administration (OSHA) [24].

2.2. Sampling and Blood Analysis

From each subject, a 50-mL blood sample was drawn from the median cubital vein in the morning, before working and without fasting. The blood sample of each subject was divided into three aliquots of 5, 10, and 35 mL. The 5-mL aliquots of whole blood, in BD Vacutainer®EDTA tube (Becton, Dickinson and Company, Franklin Lakes, NJ, USA) were assayed for Pb concentrations, using the graphite furnace atomic absorption spectrometer, AAnalyst™ 600 (PerkinElmer, Wellesley, MA, USA), available at Toxicology Laboratory, Department of Pathology, Faculty of Medicine, Ramathibodi Hospital, Mahidol University, Bangkok, Thailand. Whole Blood Metals Control Lymphochek™ Levels 1, 2 and 3 were used for quality assurance and control (Bio-Rad, Hercules, CA, USA). The coefficients of variation of blood Pb concentrations were within 10%. None of study subjects had blood Pb concentrations below the detection limit of 1.0 μg/dL [25]. The 10-mL aliquots of blood samples contained heparin as an anticoagulant were assayed for T cell subpopulations and phagocytic activity. The 35-mL aliquots of blood samples contained heparin as an anticoagulant were subjected to preparation of mononuclear cells, as detailed in Section 2.3.

2.3. Isolation of Peripheral Blood Mononuclear Cells (PBMCs)

PBMCs were isolated by the Ficoll density gradient centrifugation method [26] from 35-mL aliquots of blood samples, collected in BD Vacutainer®Lithium Heparin tubes (Becton, Dickinson and Company, Franklin Lakes, NJ, USA). Cells were counted and cell viability was determined by trypan blue staining. The PBMCs 2×10^6 cells/mL were cultured in RPMI 1640 Gibco™ culture medium

(Thermo Fisher, Waltham, MA, USA) supplemented with 15% fetal bovine serum (Merck, Darmstadt, HE, Germany) and 1% penicillin-streptomycin Gibco™ (Thermo Fisher Scientific, MA, USA).

2.4. Phagocytic Activity Assay

Phagocytosis activity was determined using the IgG-FITC Phagocytosis assay kit (Cayman Chemical, Ann Arbor, MI, USA). The instructions in the manufacturing manual were slightly modified. One milliliter of buffy coat from heparinized blood was mixed with 9 mL FACS™ lysing solution (Becton Dickinson and Company, Franklin Lakes, NJ, USA), and the samples were incubated for 15 min at room temperature. The cells were centrifuged for 5 min at 400× g at room temperature. The supernatant was carefully decanted, and cells were adjusted with PBS to a concentration of 1×10^6 cells/mL. Cells were transferred into polypropylene FACS™ tubes (Becton Dickinson and Company, Franklin Lakes, NJ, USA) and mixed with the latex beads rabbit IgG-FITC solution. Subsequently, cells were incubated in the dark in an incubator with 5% CO_2, 37 °C for 1 h. The percentages of active phagocytic cells were determined by BD FACSCalibur™ flow cytometry (Becton Dickinson and Company, Franklin Lakes, NJ, USA).

2.5. Cytokine Assay

To stimulate cytokine production, separated PBMCs were mixed with phytohemagglutinin (PHA) at a concentration of 5µg/mL (Merck, Darmstadt, HE, Germany) before they were incubated at 5% CO_2, 37 °C for 48 h [21]. Supernatants were harvested from each well and stored at −80 °C until they were measured for levels of cytokines, namely interleukin-4 (IL-4) and interferon-γ (IFN-γ), by ELISA human cytokine development kits (PeproTech, Rocky Hill, NJ, USA). Each sample was analyzed in triplicate, and controls and unstimulated blanks were analyzed simultaneously.

2.6. Proliferation Assay

A total of 2×10^6 cells/mL of PBMCs in complete medium were grown in 96-well plates and stimulated with 5 µg/mL PHA [13] and incubated at 37 °C, 5% CO_2 for 48 h. Following incubation, 3-(4-5-dimethylthaizolyl-2)-2,5-diphenyltetrazolium bromide (Merck, Darmstadt, HE, Germany) was added and the cells were incubated at 37 °C for a further 4-h period. Then, 100 µL of dimethyl sulfoxide (DMSO) was added and samples were mixed thoroughly by repeated pipetting and incubated at room temperature in the dark for 2 h. The absorbance wavelength of 570 nm and the reference wavelength of 630 nm were measured by a Thermo Scientific™ Multiskan™ GO microplate reader (Thermo Fisher Scientific, Waltham, MA, USA). Each sample was analyzed in triplicate, and controls and unstimulated blanks were analyzed simultaneously.

2.7. Determination of T Cell Subpopulations by the Flow Cytometry

Cells were stained before they were incubated with FACS lysing solution, containing paraformaldehyde for fixing cells (https://www.bdbiosciences.com/ds/is/tds/23-1358.pdf). To control for staining variability, negative isotype control was used for every sample tested. The negative isotype control ensured that the observed staining was due to specific antibody binding to the target rather than an artefact or background. The utility of Fc receptor blocking reagents was unnecessary when the negative isotype was used. For CD4 and CD8, at least 10,000 event cells were collected as the concentrations of Th and Tc cells were 800 and 500 cells/µL, respectively. For Treg cells, at least 20,000 events were collected as there was 1–2% of CD4 T cells.

2.7.1. Helper T Lymphocytes and Cytotoxic T Lymphocytes

To a 5-mL Falcon™ polystyrene tube (Becton Dickinson and Company, Franklin Lakes, NJ, USA), fifty microliters of EDTA blood was added per 10 µL of BD Tritest CD4/CD8/CD3 (Becton Dickinson and Company, Franklin Lakes, NJ, USA). The method followed the manufacturer's manual. The negative control tube was reacted with the BD FastImmune™ γ1 PE/CD45 PerCP control (Becton Dickinson and Company, Franklin Lakes, NJ, USA). Samples were analyzed by BD FACSCalibur™ flow cytometry (Becton Dickinson and Company, Franklin Lakes, NJ, USA). Cytotoxic T (Tc) cells are CD3+CD8+, while helper T (Th) cells are CD3+CD4+. The data were analyzed by BD CellQuest software version 5.0, 2002 (Becton Dickinson and Company, Franklin Lakes, NJ, USA).

2.7.2. Regulatory T Lymphocytes

To a 5-mL Falcon™ round-bottom polystyrene tube (Becton Dickinson and Company, Franklin Lakes, NJ, USA), fifty microliters of buffy coat of EDTA blood was added per 10 μL of isotype control (PE-Cy™ 7 Mouse IgG1κ isotype control (Becton Dickinson and Company, Franklin Lakes, NJ, USA) and cocktail of human regulatory T cells (CD4/CD25/CD127) (Becton Dickinson and Company, Franklin Lakes, NJ, USA) antibody in each sample. The regulatory T (Treg) cells ($CD4+CD25^{bright}CD127^{dim}$) were analyzed by flow cytometry. Events collected using a FACSCalibur™ (Becton Dickinson and Company, Franklin Lakes, NJ, USA) were analyzed using CellQuest version 5.0, 2002 (Becton Dickinson and Company, Franklin Lakes, NJ, USA).

2.8. Statistical Analysis

GraphPad Prism software version 8.01, 2018 (GraphPad Software, San Diego, CA, USA) was used to analyze data. The Mann–Whitney U test was used to determine differences in age, body mass index (BMI), and blood Pb concentration in controls versus workers. Difference in smoking history was determined by odds ratio and chi-square test. Spearman's rank correlation was used to identify the correlations between blood Pb concentration and seven measured immunologic parameters, including proliferation index, percentages of phagocytic cells, levels of cytokines, and percentages of T cell subpopulations. The result was considered statistically significant when p-values were less than 0.05 in a two-sided test.

3. Results

3.1. Characteristics of Study Workers and Controls

Table 1 provides the characteristics of the control group and worker group. Participants in the control group were men, while the worker group had nine men and five women. Half of the study workers were exposed to Pb for more than 10 years. Age, BMI, hemoglobin, hematocrit, and smoking history of both groups did not differ. Thus, demographic characteristics of the two groups were apparently homologous. The median blood Pb concentration in the worker group was 37.07 μg/dL. This blood Pb concentration was 8.7-fold higher than the controls ($p < 0.001$). It was also higher than the OSHA exposure limit for Pb-exposed workers of 25 μg/dL [24].

3.2. Profiling of Cytokine Production and Other Immunologic Parameters

Table 2 provides a profile of the immunologic parameters measured. These included the percentage of helper T (Th) lymphocytes (CD3+CD4+) together with cell proliferation index and cytokine production in response to stimulation by a mitogen. The median percentage of Th lymphocytes in workers was similar to that of controls (60.74% versus 56.31%, $p = 0.395$). In the cell proliferation and cytokine production assay, peripheral blood mononuclear cells (PBMCs) from study subjects were used, with PHA as a stimulant mitogen. The median PHA-stimulated cell proliferation index was 1.14 in workers and 1.50 in controls ($p = 0.226$). The median level of interferon-gamma (IFN-γ) generated in response to PHA stimulation was 12.14 pg/mL in workers and 20.07 pg/mL in controls ($p = 0.103$), while the median level of interleukin-4 (IL-4) was 175.58 pg/mL in workers and 155.65 pg/mL in controls ($p = 0.060$). Interestingly, the median ratio of IL-4/IFN-γ was approximately 2-fold higher in workers compared with controls (15.03 versus 7.01, $p = 0.026$). Hence, there was a shift towards humoral immune response in Pb-exposed workers, evident from an increase in IL-4 production concomitant with a decrease in IFN-γ production, which has a suppressive effect on cell-mediated immunity.

Table 1. Demographic data of control and worker groups.

Descriptors	All Subjects	Controls	Workers	Odds Ratio	p-Value [1]
Number	30	16	14		
Age, years	53.0 ± 9.7	51.5 ± 8.8	54.0 ± 11.3	-	0.595
Range, years	28–69	36–66	28–69		
BMI, kg/m^2	22.9 ± 4.1	23.7 ± 4.7	24.0 ± 4.6	-	0.874
Range, kg/m^2	16.9–32.5	19.1–32.5	16.9–30.3		
Hemoglobin, g/dL	13.9 ± 1.2	14.1 ± 1.1	13.4 ± 1.2	-	0.550
Range, g/dL	11.7–16.4	12.2–16.4	11.7–15.6		
Hematocrit, %	41.8 ± 3.2	42.4 ± 2.9	40.9 ± 3.0	-	0.698
Range, %	36.3–48	37.7–48	36.3–45.2		
Blood Pb concentration, μg/dL	16.17 ± 18.68	4.28 ± 1.12	37.07 ± 11.09	-	<0.001
Range, μg/dL	3.02–58.47	3.02–4.24	25.11–58.47		
Sex				-	-
Male	25	16	9		
Female	5	0	5		
Occupation				-	-
Caulker	10	0	10		
Fishing net worker	4	0	4		
Agriculturist	16	16	-		
Duration of Pb exposure				-	-
0 year	16	16	0		
1–5 years	3	0	3		
5–10 years	4	0	4		
>10 years	7	0	7		
Smoking history				1.158	0.282
Yes	14	6	8		
No	16	10	6		

Age, BMI, hemoglobin, hematocrit, and blood Pb concentration are presented as median ± standard deviation (SD).—means no data or not determined. [1] The p-values for age, BMI, and blood Pb were derived from the Mann–Whitney U test. The p-value for smoking history was derived from chi-square test. Significant different at p-value < 0.05.

Table 2. Profiling of immunologic parameters.

Parameters	Group	Median	SD	Range	95% CI	p-Value [1]
Th (%)	Controls	56.3	10.1	41.3–78.4	51.9–68.4	0.395
	Workers	60.7	9.3	45.8–77.2	56.9–69.9	
Proliferation index	Controls	1.50	0.35	1.06–2.41	1.22–1.66	0.226
	Workers	1.14	0.26	1.09–1.66	1.09–1.66	
IFN-γ (pg/mL)	Controls	20.1	9.3	3.2–30.0	3.2–30.0	0.104
	Workers	12.1	4.6	3.6–20.6	10.0–15.5	
IL-4 (pg/mL)	Controls	155.6	40.0	103.4–252	112.1–163	0.060
	Workers	175.6	67.2	99.2–334	114.7–215	
IL-4/IFN-γ ratio	Controls	7.0	15.6	3.5–50.4	3.5–50.4	0.026
	Workers	15.0	11.8	6.1–48.1	10.3–31.3	

[1] The p-value was derived from the Mann–Whitney U test, significant difference at p-value < 0.05.

3.3. *Effects of High Pb Exposure on Innate Immunity*

Figure 1 provides results of an investigation on innate immunity, where white blood cells separated from the buffy coats of fresh heparinized blood samples from subjects who were tested for their phagocytic activity. As the effect of smoking on the percentage of phagocytic cells was minuscule, data from non-smokers and smokers in the group of workers or controls were pooled. The median percentage of phagocytic active cells was 8.4% lower in workers than controls (89.92% vs. 98.11%, $p = 0.019$).

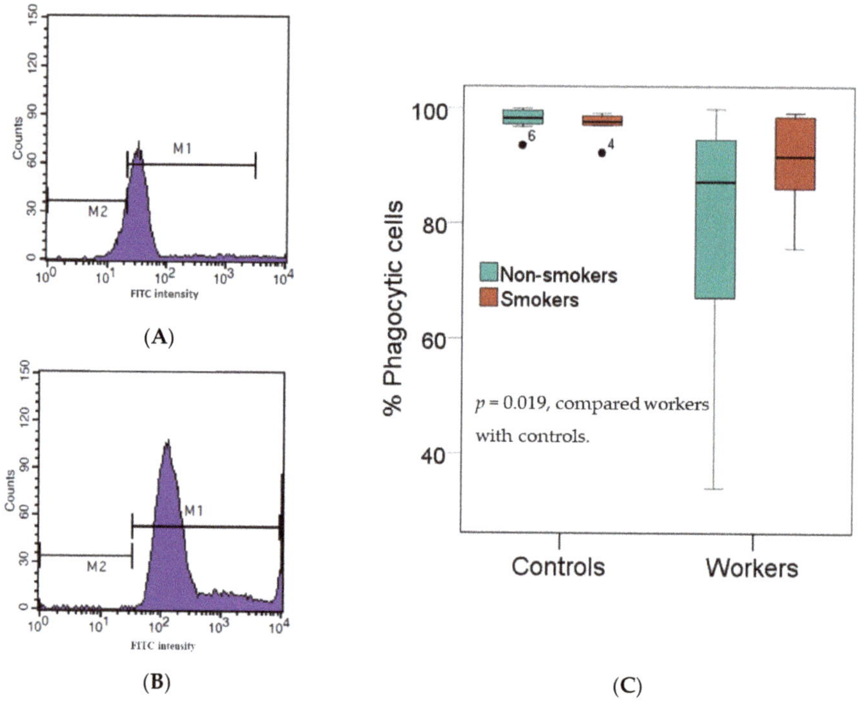

Figure 1. Effects of high Pb exposure on innate immunity. Histograms show the percentages of phagocytic cells in one Pb-exposed worker (**A**) and one control subject (**B**). Boxplots compare percentages of phagocytic cells in controls versus workers, non-smokers, and smokers included (**C**). Outliers were the data points below or above 1.5× interquartile range. The *p*-value was derived from the Mann–Whitney U test, in which outliers were included.

3.4. *Effects of High Pb Exposure on the Populations of Cytoxic and Regulatory T Lymphocytes*

Figure 2 provides boxplots that compare the percentages of cytotoxic T (Tc) lymphocytes (CD3+CD8+) in controls and workers, stratified by smoking status. As an effect of smoking on percentage of Tc lymphocyte was statistically insignificant, data from non-smokers and smokers in the group of workers or controls were pooled. The median percentage of Tc lymphocytes in the worker group was 33.9 % lower than the control group (24.30% versus 36.76%, $p = 0.004$).

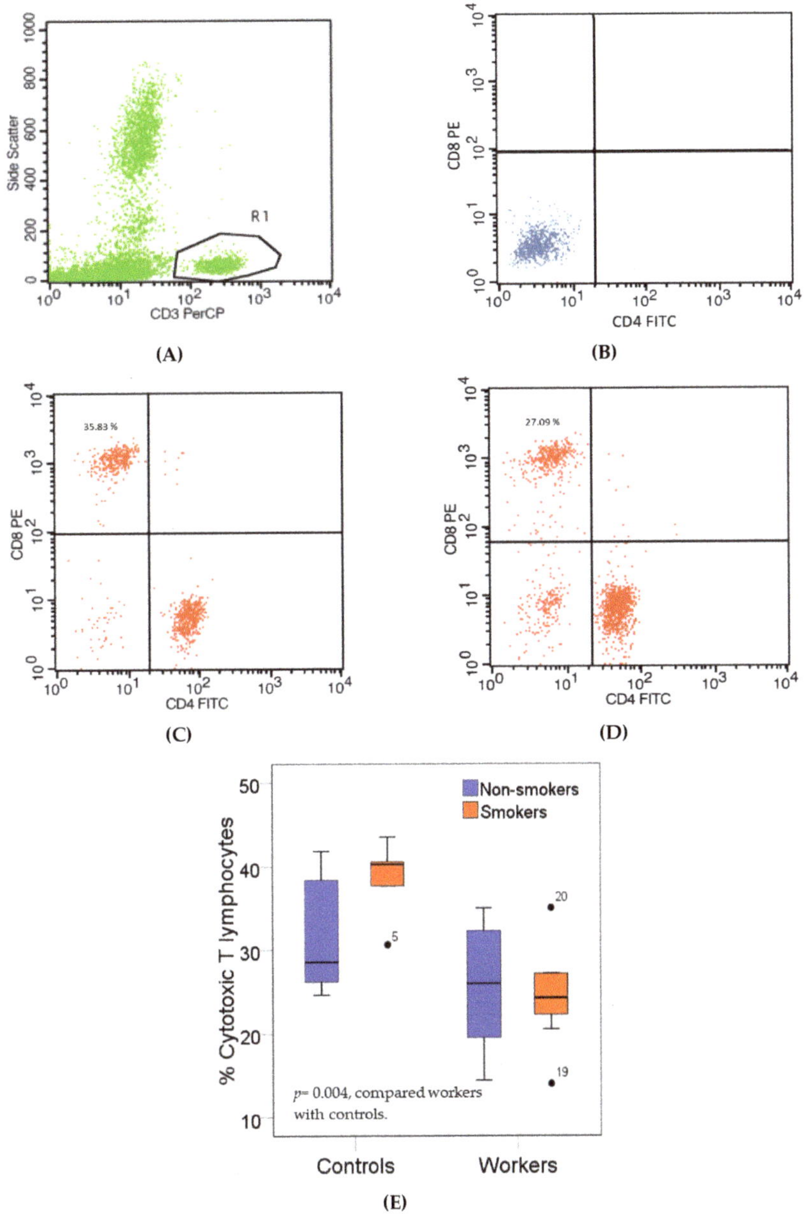

Figure 2. Effects of high Pb exposure on the percentage of cytotoxic T lymphocytes. The flow cytometry strategies (dot plots) show side scatter vs. CD3 (PerCP) (**A**), isotype control stained (**B**), the cytotoxic T (Tc) lymphocytes in one control subject (**C**), and one Pb-exposed worker (**D**). Boxplots compare percentages of Tc lymphocytes in controls versus workers, non-smokers, and smokers included (**E**). Outliers were the data points below or above 1.5× interquartile range. The *p*-value was derived from the Mann–Whitney U test, in which outliers were included.

Figure 3 provides boxplots that compare the percentages of regulatory T (Treg) lymphocytes (CD4+CD25^{bright}CD127^{dim}) in controls and workers, stratified by smoking status. As the effect of smoking on the percentage of Treg lymphocytes was statistically insignificant, data from non-smokers and smokers in the group of workers or controls were pooled. The median percentage of Treg lymphocytes in the worker group was 2.7-fold higher than the control group (6.10% versus 2.28%, $p < 0.001$). Pb-exposed workers appeared to have a decreased percentage of Tc cells concomitantly with an increased percentage of Treg cells, thereby suggesting suppression of cellular immunity.

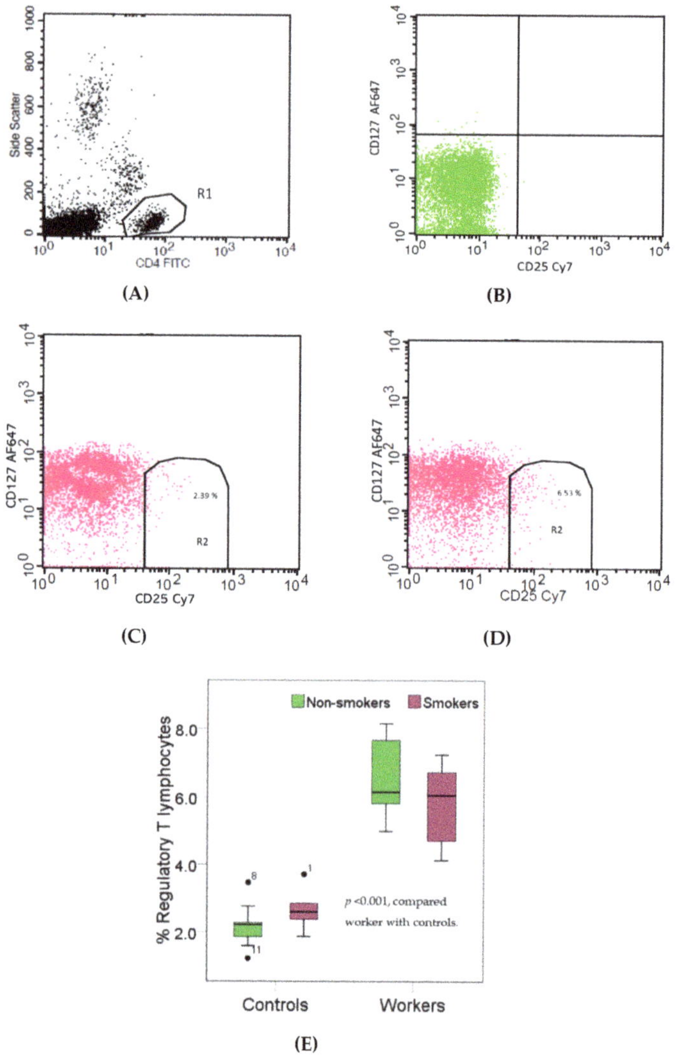

Figure 3. Effects of high Pb exposure on the percentage of regulatory T lymphocytes. The flow cytometry strategies (dot plots) show side scatter vs. CD4 (FITC) (**A**), isotype control stained (**B**), the regulatory T (Treg) lymphocytes in one control subject (**C**) and one Pb-exposed worker (**D**). Boxplots compare percentages of regulatory Treg lymphocytes in controls versus workers, non-smokers, and smokers included (**E**). Outliers were the data points below or above 1.5× interquartile range. The *p*-value was derived from the Mann–Whitney U test, in which outliers were included.

3.5. Blood Pb in Relation to Cytokines amd Immunologic Parameters

Table 3 provides results of the Spearman's rank correlation analysis of blood Pb concentration and seven immunologic parameters measured for an entire group (controls plus workers, $n = 30$). Blood Pb concentration did not correlate with phagocytic activity, proliferative response, IFN-γ, or % T helper cells ($p \geq 0.05$). However, blood Pb concentrations showed significant positive correlations with the percentages of Treg cells ($r = 0.843$, $p < 0.001$) and IL-4 ($r = 0.473$, $p = 0.041$), while showing an inverse correlation with the percentages of Tc cells ($r = -0.563$, $p = 0.015$). Thus, Pb-exposed workers were found to have elevated IL-4 production levels together with an elevated percentage of Treg cells, while having a decreased percentage of Tc cells.

Table 3. The Spearman's rank correlation analysis of blood Pb concentrations and seven immunologic parameters.

Blood Pb Versus Immunologic Parameters	Phagocytic Activity	Proliferation Index	IFN-γ	IL-4	%Th	%Tc	%Treg
Spearman's rho	−0.209	−0.329	−0.319	0.473	0.358	−0.563	0.843
p-value (two-tailed)	0.364	0.231	0.213	0.041	0.121	0.015	<0.001
Significant (α = 0.05)	No	No	No	Yes	No	Yes	Yes

4. Discussion

In this study, we investigated Pb exposure levels in occupational settings together with adverse effects of such exposure levels on the function of the body's immune system. The blood Pb concentrations in study workers showed a wide range, 25.11 to 58.47 μg/dL, while the blood Pb concentrations in age-matched farmers (a control group) were in a narrow range, 3.02 to 4.24 μg/dL. The most likely source of Pb in the control group is the diet, as Pb is present in virtually all foodstuffs [27,28]. The effects of Pb on lymphocyte proliferation, natural killer (NK) cell cytotoxicity, and IFN-γ production by PBMCs have been seen in occupationally exposed persons [29]. In parallel, some effects of Pb on the immune response have been seen in animal models, such as the innate immune system in zebra fish [30] and the humoral and cell-mediated immune responses in mice [31,32].

Compared with a former report [23], Pb exposure levels among boatyard workers in our study workers remained as high as previously observed. In addition, we observed a decrease in phagocytic activity of the neutrophils from boatyard workers. This finding agreed with a previous report [31]. The decreased phagocytic activity may be attributable to the action of IL-1, as it is known to be involved in the stimulation of neutrophils and the recruitment activated cells into the site of injury [33]. However, IL-1 was up-regulated after exposure to mixtures of Pb and arsenic [30].

IFN-γ, produced by CD8+ Th1 cells, represents a component of cell-mediated immunity known for its anti-viral and anti-parasitic propensities [34]. IFN-γ inhibits the proliferation of Th2 cells and acts in synergy with other cytokines, notably TNF-α, to impede the proliferation of normal and transformed cells [34]. In a recent review, in vivo, in vitro, and ex vivo studies have been used to confirm that IFN-γ production is inhibited by Pb [35]. It is of relevance that the levels of IFN-γ produced by PBMCs from workers showed a tendency to be lower than those from controls. In an early study [36], Pb acetate was found to be involved in immediate hypersensitivity reactions (degranulation of rat mast cells) and allergic hypersensitivity, which was mediated by Th2 [36]. Exposure to low-dose Pb led to a decrease in IFN-γ Th1 cytokine and proinflammatory cytokines TNF-α and IL-1 while inducing IL-4 and/or IL-10 to maintain a Th2 immune response [37]. It has been suggested that Pb may increase susceptibility to infection and the incidence of allergic hypersensitivity [35,37].

IL-4 is a Th2 cytokine secreted by activated Th2 and NKT cells. It is a potent inducer of naïve CD4+ T cells and directs their differentiation into Th2 effector cells. IL-4 is known as a marker of humoral immunity [38]. In the present study, PBMCs from workers showed a tendency to produce more IL-4 together with less IFN-γ than controls. Consequently, the IL-4/IFN-γ ratio produced by PBMCs from workers was 2-fold higher than the control group. This indicated toxicity of Pb on cytokine production, which is consistent with previous studies in the following ways. In BALB/c mice, levels of the *IL-4* gene were increased after exposure to heavy metals, Pb included [39]. Elevated IL-4 after Pb exposure may cause an induction of type 2 helper T (Th2) cells and M2 macrophages [40]. In effect, the increased production of IL-4 seen in boatyard workers might confer upon them increased susceptibility to infection, allergic hypersensitivity, and/or autoimmune diseases dominated by Th2.

A significant increase in Treg observed among workers in the present study is similar to previous experimental studies [41,42]. Up-regulation of IL-2RB in lymphocytes after exposure to heavy metals was observed in addition to the higher expression of Treg differentiation [43,44]. It is suggested that Pb may activate TGF-β, one of the main regulatory cytokines [41], which in turn stimulates the differentiation of regulatory T cells, promoting FoxP3 expression [45]. The link between Treg cells and cytokine suppression was confirmed by a study targeting the PI3-AKT pathway that caused the inhibition Treg proliferation [46]. In the present study, a significant reduction in Tc lymphocytes (CD3+CD8+) was observed in boatyard workers. Likewise, a significant decrease in the percentage of CD4+ Th cells was noted in a study of Pb-exposed children [47].

5. Conclusions

Herein, we have demonstrated that boatyard workers continue to be exposed to toxic high levels of Pb, as reflected by their blood Pb levels, which are 8.7-fold higher than the farmer control group. The immunological effects associated with such toxic exposure levels among study workers are reduced phagocytic activity, altered cytokine profiles (an increase in IL-4 concomitant with a decrease in IFN-γ), and deranged subpopulations of Tc and Treg cells, causing suppression of cell-mediated immunity. These findings may explain the increased risk of death from cancer and increased incidence of lung cancer and brain cancer in workers with high exposure, seen in cohort studies of Pb-exposed workers [13,14]. Public measures are required in order to reduce workplace exposure, as is a further study with a larger sample size to substantiate these important observations.

Author Contributions: Conceptualization, W.K. and S.Y.; methodology, K.P.; software, W.K.; formal analysis, K.P. and W.K.; investigation, K.P.; resources, S.Y., K.P., and W.K.; writing—original draft preparation, K.P. and W.K.; writing—review and editing, W.K. and S.Y.; supervision, W.K.; project administration, W.K.; funding acquisition, W.K. All authors have read and agreed to the published version of the manuscript.

Funding: This research was funded by the Walailak University Research Funds (grant number 18/2557 and 15/2559) and partially supported by the New Strategic Research (P2P) project, Walailak University, Thailand.

Acknowledgments: We would like to thank the Center of Excellence Research for Melioidosis (CERM) and School of Allied Health Sciences, Walailak University, Nakhon Si Thammarat 80160, Thailand, for providing the equipment.

Conflicts of Interest: The authors declare no conflict of interest.

References

1. Tchounwou, P.B.; Yedjou, C.G.; Patlolla, A.K.; Sutton, D.J. Heavy metal toxicity and the environment. *Exp. Suppl.* **2012**, *101*, 133–164. [PubMed]
2. de Souza, I.D.; de Andrade, A.S.; Dalmolin, R.J.S. Lead-interacting proteins and their implication in lead poisoning. *Crit. Rev. Toxicol.* **2018**, *48*, 375–386. [CrossRef] [PubMed]
3. Caito, S.; Aschner, M. Developmental neurotoxicity of lead. *Adv. Neurobiol.* **2017**, *18*, 3–12. [PubMed]
4. Li, X.; Gao, Y.; Zhang, M.; Zhang, Y.; Zhou, M.; Peng, L.; He, A.; Zhang, X.; Yan, X.; Wang, Y.; et al. In vitro lung and gastrointestinal bioaccessibility of potentially toxic metals in Pb-contaminated alkaline urban soil: The role of particle size fractions. *Ecotoxicol. Environ. Saf.* **2020**, *190*, 110151. [CrossRef] [PubMed]
5. Liu, J.; McCauley, L.; Yan, C.; Shen, X.; Pinto-Martin, J.A. Low blood lead levels and hemoglobin concentrations in preschool children in China. *Toxicol. Environ. Chem.* **2012**, *94*, 423–426. [CrossRef] [PubMed]
6. Hashem, M.A.; El-Sharkawy, N.I. The effects of low electromagnetic field and lead acetate combination on some hemato-biochemical and immunotoxicological parameters in mice. *Turk. J. Hematol.* **2009**, *26*, 181–189.
7. Valcke, M.; Ouellet, N.; Dubé, M.; Laouan Sidi, E.A.; LeBlanc, A.; Normandin, L.; Balion, C.; Ayotte, P. Biomarkers of cadmium, lead and mercury exposure in relation with early biomarkers of renal dysfunction and diabetes: Results from a pilot study among aging Canadians. *Toxicol. Lett.* **2019**, *312*, 148–156. [CrossRef]

8. Kim, Y.D.; Eom, S.Y.; Yim, D.H.; Kim, I.S.; Won, H.K.; Park, C.H.; Kim, G.B.; Yu, S.D.; Choi, B.S.; Park, J.D.; et al. Environmental Exposure to arsenic, lead, and cadmium in people living near Janghang copper smelter in Korea. *J. Korean Med. Sci.* **2016**, *31*, 489–496. [CrossRef]
9. Nanda, K.P.; Kumari, C.; Dubey, M.; Firdaus, H. Chronic lead (Pb) exposure results in diminished hemocyte count and increased susceptibility to bacterial infection in *Drosophila melanogaster*. *Chemosphere* **2019**, *236*, 124349. [CrossRef]
10. Jorissen, A.; Plum, L.M.; Rink, L.; Haase, H. Impact of lead and mercuric ions on the interleukin-2-dependent proliferation and survival of T cells. *Arch. Toxicol.* **2013**, *87*, 249–258. [CrossRef]
11. Chibowska, K.; Baranowska-Bosiacka, I.; Falkowska, A.; Gutowska, I.; Goschorska, M.; Chlubek, D. Effect of lead (Pb) on inflammatory processes in the brain. *Int. J. Mol. Sci.* **2016**, *17*, 2140. [CrossRef] [PubMed]
12. Baos, R.; Jovani, R.; Forero, M.G.; Tella, J.L.; Gómez, G.; Jiménez, B.; González, M.J.; Hiraldo, F. Relationships between T-cell-mediated immune response and Pb, Zn, Cu, Cd, and as concentrations in blood of nestling white storks (*Ciconia Ciconia*) and black kites (*Milvus migrans*) from Doñana (southwestern Spain) after the Aznalcóllar toxic spill. *Environ. Toxicol. Chem.* **2006**, *25*, 1153–1159. [CrossRef] [PubMed]
13. Kim, M.G.; Ryoo, J.H.; Chang, S.J.; Kim, C.B.; Park, J.K.; Koh, S.B.; Ahn, Y.S. Blood lead levels and cause-specific mortality of inorganic lead-exposed workers in South Korea. *PLoS ONE* **2015**, *10*, e0140360. [CrossRef] [PubMed]
14. Steenland, K.; Barry, V.; Anttila, A.; Sallmen, M.; Mueller, W.; Ritchie, P.; McElvenny, D.M.; Straif, K. Cancer incidence among workers with blood lead measurements in two countries. *Occup. Environ. Med.* **2019**, *76*, 603–610. [CrossRef]
15. Chaplin, D.D. Overview of the immune response. *J. Allergy Clin. Immunol.* **2010**, *125*, S3–S23. [CrossRef]
16. Zhao, Z.Y.; Li, R.; Sun, L.; Li, Z.Y.; Yang, R.L. Effect of lead exposure on the immune function of lymphocytes and erythrocytes in preschool children. *J. Zhejiang Univ.-Sci.* **2004**, *5*, 1001–1004. [CrossRef]
17. Sata, F.; Araki, S.; Tanigawa, T.; Morita, Y.; Sakurai, S.; Katsuno, N. Changes in natural killer cell subpopulations in lead workers. *Int. Arch. Occup. Environ. Health* **1997**, *69*, 306–310. [CrossRef]
18. Mishra, K.P.; Singh, V.K.; Rani, R.; Yadav, V.S.; Chandran, V.; Srivastava, S.P.; Seth, P.K. Effect of lead exposure on the immune response of some occupationally exposed individuals. *Toxicology* **2003**, *188*, 251–259. [CrossRef]
19. Massadeh, A.M.; Al-Safi, S. Analysis of cadmium and lead: Their immunosuppressive effects and distribution in various organs of mice. *Biol. Trace Elem. Res.* **2005**, *108*, 279–285. [CrossRef]
20. Fang, L.; Zhao, F.; Shen, X.; Ouyang, W.; Liu, X.; Xu, Y.; Yu, T.; Jin, B.; Chen, J.; Luo, W. Pb exposure attenuates hypersensitivity in vivo by increasing regulatory T cells. *Toxicol. Appl. Pharmacol.* **2012**, *265*, 272–278. [CrossRef]
21. McCabe, M.J., Jr.; Lawrence, D.A. Lead, a major environmental pollutant, is immunomodulatory by its differential effects on CD4+ T cells subsets. *Toxicol. Appl. Pharmacol.* **1991**, *111*, 13–23. [CrossRef]
22. Yimthiang, S.; Waeyang, D.; Kuraeiad, S. Screening for elevated blood lead levels and related risk factors among Thai children residing in a fishing community. *Toxics* **2019**, *7*, 54. [CrossRef] [PubMed]
23. Thanapop, C.; Geater, A.F.; Robson, M.G.; Phakthongsuk, P.; Viroonudomphol, D. Exposure to lead of boatyard workers in southern Thailand. *J. Occup. Health Psychol.* **2007**, *49*, 345–352. [CrossRef] [PubMed]
24. Available online: https://www.osha.gov/OshDoc/Directive_pdf/CPL_03-00-0009.pdf (accessed on 12 August 2020).
25. Trzcinka-Ochocka, M.; Brodzka, R.; Janasik, B. Useful and fast method for blood lead and cadmium determination using ICP-MS and GF-AAS; validation parameters. *J. Clin. Lab. Anal.* **2016**, *30*, 130–139. [CrossRef] [PubMed]
26. Böyum, A. Isolation of mononuclear cells and granulocytes from human blood. Isolation of monuclear cells by one centrifugation, and of granulocytes by combining centrifugation and sedimentation at 1 g. *Scand. J. Clin. Lab. Investig. Suppl.* **1968**, *97*, 77–89.
27. Shi, Z.; Zhen, S.; Orsini, N.; Zhou, Y.; Zhou, Y.; Liu, J.; Taylor, A.W. Association between dietary lead intake and 10-year mortality among Chinese adults. *Environ. Sci. Pollut. Res.* **2017**, *24*, 12273–12280. [CrossRef]
28. Wang, X.; Ding, N.; Tucker, K.L.; Weisskopf, M.G.; Sparrow, D.; Hu, H.; Park, S.K. A Western diet pattern is associated with higher concentrations of blood and bone lead among middle-aged and elderly men. *J. Nutr.* **2017**, *147*, 1374–1383. [CrossRef]

29. Koller, L.D. Effects of environmental contaminants on the immune system. *Adv. Vet. Sci. Comp. Med.* **1979**, *23*, 267–295.
30. Cobbina, S.J.; Xu, H.; Zhao, T.; Mao, G.; Zhou, Z.; Wu, X.; Liu, H.; Zou, Y.; Wu, X.; Yang, L. A multivariate assessment of innate immune-related gene expressions due to exposure to low concentration individual and mixtures of four kinds of heavy metals on zebrafish (*Danio rerio*) embryos. *Fish Shellfish Immunol.* **2015**, *47*, 1032–1042. [CrossRef]
31. Mishra, K.P. Lead exposure and its impact on immune system: A review. *Toxicol. In Vitro* **2009**, *23*, 969–972. [CrossRef]
32. Lawrence, D.A. In vivo and in vitro effects of lead on humoral and cell-mediated immunity. *Infect. Immun.* **1981**, *31*, 136–143. [CrossRef] [PubMed]
33. Queiroz, M.L.; Costa, F.F.; Bincoletto, C.; Perlingeiro, R.C.; Dantas, D.C.; Cardoso, M.P.; Almeida, M. Engulfment and killing capabilities of neutrophils and phagocytic splenic function in persons occupationally exposed to lead. *Int. Immunopharmacol.* **1994**, *16*, 239–244. [CrossRef]
34. Sen, G.C. Viruses and interferons. *Annu. Rev. Microbiol.* **2001**, *55*, 255–281. [CrossRef] [PubMed]
35. Fenga, C.; Gangemi, S.; Di Salvatore, V.; Falzone, L.; Libra, M. Immunological effects of occupational exposure to lead (Review). *Mol. Med. Rep.* **2017**, *15*, 3355–3360. [CrossRef]
36. Laschi-Loquerie, A.; Descotes, J.; Tachon, P.; Evreux, J.C. Influence of lead acetate on hypersensitivity. Experimental study. *J. Immunopharmacol.* **1984**, *6*, 87–93. [CrossRef] [PubMed]
37. Hemdan, N.Y.A.; Emmrich, F.; Adham, K.; Wichmann, G.; Lehmann, I.; El-Massry, A.; Ghoneim, H.; Lehmann, J.; Sack, U. Dose-dependent modulation of the in vitro cytokine production of human immune competent cells by lead salts. *Toxicol. Sci.* **2005**, *86*, 75–83. [CrossRef]
38. Yang, W.-C.; Hwang, Y.-S.; Chen, Y.-Y.; Liu, C.-L.; Shen, C.-N.; Hong, W.-H.; Lo, S.-M.; Shen, C.-R. Interleukin-4 supports the suppressive immune responses elicited by regulatory T Cells. *Front. Immunol.* **2017**, *8*, 1508. [CrossRef]
39. Radbin, R.; Vahedi, F.; Chamani, J. The influence of drinking-water pollution with heavy metal on the expression of IL-4 and IFN-γ in mice by real-time polymerase chain reaction. *Cytotechnology* **2014**, *66*, 769–777. [CrossRef]
40. Kasten-Jolly, J.; Lawrence, D.A. Lead modulation of macrophages causes multiorgan detrimental health effects. *J. Biochem. Mol. Toxicol.* **2014**, *28*, 355–372. [CrossRef]
41. Hernández-Castro, B.; Doníz-Padilla, L.M.; Salgado-Bustamante, M.; Rocha, D.; Ortiz-Pérez, M.D.; Jiménez-Capdeville, M.E.; Portales-Pérez, D.P.; Quintanar-Stephano, A.; González-Amaro, R. Effect of arsenic on regulatory T cells. *J. Clin. Immunol.* **2009**, *29*, 461–469. [CrossRef]
42. Gera, R.; Singh, V.; Mitra, S.; Sharma, A.K.; Singh, A.; Dasgupta, A.; Singh, D.; Kumar, M.; Jagdale, P.; Patnaik, S.; et al. Arsenic exposure impels CD4 commitment in thymus and suppress T cell cytokine secretion by increasing regulatory T cells. *Sci. Rep.* **2017**, *7*, 7140. [CrossRef] [PubMed]
43. Burchill, M.A.; Yang, J.; Vogtenhuber, C.; Blazar, B.R.; Farrar, M.A. IL-2 receptor beta-dependent STAT5 activation is required for the development of Foxp3+ regulatory T cells. *J. Immunol.* **2007**, *178*, 280–290. [CrossRef] [PubMed]
44. Andrew, A.S.; Jewell, D.A.; Mason, R.A.; Whitfield, M.L.; Moore, J.H.; Karagas, M.R. Drinking-water arsenic exposure modulates gene expression in human lymphocytes from a U.S. population. *Environ. Health Perspect.* **2008**, *116*, 524–531. [CrossRef] [PubMed]
45. Chen, W.; Jin, W.; Hardegen, N.; Lei, K.-J.; Li, L.; Marinos, N.; McGrady, G.; Wahl, S.M. Conversion of peripheral CD4+CD25− naive T cells to CD4+CD25+ regulatory T cells by TGF-beta induction of transcription factor Foxp3. *J. Exp. Med.* **2003**, *198*, 1875–1886. [CrossRef] [PubMed]
46. Abu-Eid, R.; Samara, R.N.; Ozbun, L.; Abdalla, M.Y.; Berzofsky, J.A.; Friedman, K.M.; Mkrtichyan, M.; Khleif, S.N. Selective inhibition of regulatory T cells by targeting the PI3K-Akt pathway. *Cancer Immunol. Res.* **2014**, *2*, 1080–1089. [CrossRef]
47. Li, S.; Zhengyan, Z.; Rong, L.; Hanyun, C. Decrease of CD4+T-lymphocytes in children exposed to environmental lead. *Biol. Trace Elem. Res.* **2005**, *105*, 19–25. [CrossRef]

toxics

MDPI

Article

In Vitro Evaluation of the Effects of Cadmium on Endocytic Uptakes of Proteins into Cultured Proximal Tubule Epithelial Cells

Hitomi Fujishiro, Hazuki Yamamoto, Nobuki Otera, Nanae Oka, Mei Jinno and Seiichiro Himeno *

Laboratory of Molecular Nutrition and Toxicology, Faculty of Pharmaceutical Sciences, Tokushima Bunri University, Tokushima 770-8514, Japan; donai-do@ph.bunri-u.ac.jp
* Correspondence: himenos@ph.bunri-u.ac.jp; Tel.: +81-88-602-8459

Received: 24 February 2020; Accepted: 30 March 2020; Published: 1 April 2020

Abstract: Cadmium (Cd) is an environmental pollutant known to cause dysfunctions of the tubular reabsorption of biomolecules in the kidney. Elevated levels of urinary excretion of low-molecular-weight proteins such as β_2-microglobulin (β_2-MG) have been used as an indicator of Cd-induced renal tubular dysfunctions. However, very few studies have examined the direct effects of Cd on the reabsorption efficiency of proteins using cultured renal cells. Here, we developed an in vitro assay system for quantifying the endocytic uptakes of fluorescent-labeled proteins by flow cytometry in S1 and S2 cells derived from mouse kidney proximal tubules. Endocytic uptakes of fluorescent-labeled albumin, transferrin, β_2-MG, and metallothionein into S1 cells were confirmed by fluorescence imaging and flow cytometry. The exposure of S1 and S2 cells to Cd at 1 and 3 μM for 3 days resulted in significant decreases in the uptakes of β_2-MG and metallothionein but not in those of albumin or transferrin. These results suggest that Cd affects the tubular reabsorption of low-molecular-weight proteins even at nonlethal concentrations. The in vitro assay system developed in this study to evaluate the endocytic uptakes of proteins may serve as a useful tool for detecting toxicants that cause renal tubular dysfunctions.

Keywords: kidney; endocytosis; β_2-microglobulin; metallothionein; flow cytometry; proximal tubule epithelial cells

---

1. Introduction

Cadmium (Cd) is an environmental pollutant that causes renal toxicity in animals and humans after chronic exposure in the diet [1]. Due to both the high affinity of Cd for sulfhydryl moieties in biomolecules within cells and the difficulty of excretion from cells, the biological half-life of Cd in the human kidney has been calculated to be more than 25 years [2]. The renal accumulation of Cd results in characteristic renal toxicity is known as Fanconi syndrome at the advanced stage [3–5]. Cd accumulation in the proximal tubules of the kidney has been believed to disturb the reabsorption of the luminal biomolecules, which are filtered through the glomerulus into proximal tubule epithelial cells (PTECs). Animals and humans exposed to Cd for a long time show increased urinary excretion of glucose, amino acids, and low-molecular-weight (LMW) proteins such as β_2-microglobulin (β_2-MG) and metallothionein (MT) [6–8]. Enhanced urinary levels of β_2-MG have been used as sensitive and reliable indicators of Cd-induced renal tubular damage [9,10].

The reabsorption of luminal biomolecules including β_2-MG and MT by PTECs is mediated by megalin-dependent endocytosis at the apical membrane of PTECs [11–14]. However, many studies on Cd cytotoxicity have focused on the mechanisms of cell lethality, including apoptosis caused by Cd [15–17], and only a few studies have examined Cd's direct effects on the efficiency of protein reabsorption by PTECs [18,19], especially under conditions where PTECs are surviving in the presence of Cd.

Recently, we developed an in vitro experimental system using mouse PTEC-derived S1, S2, and S3 cells, which maintain fundamental features of S1, S2, and S3 segment-specific expression of genes including metal transporters [20,21]. In the present study, we attempted to develop an in vitro experimental system for evaluating the endocytosis efficiency of LMW and high-molecular-weight (HMW) proteins into S1 and S2 cells derived from the S1 and S2 segments of proximal tubules where the reabsorption of glomerular-filtered proteins is highly active. To visualize and quantify the amounts of endocytosed proteins, we used fluorescent-labeled albumin, transferrin, β_2-MG, and MT. Here, we show that flow cytometric analyses of the incorporation of fluorescent-labeled proteins into cultured PTECs can be used to quantitatively evaluate endocytosis efficiency. By using this in vitro assay system, we detected decreases in the endocytic uptakes of β_2-MG and MT in cultured PTECs exposed to Cd.

2. Materials and Methods

2.1. Materials

Mouse anti-megalin monoclonal antibody was purchased from Abcam (Cambridge, MA, USA). Goat anti-cubilin polyclonal antibody was purchased from Santa Cruz Biotechnology (Dallas, TX, USA). Rabbit anti-transferrin receptor polyclonal antibody was purchased from Abnova (Taipei, Taiwan). Rabbit anti-β-actin polyclonal antibody, rabbit anti-Early Endosome Antigen 1 (EEA1) antibody, anti-rabbit IgG HRP-linked antibody, anti-mouse IgG HRP-linked antibody, and anti-goat IgG HRP-linked antibody were purchased from Cell Signaling Technology (Danvers, MA, USA). Alexa 555 anti-rabbit IgG antibody was purchased from Invitrogen (Carlsbad, CA, USA). Albumin-fluorescein isothiocyanate conjugate was purchased from Sigma-Aldrich (St. Louis, MO, USA), and Alexa Fluor® 488-conjugated ChromPure Mouse Transferrin was purchased from Jackson ImmunoResearch Laboratories (West Grove, PA, USA). Immortalized human renal proximal tubular epithelial cells (hRPTECs: CRL-4031) was obtained from ATCC (American Type Culture Collection, Manassas, VA, USA).

2.2. Cell Culture

S1, S2 cells, and hRPTEC were cultured in Dulbecco's modified Eagle's medium/Ham's Nutrient Mixture F12 supplemented with 5% fetal bovine serum (FBS), 1 μg/mL insulin, 10 ng/mL epidermal growth factor, 10 μg/mL transferrin, and penicillin/streptomycin under 5% CO_2 at 37 °C, as described previously [20]. Cells were used at the passages of 3–10 from the stocked original cells.

2.3. Purification of Recombinant Proteins and Their Fluorescent Labeling

The cloned mMT-I/pGEX-4T-1 plasmid and mouse β_2-MG/pGEX-4T-1 plasmid were transformed into BL21(DE3)pLysS (Promega, Madison, WI, USA). The selected transformed cells were grown in 10 mL SOB medium containing 50 μg/mL ampicillin for 16 h at 37 °C until the optical density at 600 nm reached 0.3–0.4. The expression of MT and β_2-MG proteins was induced by incubation with 1 mM IPTG for 6 h at 37 °C. The cultured cells were harvested by centrifugation at 8000 rpm for 10 min at 4 °C, and the GST-fusion proteins were purified by using MagneGSTTM Protein Purification (Promega). After a dialysis against PBS, the GST-fusion MT and GST-fusion β_2-MG proteins were digested with thrombin (GE Healthcare, Buckinghamshire, UK). The lysates were loaded onto GST GraviTrapTM gravity-flow columns (GE Healthcare) to remove GST proteins, and the lysates were loaded onto a Benzamidine Sepharose 4 Fast Flow resin (GE Healthcare) to remove thrombin.

The purified recombinant MT and β_2-MG proteins were conjugated with fluorescein isothiocyanate (FITC) by Fluorescein Labeling Kit-NH2 (Dojindo, Kumamoto, Japan). For FITC-labeled albumin and Alexa-labeled transferrin, commercially available albumin-fluorescein isothiocyanate conjugate and Alexa Fluor® 488-conjugated ChromPure Mouse Transferrin, respectively, were used.

2.4. Fluorescence Imaging of the Labeled Proteins in S1 Cells

S1 cells grown in glass-bottom dishes were incubated with each fluorescent-labeled protein and Hoechst33258 for 30 min, washed with phosphate-buffered saline (PBS), fixed with 4% paraformaldehyde in PBS for 5 min on ice, and then permeabilized with 0.5% TritonX-100 in PBS for 15 min at room temperature.

For the immunostaining of EEA1 to detect the early endosome, the fixed cells were washed with PBS and incubated with a blocking buffer containing bovine serum albumin (BSA) in PBS for 0.5 h at room temperature. The cells were then incubated with an anti-EEA1 antibody at a 1:100 dilution in blocking buffer for 1 h at room temperature. After washing with PBS, the cells were incubated with Alexa 555 anti-rabbit IgG at a 1:500 dilution in blocking buffer for 1 h at room temperature.

The distributions of FITC-albumin and Alexa-transferrin were visualized by a Nikon A1R-Si HD confocal microscope (Nikon, Tokyo, Japan), and those of FITC-MT and β_2-MG were visualized by a BZ-X700 all-in-one fluorescence microscope (Keyence, Osaka, Japan).

2.5. Assay for Sensitivity to Cd

Cells were plated on 96-well plates at a density of 3×10^3–2×10^4 cells per well, incubated for 24 h in Cd-free medium, and then treated with $CdCl_2$ for 1, 3, or 6 days. The media were not changed during the Cd exposure period. The alamarBlue® assay (Invitrogen) was used to determine cell viability. AlamarBlue solution was premixed with fresh medium and added to the 96-well plates. After incubation for 2 h, the reduction in alamarBlue by active cells was determined by absorbance at 540 nm and expressed as the percentages compared to that of control cells.

2.6. Measurement of Endocytosis Efficiency by Flow Cytometry

Endocytosis efficiency was determined by using flow cytometry (Guava easyCyte 6HT/2L; Millipore, Billerica, MA, USA). S1 and S2 cells (1×10^5 cells in 6-well dishes) were cultured with Cd at the concentrations of 10 or 15 μM for 1 day, 1 or 3 μM for 3 days, and 0.1 or 0.5 μM for 6 days. hRPTECs were cultured with Cd at the concentrations of 5 or 25 M for 3 days. After the media were changed to Cd- and serum-free ones, the cells were incubated with each fluorescent-labeled protein for 30 min, washed three times with 0.5 mL ice-cold PBS, and then harvested and subjected to flow cytometry. In order to quantify the percentages of cell populations incorporating fluorescent proteins, the populations were divided into quadrants, and the percentages of the cell populations in the lower-right section were calculated.

2.7. Immunoblot Analysis

Cells were harvested with a lysis buffer, and the extracted proteins were separated by SDS polyacrylamide gel electrophoresis (7.5–10%) and electrophoretically transferred to a polyvinylidene fluoride membrane. The transblots were preincubated with 5% nonfat dry skim milk or BSA in Tris-buffered saline (TBS, pH 7.4) and then incubated overnight with the antibody against each protein. After washing with TBS/0.05% Tween 20, the membranes were incubated with either anti-rabbit, anti-mouse, or anti-goat IgG HRP-linked antibody (1:3000). The membrane was rinsed with TBS/0.05% Tween 20, and the immunoreactive bands were developed by ECL systems (Millipore Billerica, MA, USA).

2.8. Statistical Analysis

Statistically significant differences were determined by one-way ANOVA followed by Bonferroni multiple comparisons using a Statcel 3 software (ver. 3, OMS Publication, Saitama, Japan, 2012).

3. Results

3.1. Fluorescence Imaging of Endocytic Uptakes of the Labeled Proteins into Mouse PTECs

We first confirmed the incorporation of fluorescent-labeled proteins into mouse PTECs with confocal and fluorescence microscopes. As shown in Figure 1A, the green fluorescent signals of FITC and Alexa488 were clearly detected in S1 cells 30 min after the addition of FITC-labeled albumin, β_2-MG, MT, and Alexa-labeled transferrin. The yellow fluorescent signals observed in the cells indicate the overlapping of the red fluorescence of the antibody against EEA1 and the green fluorescence of the proteins, suggesting the incorporation of the labeled proteins into the early endosomes.

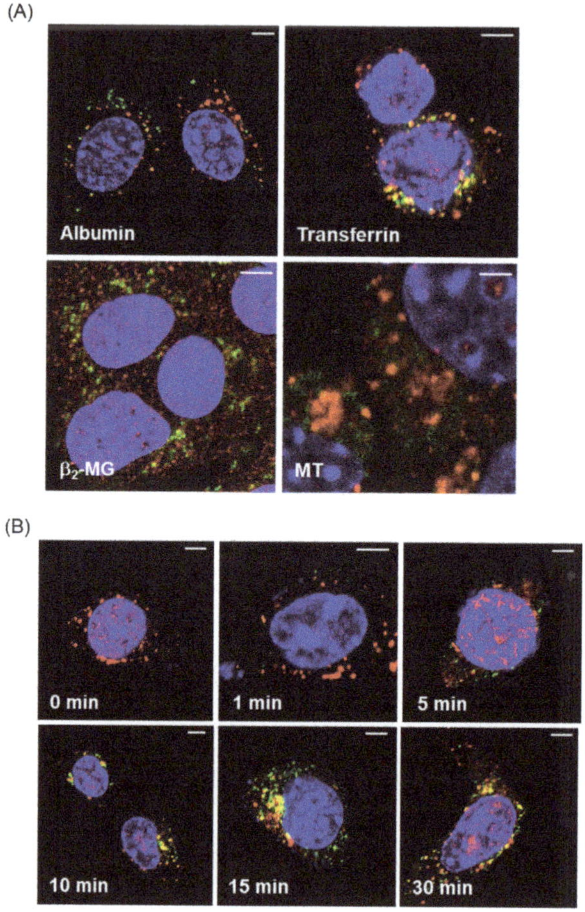

Figure 1. Fluorescence imaging of endocytosed proteins in mouse proximal tubule epithelial cell (PTEC)-derived S1 cells. (**A**) S1 cells were incubated with 50 µg/mL fluorescein isothiocyanate (FITC)-albumin, Alexa-transferrin, FITC-β_2-MG, or FITC-MT (green) for 30 min and then fixed with paraformaldehyde for immunofluorescence labeling with anti-EEA1 (red). Yellow staining demonstrates the colocalization of fluorescent-labeled proteins and early endosomes. (**B**) S1 cells were incubated with Alexa-transferrin for 1, 5, 10, 15, and 30 min. The localization of Alexa-transferrin (green) and early endosomes stained with anti-EEA1 (red) was visualized by confocal microscopy. Bars, 5 µm.

Figure 1B shows the time-dependent changes in the fluorescent signals of transferrin that showed the strongest fluorescent intensities. The green signals of transferrin began to be detected within cells 1 min after the addition of the protein. Yellow fluorescent signals, indicative of the incorporation of transferrin into the early endosomes, began to appear at 10 min and then increased up to 30 min. Thus, the results of the fluorescence imaging provided evidence for endocytic incorporation of the labeled proteins into S1 cells.

3.2. *Quantification of Endocytic Uptakes of the Labeled Proteins into Mouse PTECs*

Next, we set up a quantification system for determining the endocytosis efficiency of each protein into the cells by using flow cytometry. The cells were cultured with each fluorescent-labeled protein for 30 min, washed, harvested, and applied to flow cytometry. As shown in Figure 2, the percentages of the cell population in lower-right section in the quadrants were used as the indicator of endocytosis efficiency (%). Based on the results of preliminary experiments, the amounts of the labeled proteins were decided to be 25 μg/mL for albumin and transferrin and 50 μg/mL for β_2-MG and MT as the optimal conditions for incorporation. We used both S1 and S2 cells derived from the S1 and S2 segments of mouse proximal tubules, respectively, since both cell lines showed similar expression levels of megalin, cubilin, and transferrin receptor, which are essential for endocytosis in PTECs (Figure S1). We determined the time-dependent changes in endocytosis efficiency for each protein (Figures S2 and S3). Although these data are obtained by preliminary experiments, it was shown that the uptake rates of albumin and transferrin during 30 min were almost the same between S1 and S2 cells while those of β_2-MG and MT were lower into S2 cells than into S1 cells. Since most proteins showed maximal uptakes at 30 min, the effects of Cd exposure on the endocytic uptakes of these proteins were examined 30 min after the addition of the labeled proteins in the subsequent experiments.

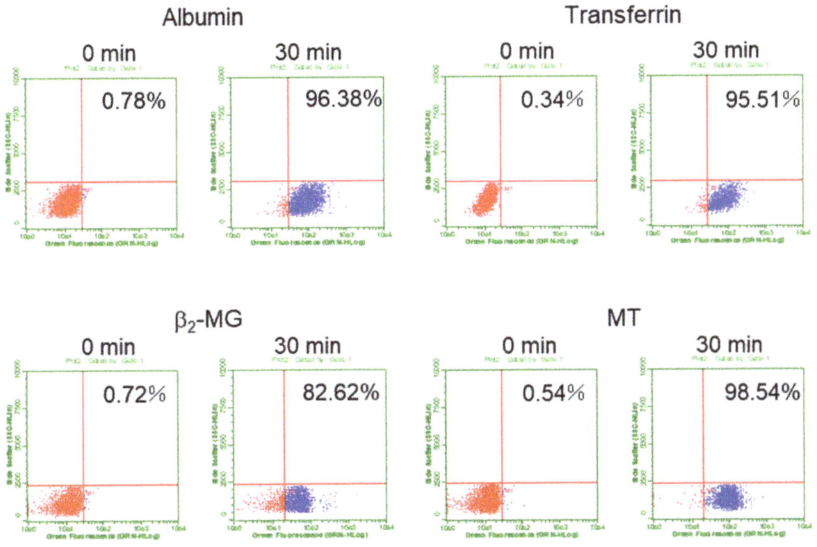

Figure 2. Evaluation of endocytosis efficiency of the fluorescent-labeled proteins by using flow cytometry. The cells were cultured with each of the fluorescent-labeled protein for 0 or 30 min and applied to flow cytometry. Typical quadrant data of each protein in S1 cells were shown here. X-axis indicates fluorescent intensity and y-axis indicates side scattering. The untreated cells (0 min) showing the auto-fluorescence were gated to be the lower-left section in the quadrants. The cell populations in the lower-right section were expressed as the percentage of total cells and used as the indicator of endocytosis efficiency (%) in the subsequent experiments.

The high efficiency of transferrin incorporation into S1 and S2 cells may be partially caused by the expression of transferrin receptor in these cells (Figure S1). It is known that the transferrin receptor in PTECs is expressed in the basolateral [22] and apical [23] membranes, whereas megalin and cubilin are expressed at the apical membrane [24], suggesting that both uptake systems for transferrin contribute to the highly efficient uptake into the endosomes in S1 cells.

3.3. *Effects of Cd Exposure on the Endocytic Uptakes of the Labeled Proteins into Mouse PTECs*

Before examining the effects of Cd exposure on the endocytic uptakes of the labeled proteins into S1 and S2 cells, we checked the lethal toxicity of Cd in S1 and S2 cells using the alamarBlue assay (Figure 3). Based on the results of this assay, we selected sublethal doses of Cd, as indicated by the arrows in Figure 3, for the subsequent endocytosis experiments. We also attempted to use much higher doses of Cd (5 μM Cd for 3 days and 1 μM Cd for 6 days), but S1 and S2 cells could not survive these concentrations of Cd when cultured in 6-well plates for endocytosis experiments. The discrepancy in cytotoxicity between the 96-well (alamarBlue® assay) and 6-well plates may be attributable to the differences in cell density. Therefore, in the endocytosis experiments we used 10 and 15 μM Cd for 1 day, 1 and 3 μM Cd for 3 days, and 0.1 and 0.5 μM Cd for 6 days. Under these conditions, very few cells were found to be detached from the plates at the end of Cd exposure, and the three-times washing of the cells with ice-cold PBS before harvesting did not result in the detachment of the cells. Thus, the effects of Cd on the endocytosis efficiencies in the following experiments were carried out with the cells including least populations of dead cells.

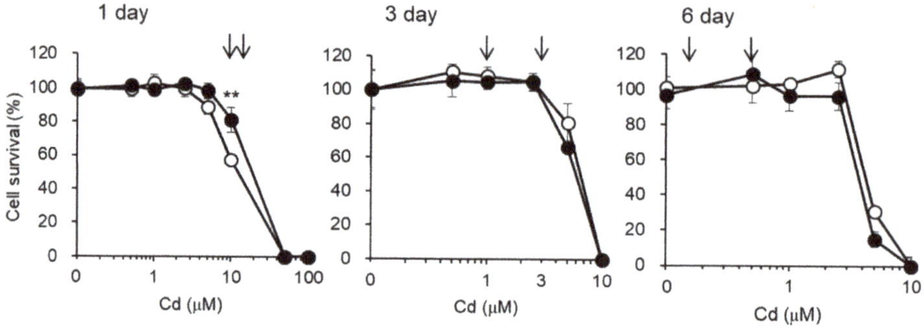

Figure 3. Cytotoxicity of Cd in S1 and S2 cells. S1 (open circles) and S2 (closed circles) cells cultured in 96-well plates were incubated with the indicated concentrations of $CdCl_2$ for 1, 3, and 6 days. Cell viability was determined by alamarBlue® assay and expressed as a percentage of the nontreated cells. From these results, the Cd concentrations to be used in the subsequent experiments were determined (arrows). Data are presented as means ± SD (n = 4–6). Statistically significant difference between S1 and S2 cells was indicated as ** $p < 0.01$.

After the exposure of S1 cells to Cd at these concentrations for 1, 3, and 6 days, the endocytic uptakes of the labeled albumin and transferrin into S1 cells were examined (Figure 4 and Figure S4). However, Cd exposure did not affect the endocytic uptake of either albumin or transferrin. On the other hand, the endocytic uptakes of β_2-MG and MT were affected by Cd exposure depending on the exposure duration (Figure 5). The 1- and 3-day exposures of S1 and S2 cells to Cd resulted in statistically significant decreases in the endocytic uptake of β_2-MG (Figure 5A), whereas only the 3-day exposure to Cd resulted in statistically significant decreases in endocytic uptakes of MT (Figure 5B and Figure S4). The 6-day exposure to Cd did not cause any significant decreases in endocytic uptakes of either β_2-MG or MT in either cells.

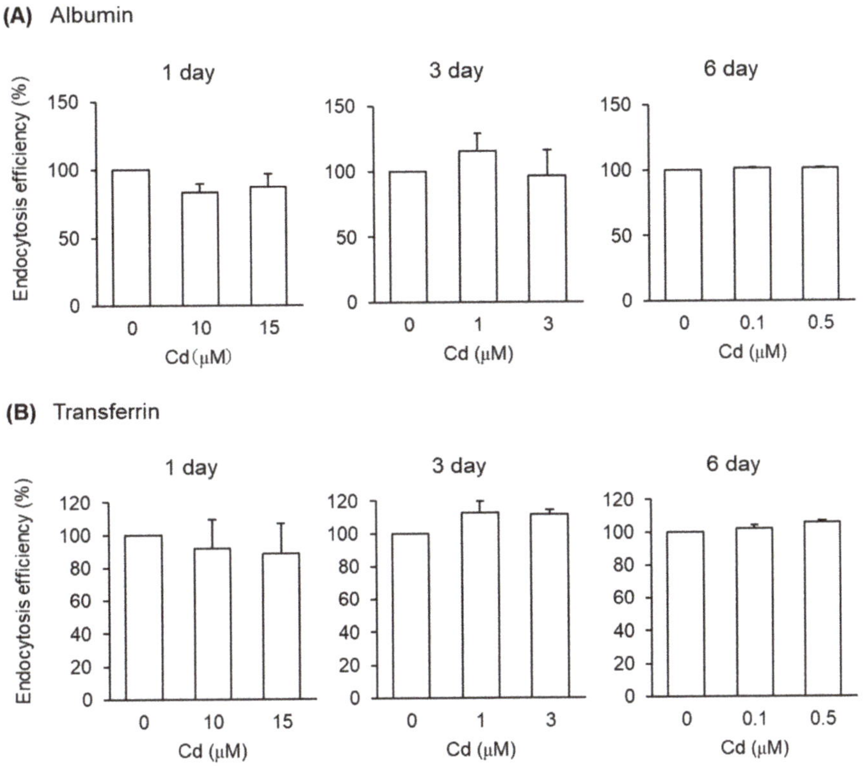

Figure 4. Effects of Cd on the endocytosis efficiencies of albumin and transferrin into S1 cells. S1 cells were exposed to $CdCl_2$ for 1, 3, and 6 days and then incubated with FITC-albumin (**A**) or Alexa-transferrin (**B**) for 30 min. The endocytosis efficiencies were determined by flow cytometry and expressed as percentages of the control cells (no exposure to Cd). Data are presented as means ± SD (n = 3–4).

3.4. Effects of Cd Exposure on the Endocytic Uptakes of the Labeled Proteins into Human PTECs

To test whether Cd exposure also affects endocytic uptakes of β_2-MG and MT in human PTECs, we utilized hRPTECs, an immortalized cell line derived from human kidney PTECs. Since the effects of Cd on the endocytic uptakes of β_2-MG and MT in mouse S1 and S2 cells were clearly detected after the 3-day exposure to Cd (Figure 5), hRPTECs were exposed to Cd for 3 days. Prior to the endocytosis experiment, we checked the sensitivity of hRPTECs to Cd. As shown in Figure 6A, hRPTECs were highly resistant to Cd compared with S1 or S2 cells. Therefore, we used 5 and 25 μM Cd for endocytosis experiments in hRPTECs. As shown in Figure 6B, the endocytic uptakes of both β_2-MG and MT were significantly reduced by 3-day exposure to Cd.

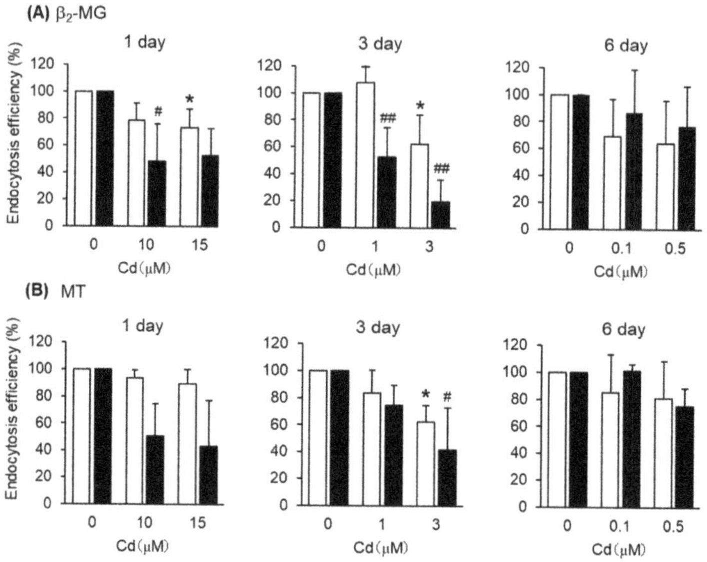

Figure 5. Effects of Cd on the endocytosis efficiencies of β_2-MG and MT into S1 and S2 cells. S1 and S2 cells were exposed to $CdCl_2$ for 1, 3, and 6 days and then incubated with FITC-β_2-MG (**A**) or FITC-MT (**B**) for 30 min. The endocytosis efficiencies were determined by flow cytometry and expressed as percentages of the control cells (no exposure to Cd). Open and closed columns represent S1 and S2 cells, respectively. Data are presented as means ± SD (n = 3–4). Statistical significance of the dose dependence determined by one-way ANOVA was detected in the following settings: day1-S1 cells ($p < 0.05$), day1-S2 cells ($p < 0.05$), day3-S1 cells ($p < 0.05$), and day3-S2 cells ($p < 0.01$) for β_2-MG (**A**), and day3-S1 cells ($p < 0.05$) and day3-S2 cells ($p < 0.05$) for MT (**B**). Statistical significances compared with the control cells determined by Bonferroni multiple comparisons are indicated as * $p < 0.05$, ** $p < 0.01$ (S1 cells) and # $p < 0.05$, ## $p < 0.01$ (S2 cells).

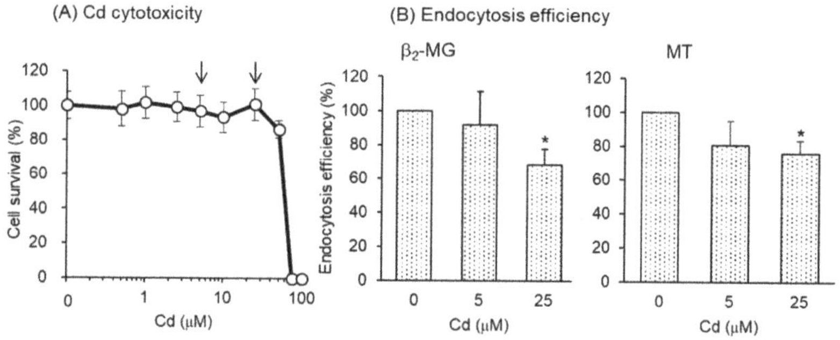

Figure 6. The effects of Cd exposure for 3 days on the endocytosis efficiencies of β_2-MG and MT into hRPTEC human renal cells. (**A**) Cell viability was determined by alamarBlue assay and expressed as the percentages of the nontreated cells. From these results, the Cd concentrations to be used in the endocytosis experiment were determined (arrows). Data are presented as means ± SD (n = 4–6). (**B**) The cells were exposed to $CdCl_2$ for 3 days and then incubated with FITC-β_2-MG or FITC-MT for 30 min. The endocytosis efficiencies were determined by flow cytometry and expressed as percentages of the control cells (no exposure to Cd). Data are presented as means ± SD (n = 3–4). Statistical significance of the dose dependence determined by one-way ANOVA was detected in both β_2-MG ($p < 0.05$) and MT ($p < 0.05$). Statistical significance compared with the control cells determined by Bonferroni multiple comparisons are indicated as * $p < 0.05$.

4. Discussion

Disturbances in the tubular reabsorption of glomerular-filtered biomolecules by PTECS in kidney are a hallmark of Cd-induced nephrotoxicity. The urinary excretion of β_2-MG has been particularly widely used as an indicator of renal tubular dysfunction among residents of Cd-polluted areas [6,9,10]. However, the precise mechanisms underlying Cd-induced dysfunctions of tubular reabsorption of LMW proteins by PTECs have not been fully investigated. This is partly due to the lack of a proper in vitro experimental system.

In the present study, we developed an in vitro experimental system for evaluating the endocytosis efficiency of fluorescent-labeled proteins into cultured PTECs derived from mouse and human kidney. The endocytic uptakes of the labeled proteins and their cellular localization were confirmed by fluorescence imaging (Figure 1). Flowcytometric analyses of the fluorescent-labeled proteins have enabled us to quantitatively evaluate the uptake rates of labeled proteins into S1 and S2 cells (Figure 2). The exposure of these cells to sublethal doses of Cd for 3 days resulted in significant decreases in the endocytic uptakes of β_2-MG and MT (Figure 5), but not in those of albumin or transferrin (Figure 4). These results demonstrated that the assay system developed in this study permitted the detection of Cd-induced declines in renal reabsorption of LMW proteins in cultured PTECs. The reason for the absence of the effects of Cd after 6-day exposure remains unknown. Possibly, more complicated factors are involved in the 6-day exposure than the 3-day exposure experiments. Although future studies are required for the mechanisms of Cd-induced decreases in the LMW protein uptakes, this assay system may be useful for screening other renal toxicants that may cause damage in tubular reabsorption.

To date, epidemiological studies in humans and experimental studies in animals have linked increases in urinary excretion of LMW proteins such as β_2-MG with the loss of functional PTECs and nephrons in the kidney at the advanced stage of Cd nephrotoxicity [25,26]. Most mechanistic studies on Cd cytotoxicity have focused on the molecular pathways leading to Cd-associated cell death and not on the direct effects of Cd on the endocytic uptakes of LMW proteins in living PTECs [15–17]. However, the effects of moderately higher, but not lethal, doses of Cd on the reabsorption efficiencies of LMW proteins by the surviving PTECs remain unclear. The results of this study demonstrated that a 3-day exposure to Cd resulted in significant declines in the endocytic uptakes of β_2-MG and MT under the conditions in which nonlethal doses of Cd were used. This could not be ascribed simply to the increase in dead cells after Cd exposure, since no effects were observed in the endocytosis efficiencies of albumin or transferrin (Figure 4) and only the surviving cells that were not detached from the plates during Cd exposure were used for flow cytometry analyses. Although a few studies have investigated the effects of Cd on the interactions of LMW proteins with megalin/cubilin systems in cultured renal cells [18,19], the present study utilized flow cytometry for quantitatively evaluating the endocytosis efficiency of the proteins and showed the effects of Cd on the uptakes of LMW proteins in cultured PTECs.

Although many epidemiological studies undertaken in Cd-polluted areas have demonstrated that urinary excretion of β_2-MG is an excellent biomarker for renal tubular dysfunctions [6,9,10], recent evidence suggested that β_2-MG plays much broader roles as a biomarker not only for tubular dysfunctions, but also for glomerular dysfunctions as well as non-renal diseases [27]. The results of our in vitro study added a piece of evidence that the decreased incorporation of β_2-MG into renal tubular cells is involved in Cd-induced kidney damages. Future studies are required to test whether the decrease in the β_2-MG incorporation into renal tubular cells is inducible specifically by Cd, or commonly by other renal toxicants using this assay system.

Compared with the uptakes of β_2-MG and MT, those of albumin and transferrin by S1 cells appear to be far less sensitive to Cd toxicity (Figure 4). Many human studies have suggested that the urinary excretion of β_2-MG, a LMW protein, reflects damage in renal tubular reabsorption, whereas the urinary excretion of albumin, an HMW protein, may reflect the dysfunction of glomeruli [28–30], although recent evidence has indicated that tubular reabsorption of albumin should not be ignored [31]. The results of this study also demonstrated that substantial amounts of albumin can be taken up by cultured

PTECs. Although the differences in the endocytic pathways between HMW albumin and LMW β_2-MG remains unclear, the higher sensitivity of β_2-MG than albumin in this in vitro assay system may reflect the in vivo observation that β_2-MG is the most sensitive indicator for renal tubular damage caused by Cd exposure [28,29]. Regarding the comparisons between HMW and LMW proteins, the differences in molecular weights, i.e., albumin and MT, could have affected the endocytosis efficiency because we used 25 μg/mL albumin and 50 μg/mL MT as the optimal conditions, not based on a molar basis, in this assay.

The strengths and limitations of this study should be noted. (1) The use of flow cytometry enabled the quantitative evaluation of the endocytosis efficiencies of fluorescent-labeled proteins, (2) the use of both mouse- and human-derived PTECs enabled the confirmation of reproducibility of Cd effects, and (3) the use of sublethal doses of Cd enabled the sensitive detection of the effects of Cd on the PTECs that survived the lethal toxicity of Cd. However, the observed effects of Cd on the endocytosis efficiencies of β_2-MG and MT were not so marked, though statistically significant, and the involvements of Cd cytotoxicity on the results of flow cytometry may not be completely excluded. Since the in vivo dysfunctions of renal tubular reabsorption generally occur under conditions where a large part of nephrons and PTECs is lost [25,26], the in vitro effects of renal toxicants on the endocytosis efficiency in the living PTECs may reflect only a part of the whole events of renal dysfunction. Nevertheless, this in vitro assay system may provide a useful tool for the future screening of other renal toxicants and for more detailed mechanistic studies.

For future applications of this assay system to the detection of possible renal toxicants damaging tubular reabsorption, the merits and disadvantages of this system should be discussed here. Since mouse S1 and S2 cells and human hRPTECs are all immortalized cell lines, they can provide reproducible and reliable results compared with the primary cultured PTECs prepared freshly from the proximal tubules of kidney. In this study, both mouse and human PTECs showed decreases in endocytic uptakes of β_2-MG and MT after the 3-day exposure to Cd. However, approximately ten times higher concentrations of Cd were required in hRPTECs than in S1 and S2 cells to produce similar detrimental effects (Figure 6) due to the high Cd resistance of hRPTECs, which is the major drawback of using hRPTECs. S2 cells showed a lower efficiency of endocytic uptakes of β_2-MG and MT than S1 cells, whereas the uptake efficiencies of albumin and transferrin were similar to those of S1 cells (Figure 2). Although both S1 and S2 cells showed significant decreases in endocytic uptakes of β_2-MG and MT (Figure 5) when exposed to Cd for 3 days, S1 cells may be more preferable for screening renal toxicants that affect the endocytic uptakes of LMW proteins, since the uptake efficiencies of LMW proteins under unexposed conditions are stable and reliable in S1 cells. We are now planning a screening study using S1 cells to test whether other renal toxicants affect the endocytic uptakes of β_2-MG.

5. Conclusions

The aim of this study was to establish an in vitro assay system for evaluating the efficiency of endocytic uptakes of LMW and HMW proteins labeled with fluorescent moiety in cultured PTECs. Flowcytometric determinations of the uptakes of the fluorescent-labeled proteins into mouse S1 and S2 cells and human hRPTECs enabled us to find that a 3-day exposure to Cd resulted decreased endocytic uptakes of β_2-MG and MT in all these cells. Thus, these cells, especially S1 cells, proved to be useful for the elucidation of the mechanisms of Cd-induced dysfunctions of renal tubular reabsorption. In future studies, this in vitro system can be used to investigate the effects of Cd exposure on the expression of megalin and cubilin at the apical membrane, the functions of mitochondria, which provide the energy for endocytosis, and other machineries required for the process of endocytosis. This system may also serve as a tool for studying the mechanisms of other toxicants causing renal tubular dysfunctions.

Supplementary Materials: The following are available online at http://www.mdpi.com/2305-6304/8/2/24/s1, Figure S1: Expression levels of the proteins involved in endocytosis in S1 and S2 cells, Figure S2: Time-dependent changes in endocytic uptakes of albumin, transferrin, β_2-MG, and MT, Figure S3: Time-dependent changes in endocytic uptakes of albumin, transferrin, β_2-MG, and MT, Figure S4: Effects of Cd on the endocytosis efficiencies of albumin and β_2-MG into S1 cells.

Author Contributions: Conceptualization, H.F. and S.H.; cell biology experiments, H.F., H.Y., N.O. (Nobuki Otera), N.O. (Nanae Oka), and M.J.; fluorescence imaging, H.Y., N.O. (Nobuki Otera), and N.O. (Nanae Oka); synthesis and purification of recombinant proteins, H.F., N.O. (Nanae Oka), and M.J.; development of flow cytometric quantification of endocytosis, H.F. and H.Y.; writing and editing, H.F. and S.H. All authors have read and agreed to the published version of the manuscript.

Funding: This work was partly supported by JSPS KAKENHI Grant Numbers 19H05770 (H.F.) and 19H01081 (S.H. and H.F.), and by the Study of Health Effects of Heavy Metals organized by Ministry of the Environment, Japan (S.H.).

Conflicts of Interest: The authors declare no conflict of interest.

References

1. Himeno, S.; Aoshima, K. (Eds.) *Cadmium Toxicity—New Aspects in Human Disease, Rice Contamination, and Cytotoxicity*; Springer Nature Switzerland AG: Basel, Switzerland, 2019; ISBN 978-981-13-3630-0.
2. Elinder, C.G.; Lind, B.; Kjellström, T.; Linnman, L.; Friberg, L. Cadmium in kidney cortex, liver, and pancreas from Swedish autopsies. Estimation of biological half time in kidney cortex, considering calorie intake and smoking habits. *Arch. Environ. Health* **1976**, *31*, 292–302. [CrossRef] [PubMed]
3. Blainey, J.D.; Adams, R.G.; Brewer, D.B.; Harvey, T.C. Cadmium-induced osteomalacia. *Br. J. Ind. Med.* **1980**, *37*, 278–284. [CrossRef]
4. Takebayashi, S.; Jimi, S.; Segawa, M.; Kiyoshi, Y. Cadmium induces osteomalacia mediated by proximal tubular atrophy and disturbances of phosphate reabsorption. A study of 11 autopsies. *Pathol. Res. Pract.* **2000**, *196*, 653–663. [CrossRef]
5. Savolainen, H. Cadmium-associated renal disease. *Ren. Fail.* **1995**, *17*, 483–487. [CrossRef] [PubMed]
6. Chan, W.Y.; Rennert, O.M. Cadmium nephropathy. *Ann. Clin. Lab. Sci.* **1981**, *11*, 229–238.
7. Tohyama, C.; Shaikh, Z.A.; Ellis, K.J.; Cohn, S.H. Metallothionein excretion in urine upon cadmium exposure: Its relationship with liver and kidney cadmium. *Toxicology* **1981**, *22*, 181–191. [CrossRef]
8. Satarug, S. Dietary cadmium intake and its effects on kidneys. *Toxics* **2018**, *6*, 15. [CrossRef]
9. Ikeda, M.; Ezaki, T.; Moriguchi, J.; Fukui, Y.; Ukai, H.; Okamoto, S.; Sakurai, H. The threshold cadmium level that causes a substantial increase in β_2-microglobulin in urine of general populations. *Tohoku J. Exp. Med.* **2005**, *205*, 247–261. [CrossRef]
10. Shiroishi, K.; Kjellström, T.; Kubota, K.; Evrin, P.E.; Anayama, M.; Vesterberg, O.; Shimada, T.; Piscator, M.; Iwata, T.; Nishino, H. Urine analysis for detection of cadmium-induced renal changes, with special reference to β_2-microglobulin. A cooperative study between Japan and Sweden. *Environ. Res.* **1977**, *13*, 407–424. [CrossRef]
11. Klassen, R.B.; Crenshaw, K.; Kozyraki, R.; Verroust, P.J.; Tio, L.; Atrian, S.; Allen, P.L.; Hammond, T.G. Megalin mediates renal uptake of heavy metal metallothionein complexes. *Am. J. Physiol. Ren. Physiol.* **2004**, *287*, F393–F403. [CrossRef]
12. Christensen, E.I.; Birn, H. Megalin and cubilin: Synergistic endocytic receptors in renal proximal tubule. *Am. J. Physiol. Ren. Physiol.* **2001**, *280*, F562–F573. [CrossRef] [PubMed]
13. Sabolic, I.; Ljubojevic, M.; Herak-Kramberger, C.M.; Brown, D. Cd-MT causes endocytosis of brush-border transporters in rat renal proximal tubules. *Am. J. Physiol. Ren. Physiol.* **2002**, *283*, F1389–F1402. [CrossRef] [PubMed]
14. Onodera, A.; Tani, M.; Michigami, T.; Yamagata, M.; Min, K.S.; Tanaka, K.; Nakanishi, T.; Kimura, T.; Itoh, N. Role of megalin and the soluble form of its ligand RAP in Cd-metallothionein endocytosis and Cd-metallothionein-induced nephrotoxicity in vivo. *Toxicol. Lett.* **2012**, *212*, 91–96. [CrossRef] [PubMed]
15. Tokumoto, M.; Lee, J.Y.; Satoh, M. Transcription factors and downstream genes in cadmium toxicity. *Biol. Pharm. Bull.* **2019**, *42*, 1083–1088. [CrossRef]
16. Fujiwara, Y.; Lee, J.Y.; Tokumoto, M.; Satoh, M. Cadmium renal toxicity via apoptotic pathways. *Biol. Pharm. Bull.* **2012**, *35*, 1892–1897. [CrossRef] [PubMed]
17. Lee, J.Y.; Tokumoto, M.; Fujiwara, Y.; Hasegawa, T.; Seko, Y.; Shimada, A.; Satoh, M. Accumulation of p53 via down-regulation of UBE2D family genes is a critical pathway for cadmium-induced renal toxicity. *Sci. Rep.* **2016**, *6*, 21968. [CrossRef]

18. Wolff, N.A.; Abouhamed, M.; Verroust, P.J.; Thévenod, F. Megalin-dependent internalization of cadmium-metallothionein and cytotoxicity in cultured renal proximal tubule cells. *J. Pharmacol. Exp. Ther.* **2006**, *318*, 782–791. [CrossRef]
19. Fels, J.; Scharner, B.; Zarbock, R.; Zavala Guevara, I.P.; Lee, W.K.; Barbier, O.C.; Thévenod, F. Cadmium complexed with β2-microglubulin, albumin and lipocalin-2 rather than metallothionein cause megalin:cubilin dependent toxicity of the renal proximal tubule. *Int. J. Mol. Sci.* **2019**, *20*, 2379. [CrossRef]
20. Fujishiro, H.; Hamao, S.; Isawa, M.; Himeno, S. Segment-specific and direction-dependent transport of cadmium and manganese in immortalized S1, S2, and S3 cells derived from mouse kidney proximal tubules. *J. Toxicol. Sci.* **2019**, *44*, 611–619. [CrossRef]
21. Fujishiro, H.; Himeno, S. Gene expression profiles of immortalized S1, S2, and S3 cells derived from each segment of mouse kidney proximal tubules. *Fundam. Toxicol. Sci.* **2019**, *6*, 117–123. [CrossRef]
22. Fuller, S.D.; Simons, K. Transferrin receptor polarity and recycling accuracy in "tight" and "leaky" strains of Madin-Darby canine kidney cells. *J. Cell Biol.* **1986**, *103*, 1767–1779. [CrossRef] [PubMed]
23. Smith, C.P.; Lee, W.K.; Haley, M.; Poulsen, S.B.; Thévenod, F.; Fenton, R.A. Proximal tubule transferrin uptake is modulated by cellular iron and mediated by apical membrane megalin-cubilin complex and transferrin receptor 1. *J. Biol. Chem.* **2019**, *294*, 7025–7036. [CrossRef]
24. Nielsen, R.; Christensen, E.I.; Birn, H. Megalin and cubilin in proximal tubule protein reabsorption: From experimental models to human disease. *Kidney Int.* **2016**, *89*, 58–67. [CrossRef] [PubMed]
25. Imura, J.; Tsuneyama, K.; Ueda, Y. Novel Pathological Study of Cadmium Nephropathy of *Itai-Itai* Disease. In *Cadmium Toxicity—New Aspects in Human Disease, Rice Contamination, and Cytotoxicity*; Himeno, S., Aoshima, K., Eds.; Springer Nature Switzerland AG: Basel, Switzerland, 2019; pp. 39–50.
26. Satarug, S.; Vesey, D.A.; Nishijo, M.; Ruangyuttikarn, W.; Gobe, G.C. The inverse association of glomerular function and urinary β_2-MG excretion and its implications for cadmium health risk assessment. *Environ. Res.* **2019**, *173*, 40–47. [CrossRef] [PubMed]
27. Argyropoulos, C.P.; Chen, S.S.; Ng, Y.H.; Roumelioti, M.E.; Shaffi, K.; Singh, P.P.; Tzamaloukas, A.H. Rediscovering beta-2 microglobulin as a biomarker across the spectrum of kidney diseases. *Front. Med.* **2017**, *4*, 73. [CrossRef] [PubMed]
28. Jin, T.; Wu, X.; Tang, Y.; Nordberg, M.; Bernard, A.; Ye, T.; Kong, Q.; Lundström, N.G.; Nordberg, G.F. Environmental epidemiological study and estimation of benchmark dose for renal dysfunction in a cadmium-polluted area in China. *Biometals* **2004**, *17*, 525–530. [CrossRef]
29. Jin, T.; Kong, Q.; Ye, T.; Wu, X.; Nordberg, G.F. Renal dysfunction of cadmium-exposed workers residing in a cadmium-polluted environment. *Biometals* **2004**, *17*, 513–518. [CrossRef]
30. Liang, Y.; Lei, L.; Nilsson, J.; Li, H.; Nordberg, M.; Bernard, A.; Nordberg, G.F.; Bergdahl, I.A.; Jin, T. Renal function after reduction in Cadmium exposure: An 8-year follow-up of residents in Cadmium-polluted areas. *Environ. Health Perspect.* **2012**, *120*, 223–228. [CrossRef]
31. Dickson, L.E.; Wagner, M.C.; Sandoval, R.M.; Molitoris, B.A. The proximal tubule and albuminuria: Really! *J. Am. Soc. Nephrol.* **2014**, *25*, 443–453. [CrossRef]

toxics

MDPI

Article

Increased Mitochondrial Fragmentation Mediated by Dynamin-Related Protein 1 Contributes to Hexavalent Chromium-Induced Mitochondrial Respiratory Chain Complex I-Dependent Cytotoxicity

Yu Ma, Yujing Zhang, Yuanyuan Xiao and Fang Xiao *

Department of Health Toxicology, Xiangya School of Public Health, Central South University, Changsha 410078, China; 196901002@csu.edu.cn (Y.M.); zhangyujing@hunnu.edu.cn (Y.Z.); xiaoyuanyuan@csu.edu.cn (Y.X.)

* Correspondence: fangxiao@csu.edu.cn

Received: 26 March 2020; Accepted: 23 July 2020; Published: 29 July 2020

Abstract: Hexavalent chromium (Cr(VI)) pollution is a severe public health problem in the world. Although it is believed that mitochondrial fragmentation is a common phenomenon in apoptosis, whether excessive fission is crucial for apoptosis remains controversial. We previously confirmed that Cr(VI) mainly targeted mitochondrial respiratory chain complex I (MRCC I) to induce reactive oxygen species (ROS)-mediated apoptosis, but the related mechanism was unclear. In this study, we found Cr(VI) targeted MRCC I to induce ROS accumulation and triggered mitochondria-related cytotoxicity. Cr(VI)-induced cytotoxicity was alleviated by pretreatment of Glutamate/malate (Glu/Mal; MRCC I substrates), and was aggravated by cotreatment of rotenone (ROT; MRCC I inhibitor). Cr(VI) induced excessive mitochondrial fragmentation and mitochondrial dynamin-related protein 1 (Drp1) translocation, the application of Drp1-siRNA alleviated Cr(VI)-induced apoptosis. The cytotoxicity in the Drp1-si plus Cr(VI) treatment group was alleviated by the application of Glu/Mal, and was aggravated by the application of ROT. Drp1 siRNA promoted the inhibition of Glu/Mal on Cr(VI)-induced cytotoxicity, and alleviated the aggravation of ROT on Cr(VI)-induced cytotoxicity. Taken together, Cr(VI)-induced Drp1 modulation was dependent on MRCC I inhibition-mediated ROS production, and Drp1-mediated mitochondrial fragmentation contributed to Cr(VI)-induced MRCC I-dependent cytotoxicity, which provided the experimental basis for further elucidating Cr(VI)-induced cytotoxicity.

Keywords: hexavalent chromium [Cr(VI)]; mitochondrial fragmentation; dynamin-related protein 1 (Drp1); mitochondrial respiratory chain complex I (MRCC I); reactive oxygen species (ROS)

1. Introduction

Chromium (Cr) widely exists in the ecological environment and can be found in pigments, chrome-plated metals, cement, detergents, and industrial Cr waste dumps [1]. Cr has a variety of oxidation states (−2 to +6), but only trivalent chromium (Cr(III)) and hexavalent chromium (Cr(VI)) are stable. The increase in industrial use, coupled with improper disposal of Cr(VI)-related waste, has led to the serious increase of Cr(VI) levels in air, water, and soil, resulting in the pollution of the environment, even the food chain [2].

Mitochondria constantly undergo a dynamic fusion/fission process, which is mainly controlled by regulatory proteins such as mitofusins (Mfns) and dynamin-related protein 1 (Drp1) [3]. This kind of dynamic balance is essential to maintain constant changes in mitochondrial shape, size, and network. Mitochondrial fission process is mainly mediated by Drp1, which exists in the cytosol and translocates to the outer membrane of mitochondrial during fission [4]. Increasing evidence suggested that the dynamic morphology of the mitochondrial network is very important. In the physiological state, the long, continuous tracks of fused mitochondria and branching networks are dominant and mainly regulated by Mitofusins (Mfns). However, upon exposure to various stresses, mitochondria undergo fission, networks become unraveled, and the fragmented morphology is more prominent (regulated Drp1). Preliminary studies have shown that Drp1 ablation declined Cyt c release and inhibited apoptosis [5]. In contrast, other studies revealed that blockage of Drp1 partially decreased [6] or had little effect [7] on Cyt c release, without affecting apoptosis.

The electron transport chain (ETC), which exists in the folded inner membranes of mitochondria, is mainly composed of four mitochondrial respiratory chain complexes (MRCC; I–IV) and two free-moving electron transfer carriers cytochrome c (cyt c) and ubiquinone. The four complexes are assembled into a specifically configured super-complex, which together with MRCC V (F1F0ATP synthase), becomes the basis of ATP generation during oxidative phosphorylation [8]. As the largest multi-subunit enzyme complex located in ETC, MRCC I is also called NADH-ubiquinone oxidoreductase, and its key role is to transfer electrons from NADH to ubiquinone [9]. The ETC is the key component of mitochondria and also known as the most important source of intracellular reactive oxygen species (ROS). ROS include oxygen-free radicals such as hydroxyl radical (OH) and superoxide anion radical (O_2^-), and non-radical oxidants such as hydrogen peroxide (H_2O_2). Due to the existence of electron leakage, not all the electrons could be successfully transferred to the final electron acceptor, O_2. Under normal conditions, 0.2–2% of the electrons do not follow the transmission order but directly leak out from ETC, and then interact with oxygen to produce ROS [10]. As a double-edged sword, ROS plays an important role in intracellular signaling pathways, but ROS accumulation can lead to cytotoxicity and even cell death.

Although it is believed that mitochondrial fragmentation is a common phenomenon in apoptosis, whether excessive fission is crucial for apoptosis progression remains controversial. Our previous studies [11,12] have demonstrated that Cr(VI) mainly targeted MRCC I and increased ROS generation to induce cytotoxicity. In addition, Cr(VI) could also cause both mitochondrial damage and apoptotic cell death during ROS-triggered cytotoxicity, but the related mechanism involved in MRCC I-dependent cytotoxicity was unclear. The present study will demonstrate the role of increased mitochondrial fragmentation mediated by Drp1 in Cr(VI)-induced MRCC I-dependent cytotoxicity, which will provide experimental evidence for further elucidating the cytotoxicity of Cr(VI).

2. Materials and Methods

2.1. Cell Culture and Cell Counts

Human L02 hepatocytes, obtained from Experimental Central of Xiangya Hospital of Central South University, Changsha, China, were cultured in 25 cm^2 culture flasks in the standard humidified incubator with the set of 5% CO_2 and 37 °C. Roswell Park Memorial Institute (RPMI) 1640 medium supplemented with 10% fetal bovine serum (FBS) (Gibco, Carlsbad, CA, USA) and 1% penicillin-streptomycin (P/S) solution was used.

Under the optimal conditions, the doubling time of L02 hepatocytes was 18–24 h, and the cells were subcultured every 2.5–3 days (d). Cell numbers were measured and recorded everyday using a hemocytometer by trypan blue exclusion method.

2.2. Drp1 SiRNA

The siRNA sequences were designed and synthesized by RibobioCo. Ltd. (Guangzhou, China). The hepatocytes were transfected with siRNA targeting Drp1 (siB121119100350-1-5) and its negative control (siB06525141910-1-5) using lipofectamine 3000 (Invitrogen, Carlsbad, CA, USA). After 4 h of transfection, the hepatocytes were changed with complete medium.

2.3. *ROS Level*

The intracellular ROS level was determined using 2′, 7′-dichlorofluorescein diacetate (DCFH-DA; Beyotime Institute of Biotechnology, Shanghai, China) by flow cytometry. L02 hepatocytes were treated with indicated chemicals and washed twice by cold PBS and loaded with 10 μM DCFH-DA at 37 °C for 40 min. After the incubation, the hepatocytes were washed again and analyzed by flow cytometry.

2.4. *Alanine Aminotransferase (ALT) and Aspartate Aminotransferase (AST) Levels*

L-02 hepatocytes were treated with different chemicals, and the supernatants were collected. ALT and AST levels were determined using the commercial kits (Jiancheng, Nanjing, China) according to the instructions. The optical density at 510 nm was measured using the multifunctional microplate reader.

2.5. *Caspase-3 Activity*

Caspase-3 activity was determined using the commercial colorimetric assay kit. The hepatocytes were treated with indicated chemicals and washed twice with PBS, followed by lysis with the Caspase-3 Assay kit (Beyotime Institute of Biotechnology, China). The centrifugation was performed at 16,000× *g* at 4 °C for 10 min. The samples were then incubated with Ac-DEVD-pNA (substrate) at 37 °C for 2 h. The absorbance was measured and recorded by a microplate reader at 405 nm.

2.6. *Apoptosis*

The cell apoptosis was determined using a commercial Annexin V-FITC apoptosis detection kit (Invitrogen, Carlsbad, CA, USA). After the treatment of different chemicals, the hepatocytes were incubated with 100 μL 1× binding buffer containing 5 μL Annexin-V-FITC and 1 μL propidium iodide (PI) for 30 min at room temperature. After the incubation, 400 μL binding buffer was added to the culture to stop the staining. The flow cytometric analysis was then performed. Data was analyzed using Flowjo 7.6 software.

2.7. *Mitochondrial Permeability Transition Pore (mPTP) Opening*

The mPTP opening was examined using the commercial kit by monitoring the release of calcein from mitochondrial. Briefly, the hepatocytes were treated with 2 μM calcein-AM and 1 mM CoCl2 for 30 min at room temperature, and washed with PBS. The culture was then incubated with 1 mM CoCl2 for an additional 20 min at 37 °C in order to specifically quench the fluorescence of free calcein in the cytosol. The fluorescence intensity of mitochondrial calcein in L02 hepatocytes was determined using a fluorescence microplate reader at 490 nm/515 nm for excitation/emission. The loss of calcein fluorescence suggested the opening of mPTP.

2.8. *Mitochondrial Membrane Potential (MMP, $\Delta\psi m$)*

The MMP of L02 hepatocytes was detected using JC-1 (Sigma, St. Louis, MO, USA). After the chemicals treatment, the cells were washed with PBS and then incubated with JC-1 for 20 min at 37 °C. The fluorescence intensity was read at the excitation/emission wavelength of 488/530 nm. The MMP is presented as % of control for the fluorescence intensity.

2.9. *qRT-PCR*

Total RNA was isolated with the TRIzol reagent (Invitrogen, Carlsbad, CA, USA) following the manufacturer's instruction. The RNA quality was verified by spectrophotometry. Later on, the cDNAs were synthesized using the ReverTra Ace qPCR RT kit (Toyobo, Tokyo, Japan). For mitochondrial DNA analyses, total DNA was extracted by a DNA extraction kit (NEP002-1, Dingguo, China) according to the manufacturer's instructions. qRT-PCR was performed using the Light Cycler®Nano SYBR Green I Master on a Light Cycler® Nano System. The PCR conditions were as follows: 10 min at

95 °C, followed by 40 cycles of 95 °C for 30 s, 56 °C for 30 s and 72 °C for 30 s. The mRNA levels were calculated using the 2−ΔΔCT method normalized to ACTB mRNA.

The Primers used in this study: Drp1, 5′-TAGTGGGCAGGGACCTTCTT-3′ (F) and 5′-TGCTTCAACTCCATTTTCTTCTCC-3′ (R); ACTB, 5′-CACCAGGGCGTGATGGT-3′ (F) and 5′-CTCAAACATGATCTGG GTCAT-3′ (R); NADH dehydrogenase subunit I (ND1), 5′-TACGCAAAGGTTCCCAACG-3′ (F) and 5′-GGTGATGGTGGATGTGGC-3′ (R); cytochrome C Oxidase Subunit IV Isoform 1 (COX4I1), 5-TAGAAACCGTCTGAACTATCC-3′ (F) and 5′- ATGATTATGAGGGCGTGA-3′ (R); β-globin, 5′-GTTACTGCCTG TGGGGCAA-3′ (F) and 5′-CAAAGGTGCCCTTGAGGTT-3′ (R). The qRT-PCR assay was designed and performed in accordance with the Minimum Information for Publication of Quantitative Real-Time PCR Experiments (MIQE) guidelines.

2.10. Mitochondria Mass

Briefly, after the treatment of different chemicals, the hepatocytes were exposed to Mito-Tracker Green (10 μM, 30 min) at 37 °C in the dark. Then the cells were thoroughly washed with pre-warmed PBS, and analyzed with flow cytometer at 490/516 nm for excitation/emission wavelengths.

2.11. ATP Level

The ATP level was examined using a luciferase-based luminescence enhanced ATP assay kit (Beyotime Institute of Biotechnology, China) following the manufacturer's instruction. The hepatocytes were washed with ice-cold PBS, lysed with 200 μL lysis buffer, and then centrifuged at 12,000× *g* for 5 min at 4 °C. ATP content in cell lysates was then determined using a luminescence plate reader.

2.12. Western Blotting

Mitochondrial fraction was isolated using the Mitochondria Isolation Kit for Cultured Cells according to the manufacturer's instructions (Beyotime Institute of Biotechnology, Nanjing, China). For total protein extraction, cells were washed twice with PBS and lysed with RIPA buffer (Beyotime Institute of Biotechnology, Nanjing, China). The homogenates were centrifuged at 12,000× *g* for 15 min at 4 °C, the supernatant was then collected. Protein concentrations were evaluated using the BCA method. Then the samples were denatured by boiling with sample buffer for 10 min, loaded to SDS-PAGE gel for separation, and then transferred onto the PVDF membrane. The membranes were blocked with 5% skim milk for 1 h at room temperature and incubated with different primary antibodies overnight at 4 °C. The membranes were then washed and incubated with secondary antibodies for 1 h at room temperature. The protein bands were visualized using the enhanced chemiluminescence (ECL) kit (Thermo, Waltham, MA, USA) and quantitated using Image J software (National Institutes of Health, USA). The band density of different proteins was normalized to the control.

ND1 (DF4214) antibody was obtained from Affinity Biosciences (Cincinnati, OH, USA). VDAC1 (55259-1-AP) antibody was purchased from Proteintech Group Inc. (Wuhan, China). Drp1 (A2586), AIF (A19536), cyt c (A4912), and caspase-3 (A11021) antibodies were purchased from ABclonal Technology (Wuhan, China). Antibody against β-actin (70-ab008-040) was obtained from MultiSciences Biotech Co. (Hangzhou, China).

2.13. MRCCs Activity

After the treatment, L02 hepatocytes were collected and suspended in 0.1 M phosphate buffer (pH 7.2). To ensure cellular disruption and after three cycles of freeze/thawing, the activities of MRCC I–V were determined spectrophotometrically as previously described [11].

2.14. Confocal Microscope

For mitochondrial morphology examination, the hepatocytes were incubated with 10 nM Mitotracker Red (Invitrogen Life Technologies, Carlsbad, CA, USA) for 45 min at 37 °C. After the indicated chemicals treatment, the hepatocytes were incubated with DAPI for another 45 min at 37 °C in the dark. The fluorescence images of each group were captured using Leica TCS SP5 II confocal spectral microscope. More than 20 clearly identifiable mitochondria were randomly selected from each treatment group. The length and density of the mitochondria were analyzed using Image J software.

To analyze Drp1 mitochondrial translocation, Cr(VI)-exposed hepatocytes were fixed with 4% paraformaldehyde for 15 min at room temperature following incubation with MitoTracker Red (10 nM, 45 min, 37 °C). The hepatocytes were then permeabilized with 0.5% Triton X-100, blocked with 5% bovine serum albumin (BSA), and incubated with primary Drp1 antibody at a 1:100 dilution at 4 °C overnight, followed by treatment with the secondary antibody. Nuclei were stained with DAPI prior to mounting. Confocal fluorescence images of each treatment group were captured with the Leica TCS SP5 II confocal spectral microscope.

2.15. Statistical Analysis

All experiments were repeated at least three times. Representative experiments or mean ± SD are shown in the figures. Statistical analyses were performed using one-way of variance (ANOVA), Student's *t*-test, using SPSS 17.0 software. A significant difference was taken as $p < 0.05$.

3. Results

3.1. MRCC I Inhibition Led to Cytotoxicity in L02 Hepatocytes

Glutamate/malate (Glu/Mal), known as the substrates of MRCC I, can directly initiate the mitochondrial main respiratory chain (NADH respiratory chain) by activating MRCC I. The inhibitor of MRCC I is rotenone (ROT). We first evaluated whether changes in MRCC I activity would affect cytotoxicity. The L02 cells were treated with different concentrations of Glu/Mal (0, 5/5, 10/10 mM; 1 h) and ROT (0, 2.5, 5 μM; 24 h). As shown in Figure 1A, the application of substrates Glu/Mal slightly inhibited ROS generation, while the application of the inhibitor ROT significantly enhanced ROS generation in a concentration-dependent manner. In most cases, the degree of ALT and AST increase was consistent with the degree of hepatocyte damage, which is the most commonly used indicator of hepatocytes/liver function. The distribution of these two enzymes in hepatocytes is different. ALT is mainly distributed in the cytoplasm, and the increase of ALT leakage indicates the membrane damage. AST is mainly distributed in both cytoplasm and the mitochondria, and the increase of ALT indicates that hepatocytes are damaged to organelle level. Compared with the control group, the treatment of Glu/Mal did not alter the leakage of ALT/AST to the culture medium, while the application of ROT increased the leakage of these two enzymes (especially ALT) in a concentration-dependent manner (Figure 1B). We further examined whether the alteration of MRCC I activity would affect cell growth and proliferation. As shown in Figure 1C, from day 2 and compared with control, Glu/Mal increased while ROT significantly decreased cell number, indicating that Glu/Mal stimulated while ROT suppressed cell growth and proliferation. Caspase-3 activity was inhibited by Glu/Mal and increased by ROT (Figure 1D). ROT treatment significantly increased the percentage (%) of apoptosis cells in a dose-dependent manner, while Glu/Mal exposure showed no effect on apoptosis (Figure 1E).

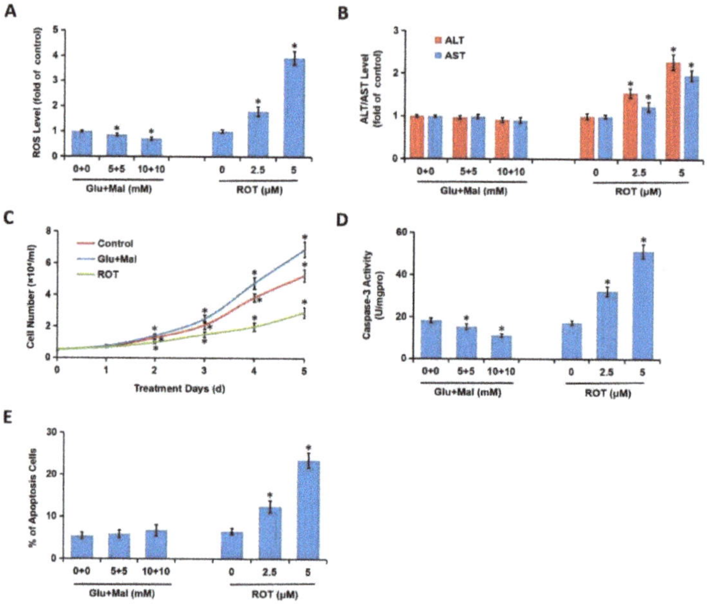

Figure 1. MRCC I inhibition led to cytotoxicity in L02 hepatocytes. (**A**) The L02 hepatocytes were either exposed to different concentrations of MRCC I substrates Glu/Mal (0, 5/5, 10/10 mM) for 1 h and then cultured for 23 h, or exposed to different concentrations of ROT (0, 2.5, 5 μM) for 24 h. ROS level was determined using the fluorescent probe DCFH-DA. (**B**) AST/ALT level was determined using the related kits. (**C**) The L02 hepatocytes were cultured for consecutive 5 days and treated with various concentrations of Glu/Mal (0, 5/5, 10/10 mM; 1 h) and ROT (0, 2.5, 5 μM; 24 h) in day 0 and day 3. The cell number, which indicated growth and proliferation of the hepatocytes, was recorded using a hemocytometer by trypan blue exclusion method. (**D**) Caspase-3 activity was examined using the commercial colorimetric assay kit. (**E**) The cell apoptosis was determined using commercial Annexin V-FITC Apoptosis Detection Kit. * $p < 0.05$, compared with the control group.

3.2. *Cr(VI) Induced Mitochondria-Related Cytotoxicity*

It is well known that mPTP and MMP are important parameters reflecting mitochondrial function. The cells were exposed to various concentrations of Cr(VI) (0, 8, 16 μM) for 24 h. Treatment with Cr(VI) caused a marked increase in mPTP opening rate (Figure 2A) and a decrease in MMP (Figure 2B) in a concentration-dependent manner, suggesting the occurrence of mitochondrial damage. The mtDNA copy number and mitochondrial mass, which might be altered during mitochondrial damage, were also detected. mtDNA encodes 13 proteins which closely related to mitochondrial function. We designed the primers for two genes encoded by mtDNA, MRCC I subunit, ND1, and MRCC IV subunit, COX4I1. The expression amount of the two genes can reflect the copy number of mtDNA. As shown in Figure 2C, both ND1 and COX4I1 mRNA levels were decreased after Cr(VI) treatment, indicating the decline of mtDNA copy number. Cr(VI) exposure also decreased mitochondrial mass (Figure 2D). Mitochondria are energy providers, generating more than 95% of the ATP required for cells. Mitochondrial damage results in the decline of the intracellular ATP level, as confirmed in Figure 2E. The mPTP opening marks the emergence of irreversible point of apoptosis, which is accompanied by the release of apoptosis-inducing factors such as AIF and Cyt C from mitochondria to the cytoplasm. Cr(VI) increased the protein levels of AIF and Cyt C (Figure 2F). As a major member of cysteinyl aspartate-specific protease (caspase) family, caspase-3 plays a vital role in apoptosis. Both the protein expression (Figure 2F) and activity (Figure 2G) of caspase-3 were enhanced by Cr(VI) treatment. Cr(VI) also increased the % of apoptosis cells in a concentration-dependent manner (Figure 2H).

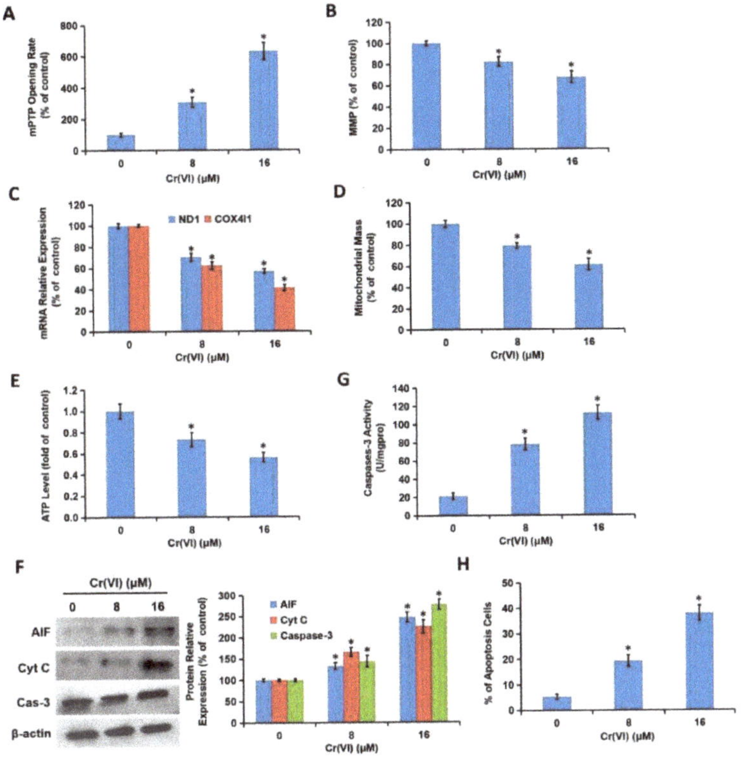

Figure 2. Cr(VI) induced mitochondrial-related cytotoxicity. L02 hepatocytes were treated with different concentrations of Cr(VI) (0, 8, 16 μM) for 24 h. (**A**) The mPTP opening was examined using the commercial kit. (**B**) The MMP was detected using JC-1. (**C**) The mRNA levels of ND1 and COX4I1, which could reflect the copy number of mtDNA were detected using quantitative real-time polymerase chain reaction (qRT-PCR). (**D**) Mitochondria mass was examined using Mito-Tracker Green by flow cytometer. (**E**) The ATP level was examined using a luciferase-based luminescence enhanced ATP assay kit. (**F**) AIF, Cyt C, and caspase-3 protein expressions were detected using Western blotting analysis. The protein bands were quantitated using Image J software. (**G**) Caspase-3 activity was determined using the commercial colorimetric assay kit. (**H**) The cell apoptosis was determined using commercial Annexin V-FITC Apoptosis Detection Kit. * $p < 0.05$, compared with the control group.

3.3. *Cr(VI) Targeted MRCC I to Induce Cytotoxicity*

We have confirmed that MRCC I inhibition led to cytotoxicity in L02 hepatocytes. Next, we verified whether Cr(VI) targeted MRCC I to induce cytotoxicity. L02 hepatocytes were treated with different concentrations of Cr(VI) (0, 8, 16 μM) for 24 h. As shown in Figure 3A, among the five complexes, the activity of MRCC I was significantly decreased while the activity of MRCC II was slightly decreased after Cr(VI) exposure. The protein expression of MRCC I subunit ND1 was also decreased by Cr(VI) in a concentration-dependent manner (Figure 3B). For the combination treatments, L02 hepatocytes were exposed to Cr(VI) (16 μM) or PBS for 24 h with or without the pretreatment of Glu/Mal (10/10 mM) for 1 h; the cells were exposed to Cr(VI) (16 μM) or PBS with or without the cotreatment of ROT (5 μM) for 24 h. The pretreatment of Glu/Mal alleviated Cr(VI)-induced increase of ALT/AST leakage, while the cotreatment of ROT significantly aggravated Cr(VI)-induced increase of ALT/AST leakage (Figure 3C). We then detected the effect of MRCC I on Cr(VI)-induced caspase-3 activation and apoptosis induction. As shown in Figure 3D,E, the pretreatment of Glu/Mal significantly alleviated Cr(VI)-induced caspase-3 activation and apoptosis induction, while the cotreatment of ROT obviously aggravated Cr(VI)-induced caspase-3 activation and apoptosis induction. The inhibiting effect of ROT on MRCC I was more obvious than the enhancing effect of Glu/Mal.

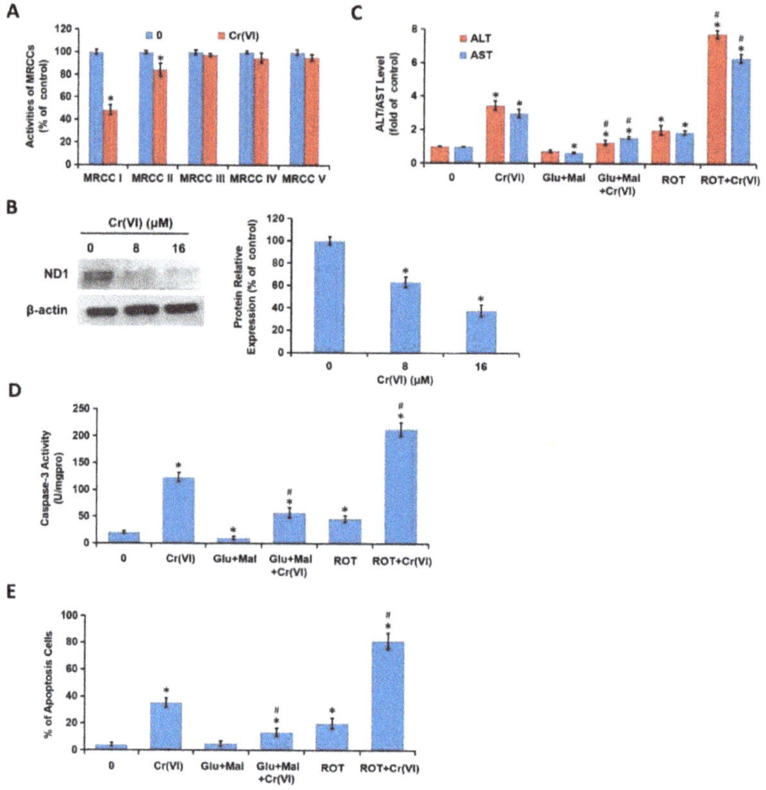

Figure 3. Cr(VI) targeted MRCC I to induce cytotoxicity. (**A**) L02 hepatocytes were treated with different concentrations of Cr(VI) (0, 8, 16 μM) for 24 h. The activities of MRCC I-V were determined spectrophotometrically using the commercial kits. (**B**) The protein expression of ND1 was determined using Western blotting. (**C**) L02 hepatocytes were exposed to Cr(VI) (16 μM) or PBS for 24 h with or without the pretreatment of Glu/Mal (10/10 mM) for 1 h; or the cells were exposed to Cr(VI) (16 μM) or PBS with or without the cotreatment of ROT (5 μM) for 24 h. AST/ALT level was determined using the commercial kits. (**D**) Caspase-3 activity was determined using the commercial colorimetric assay kit. (**E**) The cell apoptosis was determined using commercial Annexin V-FITC Apoptosis Detection Kit. * $p < 0.05$, compared with the control group. # $p < 0.05$, compared with the Cr(VI) alone treatment group.

3.4. *Cr(VI) Induced Mitochondrial Hyper-Fission via Interfering with Drp1*

Drp1, a major protein regulating mitochondrial fission in mammals, acts as an important intrinsic factor involved in mitochondria-dependent apoptosis. We then examined whether Drp1 and Drp1-related mitochondrial fission were involved in Cr(VI)-induced apoptosis. L02 hepatocytes were treated with different concentrations of Cr(VI) (0, 8, 16 μM) for 24 h. As shown in Figure 4A, the mitochondria of the control group revealed the significant large, tubular network structure, while the mitochondria of the Cr(VI)-exposed group showed the short-shaped, divided, and segmented structure, indicating that Cr(VI) induced excessive mitochondrial fragmentation. The % of cells without elongated mitochondria was also shown. Drp1 mRNA expression levels were also increased after Cr(VI) exposure in a concentration-dependent manner, indicating that Cr(VI) caused the transcriptional alteration of

Drp1 (Figure 4B). Cr(VI) up-regulated the protein expressions of both the total and mitochondrial Drp1, suggesting that in addition to inducing the translational change of Drp1, Cr(VI) also triggered the translocation of Drp1 from cytoplasm to mitochondria (Figure 4C). The mitochondrial Drp1 translocation was then observed with laser confocal microscopy. As shown in Figure 4D, Drp1 protein with a green dot-like distribution was dramatically increased after Cr(VI) treatment, and the translocation of the increased Drp1 protein to mitochondria was clearly observed.

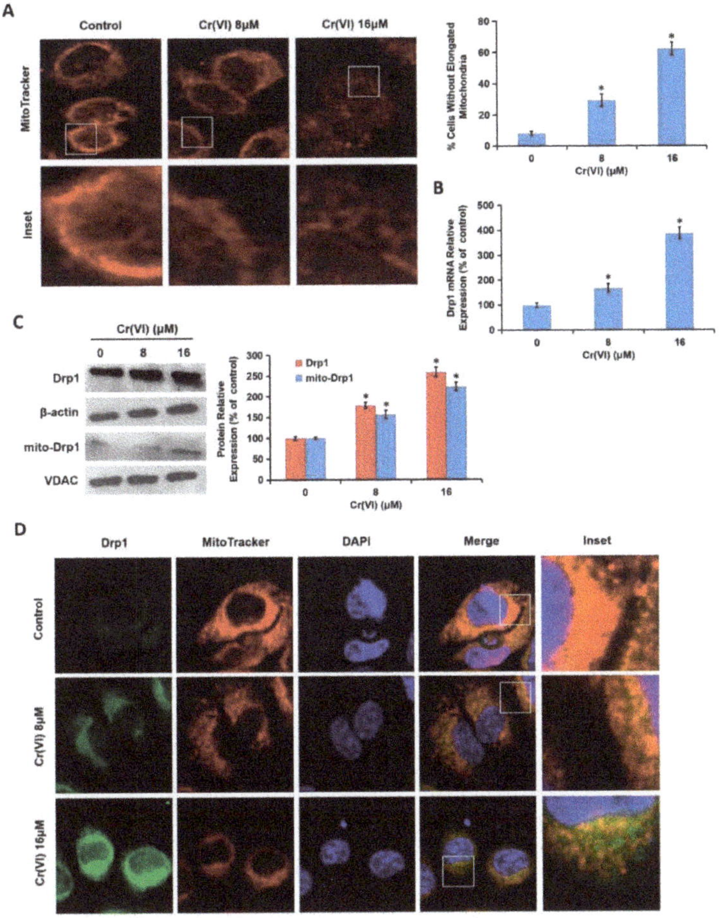

Figure 4. Cr(VI) caused mitochondrial fragmentation. L02 hepatocytes were treated with different concentrations of Cr(VI) (0, 8, 16 μM) for 24 h. (**A**) Mitochondrial morphology was determined using Mitotracker Red by confocal microscope. The % of cells without elongated mitochondria was calculated. (**B**) Drp1 mRNA expression was determined using qRT-PCR. (**C**) Total and mitochondrial Drp1 protein expressions were detected using Western blotting analysis. Voltage-dependent anion channel 1 (VDAC1) served as the loading control of mitochondrial protein. (**D**) Drp1 mitochondrial translocation was observed under a confocal microscope. * $p < 0.05$, compared with the control group.

We then explored the effect of Drp1-siRNA on Cr(VI)-induced fragmentation. We constructed Drp1-siRNA plasmid and confirmed its efficiency using qRT-PCR (Figure 5A) and Western blotting (Figure 5B). The L-02 hepatocytes transfected with Drp1-siRNA and its control (Con-si) were treated with Cr(VI) (16 μM) or PBS for 24 h. While the significantly short-shaped, divided, and segmented mitochondria were observed in the Cr(VI) exposure group, Drp1-siRNA alleviated the excessive mitochondrial fragmentation and partially restored the large and tubular network structure of mitochondria (Figure 5C).

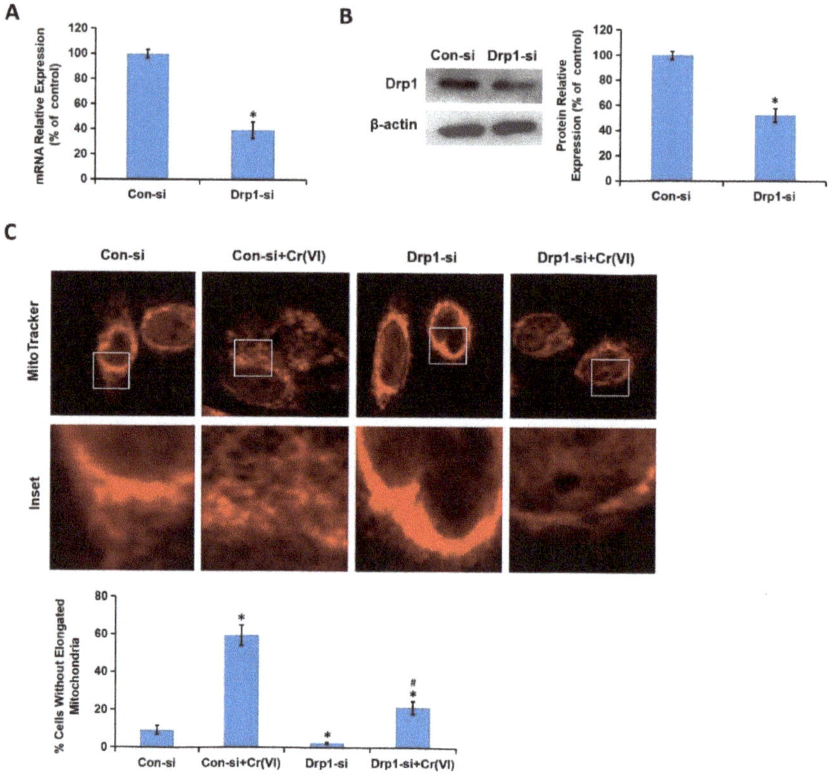

Figure 5. Cr(VI) induced mitochondrial hyper-fission via interfering with Drp1. Drp1 siRNA plasmid was constructed and verified using qRT-PCR (**A**) and Western blotting (**B**). (**C**) The L-02 hepatocytes transfected with Drp1-siRNA and its control (Con-si) were treated with Cr(VI) (16 μM) or PBS for 24 h. Mitochondrial morphology was determined using Mitotracker Red by confocal microscope. The % of cells without elongated mitochondria was calculated. * $p < 0.05$, compared with the control group. # $p < 0.05$, compared with the Con-si plus Cr(VI) treatment group.

3.5. Drp1-Mediated Mitochondrial Fragmentation Contributes to Cr(VI)-Induced MRCC I-Dependent Cytotoxicity

The effect of Drp1-siRNA on Cr(VI)-induced MRCC I-dependent cytotoxicity was further explored. The L-02 hepatocytes transfected with Drp1-siRNA and Con-si were treated with Cr(VI) (16 μM) or PBS for 24 h. The application of Drp1-siRNA alleviated Cr(VI)-induced ALT/AST leakage (Figure 6A), caspase-3 activation (Figure 6B), and apoptosis induction (Figure 6C). For the combination treatments, the hepatocytes transfected with Drp1-siRNA and Con-si were exposed to Cr(VI) (16 μM) for 24 h with or without the pretreatment of Glu/Mal (10/10 mM) for 1 h; the hepatocytes transfected with Drp1-siRNA and Con-si were exposed to Cr(VI) (16 μM) with or without the cotreatment of ROT (5 μM) for 24 h. As shown in Figure 6D,F, the ALT/AST leakage, caspase-3 activation, and apoptosis induction in Drp1-si plus Cr(VI) treatment group was alleviated by the application of Glu/Mal, and aggravated by the application of ROT. Drp1 siRNA can further promote the inhibition of Glu/Mal on Cr(VI)-induced cytotoxicity, and also can further alleviate the aggravation of ROT on Cr(VI)-induced cytotoxicity.

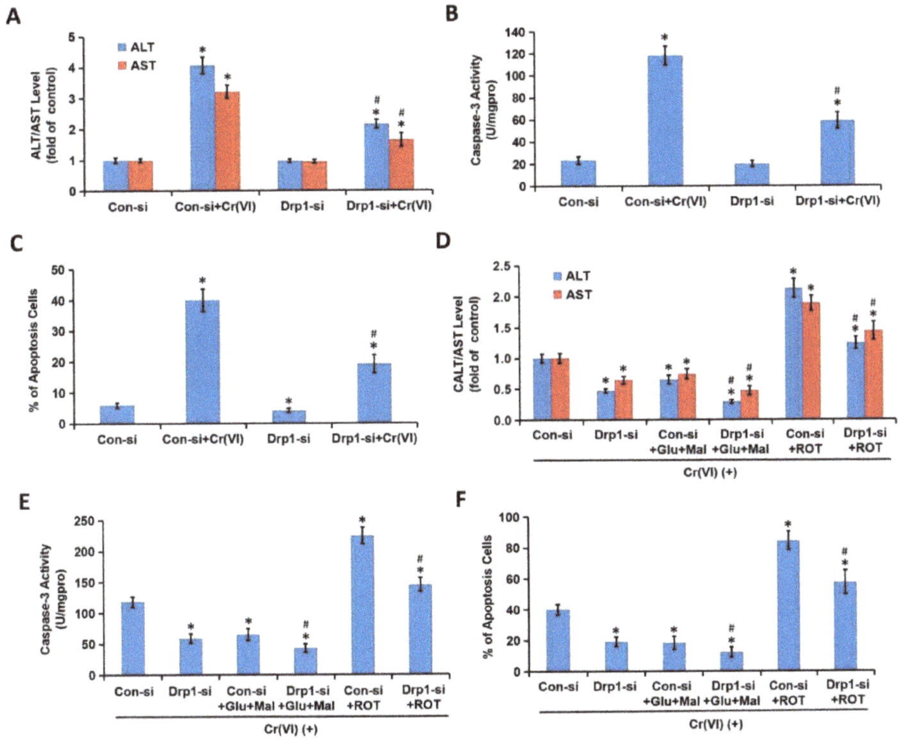

Figure 6. Drp1-mediated mitochondrial fragmentation contributes to Cr(VI)-induced MRCC I-dependent cytotoxicity. (**A**) The L-02 hepatocytes transfected with Drp1-siRNA and Con-si were treated with Cr(VI) (16 μM) or PBS for 24 h. AST/ALT level was determined using the commercial kits. (**B**) Caspase-3 activity was determined using the commercial colorimetric assay kit. (**C**) The cell apoptosis was determined using commercial Annexin V-FITC Apoptosis Detection Kit. (**D**) For the combination treatments, the hepatocytes transfected with Drp1-siRNA and Con-si were exposed to Cr(VI) (16 μM) for 24 h with or without the pretreatment of Glu/Mal (10/10 mM) for 1 h; the hepatocytes transfected with Drp1-siRNA and Con-si were exposed to Cr(VI) (16 μM) with or without the cotreatment of ROT (5 μM) for 24 h. AST/ALT level was determined using the commercial kits. (**E**) Caspase-3 activity was determined using the commercial colorimetric assay kit. (**F**) The cell apoptosis was determined using commercial Annexin V-FITC Apoptosis Detection Kit. * $p < 0.05$, compared with its relative control. # $p < 0.05$, compared with the Drp1-si plus Cr(VI) treatment group.

3.6. Cr(VI)-Induced Drp1 Modulation was Depend on MRCC I Inhibition-Mediated ROS Production

Evidence suggested that oxidative stress could activate Drp1 and promote mitochondrial fragmentation, thus we also explored whether Cr(VI)-induced accumulation of ROS could regulate Drp1. L02 hepatocytes were treated with different concentrations of Cr(VI) (0, 8, 16 μM) for 24 h. As shown in Figure 7A, Cr(VI) caused a significant increase of intracellular ROS levels in a concentration-dependent manner. The hepatocytes were exposed to Cr(VI) or PBS for 24 h with or without the pretreatment of Glu/Mal; or the cells were exposed to Cr(VI) or PBS with or without the cotreatment of ROT. Glu/Mal slightly decreased ROS level compared with the control. Cr(VI)-induced over-production of ROS was alleviated by the application of Glu/Mal, and aggravated by the application of ROT (Figure 7B), indicating that MRCC I was involved in ROS accumulation induced by Cr(VI). The hepatocytes were exposed to Cr(VI) or PBS for 24 h with or without the pretreatment of NAC for 1 h. NAC partially decreased Cr(VI)-induced increase of the mRNA level (Figure 7C), and both the total and mitochondrial protein level (Figure 7D) of Drp1, confirming that Drp1 can be regulated by ROS in both transcription and translation levels. The utilization of Glu/Mal also alleviated the increase of both total and mitochondrial Drp1 expression (Figure 7E). The above results together suggested that Cr(VI)-induced Drp1 modulation was dependent on MRCC I inhibition-mediated ROS production.

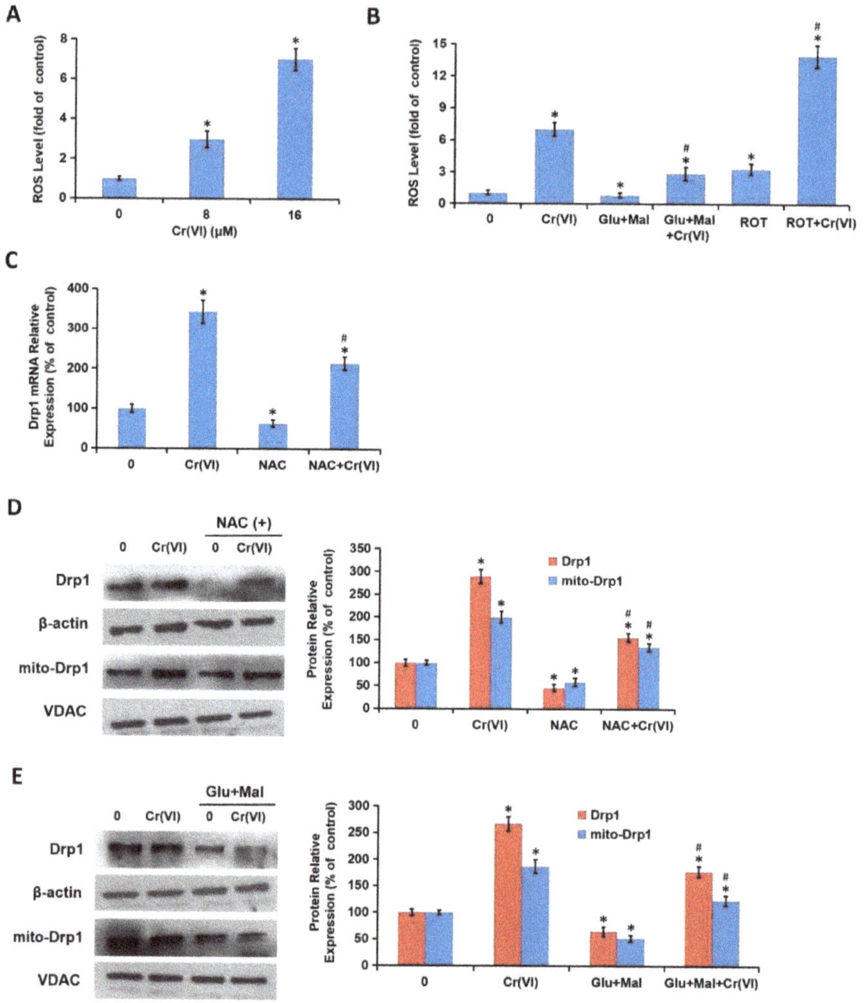

Figure 7. Cr(VI)-induced Drp1 modulation was dependent on MRCC I inhibition-mediated ROS production. (**A**) L02 hepatocytes were treated with different concentrations of Cr(VI) (0, 8, 16 μM) for 24 h. ROS level was determined using the fluorescent probe DCFH-DA. (**B**) L02 hepatocytes were exposed to Cr(VI) (16 μM) or PBS for 24 h with or without the pretreatment of Glu/Mal (10/10 mM) for 1 h; or the cells were exposed to Cr(VI) (16 μM) or PBS with or without the cotreatment of ROT (5 μM) for 24 h. ROS level was determined using the fluorescent probe DCFH-DA. (**C**) The hepatocytes were exposed to Cr(VI) (16 μM) or PBS for 24 h with or without the pretreatment of NAC (5 mM) for 1 h. Drp1 mRNA expression was determined using qRT-PCR. (**D**,**E**) Total and mitochondrial Drp1 protein expressions were detected using Western blotting analysis. * $p < 0.05$, compared with the control group. # $p < 0.05$, compared with the Cr(VI) alone treatment group.

4. Discussion

We demonstrated in the present study that MRCC I inhibition led to cytotoxicity in L02 hepatocytes, which was characterized by the increase of ALT/AST leakage, the activation of caspase-3, the inhibition of cell proliferation, and the induction of apoptosis. We then confirmed that Cr(VI) targeted MRCC I to induce ROS accumulation and then triggered mitochondrial-related cytotoxicity. Cr(VI) caused a marked increase in mPTP opening rate and decrease in MMP, declined the mtDNA copy number, mitochondrial mass, and ATP level, increased the mitochondrial release of apoptosis-inducing factors, and eventually triggered apoptosis. The pretreatment of Glu/Mal significantly alleviated Cr(VI)-induced cytotoxicity, while the cotreatment of ROT obviously aggravated Cr(VI)-induced cytotoxicity.

In theory, all four complexes (I–IV) of the ETC could generate ROS; evidence suggests that MRCC I and III are the main sites of ROS formation [13,14]. However, the ability of MRCC III to produce ROS has also been questioned, while MRCC I is considered to be the relevant major site of superoxide formation. It is reported that the formation of ROS can not be detected until MRCC III was inhibited by up to 71 ± 4%; in contrast, the small-extent deactivation of MRCC I (16 ± 2%) could lead to a significant increase of ROS generation [15]. It is also demonstrated that the production rate of endogenous H_2O_2 was much lower when Glu/Mal, the substrates of MRCC I were used as respiratory fuel; the application of ROT, the inhibitor of MRCC I, led to a significantly increasing H_2O_2 release [16]. ROT can interrupt the transfer of electrons to CoQ and enhance ROS production. The amount of ROS produced by various stimulation determines whether ROS play profitable or detrimental roles. In the physiological state, it was believed that ROS appear to be important second messengers that mediate different cell signaling pathways, while the overburdened ROS are exclusively harmful to the cells [17]. The burst generation of ROS leads to irreversible damage to mitochondria, DNA damage, lipid peroxidation, ATP exhaustion, and, eventually, cell death [18]. Although the precise mechanisms involved in ROS burst-generation and ROS-related cytotoxicity are still not clear, the application of specific ROS inhibitors such as NAC and Trolox to reduce the over-production of ROS under pathological conditions has been shown to ameliorate various diseases mediated by oxidative stress [19].

The mtDNA copy number in each mitochondrion is constant, thus, the total number of mtDNA copies reflects the total number of mitochondria in cells [20]. mtDNA is located near the ETC and its repair mechanism is incomplete, thus, mtDNA is more susceptible to damage when exposed to oxidative stress compared with the nuclear DNA [21]. The opening of mPTP represents the abrupt change in permeability of the mitochondrial inner membrane, allowing not only protons but also various ions and solutes of up to 1.5 kDa in size to freely pass through the membrane [22]. Apoptosis is initiated by the change of mitochondrial membrane permeability transition (MPT), and the opening of the non-specific mega-channel mPTP enables the membrane permeability suddenly increase, resulting in the release of the apoptosis executors including apoptosis-inducing factor (AIF), cytochrome c (Cyt c), and endonuclease G from the mitochondrial matrix to cytoplasm. The increase of mPTP opening may lead to the flow back of protons from mitochondrial membrane space to matrix, thus inhibiting MMP and ATP production, resulting in metabolic abnormalities and cytotoxicity [23]. Moreover, Cr(VI) exposure triggered over-opening of mPTP, dropped MMP, decreased mtDNA number, declined ATP synthesis, indicating that Cr(VI) can directly disrupt the structure and function of mitochondria and induce cytotoxicity. As one of the early events of apoptosis induced by various stimuli, the increase of intracellular ROS can trigger Cyt c first detaches from cardiolipin and then being released into the cytoplasm. Cr(VI) exposure disrupted mitochondrial redox homeostasis and accumulated excessive ROS, then mitochondrial function such as MMP and mPTP was severely affected, thus, L02 hepatocytes undergo mitochondria-mediated apoptosis.

Cr(VI) induced excessive mitochondrial fragmentation and mitochondrial Drp1 translocation, the application of Drp1-siRNA alleviated Cr(VI)-induced ALT/AST leakage, caspase-3 activation, and apoptosis induction. The cytotoxicity in Drp1-si plus Cr(VI) treatment group was alleviated by the application of Glu/Mal, and aggravated by the application of ROT. Drp1 siRNA can further promote the inhibition of Glu/Mal on Cr(VI)-induced cytotoxicity, and also can further alleviate the aggravation of ROT on Cr(VI)-induced cytotoxicity. The dynamic network of mitochondria can meet the energy and metabolic needs of cells. The intracellular mitochondrial morphology network represents a perfect balance between the fusion/fission events [24]. Mitochondrial dynamics is mainly regulated by Drp1, mitofusin (Mfn) 1 and Mfn2, and other mitochondrial fusion and fission-related proteins [25]. Once the damage progressed to the irreversible stage, mitochondria will reveal excessive fission and fragmentation, mass decrease, as well as membrane integrity loss. The application of Drp1 siRNA or Mdivi-1 (a specific Drp1 inhibitor) can inhibit the conversion to punctate mitochondrial phenotype, weaken the insertion and oligomerization of pro-apoptotic Bax protein, thus attenuating cell apoptosis, reducing transient focal ischemia-induced infarct and neurological deficits. Drp1 activity could be altered under all kinds of stimulation, leading to mitochondrial dynamics abnormality and cell damage [26]. It is reported that oxidative stress can enhance the activity of Drp1 and promote mitochondrial fragmentation and dysfunction mediated by Drp1, while the application of antioxidants can restore mitochondrial morphology [27,28]. Evidence suggested that the upstream transcription activator of Drp1 is p53, which could promote Drp1 transcription by binding to its promoter [29]. In the present study, we confirmed that Cr(VI)-induced Drp1 modulation was dependent on MRCC I inhibition-mediated ROS production. Taken together, this study demonstrated that Drp1-mediated mitochondrial fragmentation contributes to Cr(VI)-induced MRCC I-dependent cytotoxicity.

5. Conclusions

In summary, Cr(VI) treatment inhibited the activity of MRCC I and enhanced ROS generation in L02 hepatocytes, leading to the translocation of Drp1 from the cytoplasm to mitochondria, subsequently inducing excessive fission and fragmentation of mitochondria. The resulted imbalance of mitochondrial dynamics decreased mtDNA copy number and mitochondrial mass, and then impaired mitochondrial function, mainly manifestation as the collapse of MMP, the exhaustion of ATP, the abnormal opening of mPTP, and the mitochondrial release of apoptosis-inducing factors such as AIF and Cyt c. Eventually, Cr(VI)-cytotoxicity was characterized by the increase of ALT/AST leakage, the enhancement of caspase-3 activity, and apoptosis (Figure 8). In this process, it is not clear whether phosphorylation or other modifications of Drp 1 occurs, and this is also our next research direction.

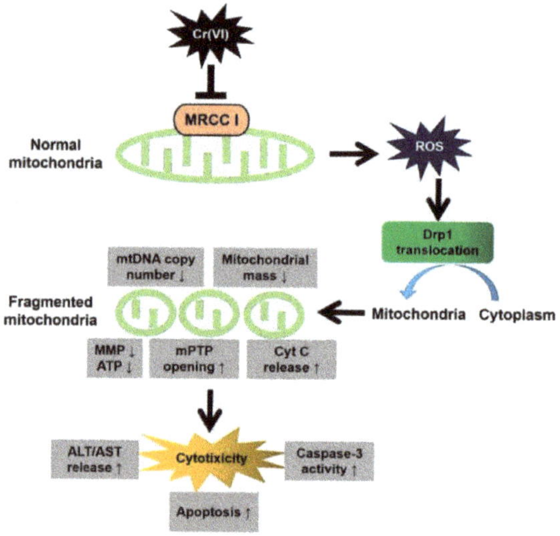

Figure 8. Summary chart of the research content of this paper. Increased mitochondrial fragmentation mediated by Drp1 contributes to Cr(VI)-induced MRCC I-dependent cytotoxicity.

Author Contributions: Conceptualization and supervision, F.X.; methodology, software, and validation, Y.M., Y.Z. and Y.X.; formal analysis and investigation, Y.Z. and Y.X.; writing—original draft preparation, F.X. and Y.Z. All authors have read and agreed to the published version of the manuscript.

Funding: The current work was supported by the National Natural Science Foundation of China (NO. 81773478) and the Natural Science Foundation of Hunan Province, China (NO. 2019JJ40402).

Acknowledgments: We thank Caigao Zhong in this laboratory for his valuable suggestions.

Conflicts of Interest: The authors declare no conflict of interest.

References

1. Chebeir, M.; Liu, H. Oxidation of cr(iii)-fe(iii) mixed-phase hydroxides by chlorine: Implications on the control of hexavalent chromium in drinking water. *Environ. Sci. Technol.* **2018**, *52*, 7663–7670. [CrossRef]
2. Gong, K.; Qian, H.; Lu, Y.; Min, L.; Guo, Z. Ultrasonic pretreated sludge derived stable magnetic active carbon for cr(vi) removal from wastewater. *ACS Sustain. Chem. Eng.* **2018**, *6*, 7283–7291. [CrossRef]
3. Chandhok, G.; Lazarou, M.; Neumann, B. Structure, function, and regulation of mitofusin-2 in health and disease. *Biol. Rev.* **2018**, *93*, 933–949. [CrossRef] [PubMed]
4. Wang, P.; Li, Y.; Yang, Z.; Yu, T.; Tang, W. Inhibition of dynamin-related protein 1 has neuroprotective effect comparable to therapeutic hypothermia in a rat model of cardiac arrest. *Transl. Res.* **2018**, *194*, 68–78. [CrossRef] [PubMed]
5. Brooks, C.; Wei, Q.; Feng, L.; Dong, G.; Tao, Y.; Mei, L.; Xie, Z.-J.; Dong, Z. Bak regulates mitochondrial morphology and pathology during apoptosis by interacting with mitofusins. *Proc. Natl. Acad. Sci. USA* **2007**, *104*, 11649–11654. [CrossRef] [PubMed]
6. Ishihara, N.; Nomura, M.; Jofuku, A.; Kato, H.; Suzuki, S.O.; Masuda, K.; Otera, H.; Nakanishi, Y.; Nonaka, I.; Goto, Y.-I. Mitochondrial fission factor drp1 is essential for embryonic development and synapse formation in mice. *Nat. Cell Biol.* **2009**, *11*, 958–966. [CrossRef] [PubMed]
7. Wakabayashi, J.; Zhang, Z.; Wakabayashi, N.; Tamura, Y.; Sesaki, H. The dynamin-related gtpase drp1 is required for embryonic and brain development in mice. *J. Cell Biol.* **2009**, *186*, 805–816. [CrossRef]
8. Beutner, G.; Porter, G.A. Analyzing supercomplexes of the mitochondrial electron transport chain with native electrophoresis, in-gel assays, and electroelution. *J. Vis. Exp.* **2017**, *124*, 55738. [CrossRef] [PubMed]
9. Jones, A.J.Y.; Blaza, J.N.; Varghese, F.; Hirst, J. Respiratory complex i in bos taurus and paracoccus denitrificans pumps four protons across the membrane for every nadh oxidized. *J. Biol. Chem.* **2017**, *292*, 4987–4995. [CrossRef]
10. Cadenas, E.; Davies, K.J.A. Mitochondrial free radical generation, oxidative stress, and aging 1 1 this article is dedicated to the memory of our dear friend, colleague, and mentor lars ernster (1920–1998), in gratitude for all he gave to us. *Free Radic. Biol. Med.* **2000**, *29*, 222–230. [CrossRef]
11. Xiao, Y.; Zeng, M.; Yin, L.; Li, N.; Xiao, F. Clusterin increases mitochondrial respiratory chain complex i activity and protects against hexavalent chromium-induced cytotoxicity in l-02 hepatocytes. *Toxicol. Res.* **2019**, *8*, 15–24. [CrossRef] [PubMed]
12. Zhang, Y.; Zhang, Y.; Xiao, Y.; Zhong, C.; Xiao, F. Expression of clusterin suppresses cr(vi)-induced premature senescence through activation of pi3k/akt pathway. *Ecotoxicol. Environ. Saf.* **2019**, *183*, 109465. [CrossRef] [PubMed]
13. Potargowicz, E.; Szerszenowicz, E.; Staniszewska, M.; Nowak, D. Mitochondria as a source of reactive oxygen species. *Postepy Hig Med. Dosw.* **2005**, *59*, 259–266.
14. Landazabal, M.A.B.; Otero, A.L.C.; Kouznetsov, V.V.; Duque, J.E.; Mendez-Sanchez, S.C. Alterations of mitochondrial electron transport chain and oxidative stress induced by alkaloid-like α-aminonitriles on aedes aegypti larvae. *Pestic. Biochem. Physiol.* **2018**, *144*, 64–70. [CrossRef]
15. Sipos, I.; Tretter, L.; Adam-Vizi, V. Quantitative relationship between inhibition of respiratory complexes and formation of reactive oxygen species in isolated nerve terminals & nbsp. *J. Neurochem.* **2002**, *84*, 112–118.
16. Ohnishi, S.T.; Shinzawa-Itoh, K.; Ohta, K.; Yoshikawa, S.; Ohnishi, T. New insights into the superoxide generation sites in bovine heart nadh-ubiquinone oxidoreductase (complex i): The significance of protein-associated ubiquinone and the dynamic shifting of generation sites between semiflavin and semiquinone radicals. *Biochim. Biophys. Acta* **2010**, *1797*, 1901–1909. [CrossRef]

17. Brand, M.D. Mitochondrial generation of superoxide and hydrogen peroxide as the source of mitochondrial redox signaling. *Free Radic. Biol. Med.* **2016**, *100*, 14–31. [CrossRef]
18. Orrenius, S.; Gogvadze, V.; Zhivotovsky, B. Mitochondrial oxidative stress: Implications for cell death. *Annu. Rev. Pharmacol. Toxicol.* **2007**, *47*, 143–183. [CrossRef]
19. Ahmad, W.; Ijaz, B.; Shabbiri, K.; Ahmed, F.; Rehman, S. Oxidative toxicity in diabetes and alzheimer's disease: Mechanisms behind ros/rns generation. *J. Biomed. Sci.* **2017**, *24*, 76. [CrossRef]
20. Medeiros, T.C.; Graef, M. Autophagy determines mtdna copy number dynamics during starvation. *Autophagy* **2018**, *15*, 178–179. [CrossRef]
21. Herbers, E.; Kekäläinen, N.J.; Hangas, A.; Pohjoismäki, J.L.; Goffart, S. Tissue specific differences in mitochondrial DNA maintenance and expression. *Mitochondrion* **2018**, *44*, 85–92. [CrossRef] [PubMed]
22. Karch, J.; Kwong, J.Q.; Burr, A.R.; Sargent, M.A.; Elrod, J.W.; Peixoto, P.M.; Martinez-Caballero, S.; Osinska, H.; Cheng, H.Y.; Robbins, J. Bax and bak function as the outer membrane component of the mitochondrial permeability pore in regulating necrotic cell death in mice. *Elife* **2013**, *2*, e00772. [CrossRef] [PubMed]
23. Ren, D.D.; Sun, J.; Chen, D.; Gao, J.; Amp, M.; Laboratory, N.; Pharmacy, S.O.; University, J. Regulation mechanism and targeted drugs of mitochondrial permeability transition pore on programmed cell death:Research advances. *Int. J. Curr. Pharm. Res.* **2017**, *44*, 415–419.
24. Matsumura, A.; Higuchi, J.; Watanabe, Y.; Kato, M.; Aoki, K.; Akabane, S.; Endo, T.; Oka, T. Inactivation of cardiolipin synthase triggers changes in mitochondrial morphology. *FEBS Lett.* **2018**, *592*, 209–218. [CrossRef]
25. Yoo, S.M.; Jung, Y.K. A molecular approach to mitophagy and mitochondrial dynamics. *Mol. Cells* **2018**, *41*, 18–26.
26. Schmitt, K.; Grimm, A.; Dallmann, R.; Oettinghaus, B.; Restelli, L.M. Circadian control of drp1 activity regulates mitochondrial dynamics and bioenergetics. *Cell Metab.* **2018**, *27*, 657–666. [CrossRef]
27. Wu, S.; Zhou, F.; Zhang, Z.; Xing, D. Mitochondrial oxidative stress causes mitochondrial fragmentation via differential modulation of mitochondrial fission-fusion proteins. *FEBS J.* **2011**, *278*, 941–954. [CrossRef]
28. Chia-Hua, C.; Ching-Chih, L.; Ming-Chang, Y.; Chih-Chang, W.; Huei-De, L.; Run-Chin, L.; Wen-Yu, T.; Tsung-Chieh, K.; Ching-Mei, H.; Jiin-Tsuey, C. Gsk3beta-mediated drp1 phosphorylation induced elongated mitochondrial morphology against oxidative stress. *PLoS ONE* **2012**, *7*, e49112.
29. Yuan, Y.; Zhang, A.; Qi, J.; Wang, H.; Liu, X.; Zhao, M.; Duan, S.; Huang, Z.; Zhang, C.; Wu, L. P53/drp1-dependent mitochondrial fission mediates aldosterone-induced podocyte injury and mitochondrial dysfunction. *Am. J. Physiol. Ren. Physiol.* **2018**, *314*, 798–808. [CrossRef]

toxics

MDPI

Article

Genotoxic Effects of Aluminum Chloride and Their Relationship with N-Nitroso-N-Methylurea (NMU)-Induced Breast Cancer in Sprague Dawley Rats

Alejandro Monserrat García-Alegría [1,2,*], Agustín Gómez-Álvarez [3], Iván Anduro-Corona [4], Armando Burgos-Hernández [5], Eduardo Ruíz-Bustos [1,2], Rafael Canett-Romero [5], Humberto González-Ríos [4], José Guillermo López-Cervantes [6], Karen Lillian Rodríguez-Martínez [7] and Humberto Astiazaran-Garcia [1,2,4,*]

1 Programa de Doctorado en Ciencias Químico Biológicas y de la Salud, Universidad de Sonora, 83000 Hermosillo, Sonora, Mexico; eduardo.ruiz@unison.mx

2 Departamento de Ciencias Químico Biológicas, Universidad de Sonora, 83000 Hermosillo, Sonora, Mexico

3 Departamento de Ingeniería Química y Metalurgia, Universidad de Sonora, 83000 Hermosillo, Sonora, Mexico; agustin.gomez@unison.mx

4 Centro de Investigación en Alimentación y Desarrollo, AC, 83304 Hermosillo, Sonora, Mexico; ivan.anduro@ciad.mx (I.A.-C.); hugory@ciad.mx (H.G.-R.)

5 Departamento de Investigación y Posgrado en Alimentos, Universidad de Sonora, 83000 Hermosillo, Sonora, Mexico; armando.burgos@unison.mx (A.B.-H.); rafacanett@gmail.com (R.C.-R.)

6 Departamento de Medicina y Ciencias de la Salud, Universidad de Sonora, 83000 Hermosillo, Sonora, Mexico; guillermo.lopez@unison.mx

7 Licenciatura en Nutrición Humana, Universidad Estatal de Sonora, Unidad Académica Hermosillo, 83100 Hermosillo, Sonora, Mexico; karenroma.ues@gmail.com

* Correspondence: monserrat.garcia@unison.mx (A.M.G.-A.); hastiazaran@ciad.mx (H.A.-G.); Tel.: +52-662-2592163(A.M.G.-A.); +52-662-2892400 (H.A.-G.)

Received: 4 March 2020; Accepted: 14 April 2020; Published: 20 April 2020

Abstract: Recently, soluble forms of aluminum for human use or consumption have been determined to be potentially toxic due to their association with hepatic, neurological, hematological, neoplastic, and bone conditions. This study aims to assess the genotoxic effect of aluminum chloride on genomic instability associated with the onset of N-nitroso-N-methylurea (NMU)-induced breast cancer in Sprague Dawley rats. The dietary behavior of the rats was assessed, and the concentration of aluminum in the mammary glands was determined using atomic absorption spectroscopy. Genomic instability was determined in the histological sections of mammary glands stained with hematoxylin and eosin. Moreover, micronucleus in peripheral blood and comet assays were performed. The results of dietary behavior evaluation indicated no significant differences between the experimental treatments. However, aluminum concentration in breast tissues was high in the +2000Al/−NMU treatment. This experimental treatment caused moderate intraductal cell proliferation, lymph node hyperplasia, and serous gland adenoma. Furthermore, micronucleus and comet test results revealed that +2000Al/−NMU led to a genotoxic effect after a 10-day exposure and the damage was more evident after a 15-day exposure. Therefore, in conclusion, genomic instability is present and the experimental conditions assessed are not associated with breast cancer.

Keywords: genotoxicity; aluminum chloride; rats

1. Introduction

Aside from the multiple industrial applications of aluminum, it has applications in different fields including a few uses related to human consumption such as a flocculant in drinking water purification processes, as an adjuvant in vaccine preparation, and as an additive in beverages, foods (e.g., sweets and cheeses), antiperspirants and deodorants, among others [1–7]. However, the soluble forms of aluminum are considered potentially toxic because of their high water solubility and genotoxic capacity and because of our exposure to these soluble forms at subacute and chronic levels on a daily basis [6,8,9]. Recent estimates from the United States denote that middle-class young adults consume an average of 105–150 mg of aluminum per day in food and drinks, indicating that individuals are constantly exposed to the frequent use or consumption of different forms of aluminum [4,5,10]. Genomic instability is an essential prerequisite for the generation of multiple carcinogenesis-related alterations and mutations [11,12]. Therefore, trace (essential) elements, metals, and heavy metals are associated with breast cancer [13–16] either because cancer decreases the levels of some trace metals or because the metals cause or are associated with the genesis of cancer [2,17]. One of these trace metals is arsenic, which is associated with genomic instability, lung cancer [18], and deficient manganese metabolism, causing mitotic deregulation associated with genomic instability in humans [19]. Iron, another trace metal, is also associated with the development of genomic instability and liver, lung, and intestinal cancers in experimental rats [20]. Moreover, copper has reportedly been linked to genomic instability, which is related to breast cancer in rats [21], whereas cadmium is related to breast cancer in women worldwide [22]. Furthermore, aluminum chloride is being investigated for its potential relationship with neurological, hepatic, bone, and hematological conditions as well as with breast cancer [23–27]. Therefore, we assessed the genotoxic effects of aluminum concentration in Sprague Dawley rats and determined whether a link could be established with N-nitroso-N-methylurea (NMU)-induced breast cancer. This will aid in the development of new strategies for addressing exposure due to the use and/or consumption of soluble forms of aluminum as well as in the elucidation of their genotoxic hazards and relationship with the genesis of breast cancer in humans.

2. Materials and Methods

2.1. Chemicals

NMU N1517-1G (lot no. SLBF6813V) reagent was purchased from Sigma Chemical Co. (St. Louis, MO, USA), TRIzol^{TM} reagent was acquired from Life Technologies (Thermo Fisher Scientific, cat. no. 1596026, (Waltham, MA, USA), and the QuantiTect Reverse Transcription Kit manufactured by Qiagen (cat. no. 205311), (Germantown, MD, USA) was obtained. In addition, the TaqMan gene expression assays were purchased from Applied Biosystems (cat. nos. 4331182 and 4308313), and aluminum chloride ($AlCl_3$) was procured from Sigma Chemical Co. (St. Louis, MO, USA). All other chemical products were of analytical grade.

2.2. Experimental Animals

We selected 32 female Sprague Dawley rats (weight between 180 and 220 g) from the biotery at the Food Sciences Graduate Studies and Research Department at the University of Sonora.

2.3. Experimental Design (Treatments)

Groups of eight rats were randomly assigned to one of the following experimental treatments: treatment A rats not fed with aluminum and with no breast cancer induction (negative control) (−Al/−NMU); treatment B rats fed with 2000 mg/L aluminum ($AlCl_3$) and breast cancer induced by NMU (+2000Al/+NMU); treatment C rats fed with 2000 mg/L aluminum ($AlCl_3$) with no breast cancer induction (+2000Al/−NMU); and treatment D rats not fed with aluminum and breast cancer induced by NMU (positive control) (−Al/+NMU). Rats not fed with aluminum ($AlCl_3$) and with no breast cancer induction (NMU) were treated with 0.98% physiological saline to match the experimental conditions. Rats were intragastrically (gavage) fed 1 mL $AlCl_3$ 5 days/week for 90 days, whereas NMU was intraperitoneally administered at 50 and 70 days of age [28,29]. A volume of 1 mL of $AlCl_3$ solution with a concentration of 2000 mg/L is equivalent to administering 2 mg of aluminum to rats, considering that the mean weight of rats is 0.2 kg. This is equivalent to a dose of 10 mg Al/day/kg of body weight.

2.4. Breast Cancer Induction in Rats

The rats were treated with NMU (N1517-1G Sigma-Aldrich, St. Louis, MO, USA) at doses of 50 mg/kg of body weight administered at 50 and 70 days of age to induce breast adenocarcinoma [30,31].

2.5. Biotery Handling Conditions

Biotery handling conditions were as follows: 12 h light/dark cycles, humidity ranging from 40% to 70%, temperature between 18 °C and 22 °C, and ad libitum access to water and food [32].

2.6. Diet

Baseline pellet diet containing 23% protein, 1% vitamins, 4% minerals, 4% fiber, 6.5% fat, 0.2% choline bitartrate, 0.2% methionine, other minor dietary components, and starch to make up to a total of 100%, was used. Maximum humidity was 12%. This rat-feed was manufactured by LabDiet, Fort Worth, TX, USA, and marketed by PetFood of México [33].

2.7. Sampling

2.7.1. Breast Tissue Samples

Samples were obtained via surgical cuts of the mammary gland of rats anesthetized in a halothane chamber and then euthanized by cervical dislocation to avoid animal suffering, as per the NOM-033-ZOO-1995 and NOM-062-ZOO-1999 Official Mexican Standards, European Medicines Agency (EMEA, Amsterdam, The Netherlands, 2009), and Food and Drug Administration (FDA, Silver Spring, MD, USA, 2014) [34–37]. After quantifying the aluminum concentration, the samples were used for histopathological evaluation and total RNA extraction to evaluate the genetic expression of *BRCA1* and *SCL11a2*.

2.7.2. Blood Samples

For genotoxicity evaluation, blood was obtained from a tail cut for micronucleus (MN) analysis and individual cells (comet assay) via alkaline electrophoresis.

2.8. Determination of Aluminum Concentration in Breast Tissues

Samples were previously digested in a TITAN MPS microwave oven [38]. Briefly, 0.4 ± 0.02 g of breast tissue was weighed and placed in 15 × 2.5 cm Teflon digestion tubes containing 7 mL of concentrated nitric acid (HNO_3). The digestion conditions were 200 °C, 35 × 10^5 Pa, and 1600 W for 47 min [39]. The resultant acidic residue was made to a total of 100 mL using deionized water for the subsequent quantification of aluminum concentration.

The determination of aluminum concentration in the standard, certified reference material, and rat breast tissue was performed using atomic absorption spectroscopy with an AAnalyst 400 automated equipment in a graphite furnace absorption atomic spectroscopy (GFAAS) or in the electrothermal absorption atomic spectroscopy (ETAAS) mode, under the operating conditions recommended by the manufacturer [40,41]. The analytical method was previously optimized and its expanded uncertainty for quantifying aluminum by FAAS (flame absorption atomic spectroscopy) and ETAAS was subsequently validated and estimated uncertainty [42–44].

2.9. Evaluation of Genomic Instability

2.9.1. Histopathological Evaluation

Morphological instability was assessed by preparing histological cuts from rat mammary glands and mounting them on fixed slides using a microtome. The preparations were stained with hematoxylin and eosin and observed under a LEICA DME optical microscope under 40× and 100× magnification [45].

2.9.2. Micronucleus Analysis

To examine MN, three female Sprague Dawley rats weighing 200 ± 20 g were used per treatment group. Peripheral blood sampling was performed according to the present regulations [34,37] at 5, 10, and 15 days of experimental treatment. Briefly, 0.5 mL of peripheral blood was collected in 1.5-mL Eppendorf tubes and three blood smears (extensions) were prepared on clean slides with blood from each rat. The smears were stained with Wright's stain [46] and MN were subsequently counted in 2000 erythrocytes (1 MN, 2 MN, or >2 MN) [28] under a LEICA DME compound microscope (Buffalo, NY, 14240, USA).

2.9.3. Alkaline Electrophoresis Test in Individual Cells (Comet Assay)

Cell viability was assessed using trypan blue dye, and cells were counted in a Neubauer chamber/hematocytometer [47,48]. The comet test was performed according to Singh's method [49] at an exploratory level. Briefly, we used three female Sprague Dawley rats from treatments A (−Al/−NMU) and C (+2000Al/−NMU), which were anesthetized in a halothane chamber, to extract 3–4 mL of blood by intracardiac puncture, and these rats were subsequently euthanized by cervical dislocation. A total of 30 µL of whole blood was added to 300 µL of 1% low melting point agarose at 37 °C. A total of 75 µL of this mixture was extracted and placed on a slide pre-coated with a 150-µL layer of 1% regular agarose, which was immediately covered with a coverslip and maintained at 4 °C for 10 min. The coverslip was removed and 75 µL of 1% low melting point agarose was added at 37 °C to create another layer and form a sandwich, which was protected with a coverslip and maintained at 4 °C for 10 min. The cells were subsequently lysed in a lysis solution (2.5 mM NaCl, 1% KOH, 100 mM EDTA, 10 mM Trizma base, 1% Triton X-100, and 10% DMSO) for 1 h at 4 °C. The samples were then placed in a dark electrophoresis chamber containing cold, alkaline running buffer at pH > 13 (300 mM NaOH, 1 nM EDTA, pH adjusted to >13). Samples were stored in the refrigerator for 20 min. The conditions of the electrophoretic run were 25 mV and 300 mA for 20 min.

Following electrophoresis, the slides were removed and washed three times with a neutralization buffer (0.4 mM Tris buffer adjusted to pH 7.5) for 5 min/wash. Finally, the slides were washed twice with anhydrous absolute ethanol for 5 min/wash. Excess alcohol was removed, and the slides were allowed to dry, following which they were then stained with 25 µL ethidium bromide (20 µg/mL in deionized water) and covered with coverslips. All stages of the comet assay were performed under indirect yellow light or in the dark. Comet observations were made under a LEICA DM2500 fluorescence microscope equipped with an excitation filter (515–560 nm) and barrier filter (590 nm). Photographs were captured with a 5-megapixel LEICA model DFC450C digital camera cooled with monochromatic light, with a C-mount adapter. The comet evaluations were performed using the TriTek CometScore software. DNA damage was reported as % Olive Tail Moment (% OTM) [50,51].

2.9.4. Genetic Expression Assay Using RT-qPCR

Chomczynski and Sacchi's method (1987) [52] was used for total RNA extraction. The mammary gland tissues (0.050 ± 0.008 g) collected from the rats was weighed and used for total RNA extraction using TRIzol. In addition, PolyTron equipment was used to homogenize the samples. Purity and concentration of the total RNA obtained was estimated by absorbance at 260/280 nm using Nanodrop equipment [53], and the integrity was determined by electrophoresis in 1.5% agarose gel under denaturing conditions and then stained with 1.5% ethidium bromide according to Jacobs Protocol

(2017) [54]. A reverse transcription reaction was performed with the RNA obtained from each sample using a QuantiTect Reverse Transcription kit to obtain the cDNA, under the operating conditions recommended by the provider (Qiagen, 2016; cat. no. 205311). PCR reactions were conducted in a T100 Thermocycler (BioRad, 2015, Hercules, CA, USA).

On obtaining the cDNA, genetic expressions of *BRCA1* and *SCL11a2* (FAM fluorophore) were evaluated using 30 ng of cDNA and TaqMan genetic expression assay (Applied Biosystems). RT-qPCR reactions were conducted in the StepOneTM v2.3 device using *GAPDH* (VIC fluorophore) as the reference gene (housekeeping gene). Duplex reactions (*BRCA1/GAPDH* and *SCL11a2/GAPDH*) were performed under the conditions recommended by the provider (Applied Biosystems 2016).

2.10. Statistical Analysis

The Kolmogorov–Smirnov test was applied to verify normality of aluminum concentrations in the mammary gland tissues; when these assumptions were not met, the data were analyzed using the Kruskal–Wallis test. Data for the variables that fulfilled the normality assumptions were assessed using one-way analysis of variance using the General Linear Model procedure (GLM ANOVA), where the experimental treatments was the main effect. Regarding the number of MNs, only counts obtained for cells with a single MN were used because no records were available for cells with ≥2 MNs. MN and genotoxicity data were analyzed using GLM ANOVA for a complete block random design. The model included the fixed effects of treatments and sampling times (blocks). Any differences observed between the means were analyzed using the Tukey–Kramer multiple comparison test. Statistical significance was considered at a 0.05 probability for type I error ($p < 0.05$). All data were processed using the NCSS statistical package, version 2007 (Kaysville, UT, USA) The research project was approved by the Commission of Bioethics in Research of the University of Sonora, ex officio CBI-UNISON 1/2015 (Approval date: 9 February 2015).

3. Results

3.1. Determining Aluminum Concentration in Breast Tissue

Table 1 denotes a significant difference ($\alpha = 0.05$) between the +2000Al/−NMU treatment and the other experimental treatments, with a value of 38.17 ± 2.49 µg of aluminum/g of mammary gland tissue.

Table 1. Concentration of aluminum (median of µg Al/g of tissue) in the mammary gland of Sprague Dawley rats quantified by graphite furnace absorption atomic spectroscopy (GFAAS).

	TREATMENTS *				
Variables	**−Al/−NMU**	**+2000Al/+NMU**	**+2000Al/−NMU**	**−Al/+NMU**	***p* Value ****
n	8	8	8	7	
Mammary gland tissue	11.395 ^{a}	12.288 ^{a}	38.17 ^{b}	17.929 ^{a}	0.0001

* = Al/NMU = ± Aluminum/± Nitrosomethylurea; ** = *p* value, Significant $p \leq 0.05$. ($\alpha = 0.05$). ^{a} or ^{b} = Different letters means statistical difference.

3.2. Evaluation of Genomic Instability

3.2.1. Histopathological Evaluation

Histopathological results (Figure 1) showed that the effect of the treatments corresponded to hyperplasia and that there was no evidence of cancer development, similar to the results obtained by some researchers [45,55,56].

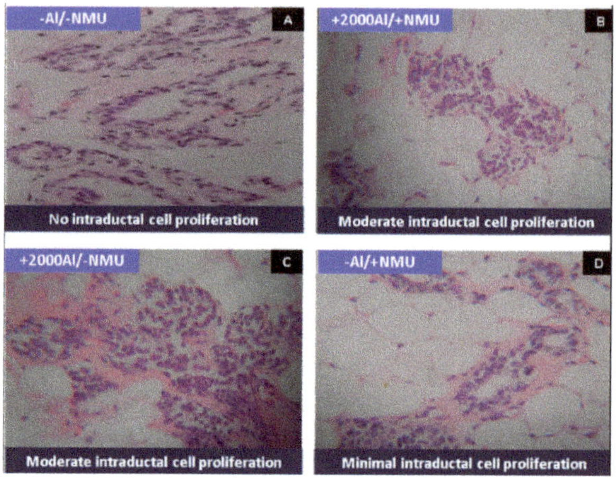

Figure 1. The histological change found in the breast tissue of Sprague Dawley rats is shown with the different treatments used. Hyperplasia of the breast ducts was minimal (**D**) to moderate (**B**,**C**). Normal/negative control (**A**). HEx400.

3.2.2. Micronucleus Analysis

MN analysis is a valuable indicator for the partial assessment of genotoxicity via ruptures in the chromosomes [57,58]. The complete MN count is shown in Table 2, which indicates that the presence of MNs was not detected in the negative control (−Al/−MNU) at 5, 10, or 15 days. This is normal to some extent because these rats were not administered aluminum solutions or NMU, a cancer inducing agent. As denoted in Figure 2, an effect from the treatment and exposure time ($p < 0.05$) was observed for counts with 1 MN. Our result suggests that there was no synergistic effect between aluminum ($AlCl_3$) and NMU, as previously noted in the results obtained for aluminum concentration in the mammary glands as well as from the histological evaluation of the breast. In the +2000Al/−NMU and −Al/+NMU treatments, a higher number of MN ($p < 0.05$) were observed. Although the average number of MN was higher for the +2000Al/−NMU treatment than for the −Al/+NMU treatment, there was no significant difference ($p > 0.05$) because of the substantial variance among the +2000Al/−NMU treatment replications. Nevertheless, the study proved that the treatment containing only aluminum could independently cause genotoxicity in rats.

Table 2. Genotoxicity caused by experimental treatments by micronucleus count (MN) in peripheral blood erythrocytes of female Sprague Dawley rats at 5, 10, and 15 days of exposure.

Treatments	5 Days			10 Days			15 Days		
	1 MN	2 MN	>2 MN	1 MN	2 MN	>2 MN	1 MN	2 MN	>2 MN
(A) −Al/−NMU	0	0	0	0	0	0	0	0	0
(B) +2000Al/+NMU	0	0	0	4	0	0	8	0	0
(C) +2000Al/−NMU	0	0	0	9.3	0	0	28.6	2.6	0
(D) −Al/+NMU	1	0	0	8	0	0	18.6	0.6	0

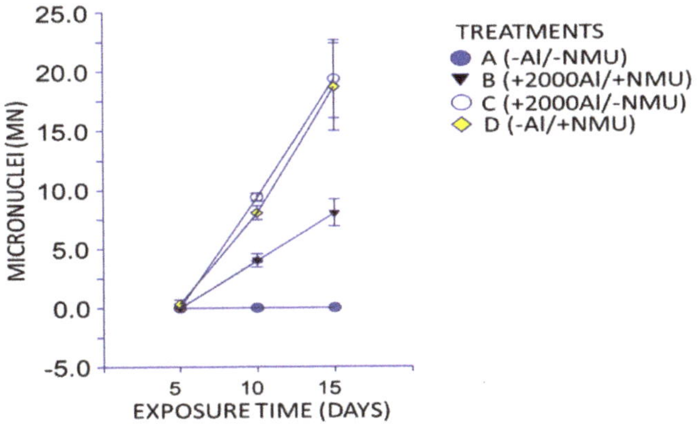

Figure 2. Genotoxicity (1 MN) caused by experimental treatments in the peripheral blood of Sprague Dawley rats at 5, 10, and 15 days of exposure.

In addition, the genotoxic effects started to significantly manifest ($p < 0.05$) on day 10 and showed greater values at day 15 (effect from exposure time), indicating a subacute effect due to aluminum bioconcentration. Additionally, the results revealed that the apparent effect was intermediate in treatments with aluminum and NMU (+2000Al/+NMU).

3.2.3. Alkaline Electrophoresis Test in Individual Cells (Comet Assay)

The 96% ± 2% cell viability identified by trypan blue was similar to the results obtained by other researchers [47,48]. This study was conducted at an exploratory level to determine whether the genotoxicity caused by aluminum in the form of $AlCl_3$ caused DNA damage or fragmentation in rat leukocytes. Only three rats were used as a negative control (−Al/−NMU) and three rats were subjected to the +2000Al/−NMU experimental treatment, thereby proving that this experimental treatment could independently induce intraductal cell proliferation in mammary glands and lead to a higher number of comet and clouds as exposure time increased. Figure 3 denotes these results, indicating that there was no genotoxic damage at 5, 10, and 15 days of exposure after the −Al/−NMU treatment (negative control). Conversely, no comets were observed in the +2000Al/−NMU experimental treatment, and only nucleoids or unrolled DNA were noted after five days of exposure. The test was consistent with the lack of genotoxicity observed in the formation of MN after five days of exposure. However, genotoxicity was distinctly observed after 10 and 15 days, when comets were observed. Although no significant differences ($\alpha = 0.05$) were observed in terms of the number of comets and % OTM after 10 and 15 days of aluminum exposure, there were significant differences in terms of cloud formation because there were three and 73 clouds per 100 comets detected at 10 and 15 days of aluminum exposure, respectively.

3.2.4. Genetic Expression Assay Using RT-qPCR

The results of genetic expression obtained for *BRCA1* and *SCL11a2* using RT-qPCR indicate that no experimental evidence demonstrating the expression of both genes was present; therefore, it can be inferred that the product of *BRCA1* does not participate in the DNA damage repair mechanism as observed in the comet test. In addition, it can be determined that the product of *SCL11a2* does not play a role in the aluminum transport process in Sprague Dawley rats under the proposed experimental conditions.

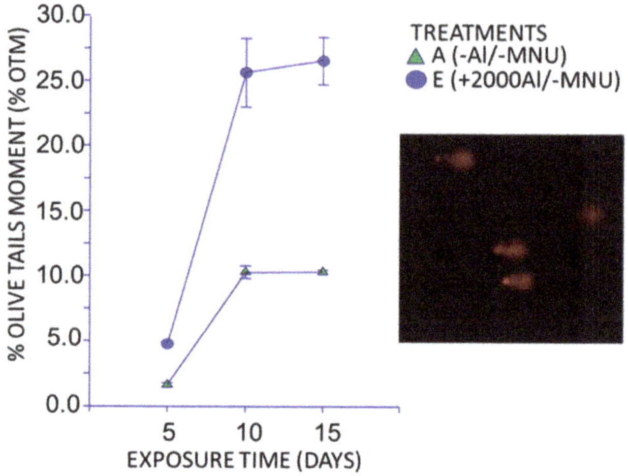

Figure 3. Genotoxic effect caused by the +2000Al/−NMU treatment in the peripheral blood of Sprague Dawley rats at 5, 10, and 15 days of exposure, evaluated by the comet test.

4. Discussion

4.1. Determining Aluminum Concentration in Breast Tissue

Oogoshi et al. (1994) reported that aluminum concentration was higher in the mammary glands of Sprague Dawley rats compared with other tissues by quantifying the concentration of various metals provided in their diet [59]. Furthermore, these results indicate that there was no synergistic effect of the treatments containing aluminum ($AlCl_3$) and NMU (+2000Al/+NMU); therefore, it can be assumed that, among the effects of NMU administration, tumorigenesis does not require aluminum as an essential microelement, or NMU leads to changes in the aluminum transportation mechanism. This effect has been observed when determining that NMU administration in rats modifies the ZnT-1 zinc transporter that causes failure in the zinc transportation mechanism [60,61].

4.2. Evaluation of Genomic Instability

4.2.1. Histopathological Evaluation

NMU induces breast cancer in laboratory rats [62–67]. However, according to the present study, this compound caused only minimal cell proliferation in the ductal epithelium (−AL/+NMU). Reportedly, adenocarcinomas appeared 140 days after NMU application [68]. Cell proliferation of the ductal epithelium was not observed in treatment A (−Al/−NMU), which was expected because this treatment represents the negative control. The most significant histopathological change caused by treatment C (+2000Al/−NMU) was ductal epithelial cell proliferation compared with the other treatments. A previous histopathological study showed that aluminum in the form of $AlCl_3$ can cause liver damage in Sprague Dawley rats when orally administered for 30 days [57].

4.2.2. Micronucleus Analysis

The present study demonstrated that NMU generates MN after 10 days of exposure under the +2000Al/−MNU treatment. A previous study assessed the genotoxicity of aluminum using the MN test and reported that genotoxic agents such as cyclophosphamide generate MN in the peripheral blood of rats within 24 h [69]. On the other hand, Balasubramanyam et al. [28,70] determined that the intraperitoneally administered nanoparticles of Al_2O_3 caused an increase in liver MN counts in female Wistar rats. Moreover, they determined that increasing the dosages (500, 1000, or 2000 mg of Al/kg of body weight) increased the number of MN when compared with the control group rats to which cyclophosphamide was administered as a genotoxic agent. This genotoxicity was corroborated by Klien and Godnić-Cvar [71]. Moreover, Türkez et al. [57,72,73] assessed liver genotoxicity caused by $AlCl_3$ solutions in Sprague Dawley rats. They observed that a sub-chronic dose of $AlCl_3$, intraperitoneally administered for 10 weeks increased the number of MN; however, this effect can be reversed using boric acid or borax. Geyikoglu et al. [58] found that $AlCl_3$ at a dose of 3 mg of aluminum/kg of body weight induced genotoxicity by forming MN in the hepatocytes of Sprague Dawley rats when aluminum was intraperitoneally administered for 10 weeks. In addition, Al-Obaidy et al. [74] demonstrated that 10, 15, and 25 mg of $AlCl_3$ solutions per kg of body weight intraperitoneally administered to male albino rats (*Rattus norvegicus*) increased the number of MN in the bone marrow, and the number of MN increased with the increase in dose. As the dose increased, the number of cells with MN decreased, and this decrease correlates with an increase in the number of cells that die due to apoptosis [75]. In the present study, we intragastrically (gavage) administered $AlCl_3$ solutions and the genotoxic effect observed was similar to that of the intraperitoneally administered aluminum solutions, as previously reported [73,74].

4.2.3. Alkaline Electrophoresis Test in Individual Cells (Comet Assay)

The results obtained in treatment C (+2000Al/−NMU) implies a greater genotoxic effect after 15 days of exposure that is irreversible and considerably greater than the effect of H_2O_2 exposure [76,77]. A previous study reported that aluminum in the form of aluminum lactate intragastrically administered for 12 weeks could cause DNA fragmentation in the brain tissue of female Wistar rats when the genotoxic effect was assessed using agarose gel electrophoresis [78]. Using comet and MN tests, correlations were determined between the genotoxic damage caused by aluminum to the DNA of human lymphocytes and an increase in the dosage and exposure time [79]. The advantage of using the alkaline comet assay over the other in vitro methods is that it can detect lesions or damage to single- or double-stranded DNA as well as breaks in labile points in the DNA of single cells [80].

4.2.4. Genetic Expression Assay Using RT-qPCR

BRCA1 is a genetic marker for breast cancer, and its role in the DNA damage repair mechanism has been demonstrated. Considering that it has undergone mutations, its expression is regulated by epigenetic modification and it is overexpressed in breast cancer [81–83]. Furthermore, the product of *SCL11a2* has been identified as a divalent metal transporter gene [84–87]. The macrophage protein associated with natural resistance, Nramp, which is a product of *SCL11a2*, has recently been linked to aluminum transportation in different organisms [88,89]. Therefore, other molecular biological approaches must be applied in an attempt to establish this genetic relationship. Indeed, other researchers have obtained similar results. For example, cadmium reportedly induces DNA fragmentation and tumorigenesis, but not the expression of genes such as *bcl-x* or *MT-1* in Wistar rat testis and prostate [90]. Rodrigues-Peres et al. [91] found no *ERBB2*, *C-MYC*, and *CCND1* gene instability when assessing the correlation between aluminum and genomic instability in cancerous human breast tissues and healthy tissues. Additionally, as previously reported, the changes were observed at extremely low or nanomolar concentrations of aluminum, with the ability to induce the expression of pro-inflammatory and pro-apoptotic genes. This may be related to some degree of genotoxicity [92,93], as observed by our research group in the present study.

5. Conclusions

This study showed that aluminum chloride causes minimum-to-moderate hyperplastic (proliferative) intraductal cell proliferation and genotoxicity. Our results indicate that the BRCA1 product is not involved in the process of DNA damage repair and infer that the SCL11a2 product does not participate in aluminum transport under the proposed experimental conditions.

Author Contributions: Performed the experiment and wrote the draft, A.M.G.-A.; Provided guidance for aluminum analysis, A.G.-Á.; Provided guidance for genomic evaluation, I.A.-C.; Provided guidance for toxicological assessment, A.B.-H.; Performed formal analysis, E.R.-B.; Performed experimental animal management, R.C.-R.; Performed statistical analysis, H.G.-R.; Provided guidance for histological analysis, J.G.L.-C.; Provided guidance for comet assays, K.L.R.-M.; Designed and supervised the study, H.A.-G. All authors have read and agreed to the published version of the manuscript.

Funding: This research was funded by Universidad de Sonora.

Acknowledgments: We acknowledge the individuals responsible for the laboratories where the experimental work was conducted.

Conflicts of Interest: The authors declare no conflict of interest. The funders had no role in the design of the study; in the collection, analyses, or interpretation of data; in the writing of the manuscript, or in the decision to publish the results.

References

1. López, F.F.; Cabrera, C.; Lorenzo, M.L.; López, M.C. Aluminium content of drinking waters, fruit juices and soft drinks:contribution to dietary intake. *Sci. Total Environ.* **2002**, *92*, 205–213. [CrossRef]
2. Darbre, P.D. Aluminium, antiperspirants and breast cancer. *J. Inorg. Biochem.* **2005**, *99*, 1912–1919. [CrossRef]
3. Kohara, I.; Tomoda, H.; Watanabe, S. New water-soluble metal working fluids additives from phosphonic acid derivatives for aluminum alloy materials. *J. Oleo Sci.* **2007**, *56*, 527–532. [CrossRef] [PubMed]
4. Yamamoto, S.; Tomoda, H.; Watanabe, S. Water-soluble metal working fluids additives derived from the esters of acid anhydrides with higher alcohols for aluminum alloy materials. *J. Oleo Sci.* **2007**, *56*, 463–469. [CrossRef] [PubMed]
5. Yokel, R.A.; Hicks, C.L.; Florenc, R.L. Aluminum bioavailability from basic sodium aluminum phosphate, an approved food additive emulsifying agent, incorporated in cheese. *Food Chem. Toxicol.* **2008**, *46*, 2261–2266. [CrossRef] [PubMed]
6. Gil, L.A.F.; Da Cunha, C.E.P.; Gustavo, M.S.G.; Salvarani, M.F.M.; Ronnie, A.; Lobato, A.F.C.; Mendonça, M.; Dellagostin, O.A.; Conceição, F.R. Production and evaluation of a recombinant chimeric vaccine against *Clostridium botulinum* neurotoxin types C and D. *PLoS ONE* **2013**, *8*, e69692. [CrossRef] [PubMed]
7. Güven, E.; Duus, K.; Laursen, I.; Højrup, P.; Houen, G. Aluminum hydroxide adjuvant differentially activates the three complement pathways with major involvement of the alternative pathway. *PLoS ONE* **2013**, *8*, e74445. [CrossRef] [PubMed]
8. Prozialeck, W.C.; Edwards, J.R.; Nebert, D.W. The vascular system as a target of metal toxicity. *Toxicol. Sci.* **2008**, *102*, 207–218. [CrossRef] [PubMed]
9. Tchounwou, P.B.; Yedjoum, C.G.; Patlolla, A.K.; Sutton, D.J. Heavy metal toxicity and the environment. *EXS* **2012**, *101*, 133–164.
10. Department of Health and Human Services. Division of Toxicology and Environmental Medicine. USA. 2008. Available online: https://www.atsdr.cdc.gov/toxprofiles/tp22.pdf (accessed on 14 April 2020).
11. Pikor, L.; Thu, K.; Vucic, E.; Lam, W. The detection and implication of genome instability in cancer. *Cancer Metastasis Rev.* **2013**, *32*, 41–352. [CrossRef]
12. Abbas, T.; Mignon, A.; Keaton, M.G.; Dutta, A. Genomic instability in cancer. *Cold Spring Harb. Perspect. Biol.* **2017**, *5*, a012914. [CrossRef] [PubMed]
13. Geraki, K.; Farquharson, M.J.; Bradley, D.A. Concentrations of Fe, Cu and Zn in breast tissue: A synchrotron XRF Study. *Phys. Med. Biol.* **2002**, *47*, 2327–2339. [CrossRef] [PubMed]
14. Al-Ebraheem, A.; Farquharson, M.J.; Ryan, E. The evaluations of biologically important trace metals in liver, kidney and breast tissue. *Appl. Radiat. Isot.* **2009**, *7*, 470–474. [CrossRef] [PubMed]
15. Silva, M.P.; Soave, D.F.; Riberiro-Silva, A.; Poletti, M.E. Trace elements as tumor biomarkers and prognostic factors in breast cáncer: A study throuh energy dispersive x-ray fluorescence. *BMC Res. Notes* **2012**, *5*, 194. [CrossRef] [PubMed]
16. Wang, Y.; Cheng, M.; Zhang, B.; Nie, F.; Jiang, H. Dietary supplementation of blueberry juice enhances hepatic expression of metallothionein and attenuates liver fibrosis in rats. *PLoS ONE* **2013**, *8*, e58659. [CrossRef]
17. Greger, J.L.; Bula, E.N.; Gum, E.T. Mineral metabolism of rats fed moderate levels of various aluminum compounds for short periods of time. *J. Nutr.* **1985**, *115*, 1708–1716. [CrossRef]

18. Hubaux, R.; Becker-Santos, D.D.; Enfield, K.S.S.; La, R.D.E.; Lam, W.L.; Martinez, V.D. Molecular features in arsenic-induced lung tumors. *Mol. Cancer* **2013**, *12*, 2–11. [CrossRef]
19. García-Rodríguez, N.; Díaz de la Loza, M.C.; Anderson, B.; Monje-Casas, F.; Rothstein, R.; Wellinger, R.E. Impaired manganese metabolism causes mitotic misregulation. *J. Biol. Chem.* **2012**, *287*, 18717–18729. [CrossRef]
20. Diwan, B.A.; Kasprzak, K.S.; Anderson, L.M. Promotion of dimethylbenz[*a*]anthracene-initiated mammary carcinogenesis by iron in female Sprague–Dawley rats. *Carcinogenesis* **1997**, *18*, 1757–1762. [CrossRef]
21. Bobrowska, B.; Skrajnowska, D.; Tokarz, A. Effect of Cu supplementation on genomic instability in chemically-induced mammary carcinogenesis in the rat. *J. Biomed. Sci.* **2011**, *18*, 95. [CrossRef]
22. Rahim, F.; Jalali, A.; Tangestani, R. Breast cancer frequency and exposure to cadmium: A meta-analysis and systematic. *Asian Pac. J. Cancer Prev.* **2013**, *14*, 4283–4287. [CrossRef] [PubMed]
23. Darbre, P.D. Underarm, antiperspirants/deodorants and breast cancer. *Breast Cancer Res.* **2009**, *11* (Suppl. 3), S5. [CrossRef] [PubMed]
24. Lambert, V.; Boukhari, R.; Nacher, M.; Goullé, J.P.; Roudier, E.; Elguindi, W.; Laquerrière, A.; Carles, G. Plasma and urinary aluminum concentrations in severely anemic geophagous pregnant women in the bas Maroni region of French Guiana: A Case-Control Study. *Am. J. Trop. Med. Hyg.* **2010**, *83*, 1100–1105. [CrossRef]
25. Wang, N.; She, Y.; Zhu, Y.; Zhao, H.; Shao, B.; Sun, H.; Hu, C.; Li, Y. Effects of subchronic aluminum exposure on the reproductive function in female rats. *Biol. Trace Elem. Res.* **2012**, *145*, 382–387. [CrossRef]
26. Zhang, C.; Li, Y.; Wang, C.; Lv, R.; Song, T. Extremely low-frequency magnetic exposure appears to have no effect on pathogenesis of Alzheimer's disease in aluminum-overloaded rat. *PLoS ONE* **2013**, *8*, e17087. [CrossRef] [PubMed]
27. Zhu, Y.; Han, Y.; Zhao, H.; Li, J.; Hu, C.; Li, Y.; Zhang, Z. Suppressive effect of accumulated aluminum trichloride on the hepatic microsomal cytochrome P450 enzyme system in rats. *Food Chem. Toxicol.* **2013**, *51*, 210–214. [CrossRef]
28. Balasubramanyam, A.; Sailaja, N.; Mahboob, M.; Rahman, M.F.; Hussain, S.M.; Grover, P. In vivo genotoxicity assessment of aluminium oxide nanomaterials in rat peripheral blood cells using the comet assay and micronucleus test. *Mutagenesis* **2009**, *24*, 245–251. [CrossRef]
29. Hirata-Koizumi, M.; Fujii, S.; Ono, A.; Hirose, A.; Imai, T.; Ogawa, K.; Ema, M.; Nishikawa, A. Two-generation reproductive toxicity study of aluminium sulfate in rats. *Reprod. Toxicol.* **2011**, *31*, 219–230. [CrossRef]
30. Gullino, P.; Pettigrew, H.; Grantham, F.N. Nitrosomethylurea is a mammary gland carcinogen in rats. *J. Natl. Cancer Inst.* **1975**, *54*, 401–414.
31. Bobrowska-Korczak, B.; Skrajnowska, D.; Tokarz, A. The effect of dietary zinc—And polyphenols intake on DMBA-induced mammary tumorigenesis in rats. *J. Biomed. Sci.* **2012**, *19*, 43. [CrossRef]
32. Chou, Y.C.; Guzman, R.C.; Swanson, S.M.; Yang, J.; Lui, H.M.; Wu, V.; Nandi, S. Induction of mammary carcinomas by *N*-methyl-*N*-nitrosourea in ovariectomized rats treated with epidermal growth factor. *Carcinogenesis* **1999**, *20*, 677–684. [CrossRef] [PubMed]
33. Rees, S.L.; Panesar, S.; Steiner, M.; Fleming, A.S. The effects of adrenalectomy and corticosterone replacement on induction of maternal behavior in the virgin female rat. *Horm. Behav.* **2006**, *49*, 337–345. [CrossRef] [PubMed]
34. Norma Oficial Mexicana. *NOM-033-ZOO-1995. Sacrificio Humanitario de los Animales Domésticos y Silvestres*; SAGARPA: México D.F., Mexico, 1995.
35. Norma Oficial Mexicana. *NOM-062-ZOO-1999. Especificaciones Técnicas Para la Producción, Cuidado y uso de los Animales de Laboratorio*; SAGARPA: México D.F., Mexico, 1999.
36. European Medicines Agency (EMEA). *Committee for Medicinal Products for Veterinary Use (CVMP). Recommendation on the Evaluation of the Benefit-Risk Balance of Veterinary Medicinal Products*; European Medicines Agency: London, UK, 2009.
37. Food and Drug Administration (FDA). *CFR—Code of Federal Regulations Title 21, Chapter I, Subchapter E, Part 511*; Revised as of April 1; Food and Drug Administration: Silver Spring, MD, USA, 2014.
38. Perkin Elmer. *Manual Operation of Equipment Microwave Furnance Model TITAN MPS*; Perkin Elmer: Waltham, MD, USA, 2014.

39. Bohrer, D.; Dessuy, M.B.; Kaizer, R.; Do Nascimento, P.C.; Schetinger, M.R.C.; Morsch, V.M.; Carvalho, L.M.; Garcia, S.C. Tissue digestion for aluminum determination in experimental animal studies. *Anal. Biochem.* **2008**, *377*, 120–127. [CrossRef]
40. Neiva, T.J.C.; Benedetti, A.L.; Tanaka, S.M.C.N.; Santos, J.I.; D'Amico, E.A. Determination of serum aluminum, platelet aggregation and lipid peroxidation in hemodialyzed patients. *Braz. J. Med. Biol. Res.* **2002**, *35*, 345–350. [CrossRef] [PubMed]
41. Perkin Elmer. *Manual Operation of Equipment Atomic Absorption Spectroscopy Model AAnalyst 400*; Perkin Elmer: Waltham, MD, USA, 2012.
42. García-Alegría, A.M.; Gómez-Álvarez, A.; Anduro-Corona, I.; Burgos-Hernández, A.; Ruiz-Bustos, E.; Canett-Romero, R.; Astiazarán-García, H.F. Optimización de las condiciones analíticas ideales para cuantificar aluminio en tejidos de ratas Sprague Dawley, mediante la técnica de absorción atómica. *Rev. Int. Contam. Ambient.* **2017**, *34*, 7–24. [CrossRef]
43. García-Alegría, A.M.; Gómez-Álvarez, A.; Anduro-Corona, I.; Burgos-Hernández, A.; Ruiz-Bustos, E.; Canett-Romero, R.; Soto-Encinas, K.K.; Astiazarán-García, H.F. Validation of analytical method to quantify aluminum in tissues of Sprague Dawley rats by FAAS and GFAAS. *Acta Univ. Multidiscip. Sci. J.* **2017**, *27*, 22–35.
44. García-Alegría, A.M.; Gómez-Álvarez, A.; Anduro-Corona, I.; Burgos-Hernández, A.; Ruiz-Bustos, E.; Canett-Romero, R.; Cáñez-Carrasco, M.G.; Astiazarán-García, H.F. Estimation of the expanded uncertainty of an analytical method to quantify aluminum in tissue of Sprague Dawley rats by FAAS and ETAAS. *MAPAN J. Metrol. Soc. India* **2017**, *32*, 131–141. [CrossRef]
45. Esendagli, G.; Canpinar, H.; Yilmaz, G.; Gunel-Ozcan, A.; Oguz-Guc, M.; Kansu, E.; Guc, D. Primary tumor cells obtained from MNU-induced mammary carcinomas show immune heterogeneity which can be modulated by low-efficiency transfection of CD40L gene. *Cancer Biol. Ther.* **2009**, *8*, 132–142. [CrossRef]
46. Hatton, C.S.R. *Hematología: Diagnóstico y Tratamiento*; El Manual Modern: México D.F., México, 2014.
47. García-Medina, S.; Razo-Estrada, C.; Galar-Martínez, M.; Cortéz-Barberena, E.; Gómez-Oliván, L.M.; Álvarez-González, I.; Madrigal-Bujaidar, E. Genotoxic and cytotoxic effects induced by aluminum in the lymphocytes of the common carp (*Cyprinus carpio*). *Comp. Biochem. Physiol. Part C* **2011**, *153*, 113–118. [CrossRef]
48. Pereira, S.; Cavalie, I.; Camilleri, V.; Gilbin, R.; Adam-Guillermin, C. Comparative genotoxicity of aluminium and cadmium in embryonic zebrafish cells. *Mutat. Res.* **2013**, *750*, 19–26. [CrossRef]
49. Singh, N.P.; Tice, R.R.; Stephensen, R.E.; Schneider, E. A microgel electrophoresis technique for the direct quantitation of DNA damage and repair in individual fibroblasts cultured on microscope slides. *Mutat. Res.* **1991**, *252*, 289–296. [CrossRef]
50. Olive, P.L.; Banáth, J.P.; Durand, R.E. Heterogeneity in radiation-induced DNA damage and repair in tumor and normal cells measured using the comet assay. *Radiat. Res.* **1990**, *122*, 86–94. [CrossRef] [PubMed]
51. Yáñez, L.; García-Nieto, E.; Rojas, E.; Carrizales, L.; Mejía, J.; Calderón, J.; Razo, I.; Díaz-Barriga, F. DNA damage in blood cells from children exposed to arsenic and lead in a mining area. *Environ. Res.* **2003**, *93*, 231–240. [CrossRef] [PubMed]
52. Chomczynski, P.; Sacchi, N. Single-step method of RNA isolation by acid guanidinium thiocyanate-phenol-chloroform extraction. *Anal. Biochem.* **1987**, *162*, 156–159. [CrossRef]
53. Desjardins, P.; Conklin, D. NanoDrop microvolume quantitation of nucleic acids. *J. Vis. Exp.* **2010**, *45*, e2565. [CrossRef]
54. Jacobs Protocol. Available online: http://www.openwetware.org/wiki/Jacobs:Protocol_RNA_Agarose_Gel (accessed on 14 April 2020).
55. Thompson, H.J.; Singh, M.; McGinley, J. Classification of premalignant and malignant lesions developing in the rat mammary gland after injection of sexually immature rats with 1-methyl-1-nitrosourea. *J. Mammary Gland Biol. Neoplasia* **2000**, *5*, 201–210. [CrossRef]
56. Perše, M.; Cerar, A.; Injac, R.; Štrukelj, B. *N*-methylnitrosourea induced breast cancer in rat, the histopathology of the resulting tumours and its Drawbacks as a model. *Pathol. Oncol. Res.* **2009**, *15*, 115–121. [CrossRef]
57. Türkez, H.; Yousef, M.I.; Geyikoglu, F. Propolis prevents aluminium-induced genetic and hepatic damages in rat liver. *Food Chem. Toxicol.* **2010**, *48*, 2741–2746. [CrossRef]

58. Geyikoglu, F.; Türkez, H.; Bakir, T.O.; Cicek, M. The genotoxic, hepatotoxic, nephrotoxic, haematotoxic and histopathological effects in rats after aluminium chronic intoxication. *Toxicol. Ind. Health* **2012**, *29*, 780–791. [CrossRef]
59. Oogoshi, K.; Yanagi, S.; Moriyama, T.; Arachi, H. Accumulation of aluminum in cancers of the liver, stomach, duodenum and mammary glands of rats. *J. Trace Elem. Electrolytes Health Dis.* **1994**, *8*, 27–31.
60. Lee, R.; Woo, W.; Wu, B.; Kummer, A.; Duminy, H.; Xu, Z. Zinc accumulation in *N*-methyl-*N*-nitrosourea-induced rat mammary tumors is accompanied by an altered expression of ZnT-1 and metallothionein. *Exp. Biol. Med.* **2003**, *228*, 689–696.
61. Lee, S.; Simpson, M.; Nimmo, M.; Xu, Z. Low zinc intake suppressed *N*-methyl-*N*-nitrosourea-induced mammary tumorigenesis in Sprague Dawley rats. *Carcinogenesis* **2004**, *25*, 1879–1885. [CrossRef] [PubMed]
62. Lee, W.M.; Lua, S.; Medlineb, A.; Michael, C.; Archer, M.C. Susceptibility of lean and obese Zucker rats to tumorigenesis induced by *N*-methyl-*N*-nitrosourea. *Cancer Lett.* **2001**, *166*, 155–160. [CrossRef]
63. Sharma, R.; Kline, R.P.; Ed, X.; Wu, E.X.; Jose, K.; Katz, J.K. Rapid in vivo taxotere quantitative chemosensitivity response by 4.23 tesla sodium MRI and histo-immunostaining features in *N*-methyl-*N*-nitrosourea induced breast tumors in rats. *Cancer Cell Int.* **2005**, *5*, 26. [CrossRef] [PubMed]
64. Vegh, I.; Enríquez de Salamanca, R. Prolactin, TNF alpha and nitric oxide expression in nitroso-*N*-methylurea-induced-mammary tumours. *J. Carcinog.* **2007**, *6*, 18. [CrossRef]
65. Goss, P.E.; Strasser-Weipp, K.; Qi, S.; Hu, H. Effects of liarozole fumarate (R85246) in combination with tamoxifen on *N*-methyl-*N*-nitrosourea (MNU)-induced mammary carcinoma and uterus in the rat model. *BMC Cancer* **2007**, *7*, 26. [CrossRef]
66. Krishnan, P.; Yan, K.J.; Windler, D.; Tubbs, J.; Grand, R.; Li, B.D.L.; Aldaz, C.M.; McLarty, J.; Kleiner-Hancock, H.E. Citrus auraptene suppresses cyclin D1 and significantly delays *N*-methyl nitrosourea induced mammary carcinogenesis in female Sprague-Dawley rats. *BMC Cancer* **2009**, *9*, 259. [CrossRef]
67. Faustino-Rocha, A.I.; Silva, A.; Gabriel, J.; Teixeira-Guedes, C.I.; Lopes, C.; Gil da Costa, R.; Gama, A.; Ferreira, R.; Oliveira, P.A.; Ginja, M. Ultrasonographic, thermographic and histologic evaluation of MNU-induced mammary tumors in female Sprague-Dawley rats. *Biomed. Pharmacother.* **2013**, *67*, 771–776. [CrossRef]
68. Rajmani, R.S.; Doley, J.; Singh, P.K.; Kumar, R.; Barathidasan, R.; Kumar, P.; Verma, P.C.; Tiwari, A.K. Induction of mammary gland tumour in rats using *N*-methyl-*N*-nitroso urea and their histopathology. *Indian J. Vet. Pathol.* **2011**, *35*, 142–146.
69. Mughal, A.; Vikram, A.; Ramarao, P.; Jena, G.B. Micronucleus and comet assay in the peripheral blood of juvenile rat: Establishment of assay feasibility, time of sampling and the induction of DNA damage. *Mutat. Res.* **2010**, *700*, 86–94. [CrossRef]
70. Balasubramanyam, A.; Sailaja, N.; Mahboob, M.; Rahman, M.F.; Misra, S.; Hussain, S.M.; Grover, P. Evaluation of genotoxic effects of oral exposure to Aluminum oxide nanomaterials in rat bone marrow. *Mutat. Res.* **2009**, *676*, 41–47. [CrossRef] [PubMed]
71. Klien, K.; Godnić-Cvar, J. Genotoxicity of metals nanoparticules: Focus on in vivo studies. *Arh. Hig. Rada Toksikol.* **2012**, *63*, 133–145. [CrossRef] [PubMed]
72. Türkez, H.; Geyikoglu, F.; Colak, S. The protective effect of boric acid on aluminum-induced hepatotoxicity and genotoxicity in rats. *Turk. J. Biol.* **2011**, *35*, 293–301.
73. Türkez, H.; Geyikoglu, F.; Tatar, A. Borax counteracts genotoxicity of aluminum in rat liver. *Toxicol. Ind. Health* **2012**, *29*, 775–779. [CrossRef]
74. AL-Obaidy, O.R.K.; Al-Samarrai, A.S.M.; Al-Samarrai, Y.S.Y. Genotoxicity of aluminum chloride ($AlCl_3$) on the albino rat *Rattus norvegicus*. *Iraqi J. Cancer Med. Genet.* **2016**, *9*, 18–24.
75. Banasik, A.; Lankoff, A.; Piskulak, A.; Adamowska, K.; Lisowsk, H.; Wojcik, A. Aluminium-induced micronuclei and apoptosisin human peripheral blood lymphocytes treated during different phases of the cell cycle. *Environ. Toxicol.* **2005**, *20*, 402–406. [CrossRef]
76. Ayala, M.C.; Hernández, Y.G.; Piñeiro, J.C.G.; González, E.P. Uso del ensayo cometa para evaluar el efecto de la temperatura sobre la reparación del daño genético inducido por peróxido de hidrógeno y la radiación ultravioleta A en células sanguíneas humanas. *Acta Farm. Bonaerense.* **2004**, *23*, 277–284.

77. Stanić, D.; Plećaš-Solarović, B.; Petrović, J.; Bogavac-Stanojević, N.; Sopić, M.; Kotur-Stevuljević, J.; Ignjatović, S.; Pešić, V. Hydrogen peroxide-induced oxidative damage in peripheral blood lymphocytes from rats chronically treated with corticosterone: The protective effect of oxytocin treatment. *Chem. Biol. Interact.* **2016**, *256*, 134–141. [CrossRef]
78. Kumar, V.; Bal, A.; Gill, K.D. Aluminium-induced oxidative DNA damage recognition and cell-cycle disruption in different regions of rat brain. *Toxicology* **2009**, *264*, 137–144. [CrossRef]
79. Lankoff, A.; Banasik, A.; Duma, A.; Ochniak, E.; Lisowska, H.; Kuszewski, T.; Góźdź, S.; Wojcik, A. A comet assay study reveals that aluminium induces DNA damage and inhibits the repair of radiation-induced lesions in human peripheral blood lymphocytes. *Toxicol. Lett.* **2006**, *161*, 27–36. [CrossRef]
80. Hartmann, A.; Schumacher, M.; Plappert-Helbig, U.; Lowe, P.; Suter, W.; Mueller, L. Use of the alkaline in vivo comet assay for mechanistic genotoxicity investigations. *Mutagenesis* **2004**, *19*, 51–59. [CrossRef] [PubMed]
81. Wu, J.; Lu, L.Y.; Yu, X. The role of BRCA1 in DNA damage response. *Protein Cell* **2010**, *1*, 117–123. [CrossRef]
82. Li, M.L.; Greenberg, R.A. Links between genome integrity and BRCA1 tumor suppression. *Trends Biochem. Sci.* **2012**, *37*, 418–424. [CrossRef] [PubMed]
83. Savage, K.I.; Harkin, D.P. BRCA1, a 'complex' protein involved in the maintenance of genomic stability. *FEBS J.* **2015**, *282*, 630–646. [CrossRef] [PubMed]
84. Jamieson, S.E.; White, J.K.; Howson, J.M.M.; Pask, R.; Smith, A.N.; Brayne, C.; Evanse, J.G.; Xuereb, J.; Cairns, N.J.; Rubinszteina, D.C.; et al. Candidate gene association study of solute carrier family 11a members 1 (*SLC11A1*) and 2 (*SLC11A2*) genes in Alzheimer's disease. *Neurosci. Lett.* **2005**, *374*, 124–128. [CrossRef] [PubMed]
85. Mims, M.P.; Prchal, J.T. Divalent metal transporter 1. *Hematology* **2005**, *10*, 339–345. [CrossRef]
86. Iolascon, A.; d'Apolito, M.; Servedio, V.; Cimmino, F.; Piga, A.; Camaschella, C. Microcytic anemia and hepatic iron overload in a child with compound heterozygous mutations in *DMT1 (SCL11A2)*. *Blood* **2006**, *107*, 349–354. [CrossRef]
87. Salazar, J.; Mena, N.; Hunot, S.; Prigent, A.; Alvarez-Fischer, D.; Arredondo, M.; Duyckaerts, C.; Sazdovitch, V.; Zhao, L.; Garrick, L.M.; et al. Divalent metal transporter 1 (DMT1) contributes to neurodegeneration in animal models of Parkinson's disease. *Proc. Natl. Acad. Sci. USA* **2008**, *105*, 18578–18583. [CrossRef]
88. Xia, J.; Yamaji, N.; Kasai, T.; Ma, J.F. Plasma membrane-localized transporter for aluminum in rice. *Proc. Natl. Acad. Sci. USA* **2010**, *107*, 18381–18385. [CrossRef] [PubMed]
89. Vanduyn, N.; Settivari, R.; LeVora, J.; Zhou, S.; Unrine, J.; Nass, R. The metal transporter SMF-3/DMT-1 mediates aluminum-induced dopamine neuron degeneration. *J. Neurochem.* **2013**, *124*, 147–157. [CrossRef] [PubMed]
90. Xu, G.; Zhou, G.; Jin, T.; Zhou, T.; Hammarström, S.; Bergh, A.; Nordberg, G. Apoptosis and p53 gene expression in male reproductive tissues of cadmium exposed rats. *Biometals* **1998**, *12*, 131–139. [CrossRef] [PubMed]
91. Rodrigues-Peres, R.M.; Cadore, S.; Febraio, S.; Heinrich, J.K.; Serra, K.P.; Derchain, S.F.M.; Vassallo, J.; Sarian, L.O. Tissue aluminum concentration does not affect the genomic stability of ERBB2, C-MYC, and CCND1 genes in breast cancer. *Biol. Trace Elem. Res.* **2013**, *154*, 345–351. [CrossRef] [PubMed]
92. Lukiw, W.J.; Percy, M.E.; Kruck, T.P. Nanomolar aluminum induces pro-inflammatory and pro-apoptotic gene expression in human brain cells in primary culture. *J. Inorg. Biochem.* **2005**, *99*, 1895–1898. [CrossRef] [PubMed]
93. Pogue, A.I.; Lukiw, W.J. Aluminum, the genetic apparatus of the human CNS and Alzheimer's disease (AD). *Morphologie* **2016**, *100*, 56–64. [CrossRef]

MDPI
St. Alban-Anlage 66
4052 Basel
Switzerland
Tel. +41 61 683 77 34
Fax +41 61 302 89 18
www.mdpi.com

Toxics Editorial Office
E-mail: toxics@mdpi.com
www.mdpi.com/journal/toxics

www.ingramcontent.com/pod-product-compliance
Lightning Source LLC
LaVergne TN
LVHW070206100526
838202LV00015B/2003
* 9 7 8 3 0 3 6 5 4 1 7 1 6 *